This is Kenton Beard's book
He is found at 3501 New Haven Rd. #155
Columbia, MO 65201
314-449-8623 after 5's

Kenton -
Thanks You for all the help in the editing of my new book. Good Luck in Path and Vet School!

Thanks!
R.G. Thom~~pson~~ whoops!

General Veterinary Pathology

second edition

R. G. THOMSON
Department of Veterinary Pathology
Western College of Veterinary Medicine
University of Saskatchewan
Saskatoon, Saskatchewan

W.B. Saunders Company
Philadelphia / London / Toronto / Mexico City / Rio de Janeiro / Sydney / Tokyo

W. B. Saunders Company: West Washington Square
Philadelphia, PA 19105

1 St. Anne's Road
Eastbourne, East Sussex BN21 3UN, England

1 Goldthorne Avenue
Toronto, Ontario M8Z 5T9, Canada

Apartado 26370—Cedro 512
Mexico 4, D.F., Mexico

Rua Coronel Cabrita, 8
Sao Cristovao Caixa Postal 21176
Rio de Janeiro, Brazil

9 Waltham Street
Artarmon, N.S.W. 2064, Australia

Ichibancho, Central Bldg., 22-1 Ichibancho
Chiyoda-Ku, Tokyo 102, Japan

Library of Congress Cataloging in Publication Data

Thomson, R. G. (Reginald G.)

General veterinary pathology.

Includes index.

Bibliography: p.

1. Veterinary pathology. I. Title. [DNLM: 1. Pathology, Veterinary. SF 769 T484g]
SF769.T46 1984 636.089'607 83–3313

ISBN 0–7216–8851–9

Listed here is the latest translated edition of this book together with the language of the translation and the publisher.

Japanese (*1st Edition*)–Gakusosha Company, Tokyo, Japan

General Veterinary Pathology ISBN 0-7216-8851-9

Last digit is the print number: 9 8 7 6 5 4 3 2

This book is dedicated to

my parents

my wife Helen

and

daughters Joanne, Carol and *Kathy*

— for their understanding of my interest in pathology.

Preface to the Second Edition

The first edition seemed to meet its objective of being a well illustrated practical and applied text for the first phase of the study of animal disease. The second edition has retained the same general format and approach. More details on specific mechanisms of disease processes, particularly in Chapter 4, have been added. There is a narrow line between not enough and too much regarding the amount of detail to provide to the intended audience. I have attempted to follow this narrow line. Many figures have been replaced and some deleted. Chapter 7 lists most of the photographs of lesions in the context of the causative agents. The appendices contain more information on applying morphologic diagnoses to lesions.

I am told that Appendix IV is very helpful to students. It is hoped that more texts will define realistically what students are expected to be able to do and to know. The volume of information in the whole veterinary curriculum demands such definitions. I would be pleased to receive constructive comments for improving the book within the context of its overall objectives.

R. G. Thomson

Acknowledgments

I am very appreciative of the comments of colleagues and students, which have brought improvements in the second edition, and for the permission by authors and publishers to use certain figures. My wife, Helen, has typed references since the last edition and also most of the changes for this edition. Jan Diederichs and Sandy Mayes also contributed substantially to the typing. Ian Shirley, Gunther Appel and Louise Stevenson printed many new photographs and were also ready and willing to assist in any way. I am grateful for the cooperation of Department Chairman Jim Mills in allowing me to use the resources of the department. The staff of the Western College of Veterinary Medicine library were always willing and able to assist with my many requests. The faculty and graduate students in the department provided many slides, suggestions and comments and provided several new figures. To all these people, I am most grateful.

The guidance, skill and assistance of Ray Kersey, Sandy Reinhardt and the staff of the W. B. Saunders Company are also much appreciated.

R. G. THOMSON

Preface to the First Edition

This book is intended as a textbook for students who are beginning the study of pathology and disease. The format and context are more or less as I have presented the material for several years in a general pathology course to second year veterinary students. A student must learn the new language of disease and how to use it. To stop after learning definitions would be to gain little because pathology is the study of dynamic processes and events. This book provides considerable factual information, but the illustrations and text are intended to convey dynamic processes, some of which are distinct entities but almost all of which are closely intertwined with other processes.

The processes and events discussed in this book are placed in the general context of what is required in general pathology at one stage of progression through the undergraduate veterinary curriculum and may not be outlined in the detail that would be required for a graduate student in pathology. Other students of disease will find the material useful but in less applied context. An effort has been made to use disease conditions in animals to illustrate or demonstrate particular points, not in the detail that would be required in special pathology but enough to whet the appetite and at the same time give the material an applied context.

Detailed supportive explanations of processes and events have been avoided in order to emphasize concepts and processes in an applied context. References are provided for additional reading on the fine detail of explanations and varying viewpoints.

It is assumed that veterinary students will have illustrated lectures and applied laboratories to stress the features of processes and lesions that relate to morphological diagnosis and especially to stimulate the students' ability to recognize, understand and describe lesions in fresh postmortem specimens. A high level of achievement in these skills is required.

Pathology is being offered more and more to students in general science and agriculture programs at the undergraduate and graduate levels as well as to students in applied health-related programs in schools of technology. Such courses are labeled "Pathobiology" or "Principles of Disease" or similar names. Departments offering such courses freely are usually overwhelmed by the student response that indicates the general student interest in disease. Why shouldn't any student learn about disease! It is hoped that this book will provide these students with the concepts and principles of disease processes and invite them to further study of disease.

The references provided are intended to lead to further information or detail and are not a complete or exhaustive list. They are likely to be more useful to graduate students than to undergraduates who choose to use the book. Some are selected because of my personal interests. Diagrams and sketches have been used from many sources. Some are very expressive and fit the context of the text so well that they have been used directly with permission. They add to the concept of dynamic processes. The Appendices reflect personal interest.

Most of the subject matter of the book is similar to that in any general pathology course but differs in the emphasis of applied features. Veterinarians are expected to have a much better working knowledge of pathology than physicians because they are required to do routine postmortem examination of animal tissues and ***must interpret the gross lesions of general pathology accurately.*** It is to this purpose that the book is directed. The stimulation for me to learn more about general pathology arose from the recognition of my lack of appreciation of the subject when I was first required to teach the course. The interest and method of presentation has evolved since then.

R. G. THOMSON

Contents

1

INTRODUCTION

WHAT IS PATHOLOGY?

Pathology is the science of the study of disease. It investigates the essential nature of disease and is usually summarized as the study of the functional and morphological changes in the tissues and fluids of the body during disease.

WHY STUDY PATHOLOGY?

The end product of a medical curriculum is a clinician whose function is the diagnosis and treatment of disease. Several main steps are involved in the evolution of a clinician. It is necessary to learn the ***normal development, structure and function*** of the body, and this occurs through the media of embryology, anatomy, histology, genetics, pharmacology, biochemistry and physiology. This step is a prelude to learning what goes wrong with the machine that is called the body. The development of ***structural and functional changes*** in cells, tissues, fluids and organs that result in malfunction and disease is studied in pathology. The ***agents*** that cause disease become known in the study of microbiology, parasitology and toxicology. With the background of knowing ***what*** goes wrong and ***how***, the next step for the prospective clinician is to learn ***how to find out what the problem is*** in the body of a sick individual and ***how to treat it*** by medical or surgical means. Better still, after all this study of disease comes the revelation that it would be easier in the long run to ***prevent*** the disease, if possible, rather than to find and treat it. Of these steps in the development of a clinician, pathology is a cornerstone, because the clinician cannot rationally diagnose and treat without understanding the disease process with which he is dealing.

WHAT IS ILLNESS?

What does it mean to be sick? If an individual is sick, it is assumed that some part of the body is not functioning properly, and it is expected that with proper diagnostic procedures the problem may be found and treated. What of the individual who was "perfectly healthy" but who died suddenly of a stroke or heart attack? There must have been a serious state of disease in some tissues even though the individual had never been "clinically" sick. In fact, some of the cells and tissues in the body of the normal individual who dies suddenly were sick and were not functioning properly. ***Pathology is the study of the molecular, biochemical, functional and morphological aspects of disease in the fluids, cells, tissues and organs of the body.*** Changes brought on by these aspects may lead to clinical illness or may be well developed but not apparent to the individual with the problem.

THE LANGUAGE OF PATHOLOGY

A number of specific terms are used in pathology and medicine and require explanation. Some of the most important are: clinical sign, lesion, etiology, pathogenesis, diagnosis and prognosis.

Suppose an individual has diarrhea. The feeling of abdominal discomfort is a ***clinical symptom*** that can be described by humans but not by animals. The animal exhibits ***clinical signs*** that are observed as diarrhea, not eating, an anxious expression and perhaps dehydration. There must be a functional derangement in the fluid transport at the cellular level in the intestinal mucosa. It may or may not be visible as a microscopic abnormality in the cell, but there is a functional problem. This problem is called a ***lesion*** and may be either ***functional*** or ***morphological*** or both. The lesion is the "abnormality" in the tissue. This word is perhaps the most commonly used word in pathology. ***Etiology*** refers to the cause of the diarrhea and might be a bacteria or virus, some unusual food or a sudden change in diet.

Pathology is the study of ***what*** happened and ***how***. The lesion is What. The sequence of events from the point at which the lesion began through its entire development is called the ***pathogenesis***. It is necessary to know the pathogenesis of lesions in order to make a rational judgment for treatment, control and prevention of disease. Pathogenesis is How—the step by step progression from the normal state through to the abnormal structural or functional state. The usual sequence is to find a lesion, to identify it and then attempt to determine the pathogenesis by investigation of the circumstances and the sequence of events that lead to the lesion.

The study of pathology involves a new language. A primary objective of that study is to master the terminology by learning the definitions, uses and limitations of the language of pathology in its role in the description of lesions and their pathogenesis and etiology. ***This is the theory of pathology but not the practice***. The practice involves being able to ***describe*** lesions, to ***recognize*** the disease process and to ***explain*** how it might have occurred. This requires practical experience, exposure to specimens and problem-solving ability. ***The theory is dangerous without the practical ability***. Depending on the objective for studying pathology, there may be good reason for just learning the words and having a general idea about specific disease processes for general interest. This may be a rewarding and satisfying experience. A license to practice, however, implies knowledge and the ability to apply it. Technical training is essential to carry out diagnostic procedures, but knowledge and practical experience are required to interpret, diagnose and provide an accurate prognosis (see Appendix IV).

In order to avoid confusion, the language of pathology must be used accurately. In general pathology, much emphasis will be placed on using proper terminology and appropriate adjectives in naming lesions. Morphological diagnosis determines the predominant lesion in the tissue, and the student is required to be proficient at making this determination. Gross lesions are described by including reference to the ***location, color, size, shape, consistency and appearance of the cut surface***. Lesions require ***quantification*** by precise measurement or by gradation, at least in general terms, such as mild, moderate or severe. Microscopic descriptions require ***orientation*** of the components of the lesion to one another and to the tissue To invert an old adage, one should start with the forest and then get to the trees in microscopic descriptions (see Appendix III).

The study of things caused must precede the study of the causes of things.

WHAT IS GENERAL PATHOLOGY?

The various types of abnormalities or lesions that may occur are grouped into categories sharing common features for purposes of study. The common categories of lesions are those associated with ***degeneration and death of cells, circulatory disorders*** common to any tissue, ***inflammation and repair***, disturbances in ***growth*** and development of ***cancer. These are the topics of general pathology***. There are features common to all inflammatory lesions, and by knowing these it is easy to apply them to a problem in the kidney, liver, brain or other tissue. All cancers have some features in common, and certain types of cancers have common features regardless of the species affected. The objective in general pathology is to learn the basic lesions and pathogenetic mechanisms associated with disease processes so that they can be applied later to the study of the lesions and pathogenesis of ***specific disease entities*** in ***special pathology***. Special pathology usually involves the ***specific diseases of organ systems***, such as the digestive, respiratory or urinary tract.

WHAT IS A PATHOLOGIST?

A ***pathologist*** is an individual devoted primarily to the study of disease processes. An experimental pathologist works principally on pathogenetic mechanisms of disease, often at the biochemical as well as the morphological level. Many different types of disciplinary experts are required in such ventures, including biochemists, geneticists, cytologists, electron microscopists and others, many of whom do not have a medical background and do not need it for their tasks as experimental pathologists. The practicing pathologist works at diagnosing disease and is the one who performs the autopsy and interprets the biopsies. The objective of the pathologist is to ***find, name and interpret*** the lesions in the tissues examined. Very often, the observations made from naturally occurring diseases are key steps in the process of determining the pathogenesis of a lesion or disease. The pathologist attempts to make a ***diagnosis***. Diagnoses may be ***morphological*** (naming the lesion), ***etiological*** (naming the cause) or ***definitive*** (naming the specific disease entity involved). For example, the lesion catarrhal enteritis, caused by ***Escherichia coli***, results in the disease colibacillosis, and the granulomatous enteritis caused by ***Mycobacterium paratuberculosis*** results in Johne's disease. It is often not possible to determine the etiology or the specific disease entity, so the pathologist records and describes the morphological lesions and then gives an ***interpretation*** of what happened (see end of Appendix I).

WHY DOES A CLINICIAN NEED PATHOLOGY?

The main role of a veterinarian is to ***diagnose, treat, prevent and control animal disease*** to reduce economic loss to society. The key to these functions is ***diagnosis***, and the key to diagnosis is ***the ability to recognize lesions in the live or dead animal, to understand their pathogenesis and, through these, to make rational conclusions and recommendations for treatment, control and prevention***. Sound diagnostic abilities must be based on comprehension of pathology—general and special—and on an understanding of their application in the diagnostic process.

An owner expects to be given a diagnosis and then an interpretation of the probable consequences of the disease in the animal or group of animals. ***Prognosis*** is the expected outcome of disease. A prognosis cannot be accurately provided without an understanding of pathogenesis and an ability to mentally visualize the disease process. The clinican must known what is likely to be the next step in that process and if it can be stopped, if it will heal well or if the probable etiology is susceptible to available therapy. The owner is usually concerned economically or emotionally and may not be as concerned with ***what the problem is*** as with ***what will happen now*** and how a recurrence of the problem can be prevented. The owner's concern is prognosis; the veterinarian's concern is diagnosis and prognosis. ***Both diagnosis and prognosis require comprehension and recognition of lesions and their pathogenesis.*** Pathology is truly the cornerstone of medicine (see Appendix II).

The objective of the chapters that follow is to discuss *general aspects of the disease process*, **to include the pathogenesis if known, to illustrate lesions and processes when appropriate and convenient and to use lesions from animal diseases as examples of particular processes. The detail of specific diseases is part of special pathology, but the examples and illustrations will be helpful and useful for other**

courses and will contribute to the cumulative exposure to animal disease. The examples used for illustration and discussion have been selected and are used in an effort to relate a particular process to a real disease and to whet the appetite for more pathology, medicine and surgery.

SUGGESTIONS FOR FURTHER READING

Pathology

Adelson, L.: The anatomy of justice. Bull. N.Y. Acad. Med., *47*:745–757, 1971.

Bertram, E., Ruf, G., and Sandritter, W.: Education of medical students in general pathology. Comparison of learning strategies: lecture, audiovisomat, self instruction. Beitr. Pathol. *152*:334–346, 1974.

Best, W. R.: Descriptive functions in disease. Biometrics, *27*:895–901, 1971.

Boyd, W.: The development of cellular pathology. Can. Med. Assoc. J., *88*:435–438, 1963.

Curran, W. J.: The medicolegal autopsy and medicolegal investigation. Bull. N.Y. Acad. Med., *47*:766–775, 1971.

Ebert, R. V., et al.: A debate on the autopsy: its quality control function in medicine. Hum. Pathol., *5*:605–606, 1974.

Feinstein, A. R.: An analysis of diagnostic reasoning. I. The domains of classical macrobiology. Yale J. Biol. Med., *46*:212–232, 1973.

Feinstein, A. R.: An analysis of diagnostic reasoning. II. The strategy of intermediate decisions. Yale J. Biol. Med., *46*:264–283, 1973.

Fletcher, O. J., and Weiser, J. R.: Evaluation of instructional methods for teaching veterinary students the components of inflammation. J. Vet. Med. Educ., *2*:2–6, 1975.

Foraker, A. G., and Houston, F. E.: Twelve characters impinging upon the pathologist. Bull. Coll. Am. Pathol., *22*:83–86, 1968.

Gardner, D. L.: The diagnosis of histopathology: senility, apathy, or disease? Hum. Pathol., *3*:445–447, 1972.

Goodale, F., and Gander, G. W.: The future of pathology: a Delphi study by pathology department chairmen. J. Med. Educ., *51*:897–903, 1976.

Gravanis, M. B., and Rietz, C. W.: The problem-oriented postmortem examination and record: an educational challenge. Am. J. Clin. Pathol., *60*:522–535, 1973.

Hudson, R. P.: The concept of disease. Ann. Intern. Med., *65*:595–601, 1966.

Innes, J. R. M.: Veterinary pathology: retrospect and prospect. Vet. Rec., *85*:730–741, 1969.

King, D. W.: The concept of pathobiology. Proc. Rudolph Virchow Med. Soc. City N.Y., *27*:247–260, 1968.

King, D. W.: Patient care, education, and research in pathology. Hum. Pathol., *5*:380–386, 1974.

King, L. S.: How does a pathologist make a diagnosis? Arch. Pathol., *84*:331–333, 1967.

Leader, R. W.: Comparative pathology—renaissance or recession. Hum. Pathol., *2*:177–179, 1971.

Prutting, J.: Lack of correlation between antemortem and postmortem diagnoses. N.Y. State J. Med., *67*:2081–2084. 1967.

Sissons, H. A.: Agreement and disagreement between pathologists in histological diagnosis. Postgrad. Med. J., *51*:685–189, 1975.

Pathology Books

Anderson, W. A. O., and Kissane, J. M. (eds.): Pathology. 7th ed. St. Louis, C. V. Mosby, 1977.

Bajusz, E., and Jasmin, G.: Methods and Achievements in Experimental Pathology. An Introduction to Experimental Pathology. Vol. 1. Chicago, Year Book Medical Publishers, Inc., 1966. Vols. 2 and 3, 1967.

Benirschke, K., et al. (eds.): Pathology of Laboratory Animals. Vols. 1 and 2. New York, Springer-Verlag, 1978.

Boyd, W.: A Textbook of Pathology. Structure and Function in Disease. 8th ed. Philadelphia, Lea & Febiger, 1970.

Cheville, N. F.: Cell Pathology. 2nd ed. Ames, Iowa State University Press, 1983.

Curran, R. C., and Jones, E. L.: Gross Pathology. A Color Atlas. New York, Oxford University Press, 1983.

Dobberstein, J., et al. (eds.): Handbuch der Speziellen Pathologischen Anatomie der Haustiere. Vols. 1 to 7. Berlin, Paul Parey, 1971.

Florey, H. W. (ed.): General Pathology. 4th ed. Philadelphia, W. B. Saunders Company, 1970.

Frei, W., et al.: Allgemaine Pathologie fur Tierarzte und Studierende der Tiermedezin. Berlin, Paul Parey, 1972.

Ghadially, F. N.: Pathology of the Cell. London, Butterworths, 1975.

Griner, L. A.: Pathology of Zoo Animals. San Diego, Zoological Society of San Diego, 1983.

Hill, R. B., Jr., and LaVia, M. F. (eds.): Principles of Pathobiology. 3rd ed. New York, Oxford Press, 1980.

Innes, J. R. M., and Saunders. L. Z.: Comparative Neuropathology. New York, Academic Press, 1962.

Jubb, K. V. F., and Kennedy, P. C.: Pathology of Domestic Animals. Vols. I and II. 2nd ed. New York, Academic Press, 1970.

Monlux, W. S., and Monlux, A. W.: Atlas of Meat Inspection Pathology. Agriculture Handbook No. 367, United States Department of Agriculture, Washington, D.C., 1972.

Montali, R. J., and Migaki, G. (eds.): Comparative Pathology of Zoo Animals. Washington, Smithsonian Institution Press, 1980.

Mouwen, J. M. V. R., and deGrout, E. C. B. M.: Atlas of Veterinary Pathology. Philadelphia, W. B. Saunders Company, 1982.

Nieberle, K., and Cohrs, P.: Textbook of the Special Pathological Anatomy of Domestic Animals. New York, Pergamon Press, 1967.

Perez-Tamayo, R.: Mechanisms of Disease. An Introduction to Pathology. Philadelphia, W. B. Saunders Company, 1961.

Ribelin, W. E., and Migaki, G. W. (eds.): Pathology of Fishes. Madison, University of Wisconsin Press, 1975.

Robbins, S. L., and Cotran, R. S.: Pathologic Basis of Disease. 2nd Ed. Philadelphia, W. B. Saunders Company, 1979.

Robbins, S. L., Angell, M., and Kumar, V.: Basic Pathology. 3rd ed. Philadelphia, W. B. Saunders Company, 1981.

Roberts, R. J. (ed.): Fish Pathology. London, Balliere Tindall, 1978.

Runnells, R. A., et al.: Principles of Veterinary Pathology. Ames, Iowa State University Press, 1965.

von Sandersleben, J., et al. (eds.): Pathologische Histologie der Haustiere. Jena, Gustav Fischer, 1981.

Sandritter, W., and Beneke, G.: Allgemaine Pathologie. Lehrbach fur Studierende und Artze. Stuttgart, F. K. Schattauer, 1974.

Sandritter, W., and Wartman, W. B.: Color Atlas and Textbook of Tissue and Cellular Pathology. Chicago, Year Book Medical Publishers, 1969.

Sandritter, W., et al.: Color Atlas and Textbook of Macropathology. Chicago, Year Book Medical Publishers, 1972.

Slauson, D. O., and Cooper, B. J.: Mechanisms of Disease. A Textbook of Comparative General Pathology. Baltimore, Williams & Wilkins, 1982.

Sodeman, W. A., and Sodeman, W. A., Jr. (eds.): Pathologic Physiology: Mechanisms of Disease. 4th ed. Philadelphia, W. B. Saunders Company, 1967.

Smith, H. A., et al.: Veterinary Pathology. 5th ed. Philadelphia, Lea & Febiger, 1982.

Thompson, S. W., and Luna, L. G.: An Atlas of Artefacts Encountered in the Preparation of Microscopic Tissue Sections. Springfield, Ill., Charles C Thomas, 1978.

Willis, R. A.: The Principles of Pathology Including Bacteriology. 3rd ed. London, Butterworths, 1972.

Animal Disease

Blood, D. C., et al.: Veterinary Medicine. A Textbook of the Diseases of Cattle, Sheep, Pigs and Horses. 5th ed. London, Bailliere Tindall, 1979.

Cooper, J. E., and Jackson, O. F. (eds.): Diseases of the Reptilia. New York, Academic Press, 1981.

Davis, J. W., et al.: Infectious Diseases of Wild Mammals. 2nd ed. Ames, Iowa State University Press, 1981.

van Duijn, C., Jr.: Diseases of Fish. Springfield, Ill., Charles C Thomas, 1973.

Ettinger, S. J. (ed.): Textbook of Veterinary Internal Medicine, Diseases of the Dog and Cat. Vols. 1 and 2, 2nd ed. Philadelphia, W. B. Saunders Company, 1982.

Goldstein, R.: Diseases of Aquarium Fish. Tropical Fish Hobbyist Publ., 1971.

Henning, M. W.: Animal Diseases in South Africa. 3rd ed. South Africa, Central News Agency Ltd., 1956.

Hofstad, M. S., et al.: Diseases of Poultry, 7th ed. Ames, Iowa State University Press, 1978.

Jensen, R., and Mackey, D. R.: Diseases of Feedlot Cattle. 3rd ed. Philadelphia, Lea & Febiger, 1979.

Jensen, R., and Swift, B. L.: Disease of Sheep. 2nd ed. Philadelphia, Lea & Febiger, 1982.

Leman, A. D., et al. (eds.): Diseases of Swine. 5th ed. Ames, Iowa State University Press, 1981.

Petrak, M. L. (ed.): Diseases of Cage and Aviary Birds, 2nd ed. Philadelphia, Lea & Febiger, 1982.

Ristic, M., and McIntyre, I.: Diseases of Cattle in the Tropics: Economic and Zoonotic Relevance. The Hague, Netherlands, M. Nijhoff, 1981.

Ruch, T. C.: Diseases of Laboratory Primates. Philadelphia, W. B. Saunders Company, 1959.

Wobeser, G. A.: Diseases of Wild Waterfowl. New York, Plenum Press, 1981.

2

DEGENERATION AND NECROSIS

Degeneration and death of cells occur at a normal rate in most tissues of the body. New cells are formed at about the same rate, keeping the mass of the tissue stable. This concept is normal for populations of animals as well as for cells. As death occurs among the aged, sick and worn-out members of a species, they are replaced by the newborn. If the death and illness rates are particularly high, the balance between those dying and the replacements is disturbed and the total group will not be able to carry out normal functions because of a lack of work force. Similarly, if too many cells become sick or die, there will be impairment of normal function in the tissue concerned. If the increased mortality occurs slowly over a long period of time, the group may adjust by increasing the birthrate, and functions may remain normal. The illness and death may occur suddenly and at a high rate, however, so that replacements would not be available soon enough to prevent disruption of function.

This chapter is concerned with ***injured, dying and dead cells: how these processes occur, how they may be recognized and their significance in disease***. The first part of the chapter involves sick cells (degeneration) and the last part deals with dead cells (necrosis), although there is some overlap. Pigmentations and chemical substances accumulating in cells or tissues undergoing degeneration or suffering from a metabolic defect are also included in this chapter, since they are to some extent degenerations.

THE NORMAL CELL

Before proceeding with illness in cells, it is appropriate to review briefly the normal structural components of cells and their functions in order to appreciate the significance of some of the degenerative changes. It is traditional to use the liver cell because it has a full complement of organelles, but it is also important to appreciate that the liver cell is used only as an example and the inferences may not be applicable to all cells in terms of structure. The function and appearance of organelles among tissues are generally similar; however, differences do occur. The general features of the cell are represented in Figure 2–1. The cell membrane controls movement into and out of the cell and in particular controls the osmotic gradients involving fluids. In addition, the cell membrane has specific receptor sites, or points of attachment, for particular chemical and biochemical compounds necessary for the function of the cell. Cell surface structure and function, including the cytoskeleton, are reviewed in detail by Rungger-Brandle and Gabbiani (1983). The mitochondria are the site of aerobic carbohydrate metabolism and are therefore the main source of energy. Glycolysis occurs outside the mitochondria in the fluid components of the cytoplasm. The endoplasmic reticulum is the center for protein production. The rough endoplasmic reticulum (RER) has ribosomes attached, and the smooth endoplasmic reticulum (SER) does not. Ribosomes may be free in the cell cytoplasm and make proteins primarily for use in the cell, whereas those proteins made in the RER are often for export. The SER is a metabolic center for breaking down or forming new compounds. The Golgi apparatus produces and often packages the secretory products made by the cell. The lysosomes contain enzymes for internal storage or digestion of unwanted products, broken-down components of organelles, or particulate matter taken into the cell. Microtubules seem to control movement of cells, some surface properties and some aspects of mitosis. The nucleus contains DNA in the chromatin granules and RNA primarily in the nucleolus, and these control the basic structure and function of the cell by directly or indirectly determining many of the functions of the organelles. Many cells have specialized structures such as cilia or microvilli for special functions. There are numerous texts of histology illustrating the structure and function of all parts of the cell in great detail.

Just as clinical illness may result when some part of the body does not function normally, sick cells result from a dysfunction in some part of the cell.

DEGENERATION

As will be mentioned on several occasions in this and later chapters, abnormal function may be associated with abnormal cell morphology, and conversely, abnormal structure may be associated with abnormal function. These abnormal morphological changes are called ***degenerations***, which in a sense implies that the cell is sick. However, these changes may arise from increased functional demands. Both causes may be within normal limits of physiological adaptation. Thus the line between normal physiological adaptation and degeneration may be ***ill defined and subjective*** if only mild or moderate morphological changes are present. Some lesions that are called degenerations are only indications of ***temporary functional changes*** or adaptations, whereas others are serious and imply ***progression toward death of the cell*** (Fig. 2–2). In general, degenerative changes are considered reversible if the functions return to normal. The nature of the biochemical and functional abnormalities cannot always be related directly to the amount or nature of morphological changes in organelles, and many abnormalities within the cell are ***nonspecific*** with regard to etiology. This is an important point to remember because there is often an attempt to relate the action of a specific agent to a specific intracellular change, but this usually cannot be determined.

The names of degenerative lesions carry the suffix ***"osis"***; for example, nephrosis and hepatosis indicate degenerative lesions in the kidney and liver, respectively.

General Intracellular Degenerative Changes

There are several general types of abnormal morphological changes found in cells. The ***cell membrane*** may alter its appearance by the formation of a variety of configurations such as folds, blebs and whorls, by separation from junctional sites with other structures or by the formation of holes. The holes are likely to be fatal to the cell because

Text continued on page 10

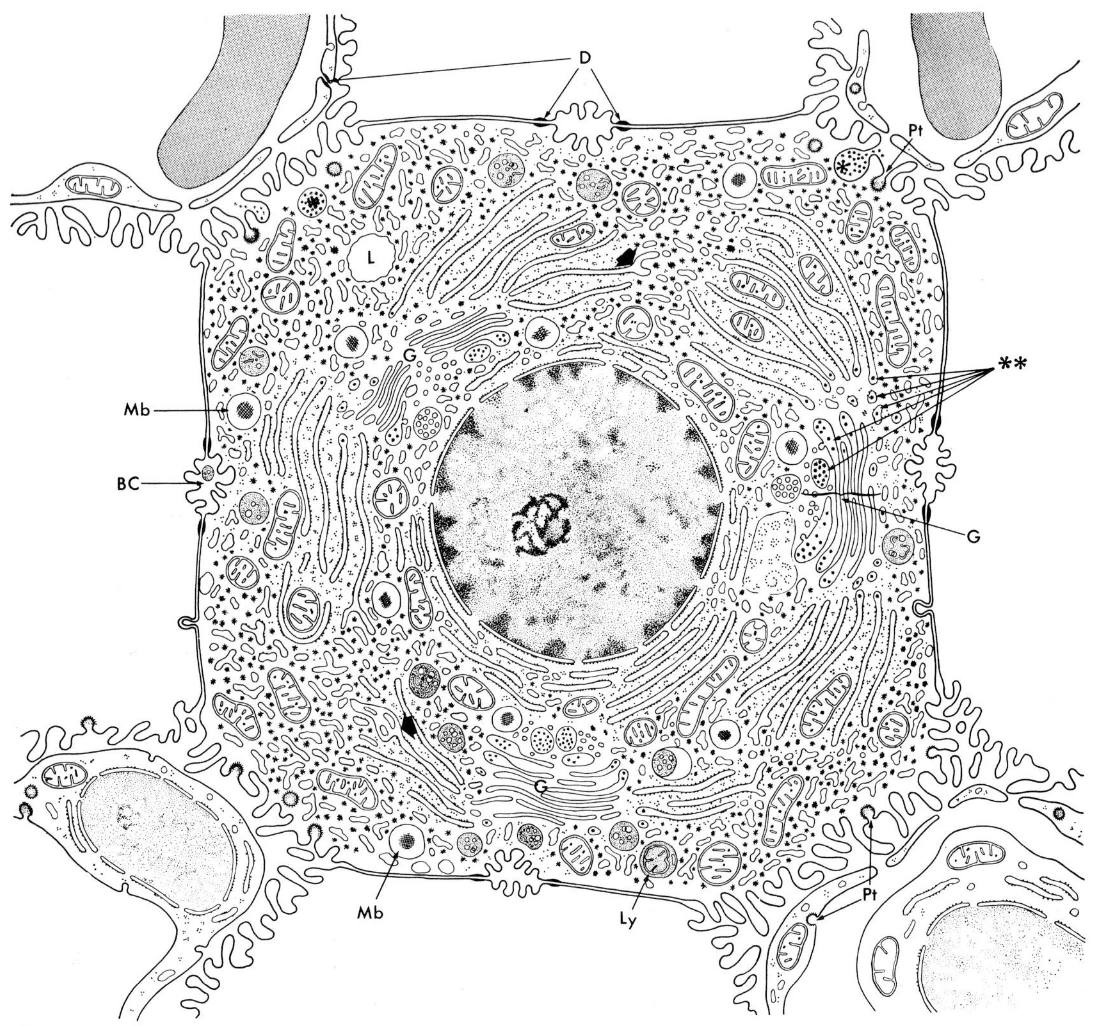
D
Pt
L
G
**
Mb
BC
G
G
Mb
Ly
Pt

Figure 2–1. The fine structure of a cell or tissue is frequently clarified by the construction of a diagram of the whole or its parts. Such constructed images represent distillations of the information gathered from the study of many micrographs. As such, they are important for the student and even more important for the investigator, who is obliged in making the diagram to clarify concepts of structural relationships that might otherwise remain confused. In representing interpretations of observations, diagrams are seldom absolutely correct in all they show and are therefore valuable only as temporary aids to understanding.

This drawing represents a single parenchymal cell of the rat liver. It is surrounded by and closely contiguous with four other hepatic cells (which are not drawn in) and four sinusoids or capillaries of the blood supply. These latter surfaces, which show several microvilli, are equivalent to the basal poles or surfaces of this epithelial cell, unusual in this instance in not being underlaid by a basement membrane. The sinusoids are limited by thin endothelial cells with openings as illustrated. Red blood cells are represented in the two at the upper right and left corners of the picture; a white cell is in the lower right.

The student should have no difficulty in recognizing such prominent constituents of the cell as nucleus, mitochondria and the long slender profiles of cisternae belonging to the endoplasmic reticulum, or ER. Small particles or ribosomes are abundant on the surfaces of the latter and in the ground substance between them. The cisternae are ordinarily arranged in stacks of 6 to 12 units. One margin of such an assemblage frequently lies adjacent to the Golgi complex, and it will be noted that small granules of a particular type occupy the ends of these cisternae and the vesicles intervening between ER and Golgi, as well as the expanded ends of cisternae and spherical vesicles belonging to the Golgi proper (G). These images (**) are designed to show the mechanism of protein transport from ER to Golgi where packaging for export takes place (see * in upper right corner). The other margin of the stacks of ER cisternae borders on masses of glycogen and associated vesicles belonging to the so-called smooth endoplasmic reticulum, or SER. These two forms are often continuous as though the smooth form may develop from the rough. Such continuities are indicated by thick arrows. It is thought by some, on incomplete evidence, that the SER is involved in the transport of glucose from the liver cell during glycogenolysis. Other prominent components of the hepatic cell cytoplasm include lysosomes (Ly), containing remnants of organelles and ground substance apparently set aside for hydrolysis, and microbodies (mb) of uncertain significance, though probably rich in enzymes. A single lipid granule is indicated at L.

Various differentiations of the cell surface are shown, though their full functional meaning is not completely clarified as yet. The surface adjacent to and limiting the bile canaliculus is increased in area by many microvilli. This represents the free surface of this cell, and as is common in epithelial cells, it is limited by tight junctions and desmosomes (D). Besides showing numerous microvilli on its sinusoid surface, the liver cell possesses peculiar pits (Pt) or spherical depressions with what appear as short bristles on their cytoplasmic surfaces. These same structures are present on the endothelial cells and Kupffer cells lining the sinusoids. They are thought to be involved in the selective uptake of proteins and possibly other macromolecules from the circulating blood plasma. (From Porter, K. R., and Bonneville, M. A.: An Introduction to the Fine Structure of Cells and Tissues. Philadelphia, Lea & Febiger, 1964. Reprinted by permission.)

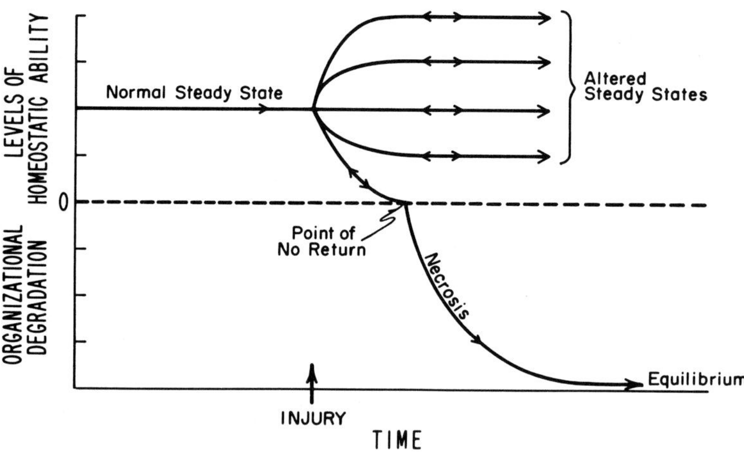

Figure 2–2. Conceptualization of cell injury. Following injury, a cell that was previously in a normal steady state can be considered to enter a phase in which the homeostatic mechanisms are altered, resulting in new or altered steady states, such as fatty metamorphosis, hypertrophy or atrophy. The cell may remain in this new steady state for long periods of time while the injury is continued. In the case of lethal injuries, on the other hand, the cell can eventually be assumed to pass a point, shown as zero level of homeostatic ability, beyond which it is unable to restore equilibrium even if the injury is eliminated. The zero level of homeostatic ability may be referred to as the *point of no return* or the *point of cell death*. Beyond this, the cell undergoes a series of degradative reactions leading to the production of cell debris or a state of physicochemical equilibrium. (From Trump, B. F., and Ginn, F. L.: The pathogenesis of subcellular reaction to lethal injury. *In* Bajusz, E., and Jasmin, G. [eds.]: Methods and Achievements in Experimental Pathology. Vol. 4. Chicago, Year Book Medical Publishers, 1969. Reprinted by permission.)

of osmotic swelling, as in injury by complement. Peroxidation of unsaturated lipids in all membranes by free radicals is a common injury and may lead to configurational changes or breakdown. The free radicals lead to degeneration of the phospholipid layer and eventually the protein components of the cell membrane. Parts of the normal membrane may bud off as external blebs, a process called ***exocytosis or exotropy,*** or particles and fluids may be taken in by internal blebs in a process called ***endocytosis or esotropy.*** These processes may be accentuated in injury. The cell membrane separates the internal from the external constituents of the cell by control of membrane permeability, membrane-associated enzyme or carrier systems, the electrochemical gradient and the energy supply. Each of these may be upset by a particular injury. Cell volume is particularly significant. Water movement is passive and controlled largely by potassium and sodium transport. Injury to the sodium pump results in movement of sodium and chloride into the cell together with water.

Mitochondria may be altered into a variety of configurations, as indicated in Figure 2–3. ***Endoplasmic reticulum*** may lose ribosomes, break up or become greatly dilated into vesicular structures or may form dense whorls when injured (Fig. 2–4). ***Lysosomes*** may become quite prominent for a number of reasons: the need for digestion, the removal of particles brought into the cell by the process called ***heterophagy*** or the removal of degenerate components within the cell by the process of ***autophagy*** (Fig. 2–5). Lysosomes may have a variety of shapes and sizes, depending on their work requirements or the degree of degeneration of other cellular components. Some intended secretions are transferred to lysosomes for disposal. Lysosomes represent a system of channels and cavities in the cell that include phagosomes, secondary lysosomes, the Golgi apparatus, and the endoplasmic reticulum. This system serves in the digestion of constituents, such as macromolecules taken into the cell by endocytosis, as well as in the digestion of cellular components, such as mitochondria and other membranous structures sequestered from the remainder of the cell by autophagocytosis. The process of digestion involves bringing substrate and acid hydrolases into contact within the digestive vacuole. Typically, this occurs by fusion of a heterophagosome or autophagosome with a primary or secondary lysosome containing acid hydrolase. The acid hydrolases typically have long half-lives and may be used for many digestive events. Synthesis of acid hydrolases appears to occur on polysomes of the rough endoplasmic reticulum with transport via the reticular cisternae to the Golgi apparatus, where packaging into the primary lysosomes or Golgi vesicles occurs. While within the digestive vacuoles, the digestive enzymes do not have access to other sub-

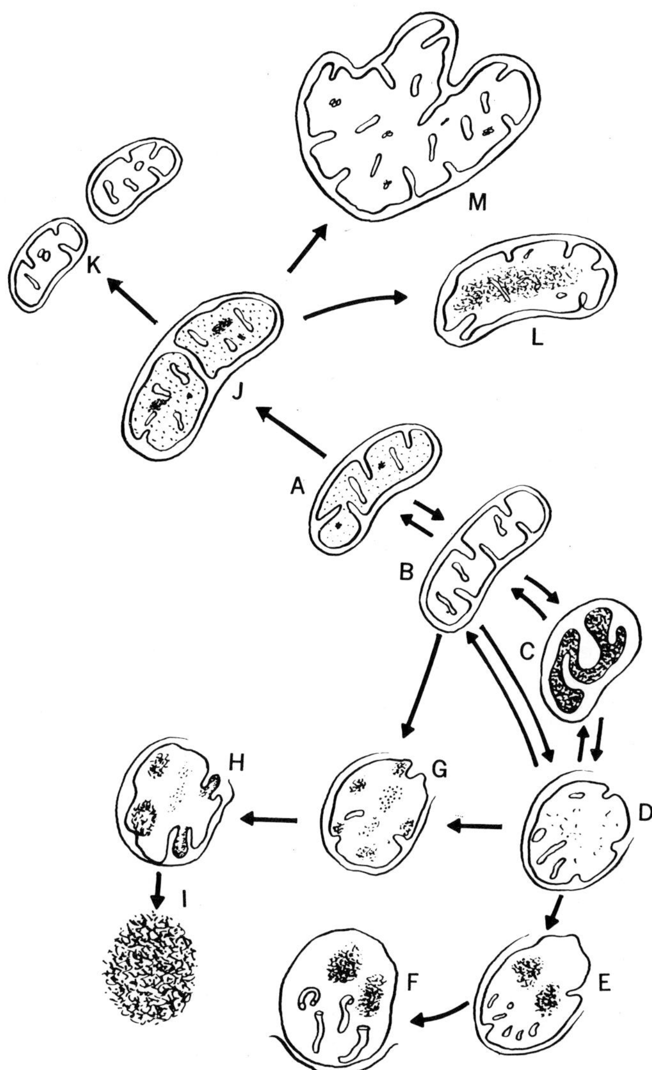

Figure 2–3. Diagram of progressive mitochondrial changes in cell injury. (From La Via, M. F., and Hill, R. B.: Principles of Pathobiology. New York, Oxford University Press, 1971. Reprinted by permission.)

A Typical normal mitochondrion.
B The mitochondrial granules are lost, presumably owing to decrease in ATP.
C Condensed mitochondrion in which the matrix is contracted, possibly the result of condensation of matrix proteins following changes in ADP/ATP ratio. Increased levels of ADP often produce contraction.
D This shows high-amplitude swelling after ion and water movements into the mitochondrion with rupture of the outer membrane.
E Fluffy deposits that probably represent aggregations of denatured proteins are seen; at this stage, mitochondria are severely damaged, and P/O ratios approach zero.
F Tubular forms have arisen from the inner membrane.
G Deposits of apatites occur following calcium and phosphate accumulation by mitochondria.
H The calcium deposits are in annular patterns adjacent to the inner membrane.
I The entire mitochondrion has calcified.
J Beginning mitochondrial division with a septum separating the inner compartment into two phases, each of which contains clumped mitochondrial DNA in the matrix.
K The division is completed.
L A paracrystalline aggregate in the mitochondrial matrix, as seen in human livers.
M A megamitochondrion that may arise from defective mitochondrial division or from fusion.

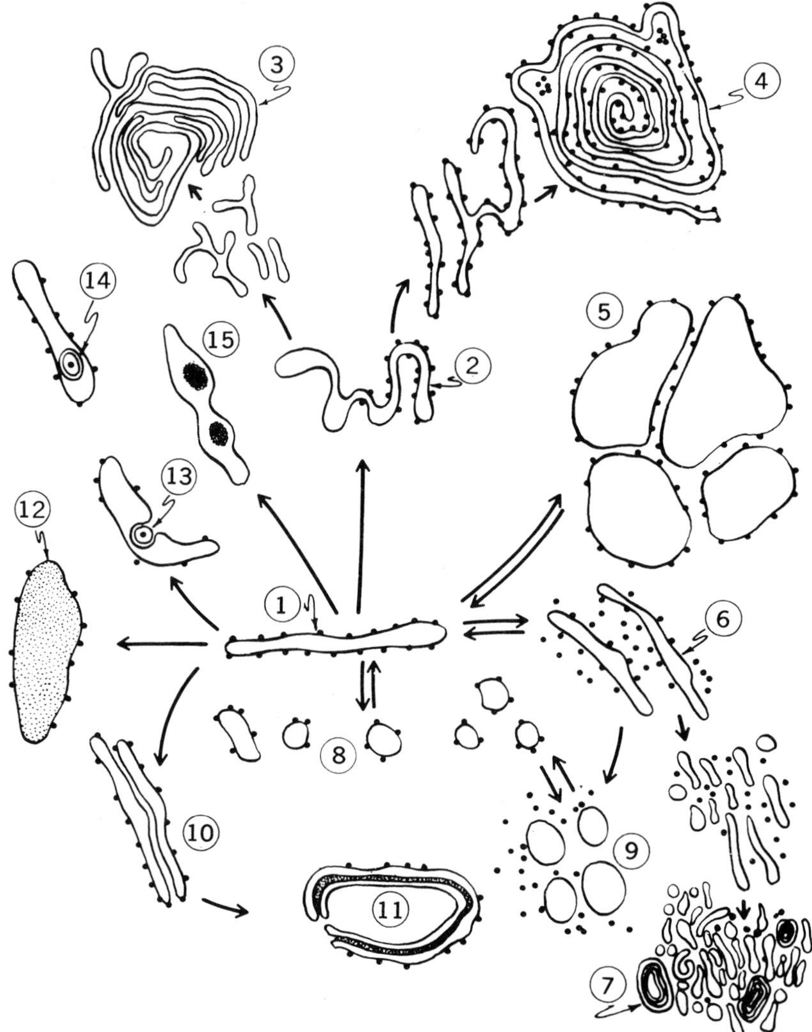

Figure 2–4. Conformational changes in rough endoplasmic reticulum. *1,* Normal conformation. *2,* Stimulated synthesis of rough and smooth ER membranes results in proliferations of smooth ER (*3*), as after phenobarbital-induced detoxification, and complex proliferations of rough ER (*4*). *5,* Dilatation of endoplasmic cisternae is caused by mild injuries with changes in ion and water movements. *6,* Degranulation (loss of polysomes from the endoplasmic reticulum) is a common response to injury. *7,* Peroxidation results in changes of membrane conformation and accumulation of densities. *8, 9,* Progressive fragmentation of ER results in smooth vesicles and detached polysomes. *10, 11,* Paired cisternae are formed after treatment with certain hormones, including cortisone. *12,* Materials such as glycoproteins may accumulate with ER cisternae. *13, 14,* Exotrophy of naked virions into the endoplasmic reticulum cisternae results in an enveloped virus within ER. *15,* Lipoprotein may accumulate in ER. (From La Via, M. F., and Hill, R. B.: Principles of Pathobiology. New York, Oxford University Press, 1971. Reprinted by permission.)

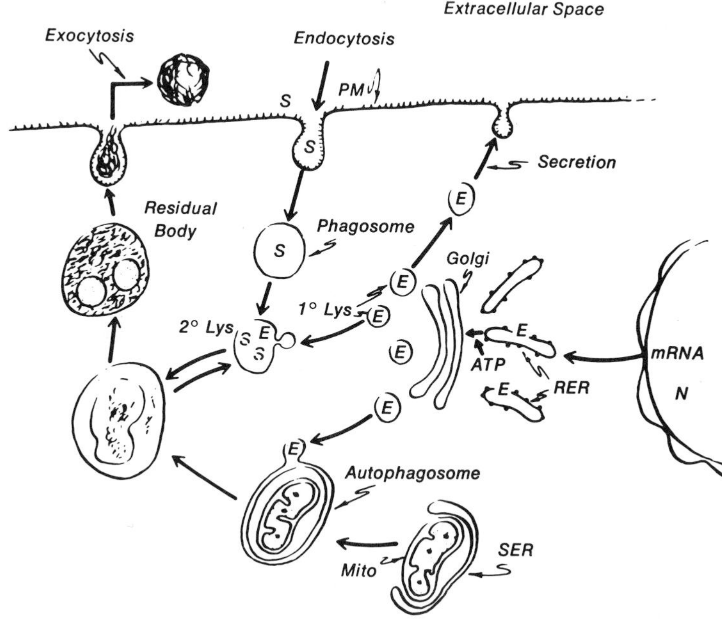

Figure 2–5. Diagram showing relation of the lysosome system. *E,* Acid hydrolase; *RER,* rough endoplasmic reticulum; *mRNA,* messenger RNA; *N,* nucleus; *SER,* smooth endoplasmic reticulum; *PM,* plasma membrane; *S,* substrate; broken *S,* partially digested substrate; *1° Lys,* primary lysosome; *2° Lys,* secondary lysosome; *Mito,* mitochondrion. (From Scarpelli, D. G., and Trump, B. F.: Cell Injury. Kalamazoo, Michigan, The Upjohn Company, 1964. Reprinted by permission.)

strates in the cell. Damage to the lysosomal membrane, however, tends to promote increased permeability, as noted earlier. This ultimately permits other substrates to enter the lysosome; if the damage is sufficiently severe, it permits the acid hydrolases to leave the lysosome and attack other substrates within the cell. Autophagic vacuoles may be prominent in vitamin E deficiency. Some compounds, such as hemosiderin, are stored in lysosomes. Internal release of the enzymes from lysosomes is likely to be fatal to the cell and is named ***autolysis***. A summary of intracellular reactions to chronic cell injury is included in Figure 2–6.

Stenger (1970) illustrates the ***nonspecific nature of the actions of many agents on the cell and the difficulty in making firm statements about specificity or even generalizations about actions of groups of agents***. Cheville (1983) classifies many cellular degenerations of organelles according to types of etiological agents and gives examples of agents that cause certain lesions in organelles. These references are useful for more detailed consideration of organelle lesions than is appropriate here.

Morphological changes in cell membranes and organelles are only visible in detail at the ultrastructural level and by light microscopy appear as vacuoles, droplets or inclusions that are sometimes rather vague. The emphasis here will be on light microscopy in prominent lesions, and it must be remembered that the specific definition of any cellular lesion must be made by electron microscopy and that any lesion visible by light microscopy will be prominent by electron microscopy. The use of electron microscopy is becoming routine in some diagnostic functions and particularly in long-term drug evaluation and testing for cancer-inducing agents. Even in these studies, however, interpretation is still difficult because many agents produce similar morphological changes. ***Examine Figures 2–1 to 2–6 and their legends in detail.***

The liver cell has been studied in detail to determine the sequence of events in cell degeneration and death. Many agents have been used to induce cell injury, including ethionine, which primarily causes depletion of adenine and nucleotides; galactosamine, which depletes the supply of uridine nucleotides; carbon tetrachloride, which disrupts membranes by free radical formation; and acute anoxia, which allows excess calcium into the cell because of cell membrane changes. In general, RNA deficiency, ATP deficiency, reduced protein synthesis, mitochondrial calcification and rupture of lysosomes are late events in the process of cell death and none is specific as being the key limiting factor. Actually it is not easy to separate cause from effect in the sequence of events and it may be erroneous

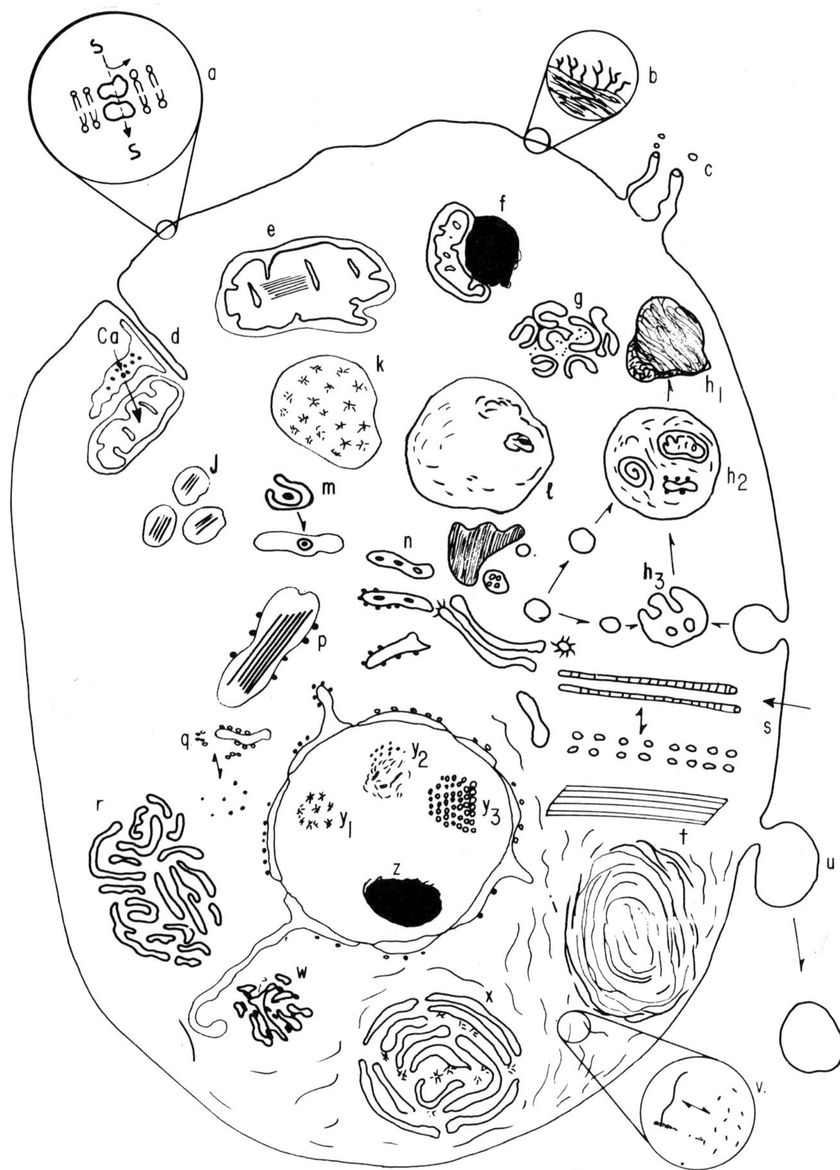

Figure 2–6. Diagram showing chronic reactions to cell injury. The letters in sequence are as follows: *a,* Alteration of transmembrane transport processes; *b,* alteration of cell surface coat, e.g., neoplastic transformation; *c,* alterations of cell surface activity, e.g., tubular forms; *d,* calcium shift from sarcoplasmic reticulum to mitochondria in heart failure; *e,* megamitochondria; *f,* lipid droplet; *g,* exotropy induced by poliomyelitis virus; h_1, lipofuscin; h_2, autophagic vacuole; h_3, multivesicular body; *i,* alcoholic hyalin; *j,* formation of new peroxisomes; *k, l,* lysosomal storage; *m,* virus budding into ER; *n,* lipoprotein in ER; *o,* storage in dilated ER cisterna; *p,* protein crystals in ER, e.g., Russell bodies; *q,* separation of polyribosomes from membrane; *r,* proliferation of SER; *s,* microtubule—disassembly; *t,* microtubules—crystal formation; *u,* exotropy at surface; *v,* microfilament—disassembly; *w,* peroxidation lesions of ER; *x,* glycogen body; y_1, virus production; y_2, stratification of elements in nucleolus; y_3, crystalline virus inclusion; *z,* protein inclusion in nucleus, e.g., Pb poisoning. (From Zweifach, B. W., et al. [eds.]: The Inflammatory Process. New York, Academic Press, 1965. Reprinted by permission.)

to assume there is one common path to cell necrosis. Attention centers on the key point of determining the event that is considered to be the point of irreversibility and is perhaps the most important. Farber and coworkers emphasize the ***influx of calcium ions*** in ischemia as the critical event. Ischemia causes degradation of phospholipids in internal and cell wall membranes, which disrupts the ionic permeability barriers, allowing calcium ions into the cell. The accelerated phospholipid degradation is probably a consequence of the activation of endogenous phospholipases as a result of disturbed calcium homeostasis, which in part is an intracellular redistribution of calcium ions.

Blockage of the blood supply to a liver lobe for three hours causes no alteration in hepatocyte structure, but when the circulation is resumed, lesions of acute degeneration and necrosis follow, primarily because of calcium influx into the cells. The switch to ***anaerobic metabolism*** because of anoxia is also significant in altering intracellular pH. Figure 2–7 provides an overview of cellular events caused by anoxia. Cheville provides many electron micrographic illustrations of degenerative changes in cells.

Robbins and Cotran identify the following sequence of events in ***hypoxia***: reduced ATP, stimulation of phosphofructokinase and anaerobic glycolysis, reduced intracellular pH, clumping of nuclear chromatin, cell swelling caused by a defective sodium pump, dilated smooth endoplasmic reticulum, detachment of ribosomes, bleb formation in membranes, myelin figure formation, swelling and vacuolation of mitochondria with formation of flocculent densities, calcification of mitochondria, release of lysosomal enzymes internally and cellular enzymes externally, continuing disruption of membranes and finally, breakup of the cell.

Important causes of degeneration or necrosis include mechanical injury, such as trauma, ischemia, toxins, lipid peroxidation, some bacterial, parasitic and viral infections, immune cytotoxicity and metabolic suppression or derangement.

Free radicals are capable of reacting with nearly all macromolecules of the cell and thereby potentially cross linking and denaturing DNA and enzymes, or causing lipid peroxidation of organelle membranes and disrupting metabolism.

Complete reduction of oxygen results in formation of intermediates in the form of the superoxide anions, hydrogen peroxide and the hydroxyl radical. Formation of free radicals is a major component of radiation injury. These radicals are dangerously reactive and must be neutralized. The superoxide radical is eliminated by ***superoxide dismutases,*** which catalyze its conversion to hydrogen peroxide plus oxygen. The hydrogen peroxide is removed by catalases, which convert it to water plus oxygen, and by peroxidases, which reduce it to water. The superoxide radical, O_2^{-} can induce lipid peroxidation, damage membranes and kill cells. The O_2^{-} radical is used by neutrophils to kill bacteria taken into phagosomes. Also, death of activated neutrophils may release this potent toxin into tissue and cause necrosis.

Vitamin E is one of the main ***antioxidant*** protective mechanisms for lipid membranes of the cell. It acts by donating hydrogen to peroxides that form in lipid membranes and thus limits their reaction with neighboring polyunsaturated fatty acids. This process confines lipid peroxidation chain reactions and resultant membrane damage.

Figure 2–8 conveys events leading to cell death caused by acute toxicity, such as that caused by carbon tetrachloride. Figure 2–9 provides a view of some of the morphological events leading to cell death. ***These should be examined in detail.***

Specific Types of Intracellular Degenerative Changes

A number of specific degenerations will be discussed. There is not necessarily a relationship between them, other than being examples of changes that occur in tissues or cells and that have been given names. Confusion may occur because they are not necessarily related to each other. ***They should be regarded as separate, sometimes unrelated, examples of lesions*** in cells and tissues. Some of the names have come from Virchow's time and now have a somewhat different context than when he used them. All, however, are abnormalities, and each can be caused by a variety of etiological agents or functional abnormalities.

Text continued on page 18

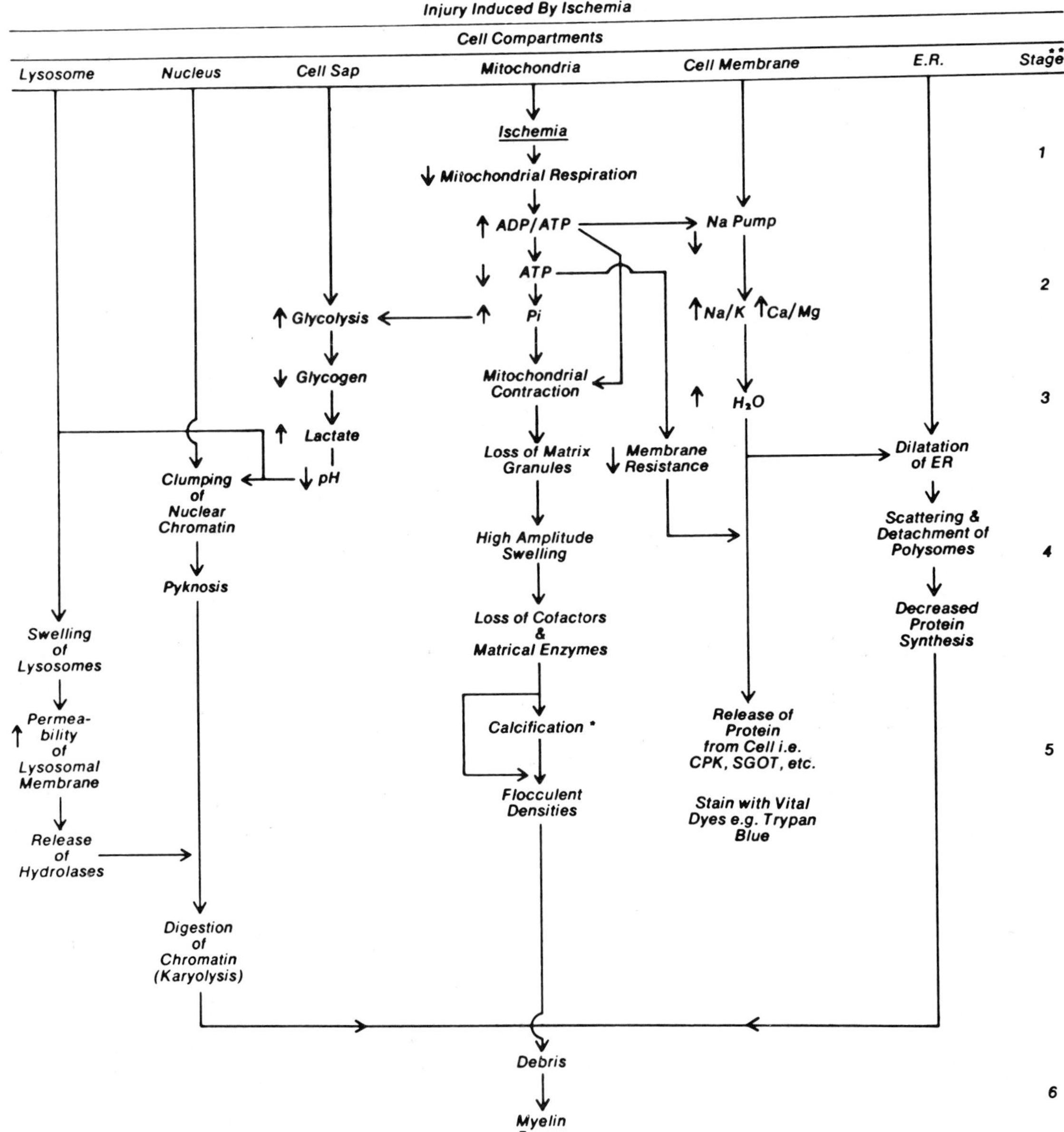

Figure 2–7. Pathogenesis of ischemic cell injury. (From Scarpelli, D. G., and Trump, B. F.: Cell Injury. Kalamazoo, Michigan, The Upjohn Company, 1964. Reprinted by permission.)

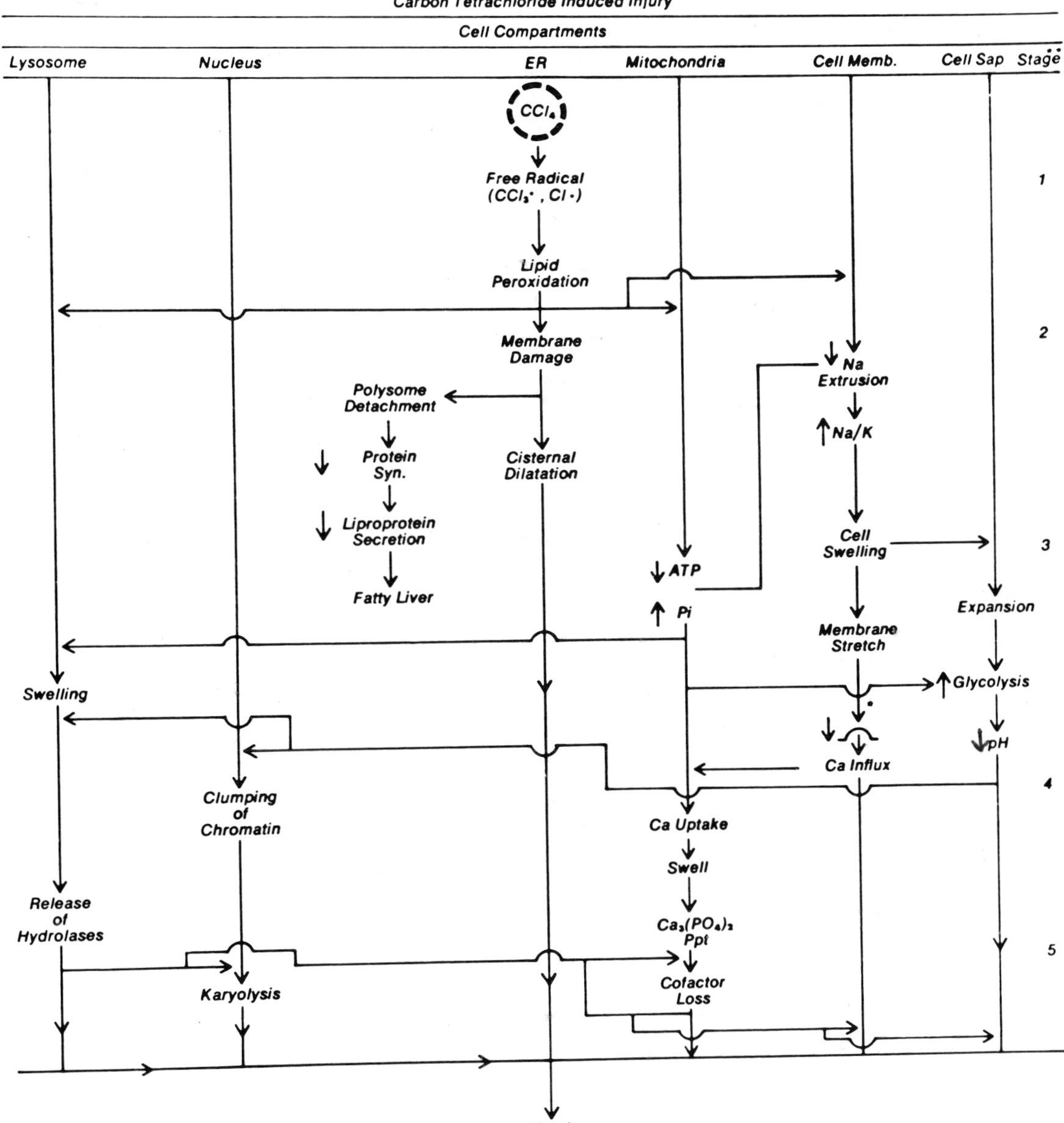

*Electrical Resistance of Membrane.

**Numbers at the right correspond to the temporal sequence of events.

Figure 2–8. Pathogenesis of carbon tetrachloride induced injury. (From Scarpelli, D. G., and Trump, B. F.: Cell Injury. Kalamazoo, Michigan, The Upjohn Company, 1964. Reprinted by permission.)

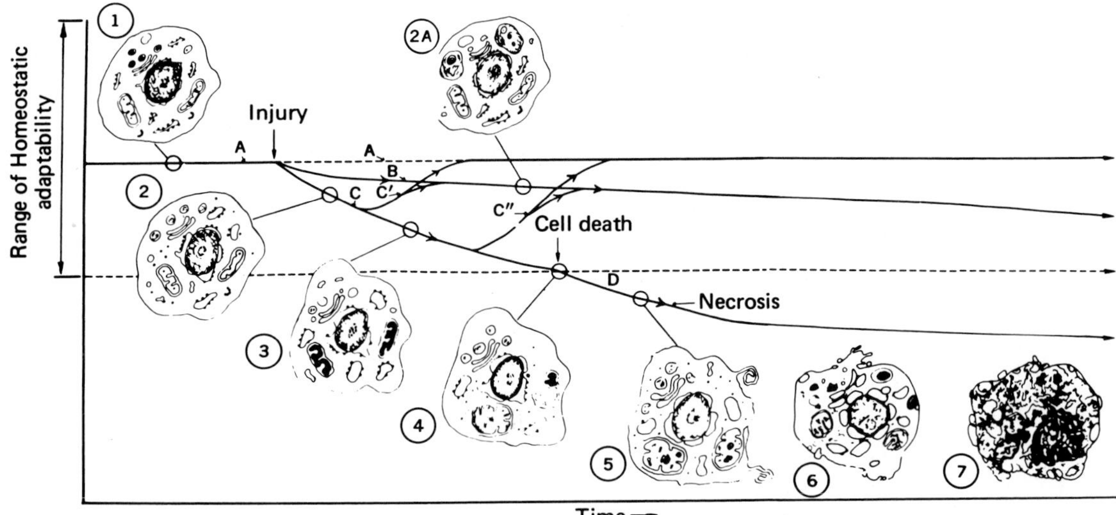

Figure 2–9. Stages of cell injury. Plotted along the abscissa is time, and along the ordinate is range of homeostatic ability.

Stage 1 shows a cell in a normal steady state (curve A). At the arrow an injury is applied which may be acutely lethal or sublethal. In the case of the lethal injury, the cell loses homeostatic ability along curve C. Prior to the point of cell death, however, recovery can occur if the injurious stimulus is removed. Such recovery might proceed along curve C′ or curve C″. In stage 2 the principal change consists of dilatation of the ER and slight clumping of the nuclear chromatin, though some ribosomes may be detached from the endoplasmic reticulum, and the entire cell may be slightly swollen. In stage 3 the mitochondria are condensed, the cell is more swollen, and blebs begin to appear along the cell membrane. After the point of cell death, recovery cannot occur, even if the injurious stimulus is removed; the cell is said to enter the phase of necrosis. During this transitional period, stage 4 is seen, and in it changes similar to those in stage 3 occur, except that some mitochondria are markedly swollen, while in others portions of their inner compartments are condensed and other portions are swollen. The lysosomes remain intact; there is increased ribosomal scattering and increased cell swelling. During the phase of necrosis, the cell undergoes degradation by autolysis and denaturation, and a typical morphologic picture occurs as in stage 5. In stage 6 the secondary and primary lysosomes in the cell begin to disappear, and large gaps and irregularities in the cell surface membrane can be seen.

In stage 7 the membrane debris resulting from fragmentation and distortion of organelles begins to be converted to large myelin figures that occupy large areas of the cytoplasm and represent formation of bilayer configurations from the altered and hydrated lipid derivatives.

Stage 2A represents a common sublethal adaptation, one in which numerous secondary lysosomes filled with digestive debris can be seen. Note that the other organelles appear well preserved. Note also that incomplete recovery during the reversible phases after a lethal injury might result also in a new steady state, depicted by the right hand limb of curves C′ and C″. (Modified from Trump, B. F., et al.: Cellular change in human disease. A new method of pathological analysis. Hum. Pathol., 4:89, 1973.)

CELL SWELLING

Swelling of the cells is the most common and most important response to cellular injuries of all types, including mechanical, anoxic, toxic, lipid peroxidation, viral, bacterial and immune mechanisms. It is observed most readily in epithelial and endothelial cells by light microscopy. If generalized cell swelling occurs in an organ such as the liver or kidney, the organ will be somewhat enlarged. An objective interpretation of such a lesion on gross examination of the organ would be difficult, however.

By light microscopy, the cells appear crowded, with a diluted, dispersed or indistinct appearance of the cytoplasm. The cell membranes develop large surface extrusions or blebs, and specialized structures such as microvilli are distorted. Within the cytoplasm there is expansion but no increase in organelles. The cytoplasm appears dilute or rarefied, and combinations of mitochondrial swelling, vesiculation and fragmentation of endoplasmic reticulum and lysis of the protoplasm of the cell occur either focally or diffusely. The degree of response in the parts of the cell varies with the agent causing the swelling and the severity of injury. It is not possible to differentiate the various changes within the cell organelles by light microscopy. In severe injury, it is usually the greatly dilated and distorted endoplasmic reticulum that gives the appearance of pale areas within the cell observed with light microscopy.

The nucleus responds to injury with swelling, dispersion of chromatin, disruption of nucleoli and, if severely injured, disruption of membranes. Minor injuries to the nucleus may affect chromosomes and alter the genetic coding of the cell, which may have such long-term effects as the generation of cancerous cells.

Cloudy swelling is an old term for a swollen cell in which the cytoplasm has a uniformly swollen, cloudy appearance. Virchow used the name in reference to unstained tissues, so it has little direct connection to the usage today. The change is nonspecific and usually occurs in the liver and kidney. ***Autolysis results in a similar light microscopic appearance,*** creating difficulties in interpretation. The term should not be used for gross lesions and should be used with considerable caution in light microscopy. A tissue could be swollen grossly by enlargement of cells, as in cloudy swelling, but this would be most difficult to differentiate from diffuse accumulation of fluid or other materials in the tissue. ***Cell swelling*** is really a more appropriate term.

Hydropic degeneration is another term used to describe swelling of cells and is considered to have causes similar to those of cell swelling but to be a more advanced lesion. It is also called ballooning degeneration. There is a clear vacuole in the cytoplasm of the cell, perhaps beside or around the nucleus, and the cell is swollen. The term should not be used for gross lesions and microscopically must be ***differentiated from cell swelling, fatty degeneration, glycogen, autolysis and artifact***. Hydropic degeneration is usually associated with epithelial lesions and has particular associations that are clues to the diagnosis of specific diseases; for example, it is associated with inclusion bodies in the urinary tract epithelium of dogs with distemper, in cells infected with virus in many diseases and in the rumenal epithelium in cattle with carbohydrate rumen overload. In the last case, the hydropic changes in the squamous epithelium progress to bursting and coalescence to form ***microvesicles*** within the epithelium (Figs. 2–10 and 2–11). The excess carbohydrate ferments rapidly to produce lactic acidosis, which increases the osmotic pressure in the rumen. The animal becomes very dehydrated as fluid from the blood enters the rumen, and the epithelium is injured by either the acidity or osmolarity or both. The epithelium may be completely

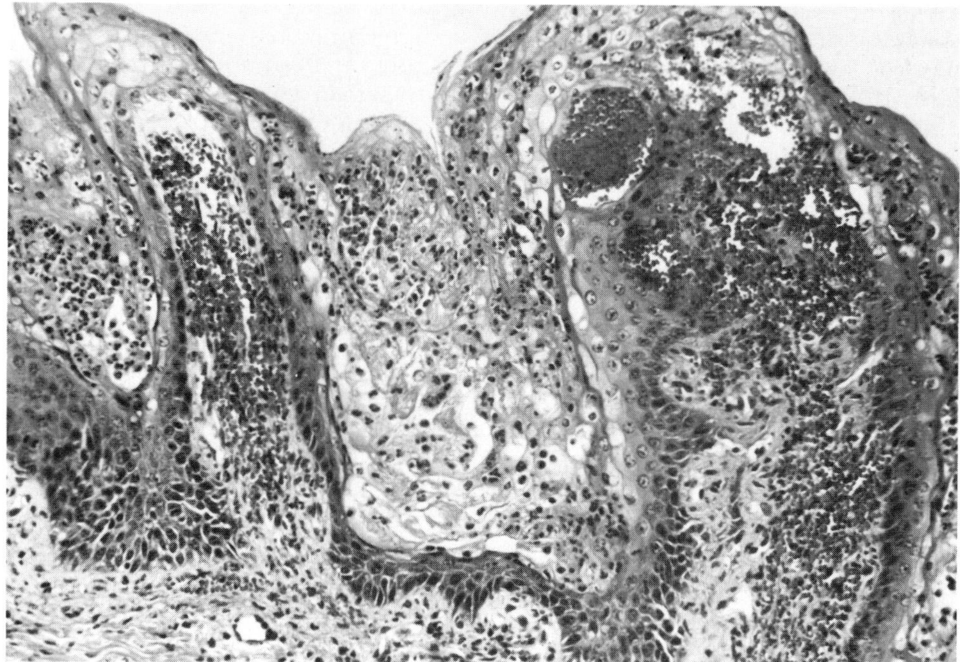

Figure 2–10. Hydropic degeneration in the rumen epithelium in a case of grain overload in a steer. The cells in the mid-layers of the epithelium are vacuolated and ballooned. There are many red blood cells in the lamina propria.

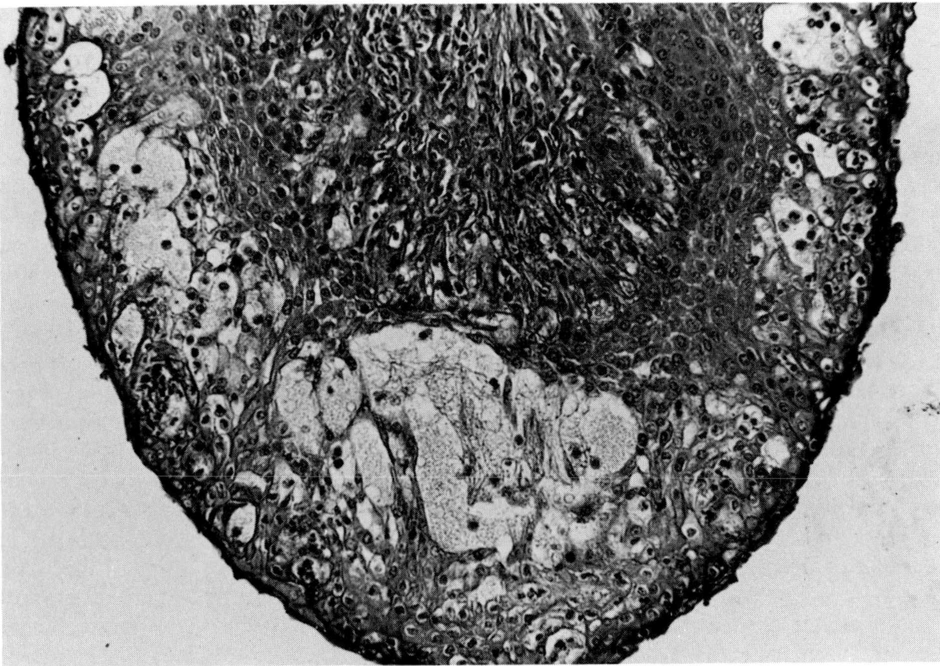

Figure 2–11. Variation in hydropic cells and microvesicles in a lesion similar to that in Figure 2–10. Infection of these lesions, when they ulcerate, leads to the large number of liver abscesses in feedlot cattle by embolic transport of organisms to the liver. Fungal infection can also occur and results in mycotic rumenitis, often with spread to the liver and other organs.

ulcerated and secondary bacterial infection may occur. In this disease, it is the localized infection in the rumen that spreads in the venous blood to the liver and is the basis of the high incidence of liver abscesses in feedlot cattle. Secondary involvement with fungi leads to the well-known condition of mycotic rumenitis as a sequel to the overload.

The terms cloudy swelling and hydropic degeneration are used less and less because of their lack of specificity, and they are nearing obsolescence. However, they can convey significant lesions in fresh well-fixed tissue.

Virchow's original descriptions and definitions have been translated into English.

DEGENERATION INVOLVING FAT

1. Fatty Degeneration. ***Fatty degeneration*** is the abnormal accumulation of fat in the cytoplasm of parenchymal cells. The liver is the best known location of the lesion, but it also occurs in renal tubular epithelium and myocardial cells, as well as in some other places. The liver will be used here as the focus of the discussion.

The generalities of normal processing of fat in the liver are as follows. Fatty acids arrive in the liver via the plasma from two sources: as triglycerides from fat depots and as chylomicrons from the intestine. They either are used in the liver in metabolic processes or are bound to protein produced in the endoplasmic reticulum and secreted from the liver into the plasma. They may also leave as phospholipid or cholesterol compounds. Problems in these processes of synthesis or secretion may lead to accumulation of visible fat droplets in the hepatocytes.

The following mechanisms for the lesion may occur: (a) Specific or nonspecific damage to the hepatocyte and certain nutritional deficiencies may interfere with protein production in the endoplasmic reticulum; lipoproteins cannot be formed and, as a result, the lipid cannot be secreted from the cell and therefore accumulates; (b) interference with the release of lipoproteins from the cell; (c) impaired combination of lipid with protein; (d) blockage of oxidation of fatty acid; (e) higher than normal amounts of fatty acid presented to the liver by absorption from the intestine or release from adipose tissue. These processes are outlined in Figure 2–12.

The liver is considered the nutritional guardian of the body, but ***dietary, toxic*** or ***hypoxic*** factors may interfere with this general function. In animals, fatty liver is well known in diabetes, particularly in dogs, and in ***ketosis,*** particularly in cows. In both conditions, utilization or availability of glucose is impaired, lipids are mobilized as an energy source and the liver is functionally overloaded. In mild anoxia or toxicity, the hepatocytes in the periacinar areas become fatty. This occurs because they are the least oxygenated, being farther from the source of nutriment. Their capacity to metabolize lipid may therefore be reduced. The periacinar distribution is the most common expression of fatty liver. A focal distribution involving groups of lobules occurs in dogs, usually associated with consumption of high fat-low protein diets.

The ***microscopic*** appearance of the fat is as large, clear, discrete droplets or as many tiny droplets with a foamy appearance. The amount of fat may be minor or so extensive as to displace the nucleus of the hepatocyte and give the tissue the appearance of adipose tissue. In either state, the droplets may be free in the cytoplasm or membrane-bound (Fig. 2–13 through 2–16). This difference has no known specificity in animals; but in humans, large unbound droplets, which may fuse, are associated with choline deficiency and alcoholism, whereas small membrane-bound droplets, which do not fuse, are associated with excess fat intake.

The gross appearance of fatty liver is yellow, with the degree of yellow corresponding to the extent of fat accumulation in hepatocytes. In severe cases, the liver is enlarged and uniformly yellow and has a greasy texture on cut surface (Fig. 2–17). When the periacinar pattern predominates, there will be a mixed pattern of pale to yellowish combined with normal brown, the yellow being around central veins and the brown around portal triads. Dogs may have groups of lobules affected, which are sometimes called fatty cysts.

Special stains will specifically identify the fat, if necessary, but usually vacuolation in the cytoplasm of hepatocytes is considered to be fatty degeneration. Hydropic degen-

Text continued on page 24

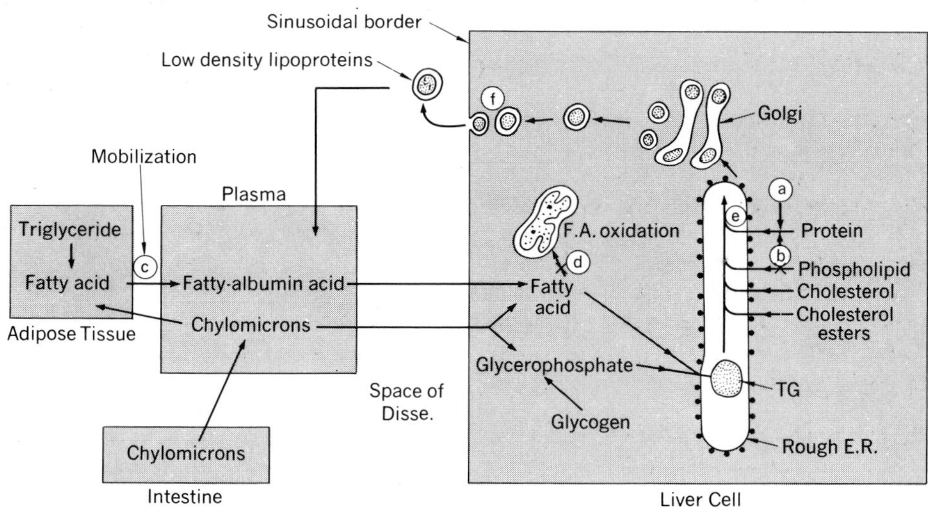

Figure 2–12. Pathogenesis of fatty liver. The letters indicate points at which some specific mechanisms act. Specific mechanisms by specific agents are indicated in the figure. See text for discussion of general mechanism. (From La Via, M. F., and Hill, R. B.: Principles of Pathobiology. New York, Oxford University Press, 1971. Modified from Lombardi, 1965.)

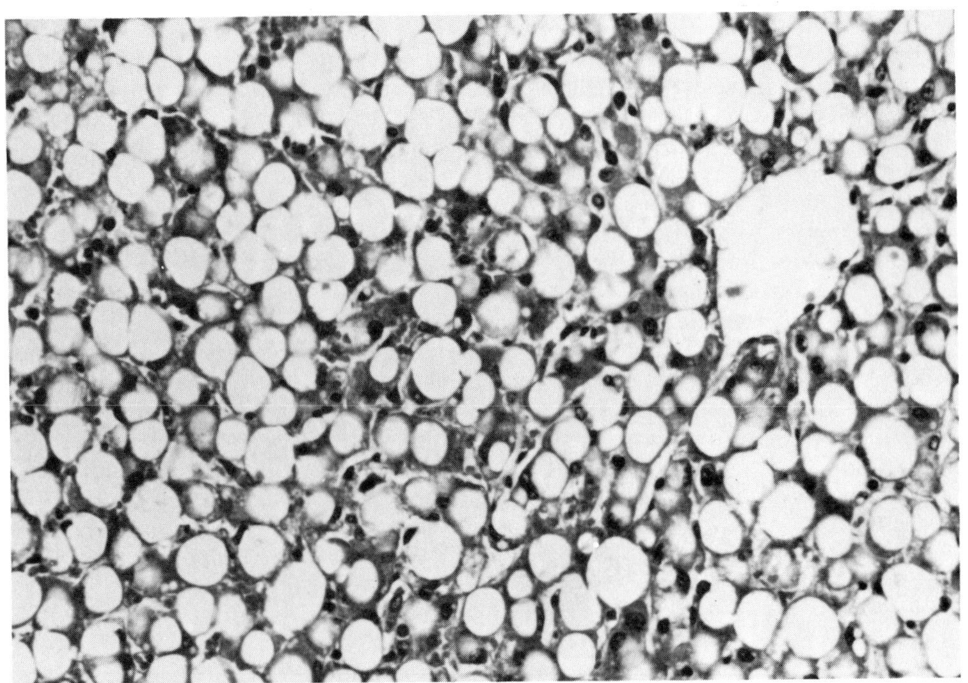

Figure 2–13. Fatty liver with discrete vacuoles in hepatocytes.

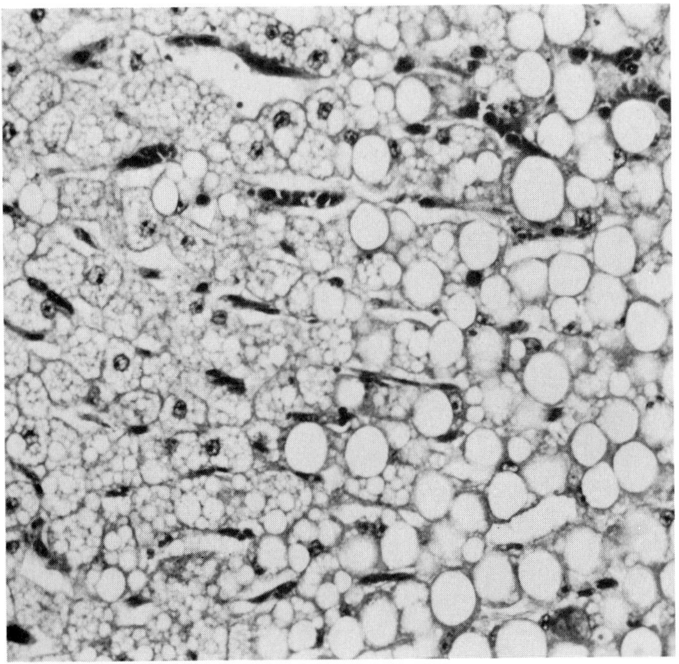

Figure 2–14. Fatty liver. Note the variation in size of fat vacuoles. The largest are nearer the central vein.

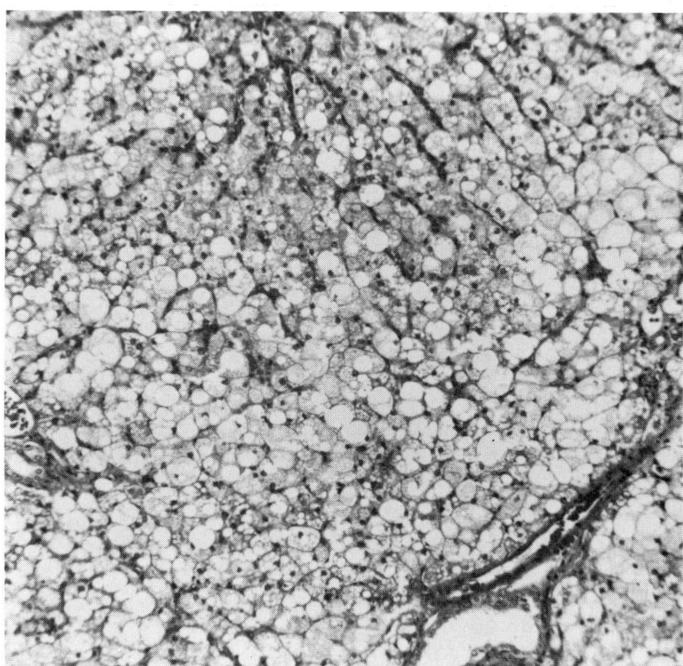

Figure 2–15. Fatty liver with variably sized vacuoles in a case of fatty liver syndrome in a mink.

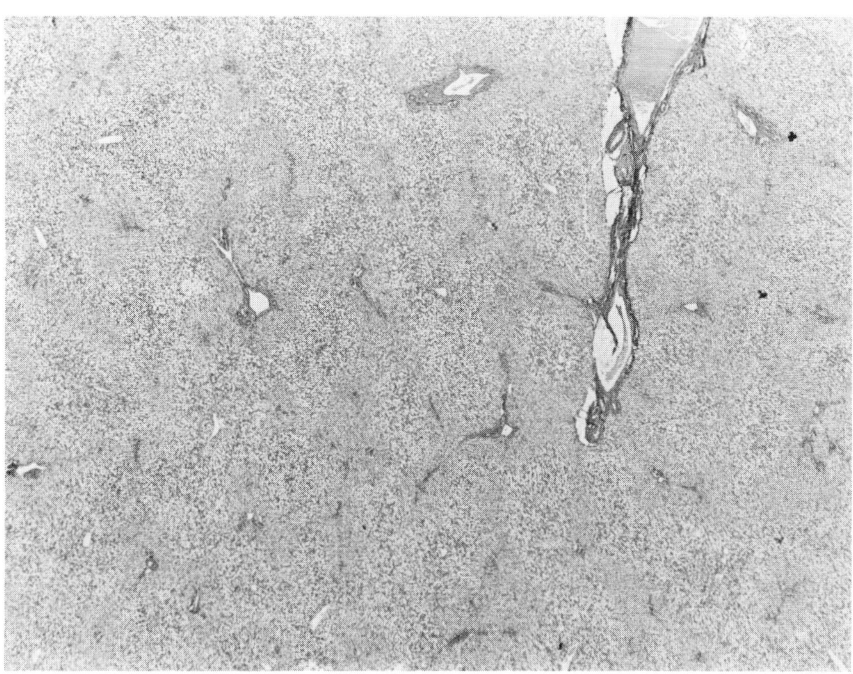

Figure 2–16. Low-power view of a fatty liver to demonstrate how extensively the liver may be affected in a case of bovine ketosis.

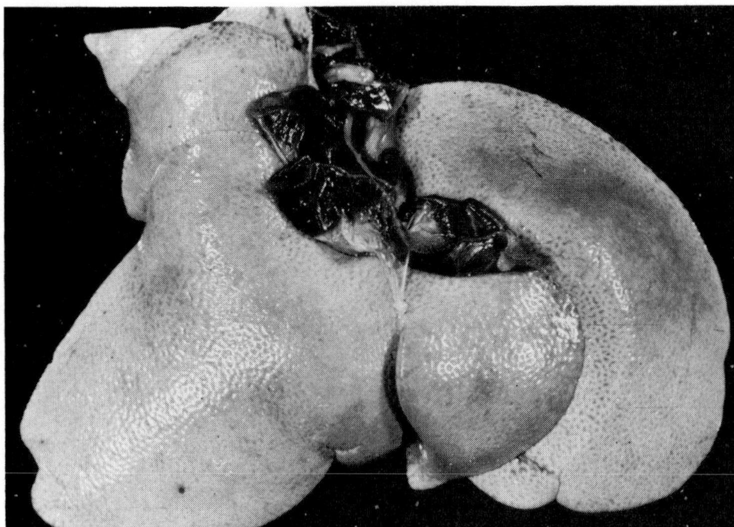

Figure 2–17. Extremely fatty liver from a cat, which probably was diabetic.

eration or the presence of glycogen must be considered, however. Special stains are always required in the myocardium and preferably in the kidney. The lesion in the myocardium is seldom recognized microscopically, although it may be common. It is also difficult to recognize grossly and microscopically, as well as to differentiate this lesion from postmortem change. Cats normally have large amounts of fat in their renal tubular epithelium and therefore have quite pale kidneys.

Fatty degeneration is considered reversible if the causes are removed, but many cells burst and die. In general, fatty degeneration is a common nonspecific indication of injury, although the locations and circumstances in which the lesion is found *may* be quite suggestive of a particular pathogenetic mechanism or specific disease (Fig. 2–18).

2. Fatty Infiltration. ***Fatty infiltration*** is included here under the subject of fat but is not really an intracellular degeneration. The lesion consists of the accumulation of adipose cells in tissue in which they are not normally present. Usually, they seem to be replacing some of the atrophied tissue (Fig. 2–19). The term ***fatty replacement*** is sometimes used. The lesion occurs in myocardial and skeletal muscle, as well as in the pancreas, but is not common. The reason for the presence of fat is not known, nor is it known whether it is present as an active or passive process. It is not clear why fat would be present rather than a scar or a simple collapse and condensation of the affected tissue. A form of this lesion is known as ***steatosis*** (Figs. 2–20 and 2–21), in which large areas of muscle have a pale or mottled color caused by fatty infiltration. It occurs in the heavy muscle of the hind leg, loin and shoulder in cattle and pigs, but no clinical signs are evident.

Glycogen may accumulate in abnormal amounts in the cytoplasm of cells and appears as clear vacuoles. This is not common but occurs in prolonged hyperglycemia, particularly in diabetes. It occurs in renal tubules when glycogen is reabsorbed and stored. The liver normally contains some glycogen, but the amounts are markedly increased in diabetes. Glycogen storage diseases occur when there is a congenital absence of an enzyme required to metabolize carbohydrate.

INTRACELLULAR INCLUSIONS

The following are examples of abnormalities in the appearance of cells caused by abnormal accumulation of material ***intracellularly***. Pigments may also be intracellular and will be discussed later.

Hyaline droplets are small eosinophilic structures in the cytoplasm of cells. The resulting lesion is sometimes called hyaline droplet degeneration. This is more likely a compensatory functional change caused by accumulation of secretion or increased intake of compounds by endocytosis (Fig. 2–22). One example is the presence of hyaline

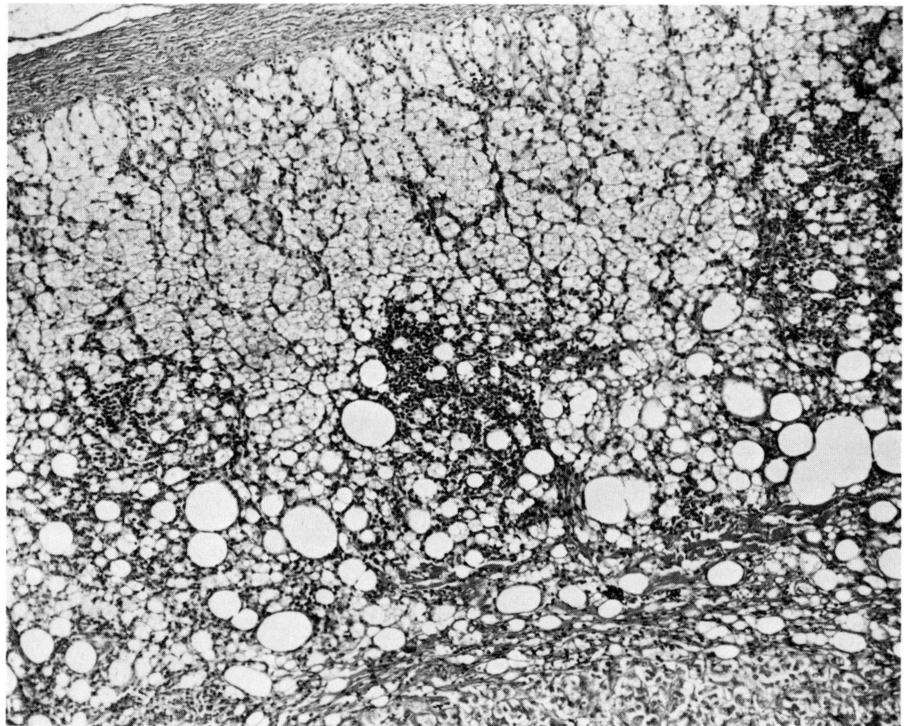

Figure 2–18. Extensive fatty degeneration of the adrenal cortex in a dog. Note the similarity to the liver lesions. The lymphocytes are suggestive of an autoimmune reaction within the adrenal gland.

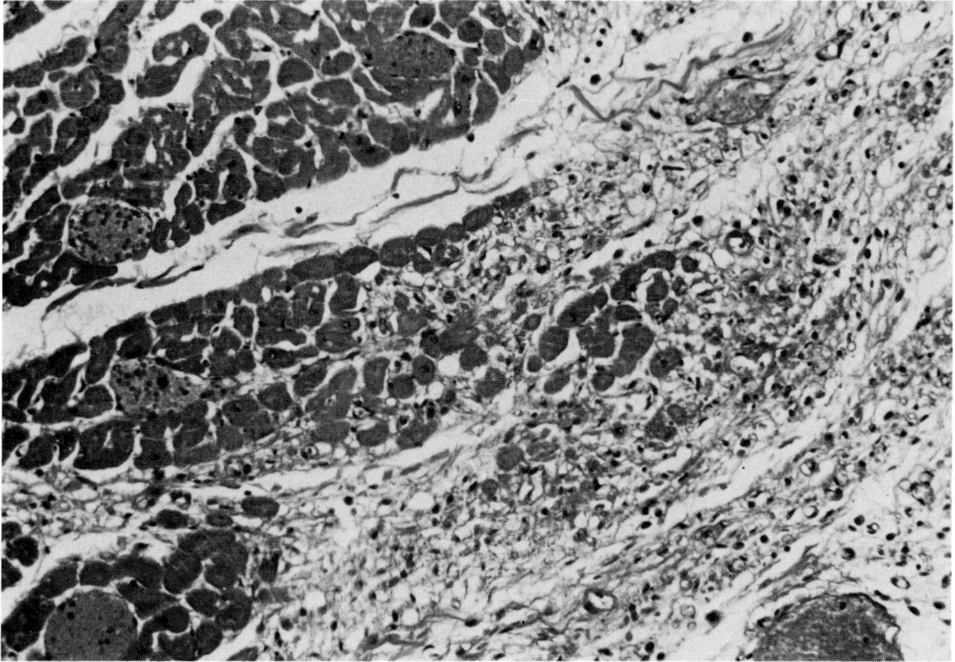

Figure 2–19. Fatty infiltration in the myocardium in which the muscle fibers become small and disappear. The pathogenesis is not clear, but such pale areas observed grossly must be differentiated from other gross lesions that are pale.

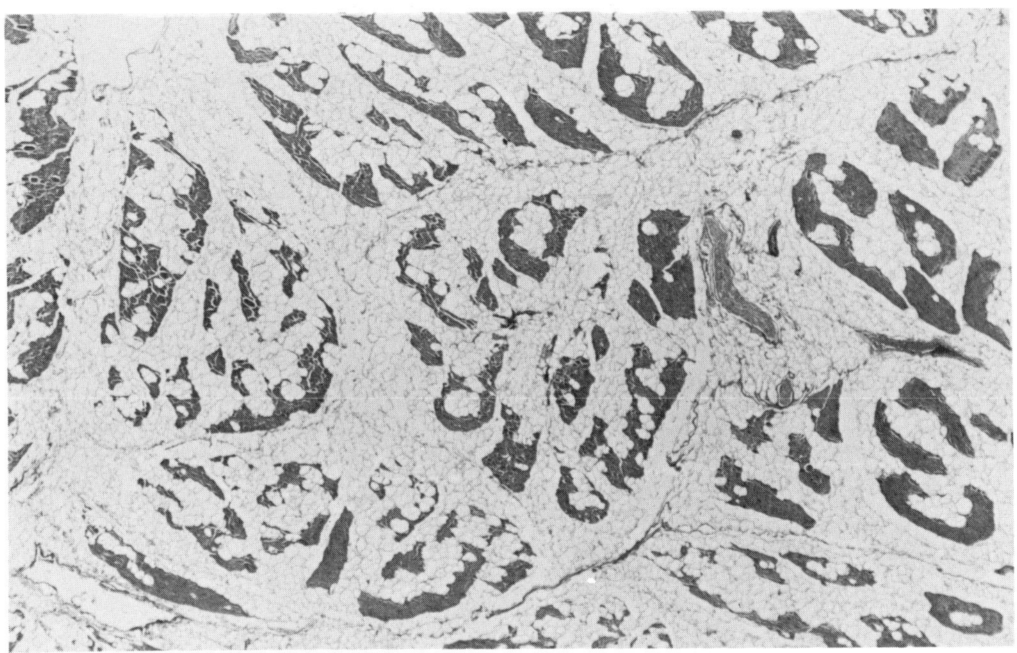

Figure 2–20. Extensive steatosis in skeletal muscle.

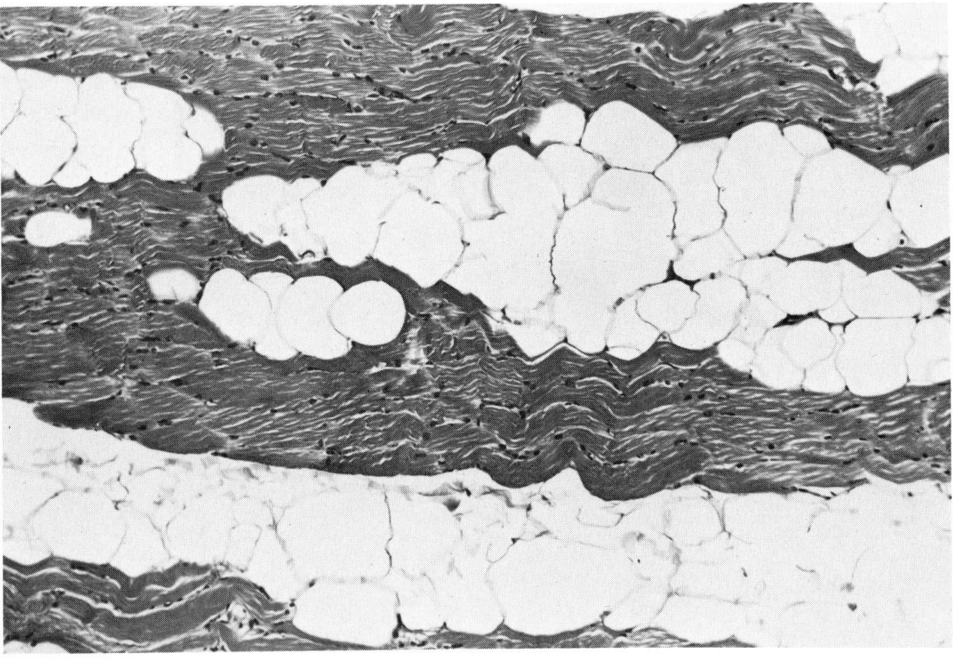

Figure 2–21. Higher power view of the lesion in Figure 2–20.

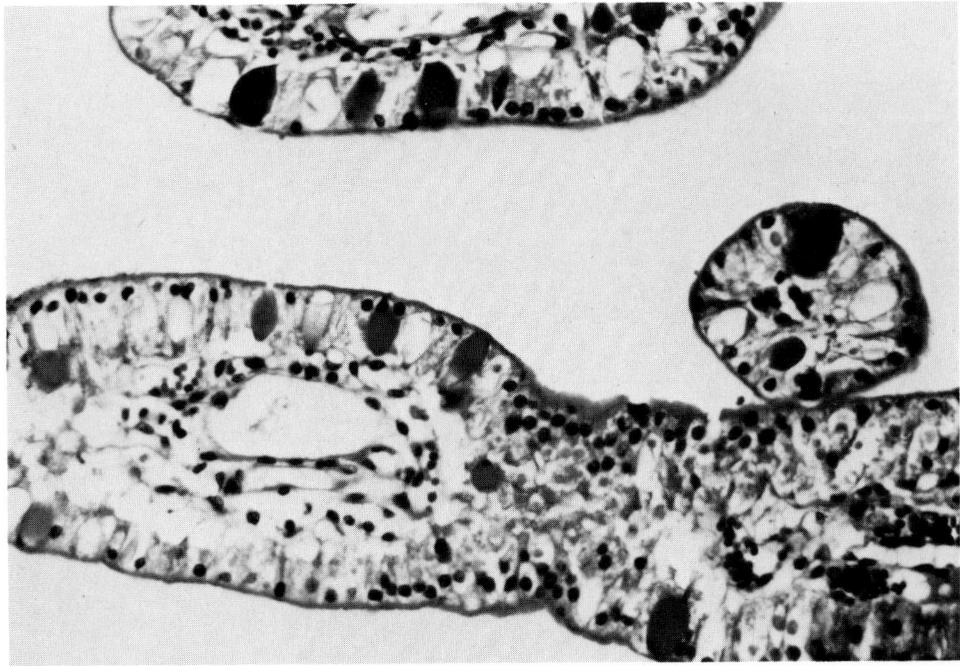

Figure 2–22. Large eosinophilic droplets in the intestinal epithelium from absorption of colostrum in a neonatal animal.

droplets in renal tubular epithelium from uptake of protein from the lumen when the glomeruli allow proteins to pass (Fig. 2–23). A number of other lesions may show up as eosinophilic droplets, either single or multiple, large or small. They usually consist of concentric layers of paired membranes of endoplasmic reticulum. They may form ***myelin bodies***, which are very tightly packed layers of membrane, or ***fingerprints***, which are loosely arranged. Such structures are common in various degrees of degeneration in cells but only become visible by light microscopy if they are very large.

Various ***inclusions*** occur in cells and may be very prominent, such as inclusion bodies induced by viral infection of cells. These may be intranuclear, intracytoplasmic and either eosinophilic or basophilic, single or multiple (Figs. 2–24 through 2–34). Intranuclear inclusions, which may be detected by acid-fast stains, occur in renal tubular epithelium in some cases of lead poisoning. So-called "bricks" occur in renal tubular cells in dogs and, although striking in appearance, have no known significance (Fig. 2–35). Nuclear inclusions occur in many isolated, unrelated lesions of various types not identified with viral infection, including tumors and intoxications in various tissues. These are cytoplasmic invaginations into the nucleus and are bound by cytoplasmic membranes. The genesis may be related to cytoplasmic swelling.

In some congenital metabolic disorders, lipids accumulate in the cytoplasm of parenchymal cells and appear as clear or cloudy vacuoles. These are well known in diseases affecting neurons and are called ***lipid storage diseases***, which occur in several species (Fig. 2–36). A key enzyme is defective or missing and, as a result, a lipid is not metabolized and therefore accumulates. The deposits are usually composed of gangliosides or sphingomyelin.

Certain ***parasites*** are found in intracellular locations, usually as dark dots or round vesicular structures. These are numerous and usually involve stages in the life cycle of the organism. Examples of diseases caused by these include coccidiosis, toxoplasmosis (Fig. 2–37), malaria, theileriasis and many others, and they are discussed in courses on parasitology. These agents usually cause death of the cell in which they spend part of their lives.

Text continued on page 35

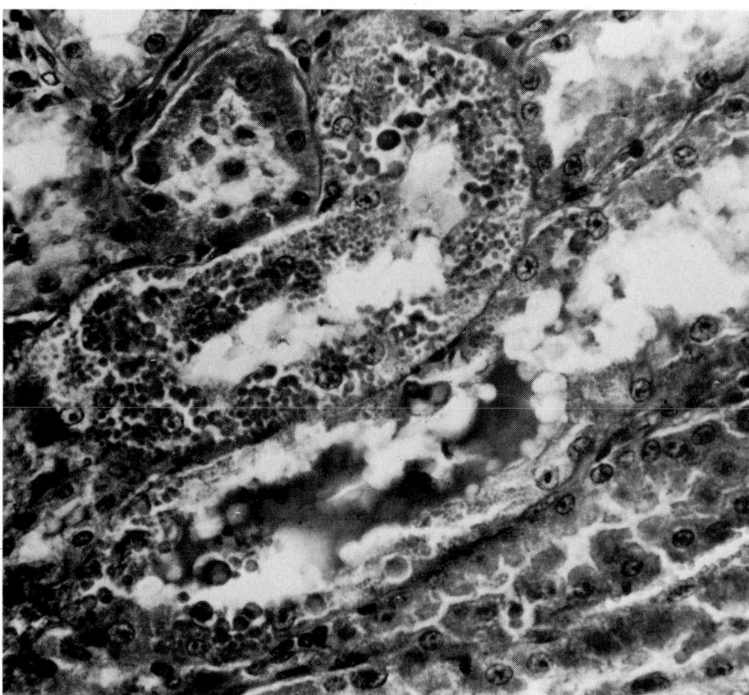

Figure 2–23. Hyaline droplets in renal tubular epithelium due to reabsorption of protein that has leaked through the glomerulus. This is really a compensatory functional change on the part of the epithelial cells.

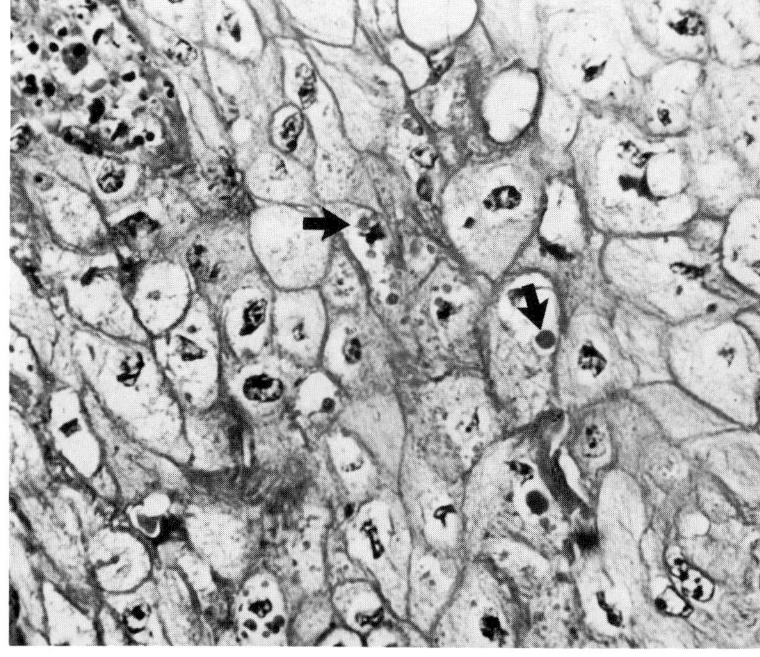

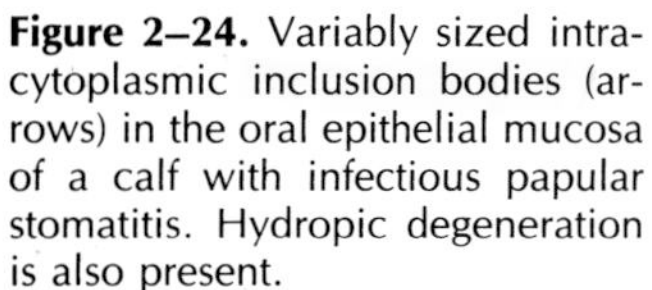

Figure 2–24. Variably sized intracytoplasmic inclusion bodies (arrows) in the oral epithelial mucosa of a calf with infectious papular stomatitis. Hydropic degeneration is also present.

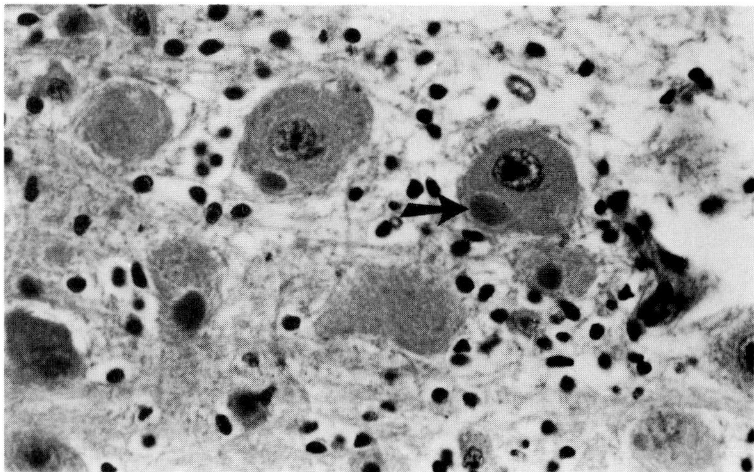

Figure 2–25. Large intracytoplasmic inclusion bodies (arrow) in Purkinje cells of the cerebellum in rabies.

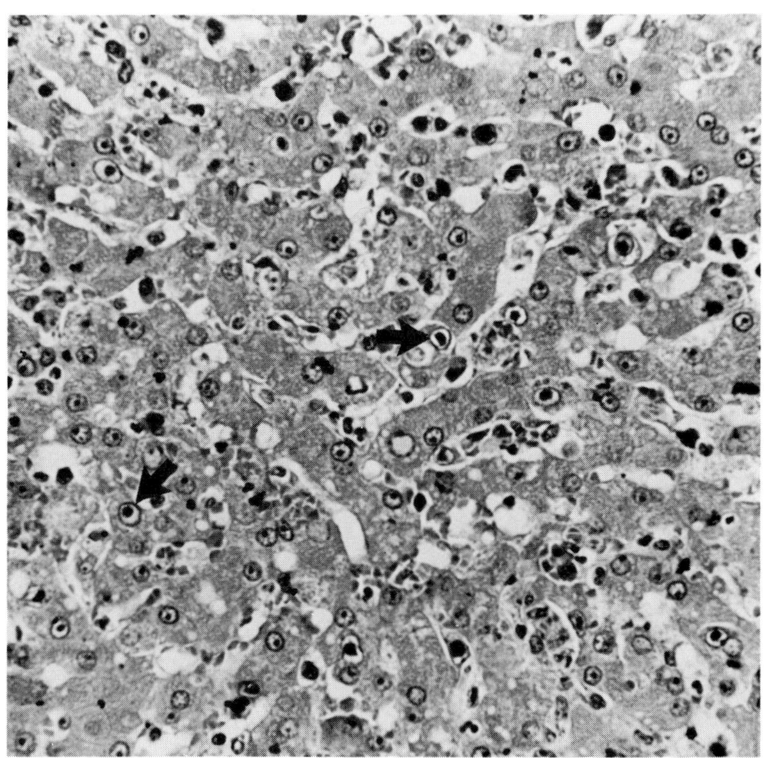

Figure 2–26. Intranuclear inclusion bodies (arrows) in hepatocytes in infectious canine hepatitis.

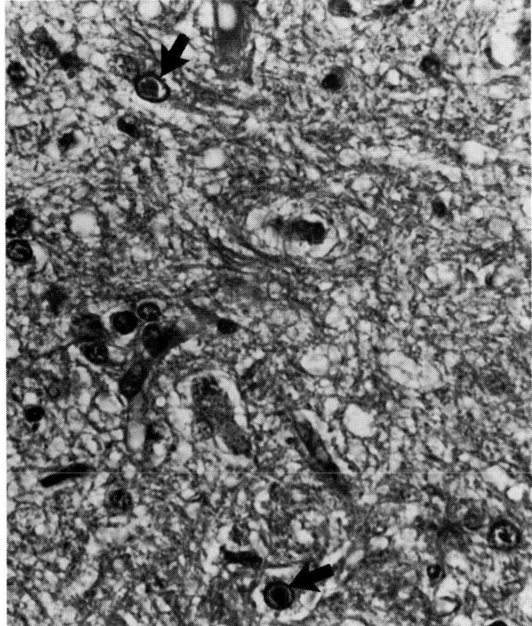

Figure 2–27. Distemper inclusion bodies (arrows) in the nuclei of astrocytes that have dense nuclear membranes.

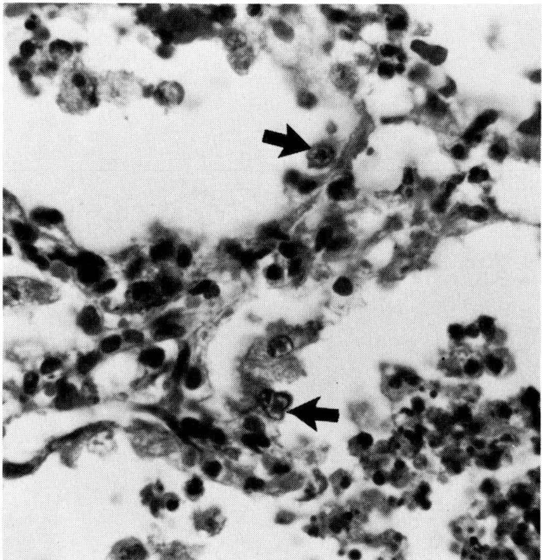

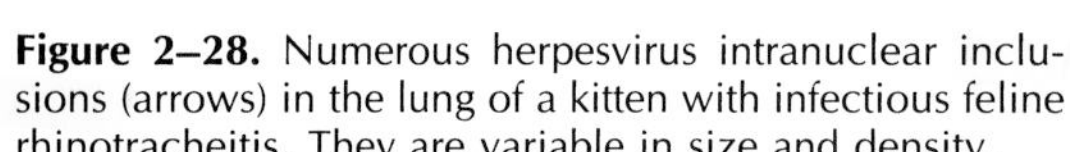

Figure 2–28. Numerous herpesvirus intranuclear inclusions (arrows) in the lung of a kitten with infectious feline rhinotracheitis. They are variable in size and density.

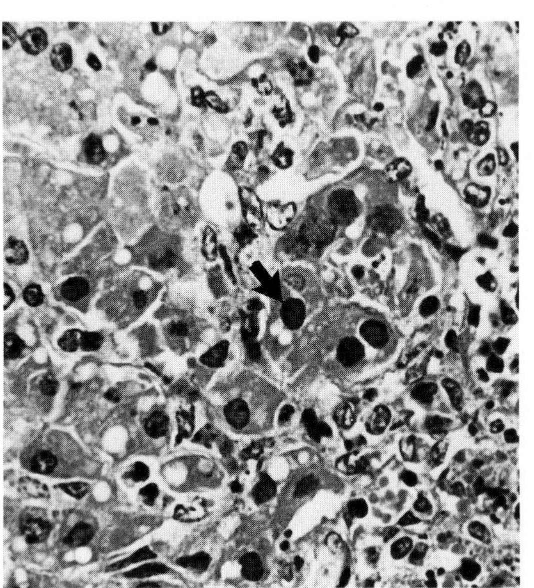

Figure 2–29. Large dense intranuclear inclusion bodies (arrow) in the liver of an aborted bovine fetus with infectious bovine rhinotracheitis. Note the destruction of cells to the right.

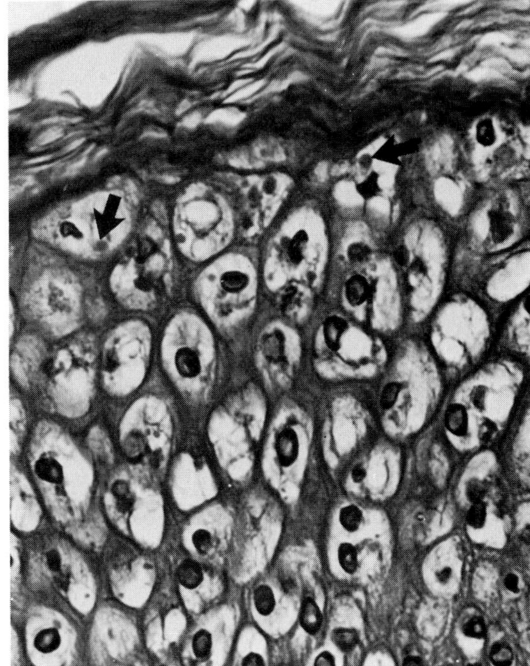

Figure 2–30. Rather indiscrete intracytoplasmic inclusions (arrows) in swine pox. See also Figure 2–31.

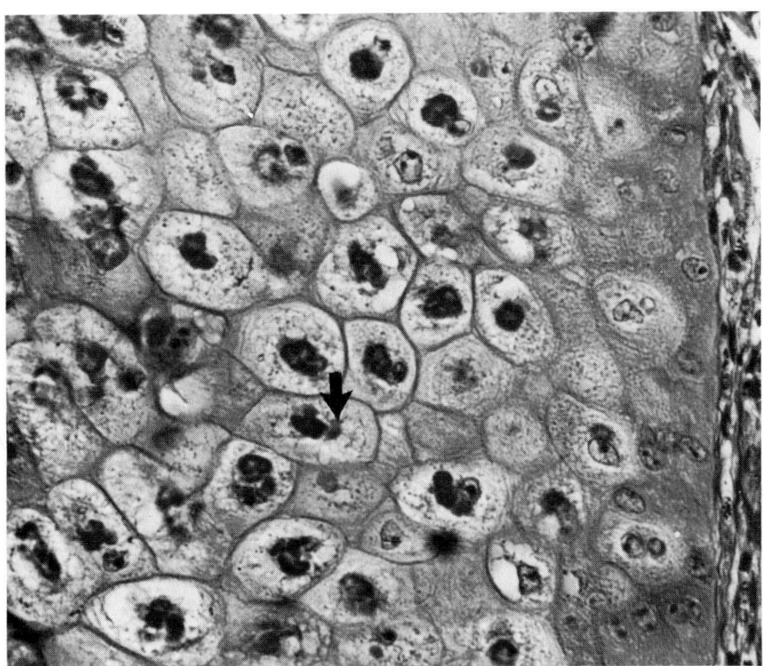

Figure 2–31. Large multiple intracytoplasmic inclusions (arrows) in fowl pox. See also Figure 2–30.

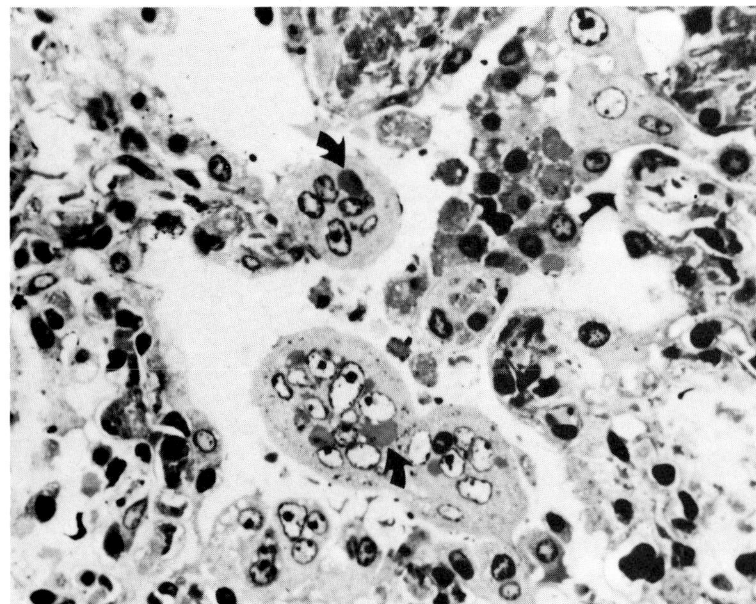

Figure 2–32. Parainfluenza-3 viral inclusion bodies (arrows) in giant cells in a calf's lung.

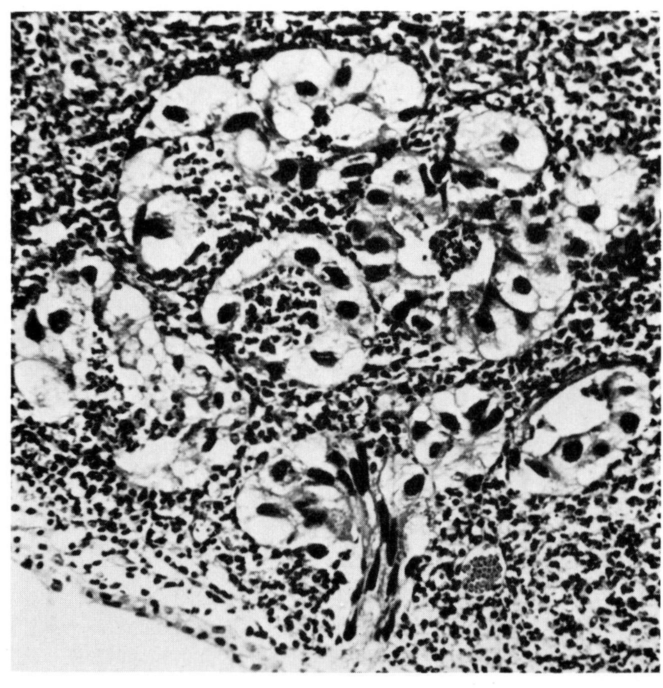

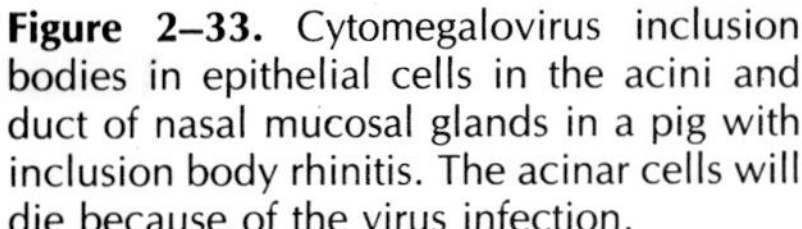

Figure 2–33. Cytomegalovirus inclusion bodies in epithelial cells in the acini and duct of nasal mucosal glands in a pig with inclusion body rhinitis. The acinar cells will die because of the virus infection.

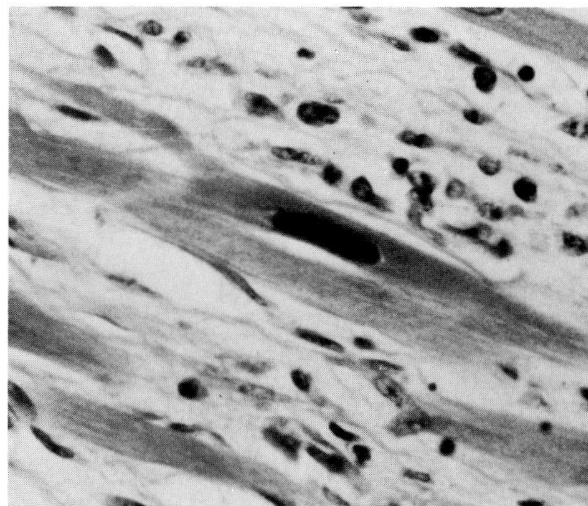

Figure 2–34. Parvoviral inclusion body in the nucleus of a dog's myocardial fiber.

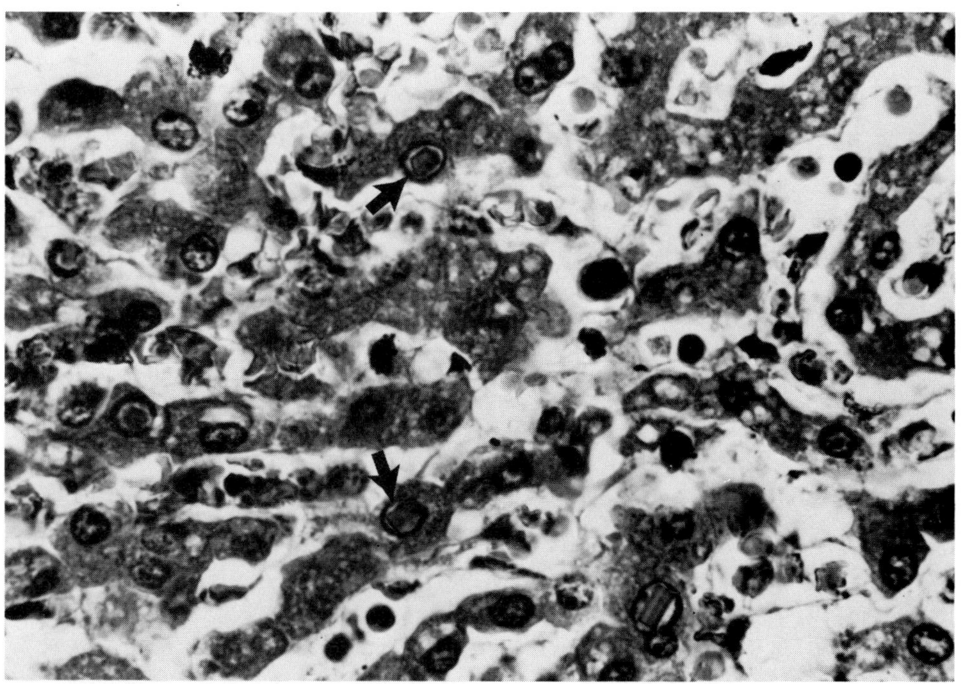

Figure 2–35. Intranuclear inclusions (arrows) occasionally are found in the liver and kidney of old dogs. The inclusions vary in size and shape but often are shaped like bricks. They do not seem to have clinical significance.

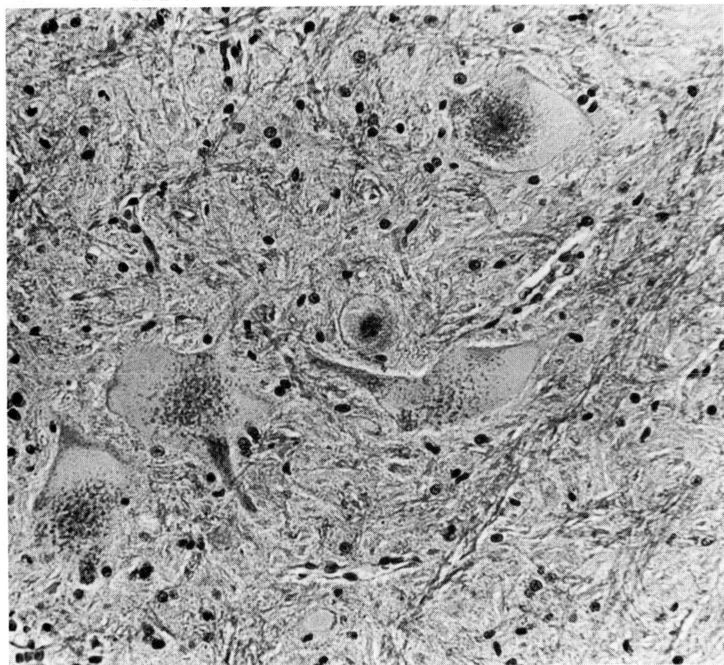

Figure 2–36. Lipid storage disease with accumulations of ganglioside GM_1, in neuronal cytoplasm in a 5-month-old mixed-breed dog. The Nissl substance is pushed aside and the lipid accumulates because of the congenital absence of an enzyme to metabolize the lipid. In this case, the neurons are deficient in beta-galactosidase.

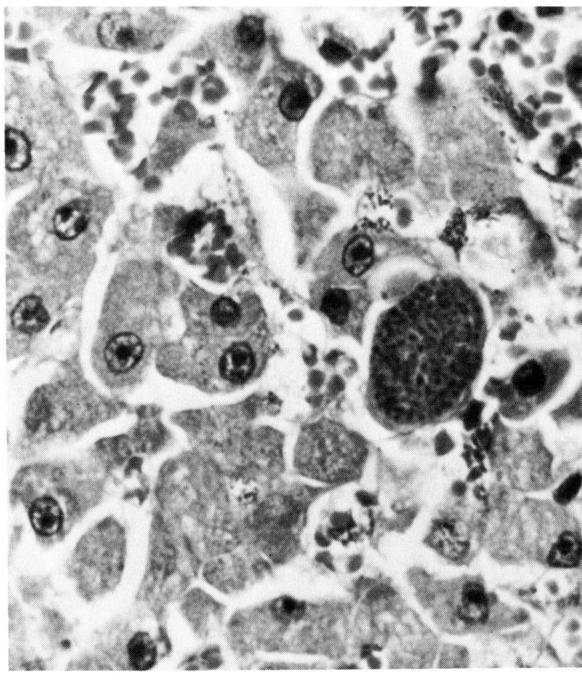

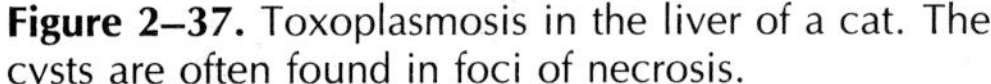

Figure 2–37. Toxoplasmosis in the liver of a cat. The cysts are often found in foci of necrosis.

Specific Types of Extracellular Degenerative Changes

Abnormal materials also may occur ***extracellularly*** in tissues, and these are also called degenerations (although this stretches the use of the word somewhat). They are not necessarily related to each other and are discussed here as ***isolated examples of specific abnormalities that occur in tissues***.

HYALINIZATION

Hyalinization or ***hyalinized*** is a term used to describe the change from normal to variable degrees of smooth eosinophilic appearance in the ***microscopic*** examination of tissue. The eosinophilia indicates the presence of protein. It can be present in many tissues but usually involves connective tissue or basement membranes. In connective tissue, it may be a change in ratio between nuclei and collagen, so that eosinophilia predominates, as in a scar or an atretic graafian follicle. The word is used to describe the ***appearance*** of an abnormality, not a specific pathogenetic mechanism or disease. ***Hyalin*** is sometimes used as a noun, but it is a physical state of the tissue, not a specific chemical compound. Thickening of basement membranes, as in some glomerular disorders, is called hyalinization and is an indication of glomerular disease (Fig. 2–38). The smooth eosinophilic content of coagulated protein in renal tubules is called ***hyaline casts*** in diseases in which protein leaks through glomeruli (Fig. 2–39). Hyaline droplets in some cells are foci of proliferation of endoplasmic reticulum and may be an indication of excess function or toxicity. Smooth, shiny red capillary thrombi are called ***hyaline thrombi*** (see Figs. 3–75 and 3–76).

FIBRINOID

Fibrinoid is an amorphous, bright, eosinophilic material found particularly in the walls of blood vessels of various sizes. Fibrin is a major component along with serum proteins, particularly immunoglobulins. There is a strong association between the presence of fibrinoid and acute immunologically based lesions, such as the Arthus reaction. These lesions involve antigen-antibody complexes and complement, and the combination causes severe injury to the vessel wall and leakage of plasma protein into the lesion (Figs. 2–40 and 2–41). Fibrinoid may also be associated with severe injury in connective tissue, as sometimes occurs in mast cell tumors.

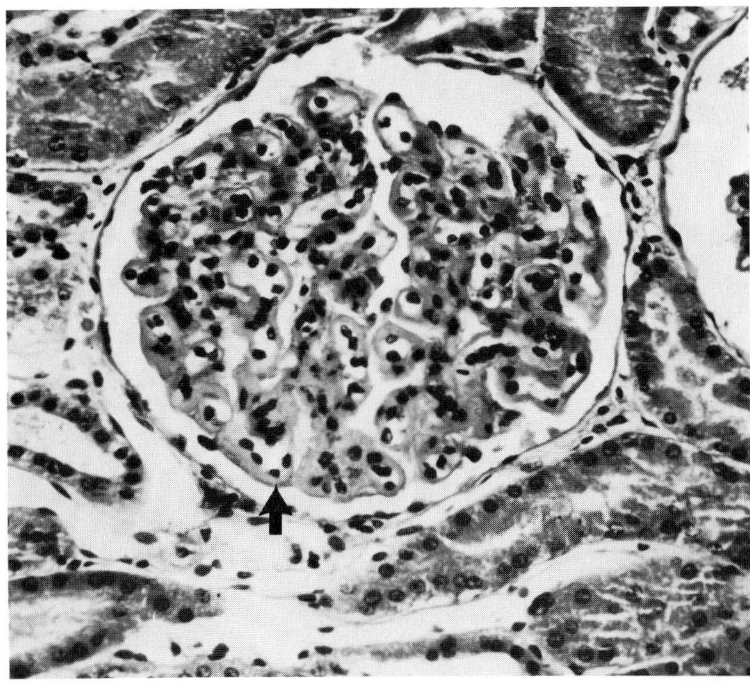

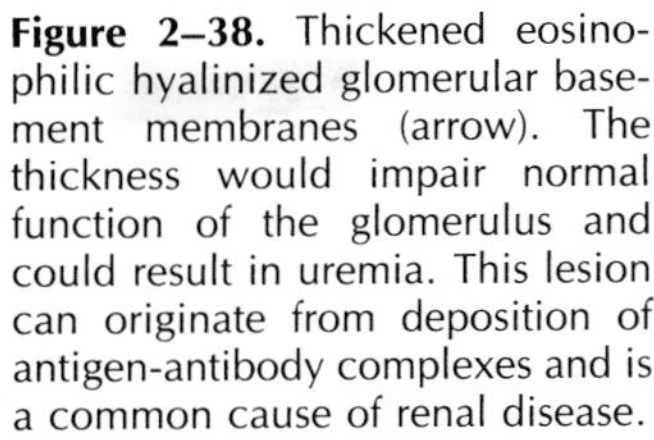

Figure 2–38. Thickened eosinophilic hyalinized glomerular basement membranes (arrow). The thickness would impair normal function of the glomerulus and could result in uremia. This lesion can originate from deposition of antigen-antibody complexes and is a common cause of renal disease.

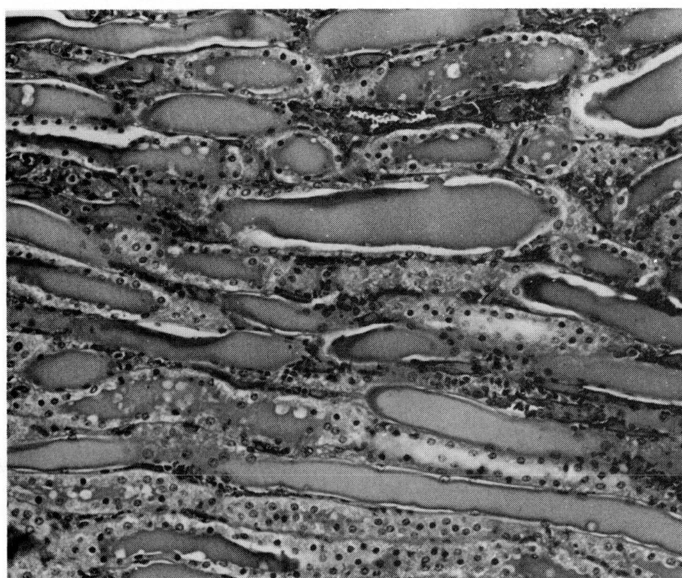

Figure 2–39. Proteinaceous eosinophilic hyalinized casts of variable density in renal tubules caused by leaky glomeruli. The staining density of the casts varies with the concentration of protein. The animal had proteinuria.

GOUT

Gout is the name of the disease that occurs when uric acid and urate crystals are deposited in tissue as a result of defects in purine metabolism. This tends to occur in joint spaces or on other serous membranes (Figs. 2–42 and 2–43), such as pleura or peritoneum, or in renal tubules. The condition is known in humans and in avian species and is named articular or visceral gout. The crystals cause irritation, pain and chronic inflammation (Figs. 2–44 and 2–45). The cause is incomplete metabolism of purine derivatives, and the crystals can be specifically identified in tissues. More specifically, active uric acid excretion is interfered with in the kidney by peritubular lesions, such as chronic renal inflammation. High protein diets may increase the amount excreted and compound the problem. In addition, there seems to be individual variation in the level of blood urates at which the crystals begin to precipitate. The disease is most common in avian species.

CHOLESTEROL CLEFTS

Cholesterol may collect as crystals in tissue after severe tissue damage or hemorrhage (Fig. 2–46). The crystals have a characteristic appearance called clefts and occur in picket fence–type groups. They have no significance other than to indicate that there has been tissue injury or hemorrhage or both. They often occur in tumors. There is a condition in avian species called ***xanthomatosis*** that results from massive accumulation of lipids in macrophages. Cholesterol clefts are often found in these lesions (Fig. 2–47).

CORPORA AMYLACEA

Corpora amylacea are circular laminated concretions found in glandular tissue or free in secretions. They stain blue to pink, are common in normal mammary glands and are usually an incidental finding. They are considered concretions formed from a nidus of debris, with successive layers of debris forming strata. Occasionally, they occur in brain, lung and seminal vesicles in which they may be an indication of old lesions in which tissue debris or secretions have accumulated (Figs. 2–48 and 2–49).

AMYLOID

Amyloid has an amorphous eosinophilic appearance, is usually located on basement membranes or vessel walls, and occurs in several organs in several species. Until recently, amyloidosis was considered to be one disease with different manifestations in different individuals. It is now apparent that amyloidosis is really several different diseases, each with a different pathogenesis, but with one common factor, that

Text continued on page 42

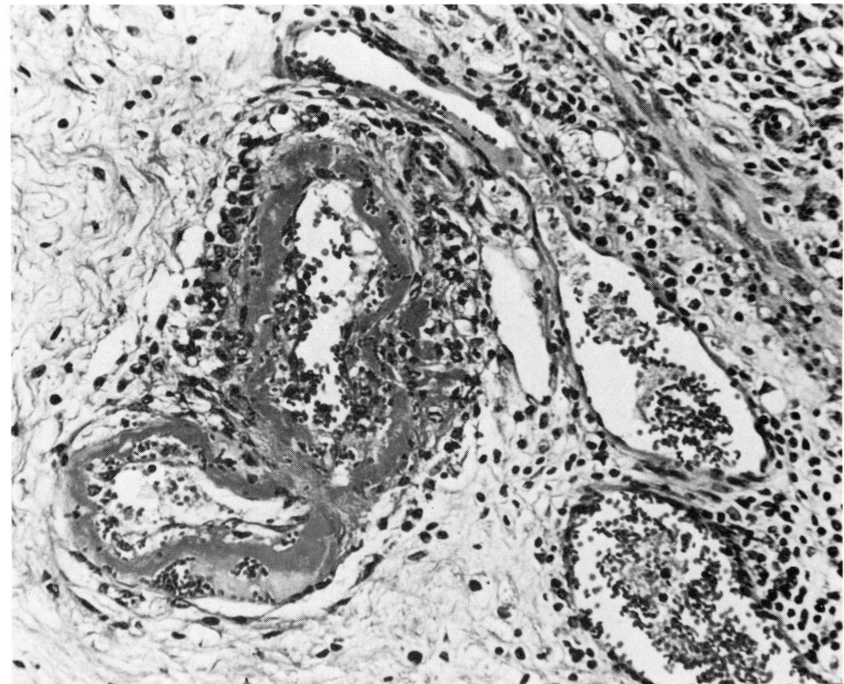

Figure 2–40

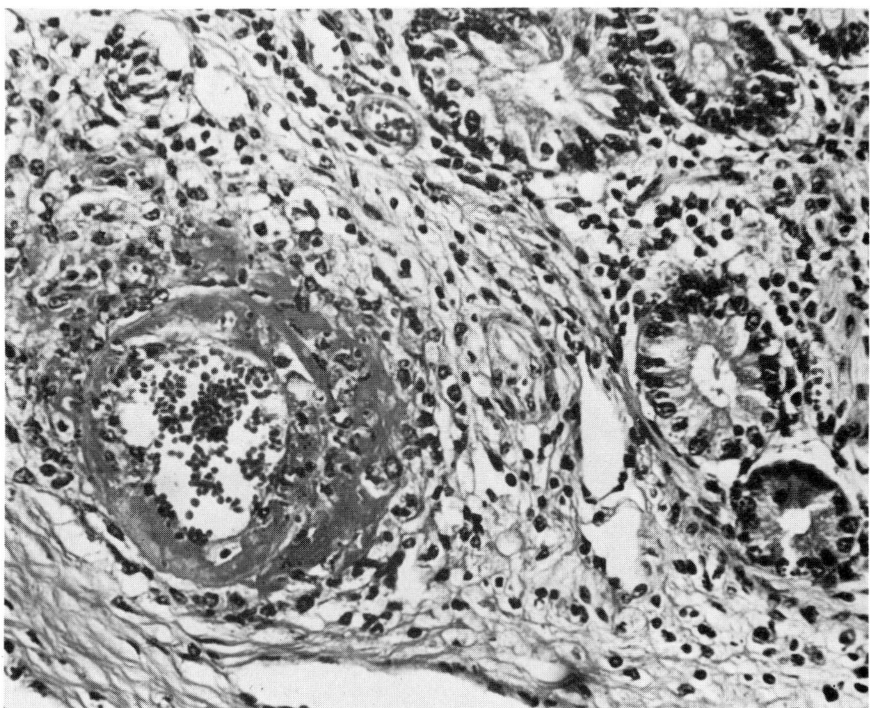

Figure 2–41

Figures 2–40 and 2–41. Fibrinoid in the walls of blood vessels in the intestine of a calf. The eosinophilic fibrinoid accumulates in varying degrees within or just outside the vessel wall, usually causing destruction of the vessel wall, edema and inflammation. These lesions are often caused by deposition of antigen-antibody complexes in the vessel wall, causing acute inflammation.

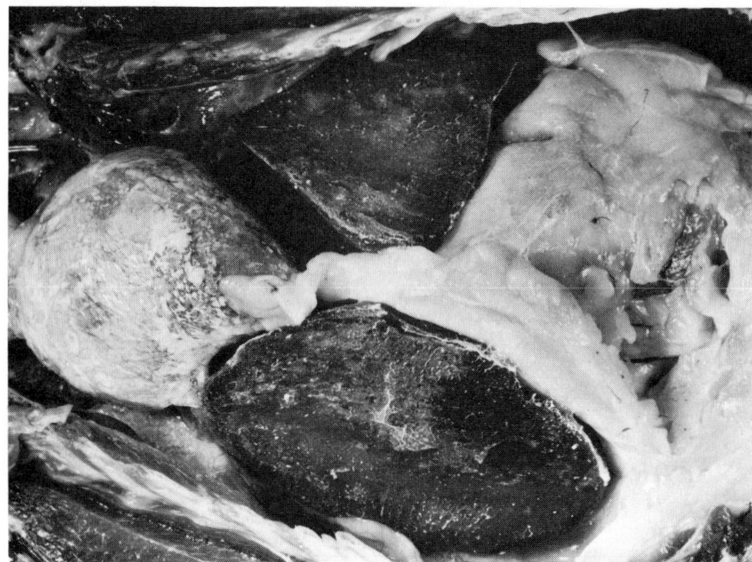

Figure 2–42. Visceral gout in a wild duck. Note the white crystals on the serous surfaces. (From Wobeser, G.: Diseases of Wild Waterfowl. New York, Plenum Press, 1981. Reprinted by permission.)

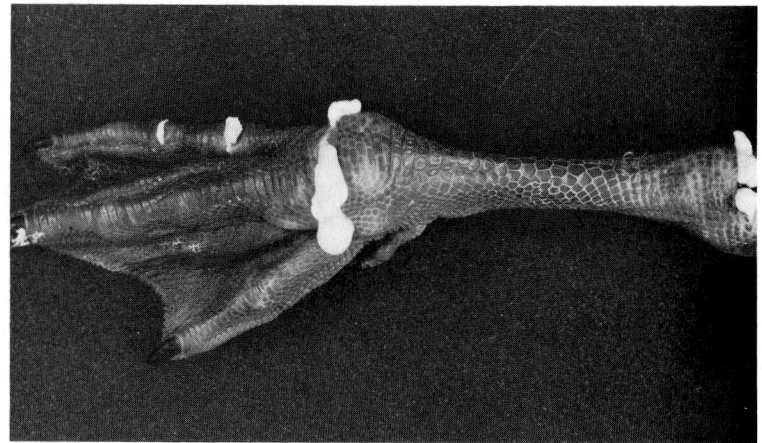

Figure 2–43. Semisolid white urates flow from an incised joint in a bird with articular gout. (From Wobeser, G.: Diseases of Wild Waterfowl. New York, Plenum Press, 1981. Reprinted by permission.)

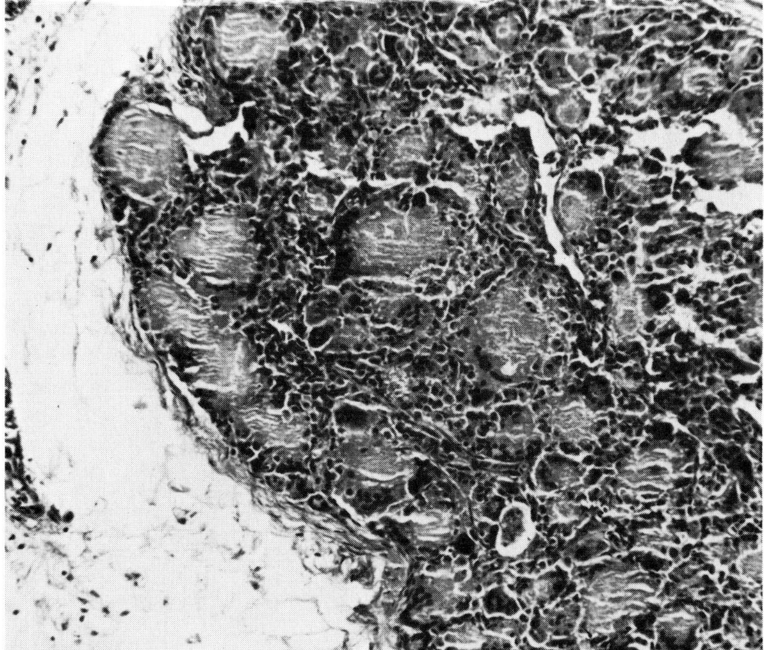

Figure 2–44. Gout in the joint space of the knee of a bird. The amorphous granular material consists of the crystals of urates and uric acid, and there is a marked cellular reaction because the crystals are irritating. The reaction causes much pain.

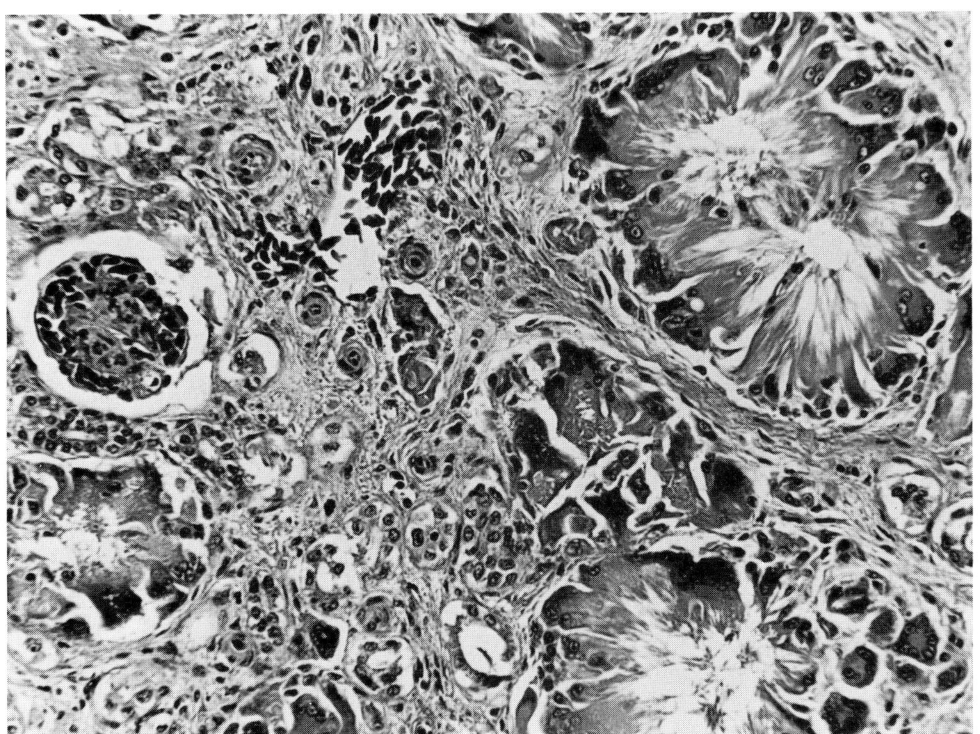

Figure 2–45. Giant cell reaction in renal tubules that contain urate crystals. There is extensive damage to the kidney caused by the reaction to the crystals.

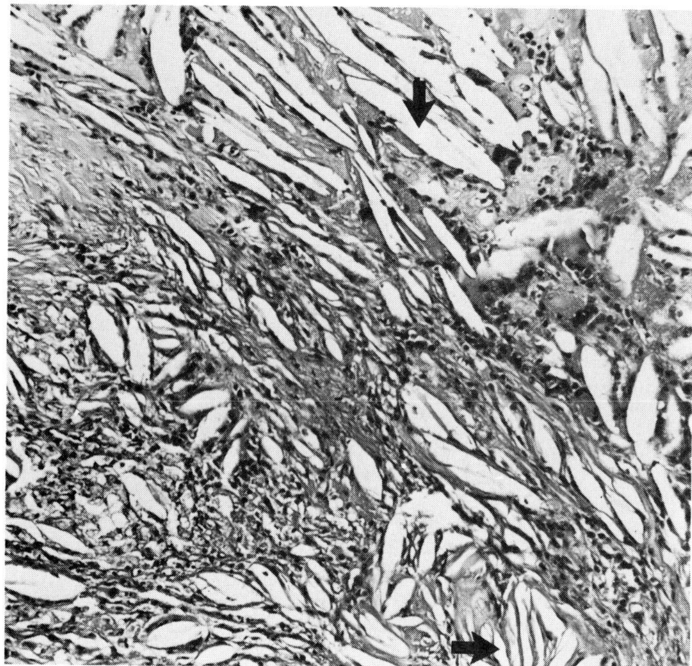

Figure 2–46. Variably sized and shaped cholesterol clefts (arrows) in a canine mammary tumor.

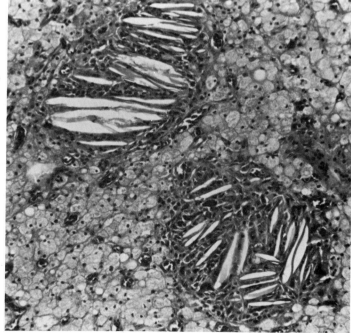

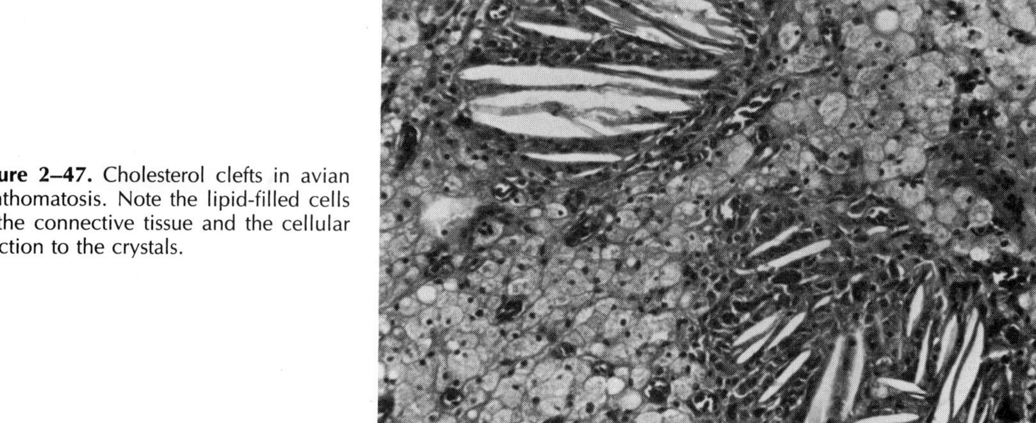

Figure 2–47. Cholesterol clefts in avian xanthomatosis. Note the lipid-filled cells in the connective tissue and the cellular reaction to the crystals.

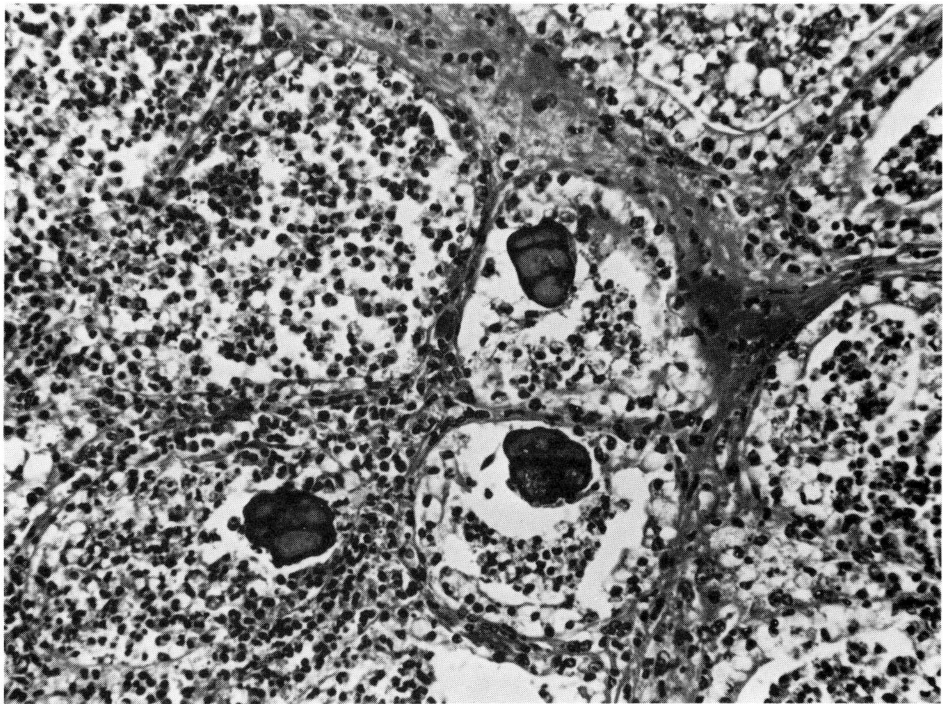

Figure 2–48. Irregularly shaped corpora amylacea in a mammary gland of a cow with mastitis.

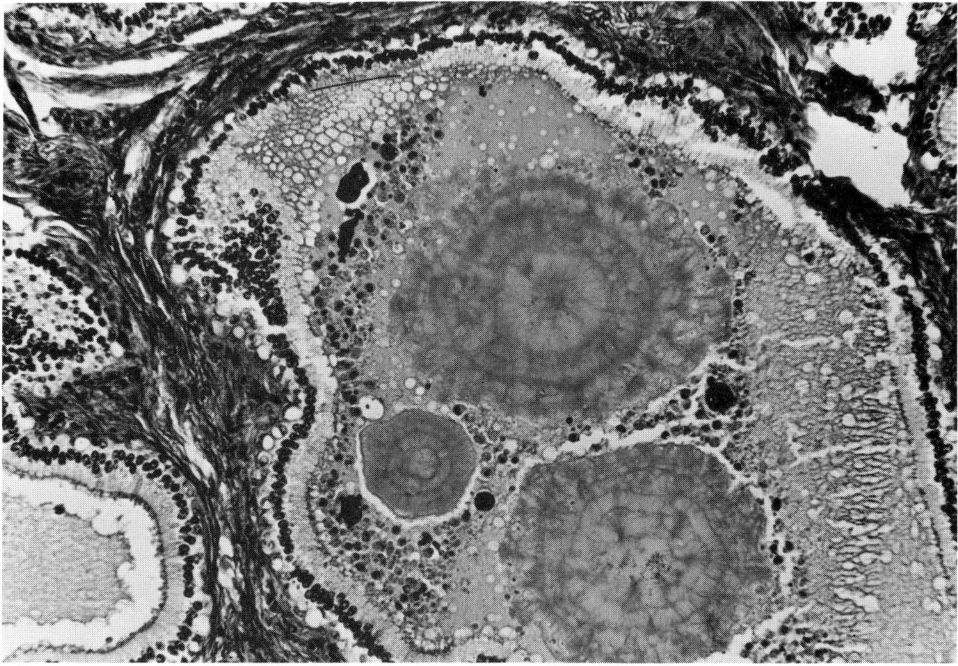

Figure 2–49. Large lamellated corpora amylacea in the seminal vesicles of a bull. Note the variation in size and internal structure, as well as the small dark concretions near the large ones.

being the presence of very distinctive extracellular fibrils called β-pleated sheet fibrils. Several different proteins can form these sheets and several clinical syndromes result from the location and composition of these abnormal deposits. The primary event is overproduction of a precursor protein which can be processed and deposited as amyloid fibers. These are rather inert fibrils, which can cause pressure atrophy and eventually necrosis, as well as marked disturbance of normal physiological processes. The eventual inactivation of a vital function caused by the presence of the amyloid leads to clinical disease and death. Some syndromes are generalized and some are localized to specific organs.

The terms primary and secondary amyloidosis are becoming outdated. The main groups are (1) ***acquired systemic amyloidosis***, the cause of which is abnormal production of immunoglobin unrelated to any infectious process; tumors or dyscrasias of plasma cells in bone marrow are causes in this group; (2) ***reactive acquired amyloidosis,*** resulting from chronic infectious disease; (3) ***organ limited amyloidosis***, particularly skin, cerebrum, and heart, which seems to occur without an obvious cause; and (4) ***localized amyloidosis***, caused by localized tumors of plasma cells in various tissues (see the recent review by Glenner [1980].)

Detailed classification of the disease into types in animals has not yet been accomplished. Amyloid is best known in animals as a primary cause of uremia (Figs. 2–50 and 2–51), as a cause of diabetes when it replaces pancreatic islets, for its interference with the immune response when it replaces splenic white pulp (Fig. 2–52), as a cause of less specific effects when it forms in the walls of small arteries, and as a space-occupying lesion in hepatic sinusoids, interfering with hepatic function (Fig. 2–53). Wild waterfowl frequently develop hepatic and splenic amyloidosis. Amyloid also seems to have a relationship to abnormal products of certain endocrine glands of animals, such as thyroid and pancreas, in which amyloid fibrils form. Examples are amyloidosis of the islets of Langerhans in some cases of diabetes and also some thyroid tumors. The Lugol's iodine test will identify renal amyloidosis affecting glomeruli in relatively advanced cases by applying the iodine to the fresh gross specimen (Fig. 2–54). The disease is readily reproduced experimentally by repeated injection of highly antigenic material such as casein. Historically, the disease is best known as a cause of renal failure in horses used for repeated antiserum production.

Calcification

Calcification refers to the deposition of calcium salts ***in soft tissues.*** If enough is present to be grossly visible, the deposit is white. The lesion occurs in quite a variety of circumstances and requires proper interpretation. Special stains can specifically identify calcium in tissue. It stains blue with hematoxylin-eosin and can be confused with bacteria. Pathological calcification should be clearly separated from bone production. Ectopic or metaplastic bone formation does occur, but calcification in the context used here refers to deposition of phosphate and carbonate salts of calcium in soft tissues, not bone formation. Mineralization of ligaments and tendons is a form of metaplasia (Chapter 5), rather than merely calcification.

There are two classic types of calcification: dystrophic and metastatic. ***Dystrophic*** implies tissue damage, degeneration or death of cells or denaturation of protein in tissues, which allows the salts of calcium to precipitate. Calcium enters rapidly into most degenerating cells, but some tissues seem to have an affinity for taking up calcium. Muscle has this particular affinity, and the calcium contributes to the color in white muscle disease. Dystrophic calcification may be prominent in some chronic tissue-destructive lesions such as tuberculosis in cattle or nodular worm infection in sheep (Fig. 2–55). Calcification of degenerate nucleus pulposus occurs in disc disease in dogs (Figs. 2–56 to 2–58) and can be visualized in radiographs. Thus dystrophic calcification has an association with some specific diseases but also occurs in nonspecific degenerative or necrotic lesions (Fig. 2–59).

Metastatic calcification occurs as a deposition on basement membranes and elastic fibers in several organs, particularly arteries, and implies high levels of serum calcium, excess vitamin D or hyperparathyroidism (Fig. 2–60). The deposit may be smooth on all basement membranes or irregular in distribution. If intracellular, the

Text continued on page 46

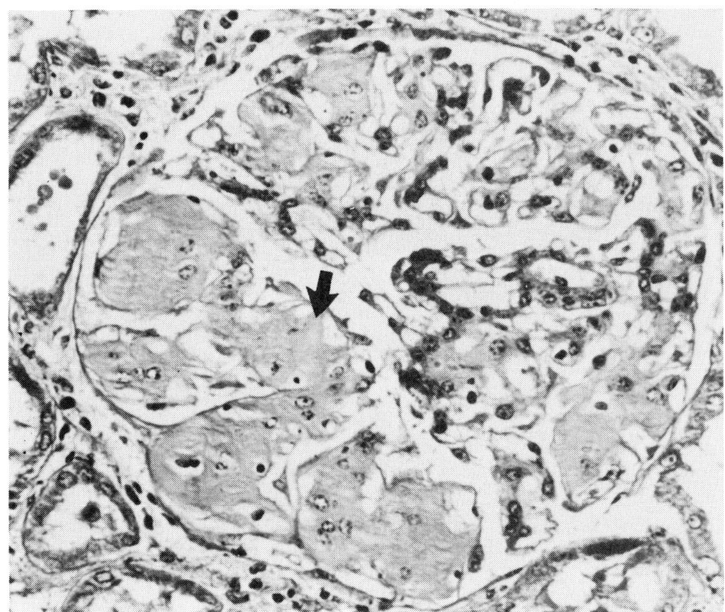

Figure 2–50

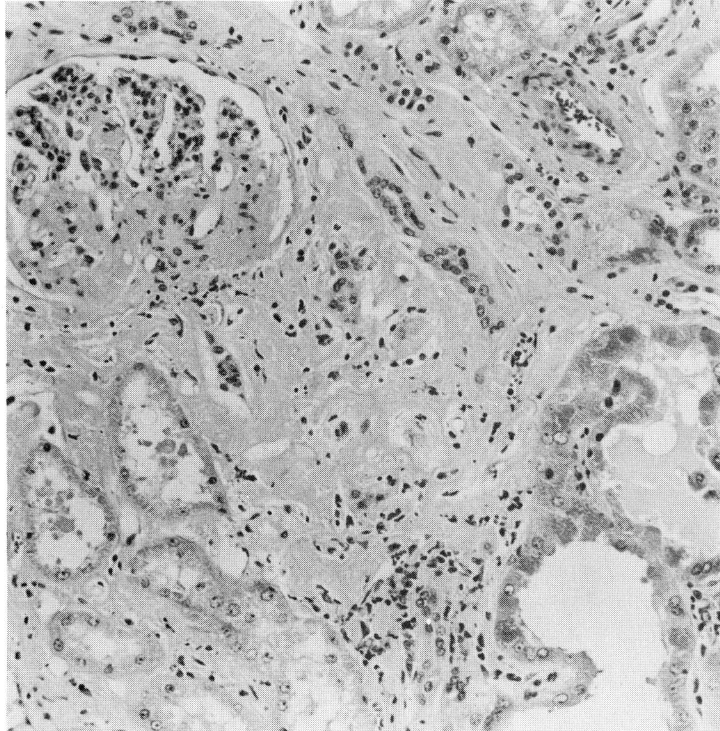

Figure 2–51

Figures 2–50 and 2–51. Amyloid accumulation in a glomerulus (arrow) in which capillaries have been partially obliterated. Less often amyloid also accumulates in interstitial tissue around tubules (Fig. 2–51).

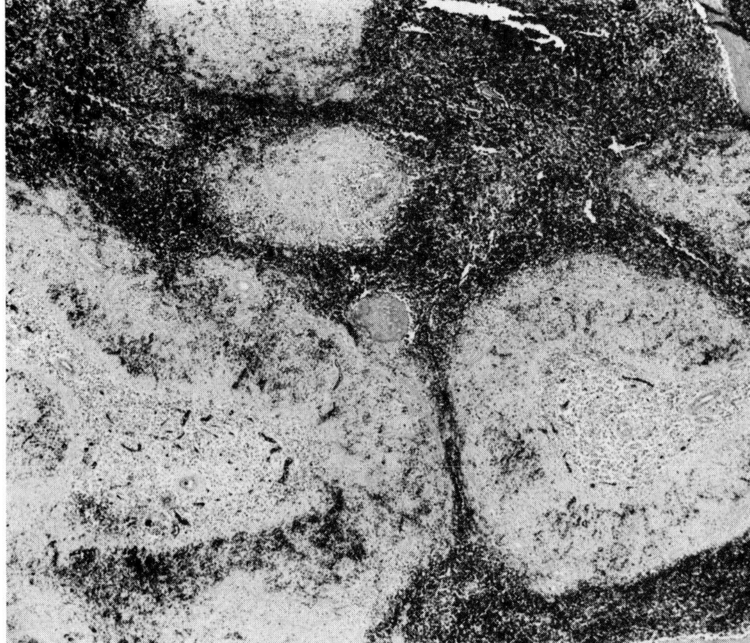

Figure 2–52. Extensive replacement of lymph follicles by amyloid. This lesion is relatively common in wild waterfowl.

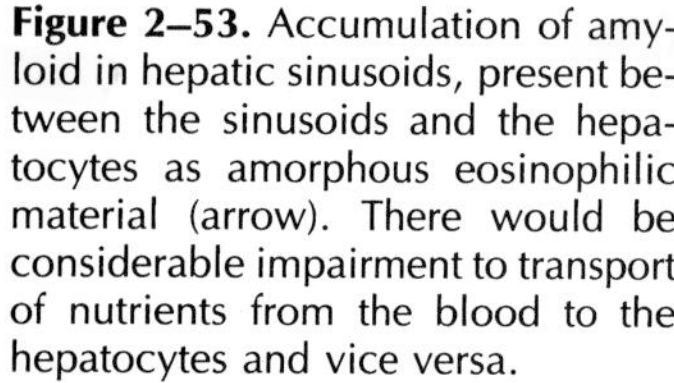

Figure 2–53. Accumulation of amyloid in hepatic sinusoids, present between the sinusoids and the hepatocytes as amorphous eosinophilic material (arrow). There would be considerable impairment to transport of nutrients from the blood to the hepatocytes and vice versa.

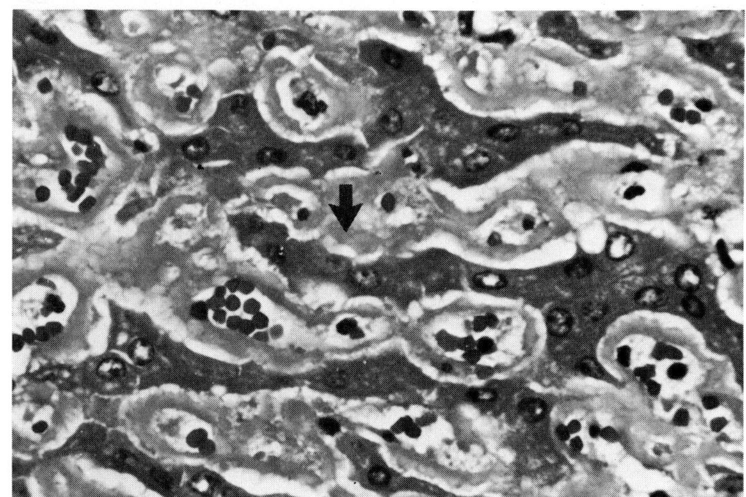

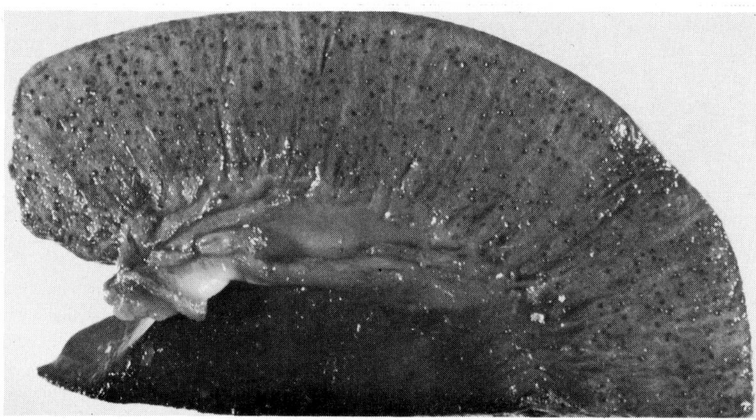

Figure 2–54. Positive Lugol's iodine test for renal glomerular amyloidosis.

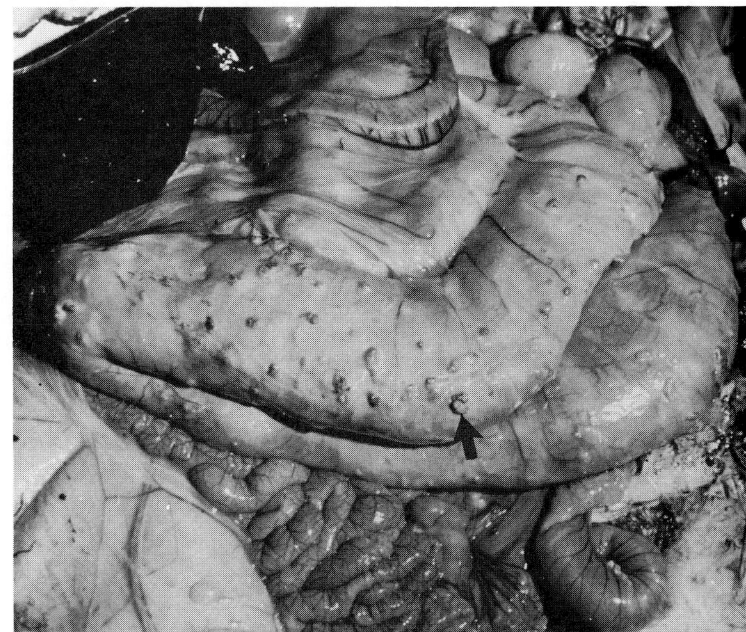

Figure 2–55. Calcified nodules (arrow) in the intestinal serosa in a sheep. The nodules are dead stages of *Oesophagostomum* worms. These are hard and gritty but of little clinical significance.

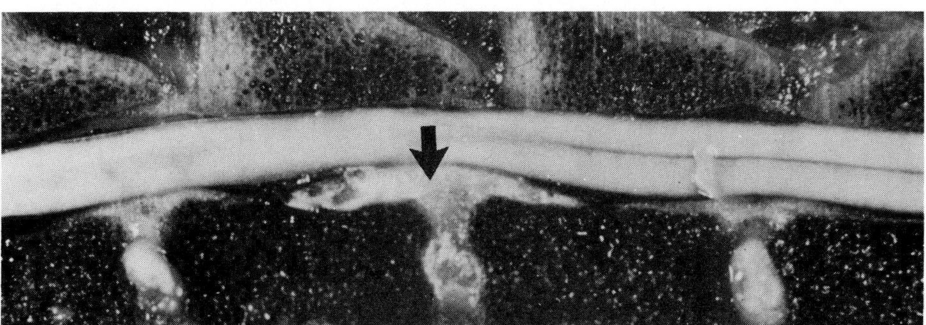

Figure 2–56. Calcified degenerate nucleus pulposus from the intervertebral disc of a dog has prolapsed dorsally into the spinal canal to form a space-occupying lesion (arrow) that will lead to posterior paralysis. The discs on either side are also somewhat calcified but have not prolapsed yet.

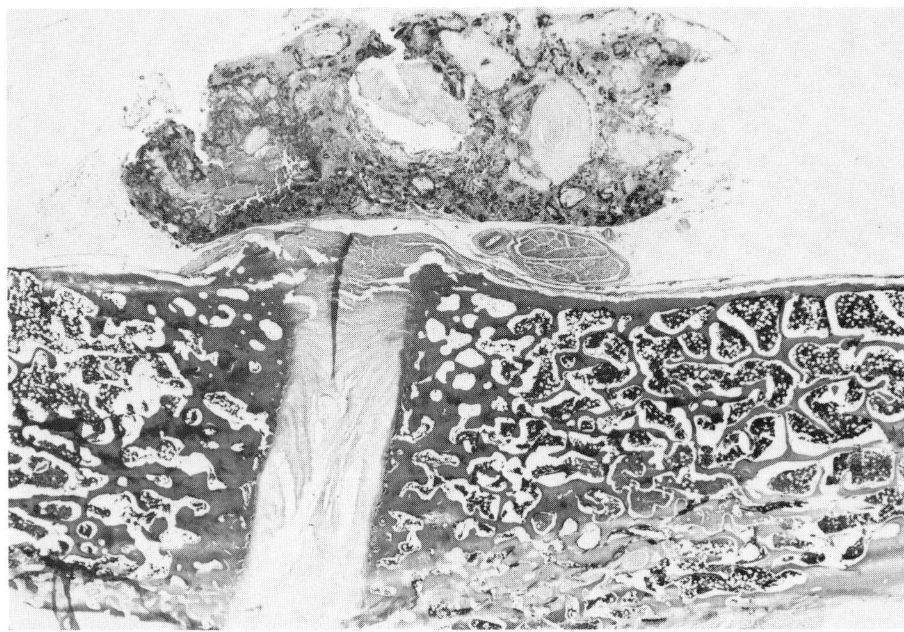

Figure 2–57. This lesion is similar to that in Figure 2–56. The dark areas in the mass lying above the intervertebral space and in the spinal canal are calcified. Remnants of cartilage from the nucleus pulposus are present in the mass.

calcification tends to be deposited on organelles, particularly mitochondria. The term ***calcinosis*** is sometimes used to describe extensive metastatic calcification.

Microscopically, the appearance of calcium will vary from a smooth, shiny blue color along basement membranes, through tiny stippling, to dense, dark blue clumps, depending on the location and type of calcification (Figs. 2–61 and 2–62). The lesion is usually seen grossly but may not be palpable. There is an association between metastatic calcification of the kidney and uremia. In addition, calcification of the subpleural intercostal muscles and ventral surface of the tongue (Fig. 2–63) in dogs is highly suggestive of uremia, as is subendothelial calcification of small vessels in several locations. Calcification is visible grossly in testes in cases of extensive tubular degneration (Fig. 2–64). In white muscle disease, the tissue is streaked or mottled with white but there is no change in texture (Fig. 2–65). The calcification may change the texture, however, if extensively present, to form hard gritty lumps as in the dystrophic calcification of tuberculosis in cattle or sometimes in the metastatic calcification of enzootic calcinosis in cattle (Fig. 2–66). The latter is restricted to certain areas where a particular forage is available that apparently contains excess vitamin D. The lesions become so extensive that the large vessels become white, thick and rigid, the lung comes to have the texture seen in asbestosis and the joints become painful. The disease has particular names, depending on where it occurs, such as Manchester wasting dis-

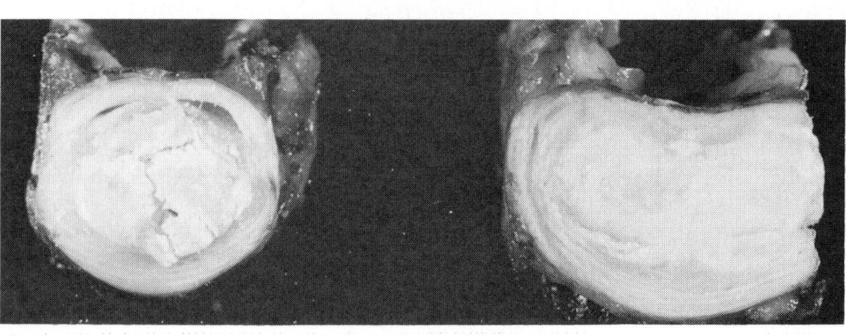

Figure 2–58. Varying degrees of dystrophic calcification in canine intervertebral discs. The lesion on the left is advanced.

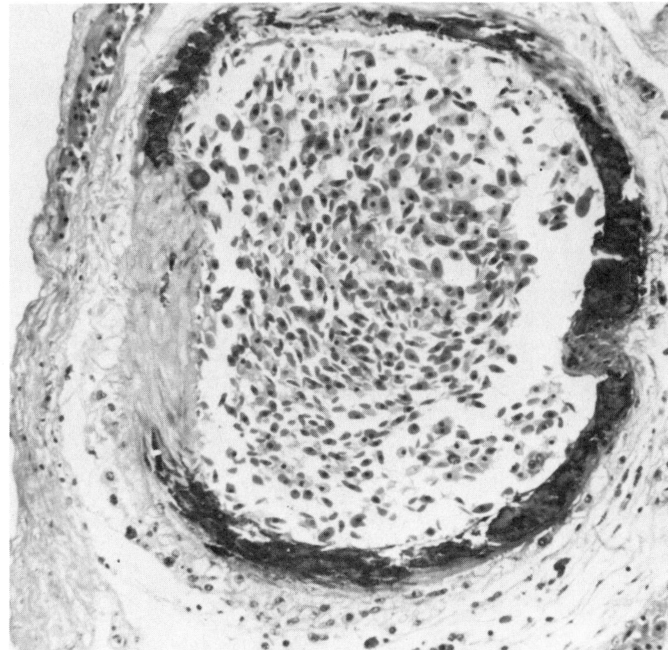

Figure 2–59. Dystrophic calcification of the media of an artery in a turtle.

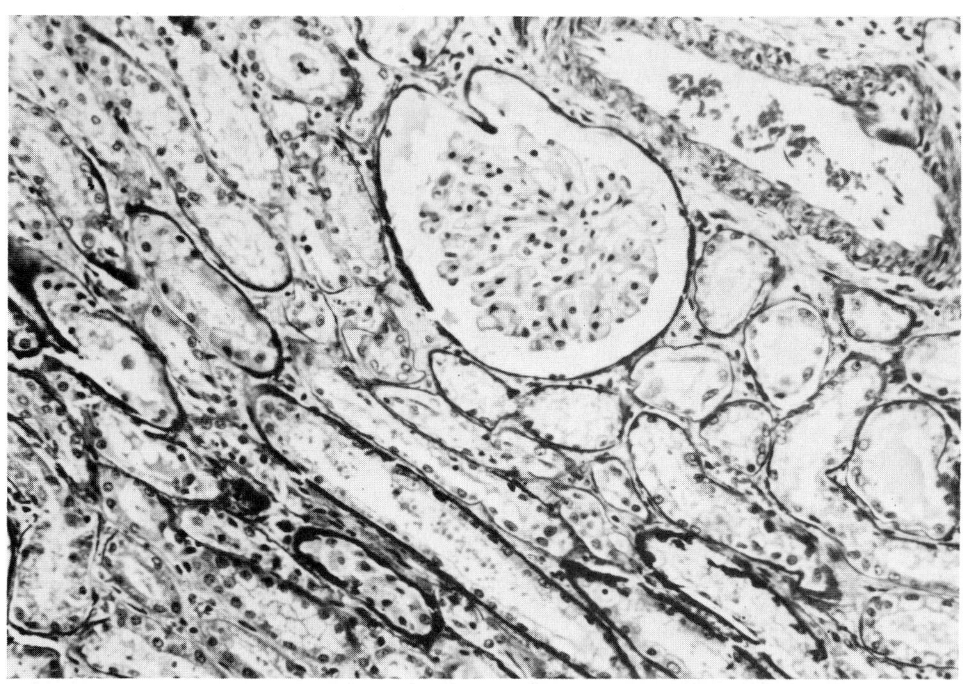

Figure 2–60. Diffuse metastatic calcification in a canine kidney. Note the deposition of calcium along basement membranes (arrow).

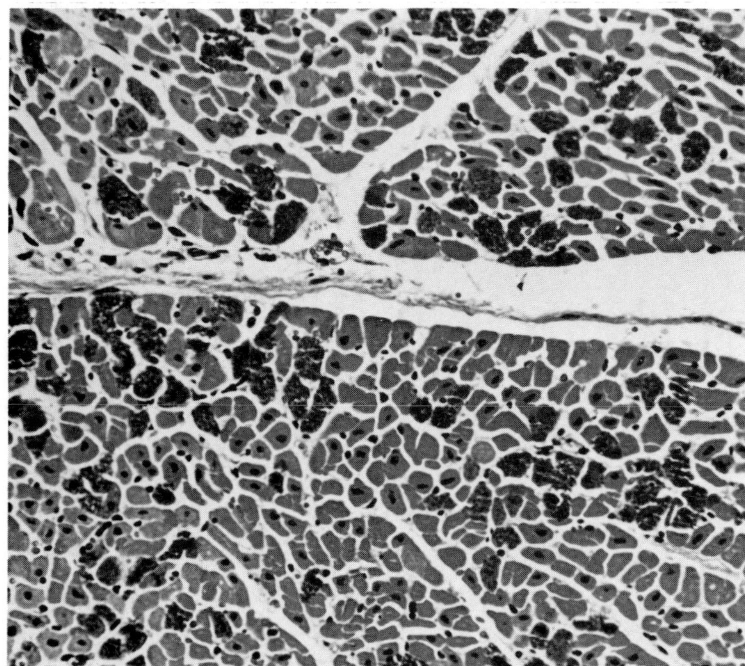

Figure 2–61. The dark areas in the muscle fibers are due to dystrophic calcification in acutely degenerate fibers in white muscle disease in a calf. These areas would stain bluish-purple with a von Kossa stain.

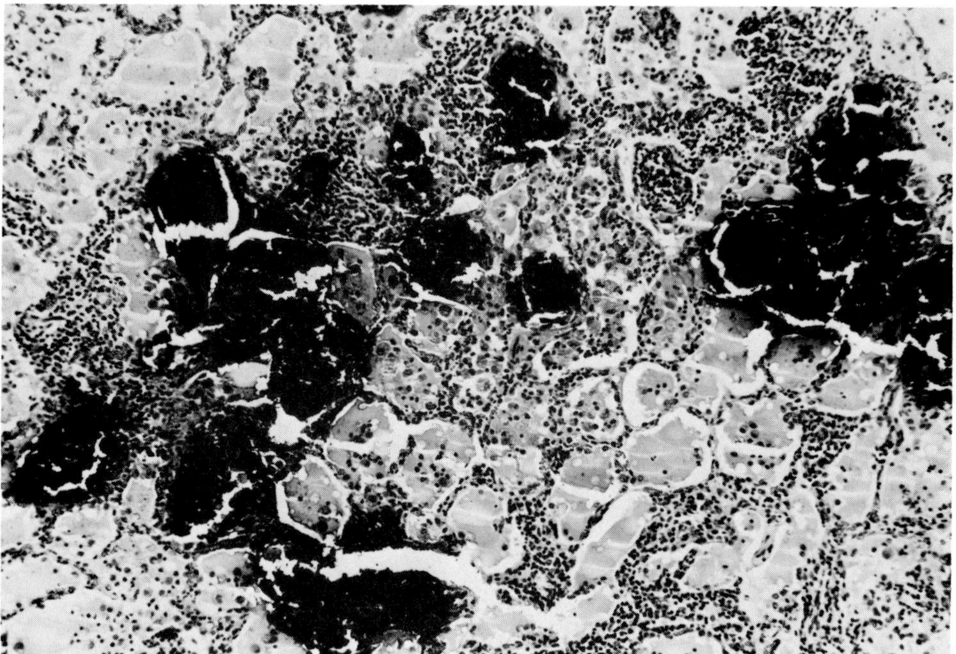

Figure 2–62. Dystrophic calcification in a sheep's lung, probably related to the presence of dead lungworms. The dark areas of calcification tend to shatter when cut by the microtome.

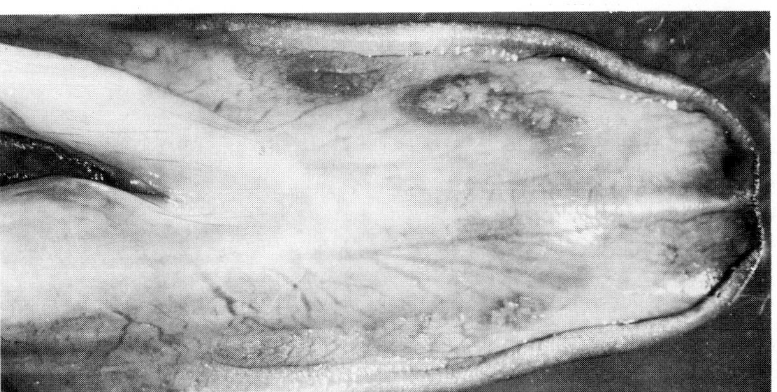

Figure 2–63. Dystrophic calcification, sometimes called "frosting," on the ventral surface of a uremic dog's tongue.

ease in Jamaica, enteque seco in Brazil, and naalehu in Hawaii.

Calciphylaxis is a term derived by Selye to described widespread deposition of calcium in tissues of individuals treated with a calcium sensitizer. The sensitizer may be vitamin D, parathyroid hormone or iron. The lesion develops after these have been applied and is precipitated by availability of quantities of calcium or by trauma. It is considered an experimental condition but may well occur naturally in circumstances related to overfeeding of minerals and vitamins.*

NECROSIS

Necrosis refers to the rapid death of a limited portion of an organism and is considered to be the final stage in ***irreversible degeneration. Necrobiosis*** is the term used for the entire process of degeneration and death of cells. Before proceeding, some discussion of death is in order. Individuals who die suddenly in traumatic accidents can sometimes be said to have ***died instantly.*** It is possible, however, to take organs from such individuals and transplant them to other individuals or culture the cells of the organ in tissue culture. Kidneys may be placed in a cooler overnight and prepared for tissue culture the next day. Ciliary activity can be demonstrated on a dead calf's nasal mucosa by spreading carbon particles on the mucosa and watching the carbon move for several hours. The head may be placed in a cooler overnight and brought out the next day and the exercise repeated. How can this be, when the electron microscopist says that irreversible changes occur in cells minutes after death? The medicolegal community is being pressed to ***define death,*** particularly for transplantation of organs when those carrying out the procedure must wait until the donor is officially dead. The definition of death of the entire body seems to relate in the final analysis to the extent of activity recorded on an electroencephalogram. (And then there was Lazarus!) The definition has different meanings for different people, depending upon their particular interest in a given situation. The veterinary pathologist is usually presented with an animal that clearly is dead. The owner knows it is dead and so does the clinician.

It was mentioned previously that there is a normal pattern of death and replacement of cells in most tissues and organs. This process proceeds so gradually that these dead cells are seldom observed in normal tissue sections. If the death rate increases, however, then the remnants of the dead cells will be visible. The difference will be easier to recognize if the loss occurs suddenly in one small area and can be compared with normal tissue nearby. Necrosis to the pathologist means that the ***tissue was dead prior to the time of removal from the***

Text continued on page 52

---

*Lesions caused by or related to nutritional and metabolic diseases are usually degenerative processes and are illustrated in the following figures.

Chapter 2: Figures 2–10, 2–11, 2–16, 2–17, 2–18, 2–35, 2–36, 2–42, 2–43, 2–44, 2–45, 2–47, 2–50, 2–51, 2–52, 2–53, 2–54, 2–60, 2–61, 2–63, 2–65, 2–66, 2–78, 2–79, 2–80, 2–81, 2–82, 2–83, 2–126, 2–129, 2–130, 2–132, 2–133.

Chapter 3: Figure 3–49.

Chapter 4: Figure 4–154.

Chapter 5: Figures 5–4, 5–7, 5–8, 5–9, 5–15, 5–16, 5–26, 5–27, 5–28, 5–33, 5–35, 5–38, 5–41, 5–42, 5–43, 5–45.

Chapter 6: Figure 6–14.

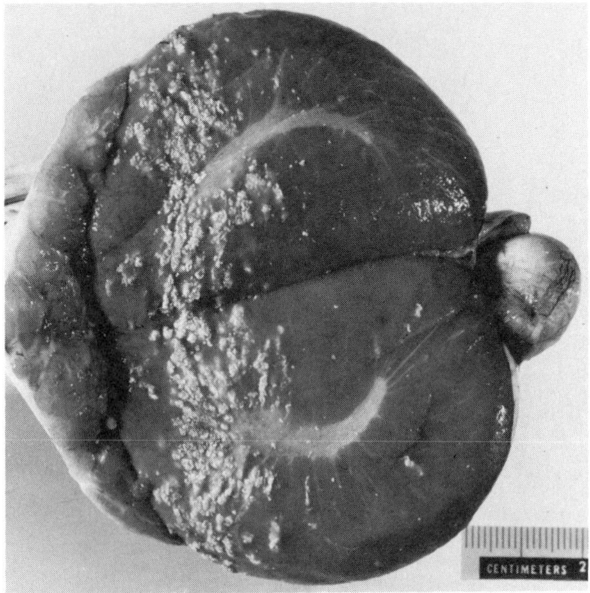

A

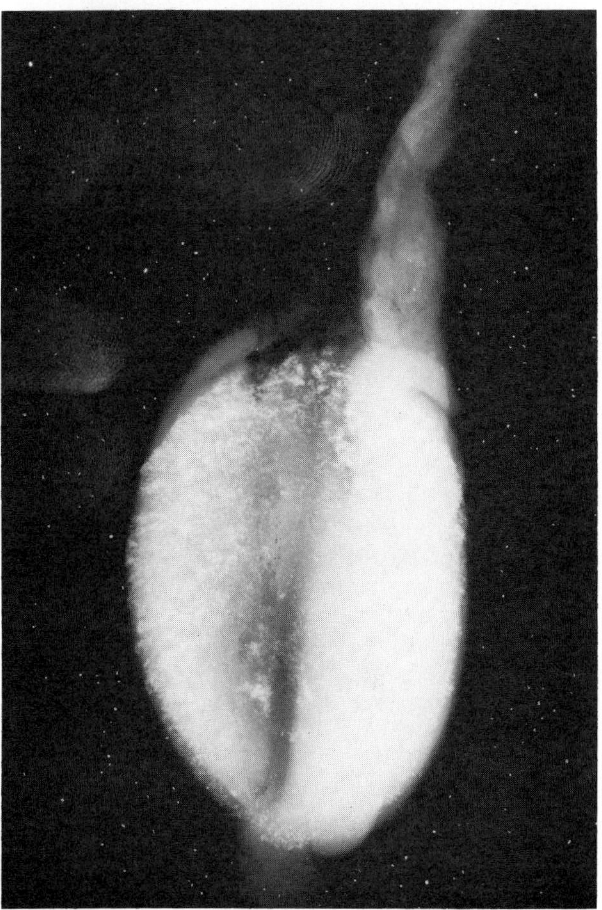

B

Figure 2–64. *A,* White granular foci of dystrophic calcification in testicular degeneration in a ram. *B,* A radiograph shows a much more extensive lesion. (Courtesy of C.A.V. Barker.)

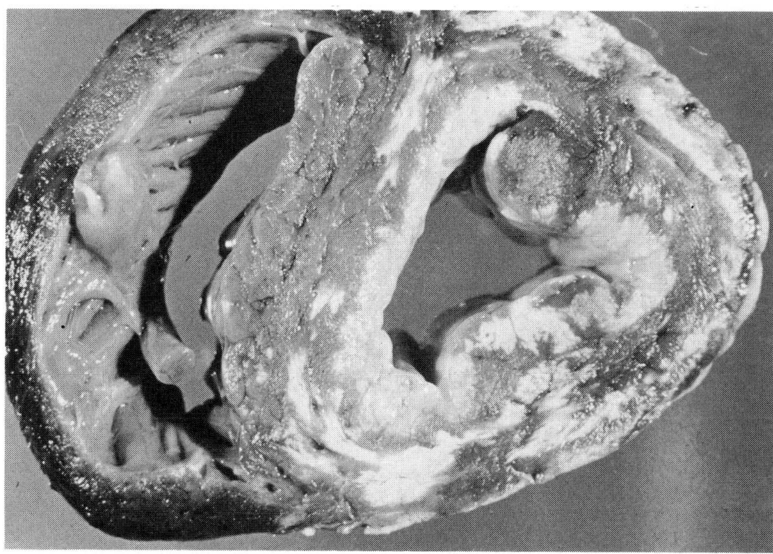

Figure 2–65. Cross section of both ventricles in the heart of a calf with white muscle disease. The dystrophic calcification is very pronounced in this case. Note the three shades of color in the myocardium—normal, pale, and white.

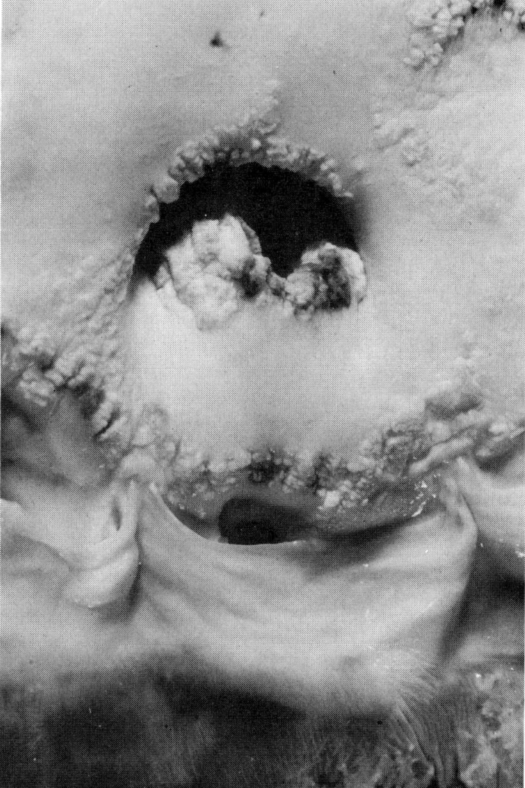

Figure 2–66. White raised areas of metastatic calcification around the valves and coronary artery orifice in the heart of a cow with diffuse calcinosis. (Courtesy of D. Read.)

live body or prior to the time of the animal's death: thus the definition ***rapid death of a limited area of tissue.*** Necrosis is recognized by specific types of changes in cells and tissues that will be present along with some of the degenerative changes discussed earlier. Some features are distinctive on gross examination and some on microscopic examination. The recognizable changes occur in the nucleus, cytoplasm and cell as a whole. The features of necrosis that may be recognized in individual cells take six to eight hours to develop after the death of the cell, and the pale color of a necrotic area observed on gross examination may be evident earlier than the microscopic changes.

Cellular Characteristics of Necrosis

Four types of nuclear changes may occur: ***pyknosis,*** the condensation of nuclear chromatin into a dark, round, homogeneous mass smaller than in a normal nucleus; ***karyorrhexis,*** the splitting of the nucleus into numerous pieces; ***karyolysis,*** dissolution of nuclear chromatin, leaving a hollow, large, round, ghost form of the nucleus. Karyolysis develops following initial clumping of chromatin and need not pass through or be related to stages of pyknosis or karyorrhexis, which apparently require reduction in nuclear volume or nuclear fragmentation. These changes may be present in individual cells in the same lesion or one type may predominate (Fig. 2–67). Karyorrhexis tends to imply a more severe sudden insult. The various nuclear changes are illustrated in Figures 2–68 through 2–72. When necrosis is extensive, clumps of scattered ***nuclear debris*** will be present, including pyknotic and karyorrhectic remnants, sometimes in quite concentrated amounts, indicating death of many cells (Figs. 2–73 and 2–74). The process of necrosis may go on in an area for an extended period with the result that all degrees and types of nuclear changes, including large accumulations of nuclear debris, may be present.

The cytoplasmic indications of necrosis are increased ***acidophilia,*** which is most common, or ***lysis*** of the cytoplasm, giving a pale vacuolated appearance. The cell as a whole loses its outline, and there are reduced differential staining of nucleus and cytoplasm and complete loss of cells. The progression in cytological changes is illustrated in Figure 2–75, which supplies more detail than in Figure 2–9. ***All of these nuclear and cytoplasmic changes can occur in autolysis.*** Therefore, it is usually necessary to have viable tissue present in a lesion for comparison with a necrotic area in order to recognize necrosis.

Gross Characteristics of Necrosis

The ***gross*** indications of necrosis are loss of color or ***paleness*** of the tissue, ***loss of strength*** of the tissue as it softens, a definite ***zone of demaracation*** between necrotic and viable tissue and in some instances the location or ***pattern*** of the lesion (Figs. 2–76, 2–77, 2–78).

However, if a tissue is very congested or if hemorrhage has occurred prior to necrosis, the tissue may be very dark or almost black. Therefore, the color changes that occur with necrosis can be confusing. Sometimes the term hemorrhagic necrosis is used when both occur in the same lesion. It is best to state what can be observed and say hemorrhage *and* necrosis. This problem is further compounded when such a lesion also involves inflammation; thus the need to be as precise as possible in the interpretation of lesions.

Recognition of the pattern of a lesion suggestive of necrosis comes with experience and will be assisted by the knowledge of how particular agents cause lesions in particular tissues in particular species. The line of demarcation between viable and necrotic tissue is the most useful and reliable means of recognition of necrosis, but it takes two or three days to develop. Loss of strength and all other indications are evident in several days. The pale appearance of necrosis in tissue may be difficult to interpret, ***particularly in an early lesion,*** and other lesions appear to be similar and cause confusion in interpretation. Pressure from other viscera may cause the blood to be unevenly distributed on the surface of an organ and lead to an uneven pale and dark color. This may be a postmortem change (see later in this chapter) and not degeneration or necrosis. The blood flow through an organ may not be uniform prior to death, and there may be some areas that are congested and some that are relatively

Text continued on page 60

Figure 2–67. Diagram of the different manifestations of nuclear destruction. (From Sandritter, W., and Wartman, W. B.: Color Atlas and Textbook of Tissue and Cellular Pathology, 3rd ed. Chicago, Year Book Medical Publishers, 1969. Reprinted by permission.)

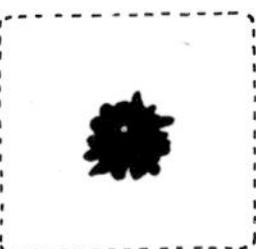

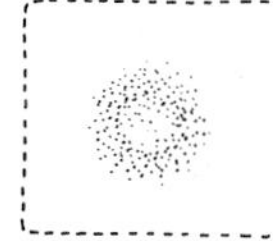

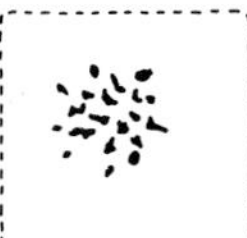

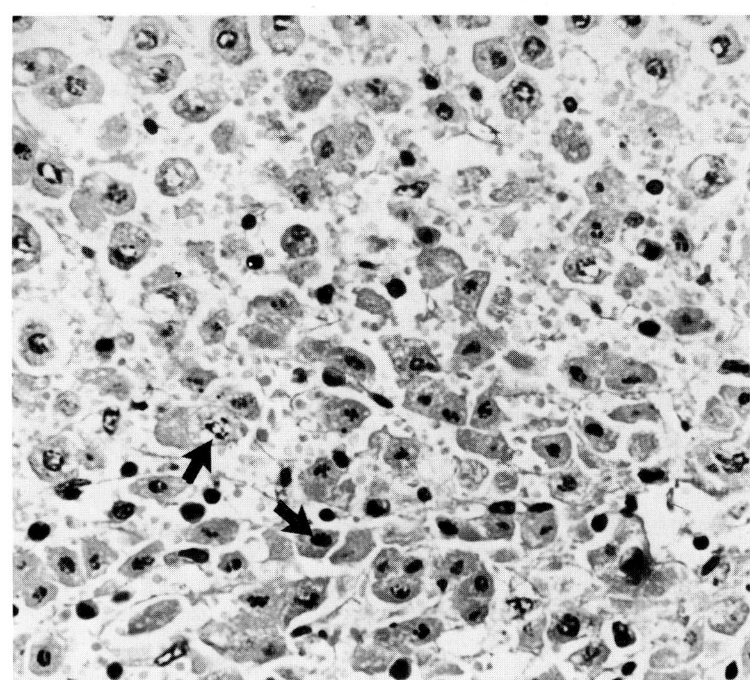

Figure 2–68. Pyknosis and karyorrhexis (arrows) in hepatocytes in a calf with acute chlorinated hydrocarbon toxicity. The increased density and eosinophilia of the cytoplasm are apparent near the central vein, and the cells have separated from their normal structure in cords.

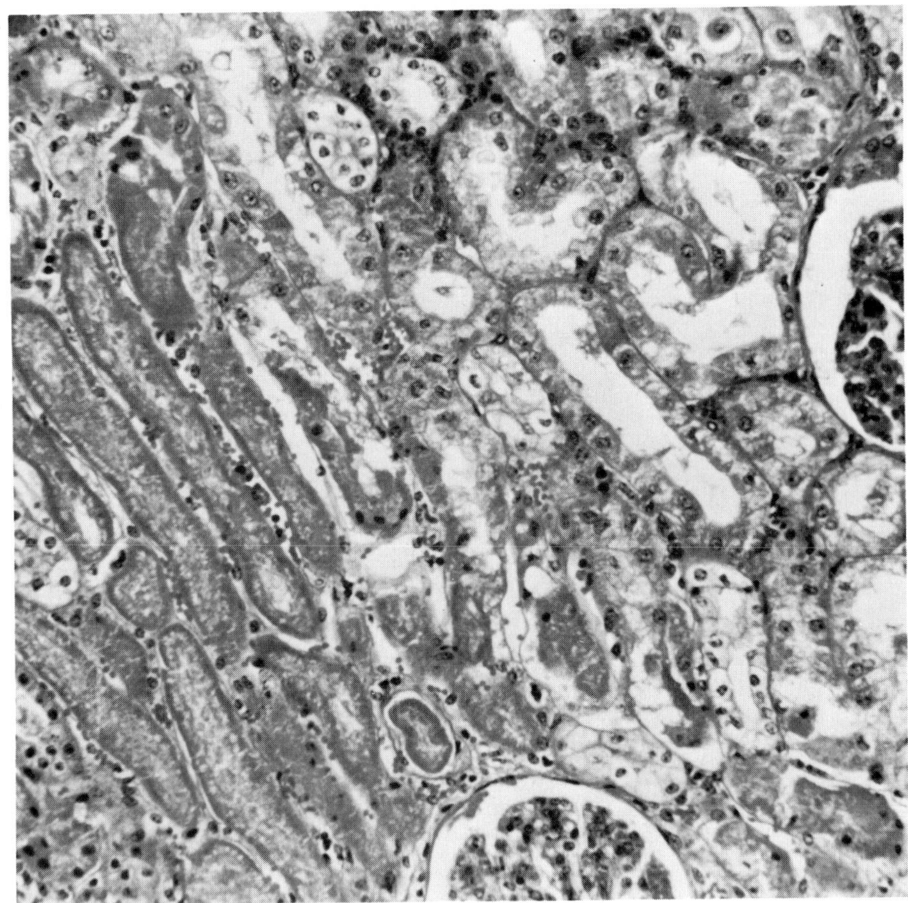

Figure 2–69. On the left there is complete absence of nuclei in tubules, which have undergone necrosis. The cells at the upper right appear more normal. The lesion could be caused by acute anoxia, such as an obstruction of blood flow, or by a toxin acting in an area of the tissue, which was well supplied with blood and functioning well at the time the toxin struck.

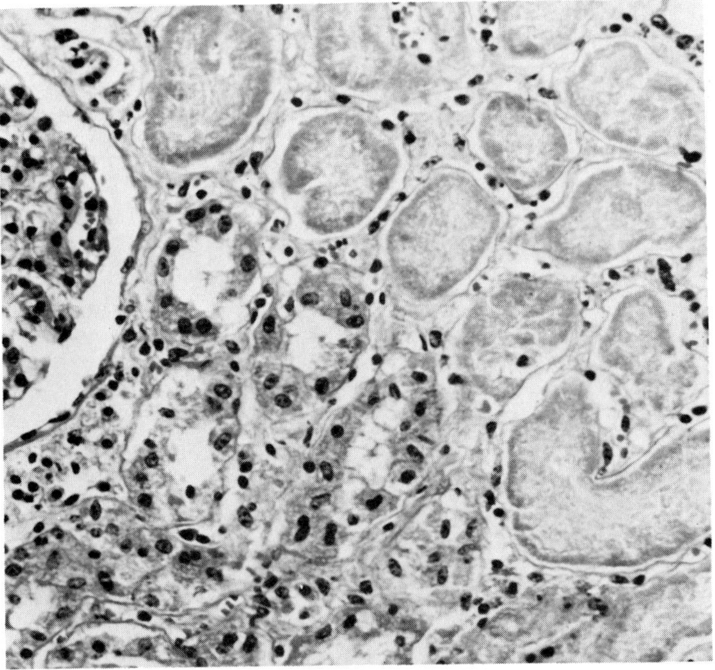

Figure 2–70. Closer view of renal tubules with necrotic ischemic tubules to the upper right indicated by absence of nuclei. Note how closely the necrotic tubules are located to more normal tubules.

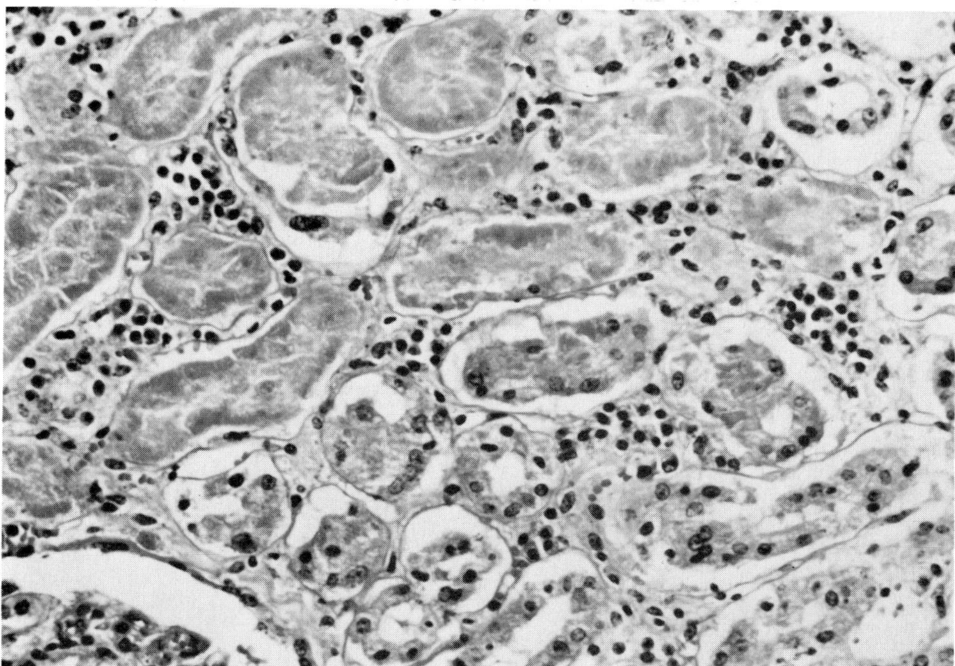

Figure 2–71. Lesion similar to Figure 2–70. Note absence of nuclei in some tubules and degenerate pyknotic nuclei in some individual cells in tubules toward the bottom, indicating progression of the lesion. Also note for later reference the increase in number of cells between the tubules. Lesions of the type in the last three figures would appear pale grossly.

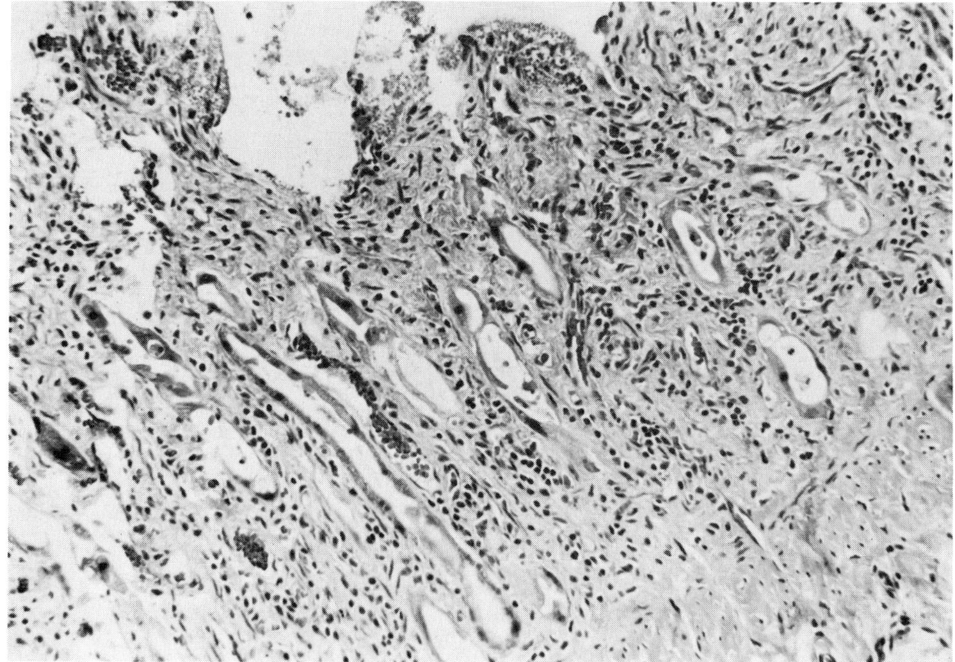

Figure 2–72. Intestine of a dog with marked loss of epithelial cells due to necrosis and collapse of villi and crypts. The absence of epithelial lining cells is indicative of extensive necrosis, in this case due to irradiation. Some viral agents cause a similar type of destruction of intestinal epithelium.

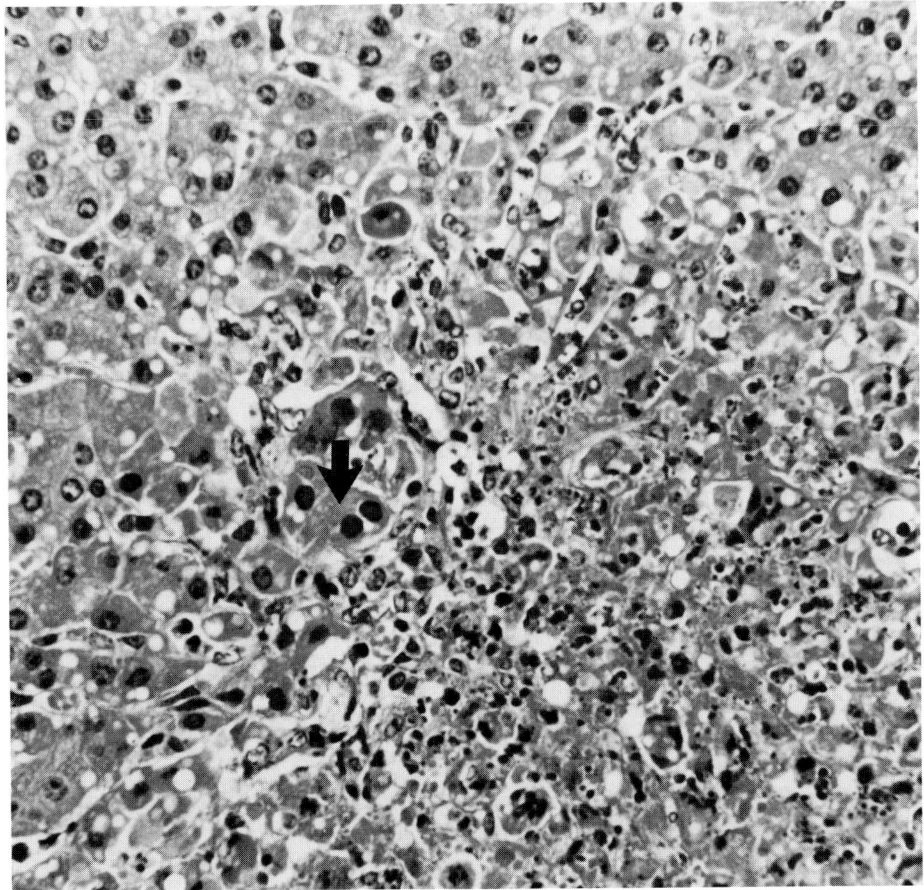

Figure 2–73. Necrosis in the liver in infectious bovine rhinotracheitis. Nuclear debris to the lower right indicates necrosis of hepatocytes. This area would appear as a pale focus grossly. Note the inclusion bodies (arrow).

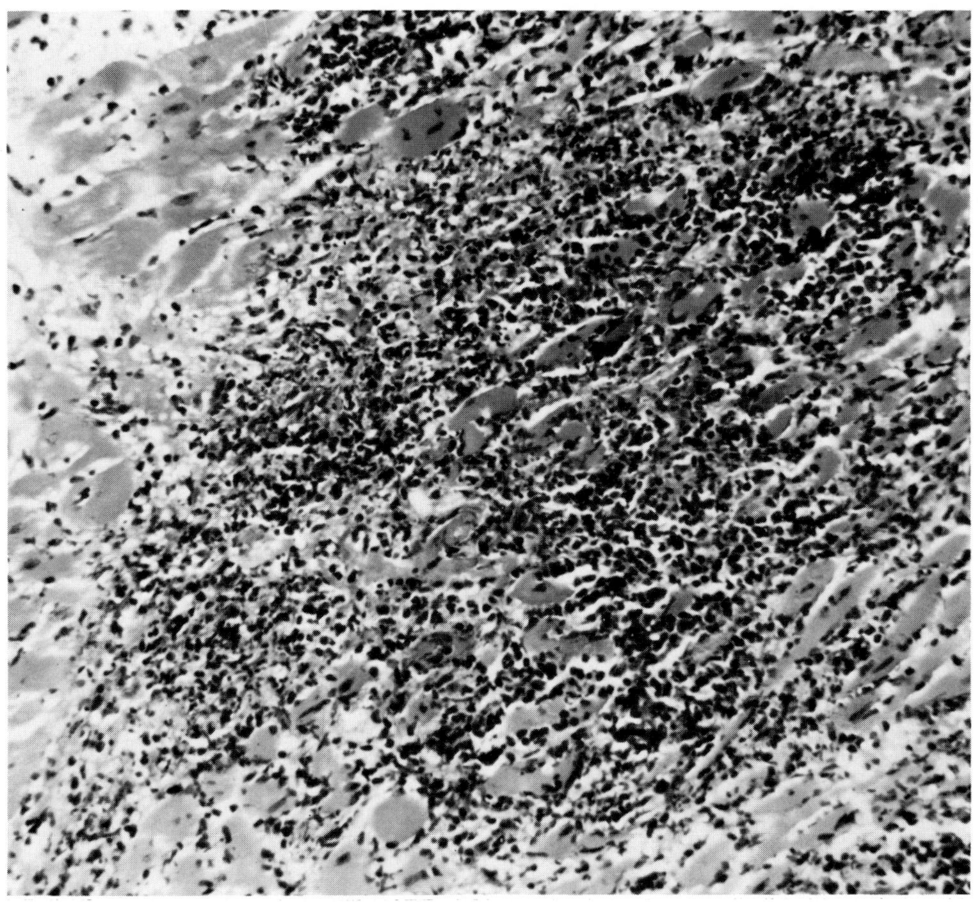

Figure 2–74. Necrosis in muscle as indicated by the nuclear debris that has accumulated between muscle fibers and by the loss of fibers from the area. This lesion would appear pale in the gross lesion because of the concentration of nuclei, mainly neutrophils, which have been drawn to the area of necrosis. The lesion could be the result of injection of an irritating substance into the muscle.

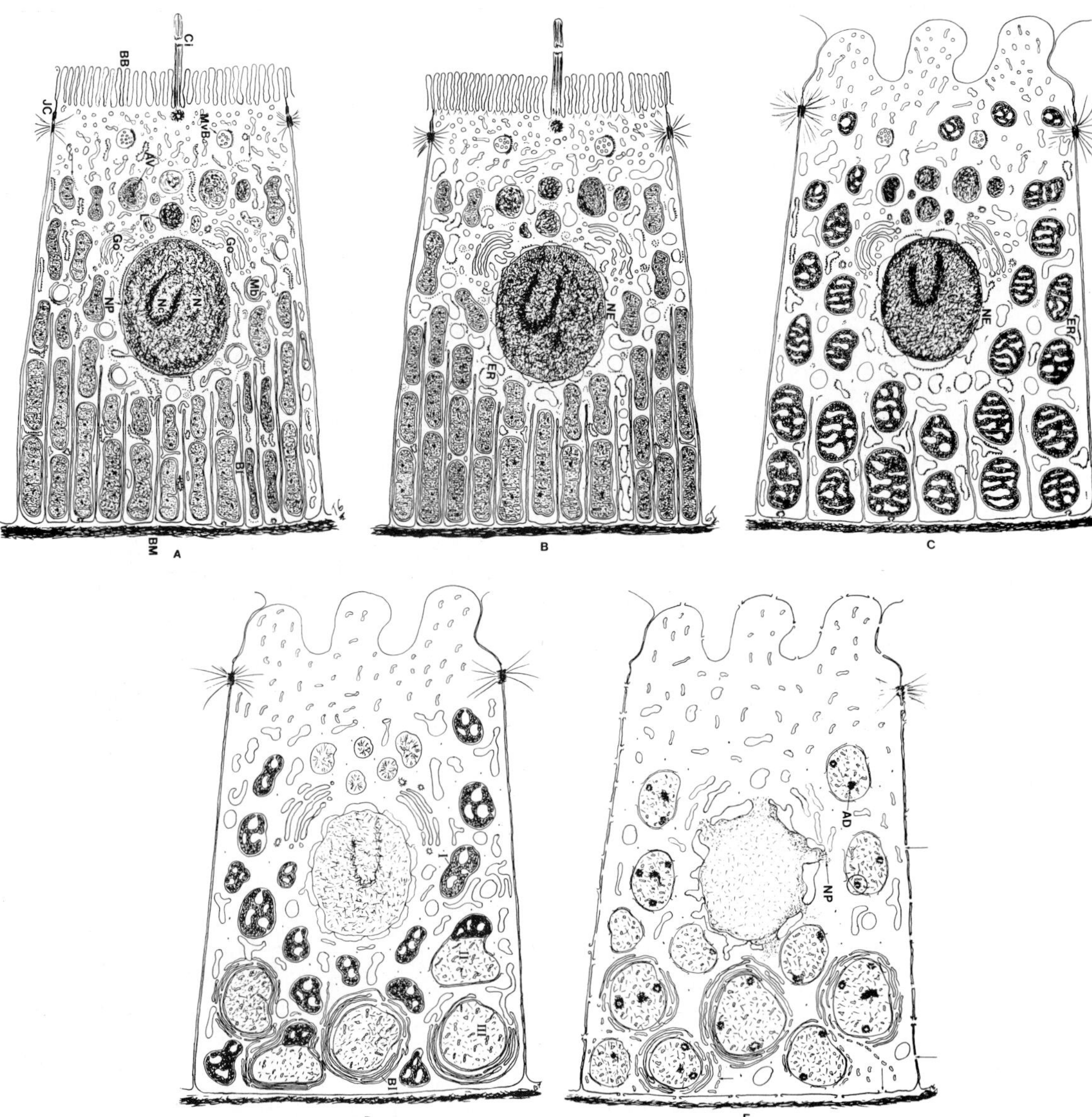

Figure 2–75. This series of diagrams depicts stages of loss of cell volume regulation leading from a normal to a necrotic cell.

A, A normal renal tubule cell. Ci, cilium; BB, brush border; JC, junctional complex; L, secondary lysosomes; AV, autophagic vacuoles; Go, Golgi apparatus; N, nucleus; Nc, nucleolus; NP, nuclear pores; Mb, microbodies; arrows, face-on view of rough-surfaced endoplasmic reticulum; BI, basilar invaginations; BM, basement membrane.

B, The only change visible is dilatation of the endoplasmic reticulum (ER) and nuclear envelope (NE).

C, Condensation of the mitochondrial inner compartment with relative expansion of intracristal spaces and swelling of the cell sap. The brush border swells and becomes distorted.

D, Some mitochondria (I) are still condensed like those in C. Others (II) have a condensed portion and a portion in which the matrix is greatly expanded, while some (III) show only expansion of the inner compartment. Basilar infoldings often form circumferential scrappings around mitochondria. Polysomes are infrequent or absent. Lysosomes are pale; the nucleoplasm is dispersed and indistinct.

E, The state of necrosis. All mitochondria are swollen and contain two types of densities: an amorphous type (AD) and a microcrystalline density in apposition to the inner membranes (encircled areas). Interruptions occur in the continuity of the plasma membrane and basilar infoldings (arrows). The nucleus is disintegrating. NP, Nuclear pore. From Ginn, F. L., Shelburne, J., and Trump, B. F.: Disorders of cell volume regulation. I. Effects of inhibition of plasma membrane adenosine triphosphatase with ouabain. Am. J. Pathol., *43*:1041–1071, 1968. Reprinted by permission.)

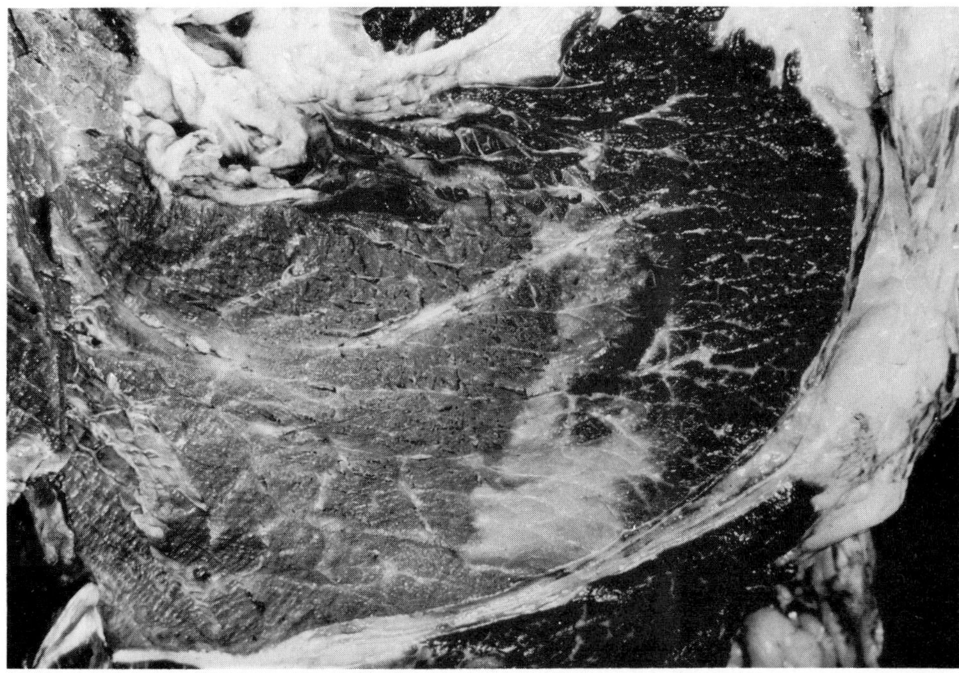

Figure 2–76. Large pale area of ischemic necrosis in the hamstring muscles of a downer cow. Normal muscle is to the right.

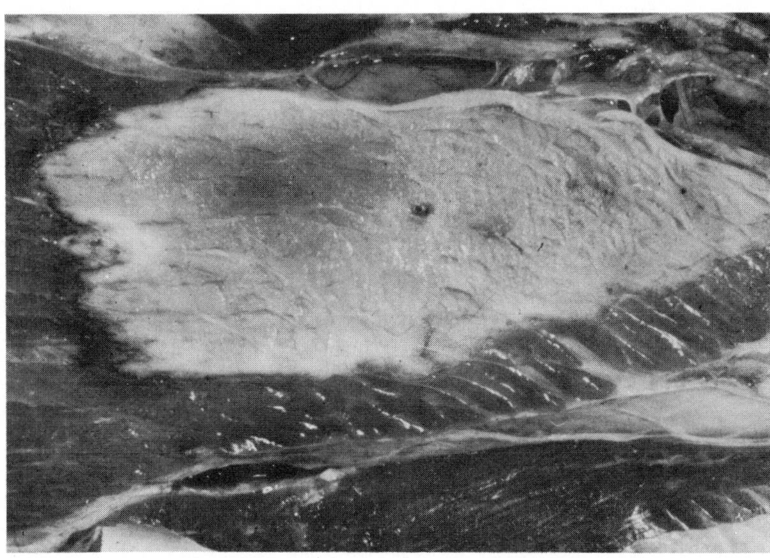

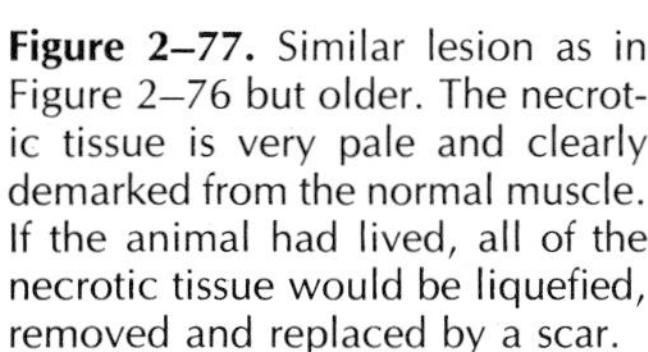

Figure 2–77. Similar lesion as in Figure 2–76 but older. The necrotic tissue is very pale and clearly demarked from the normal muscle. If the animal had lived, all of the necrotic tissue would be liquefied, removed and replaced by a scar.

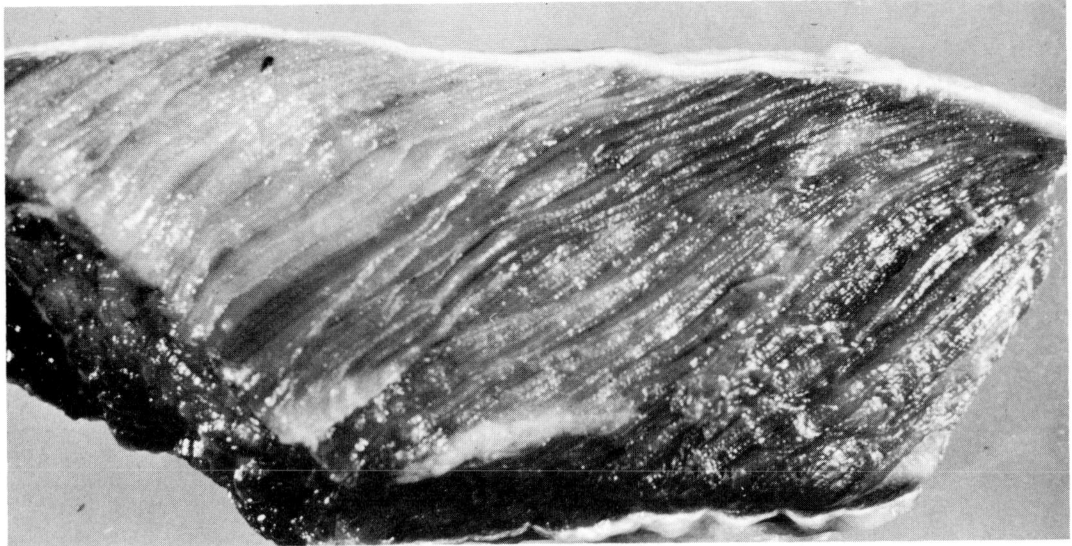

Figure 2–78. Pale areas of degeneration and necrosis in skeletal muscle of a calf.

ischemic. This situation may lead to a mottled appearance on the surface that extends into the tissue. The kidney often presents this color change. Necrosis in the liver and lung may appear dark red initially because of the double circulation in these organs.

Degeneration also is pale in most tissues such as heart, liver, kidney and muscle. Degenerate muscle, as in white muscle disease caused by vitamin E deficiency, is pale from degeneration and becomes white because of secondary dystrophic calcification (Figs. 2–79 through 2–83).

Considerable experience and careful observation are required in the recognition of the gross lesions of degeneration and necrosis in various tissues. ***The recognition of necrosis in gross lesions will be one of the most difficult practical aspects of general pathology to master.*** **Unfortunately, the problem is often carried into all other courses in pathology. The definition and description given here seem simple enough, but not so. Wait and see.**

Types of Necrosis

Necrotic tissue may have a variety of gross and microscopic characteristics, depending on the etiological agent or pathological process involved as well as the site and distribution of the dead tissue. A classification of the morphological expressions of necrosis is very useful.

Necrosis is divided into two main types, coagulation and caseation, based on gross and microscopic appearance, and ***both have implications relating to etiology and pathogenesis.***

Coagulation necrosis refers to an area of necrosis in which the gross and microscopic architectures of the tissue and some of the cells are recognizable. If acute, it may be recognized by nuclear changes, acidophilia of cytoplasm and reaction in surrounding tissues, perhaps in the form of edema or hemorrhage. This type is usually caused by acute anoxia, such as obstruction to blood flow, or very acute toxicity (Figs. 2–84 through 2–89).

Caseation necrosis is manifested by loss of recognizable architecture and will contain combinations of much dark nuclear debris and amorphous eosinophilic cytoplasmic debris, perhaps mixed with components of blood clots, hemorrhage, thrombi and calcification. The implication is that an etiological agent has caused severe local destruction (Figs. 2–90 through 2–96). The name ***caseous*** implies curdled or cheesy, which is suggested by the gross appearance and texture.

Liquefactive necrosis is another morphological type of necrosis and suggests a semisolid or fluid mass that has been present for some time, undergoing self-digestion.

Text continued on page 69

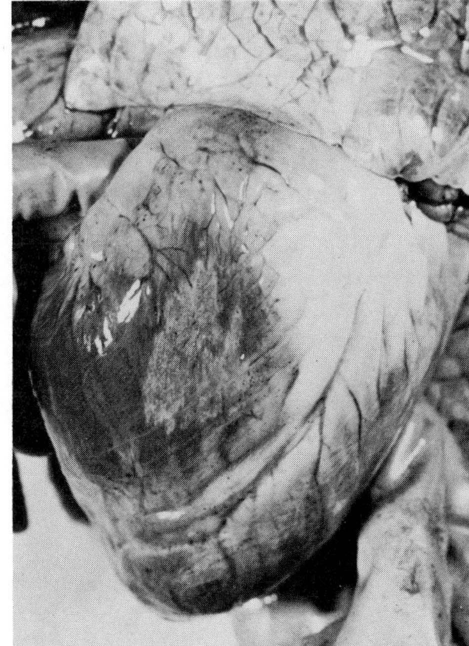

Figure 2–79. Pale areas of degeneration in myocardium of a pig with vitamin E deficiency.

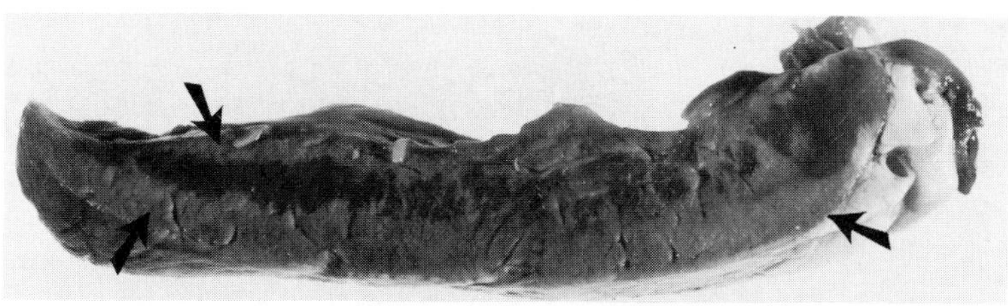

Figure 2–80. Pale areas of degeneration (arrows) in myocardium of a calf with white muscle disease. The dark areas toward the top were more normal.

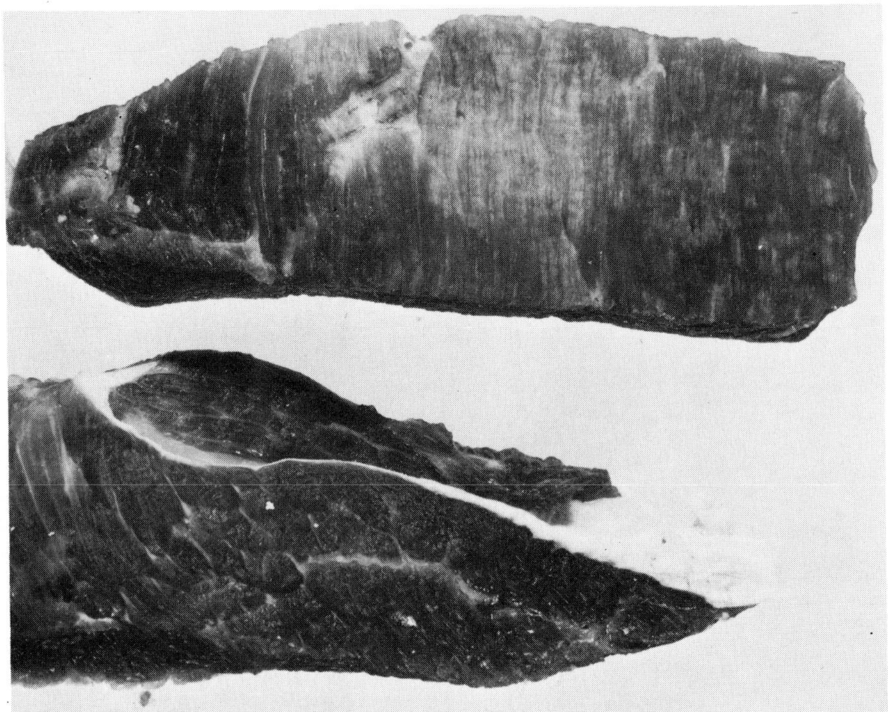

Figure 2–81. Pale areas of degeneration in skeletal muscle of a steer (lower tissue is normal in color).

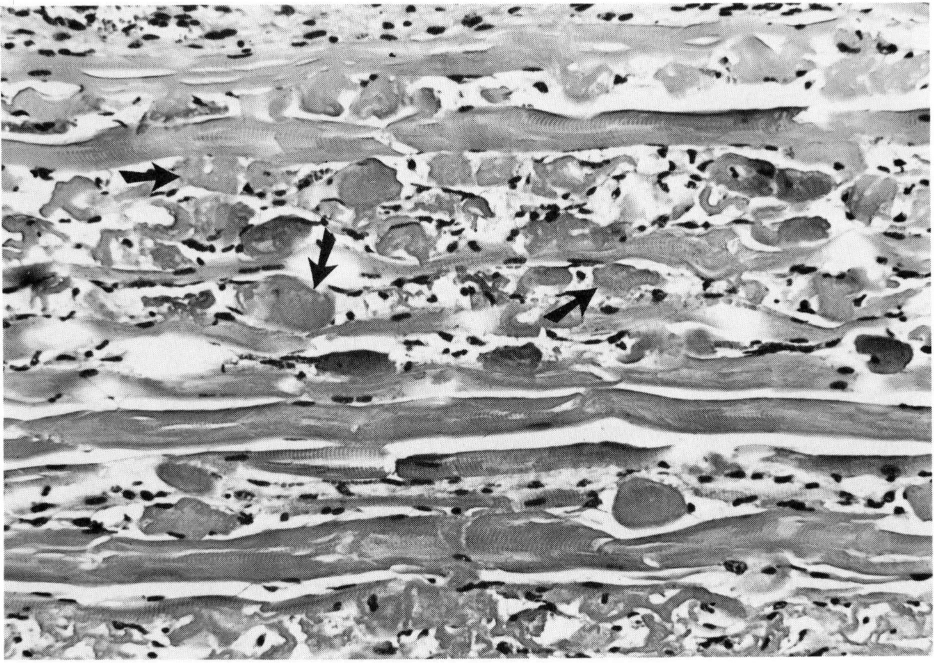

Figure 2–82. The paleness in the muscle lesion is due to degeneration, as shown in this illustration by the clumping of sarcoplasm of myofibers (arrows). When dystrophic calcification occurs in these degenerate fibers (Fig. 2–83), the muscle becomes white on gross examination, leading to the name white muscle disease, which is a vitamin E deficiency syndrome in calves, lambs and some other species. Note the variation in diffuseness or discreteness of the gross lesions. In the calf in Figure 2–80, only the left ventricle was affected, whereas in the steer in Figure 2–81, muscle throughout the body was diffusely affected. Calcification gives the dark granular appearance within fibers (Fig. 2–83).

Figure 2–83. See the legend for Figure 2–82.

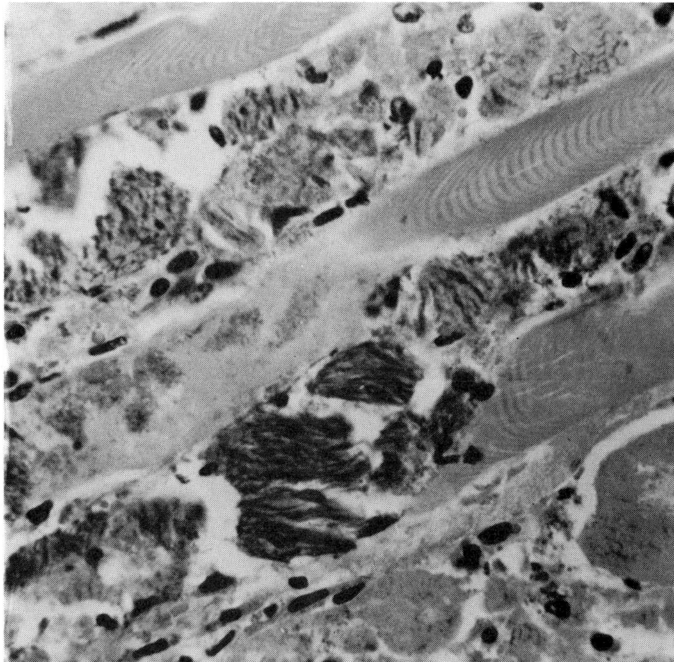

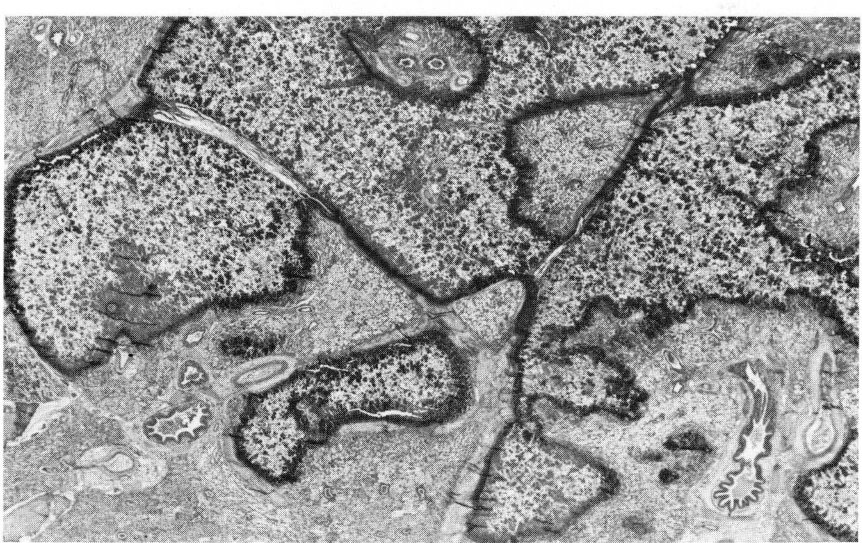

Figure 2–84. Irregular areas of coagulation necrosis toward the top in the lung of a steer with pasteurellosis. Note the clear demarcation from the normal tissue outlined by a concentrated rim of nuclei, which are mainly from neutrophils and macrophages. The areas of necrosis and the ring of nuclei would appear pale grossly.

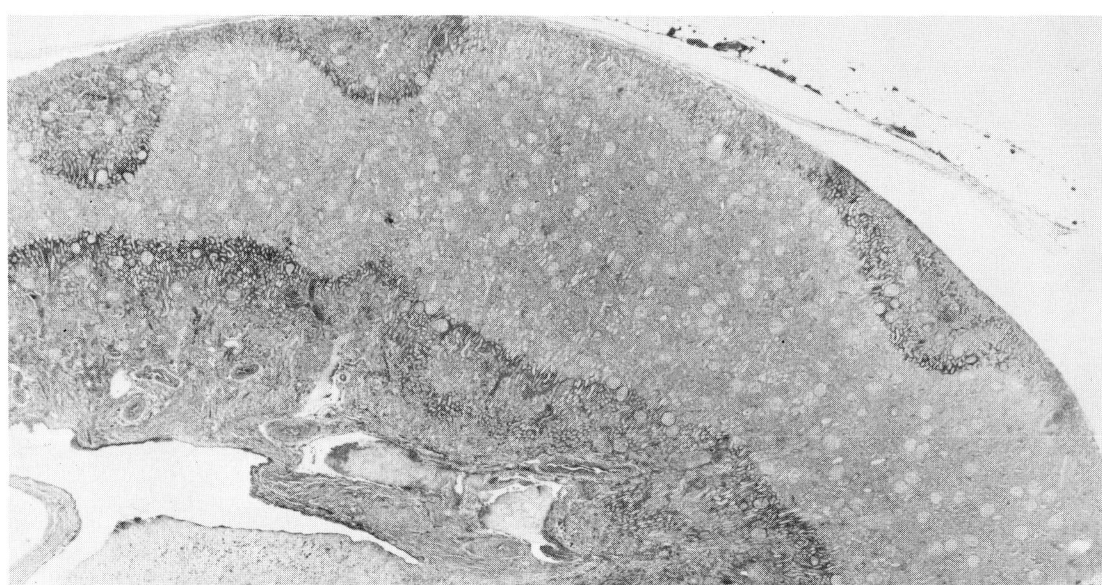

Figure 2–85. Pale area of coagulation necrosis due to ischemia in a kidney with demarcation by neutrophils beginning. This area would appear pale, surrounded by a white line, on gross examination.

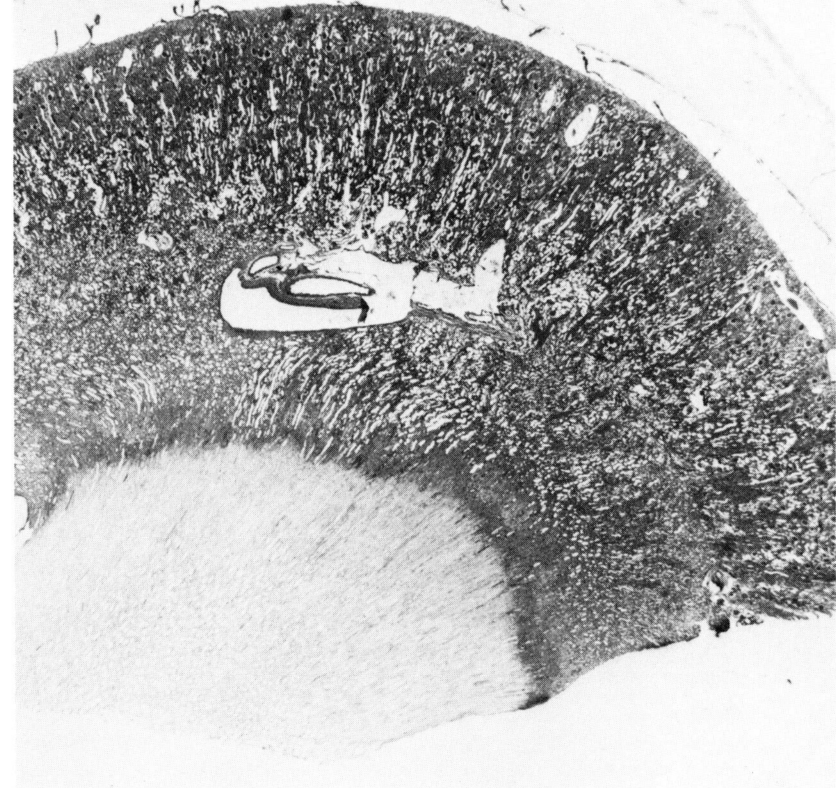

Figure 2–86. Acute renal medullary necrosis in a dog. Note the clear line of demarcation between the pale medulla and dark cortex.

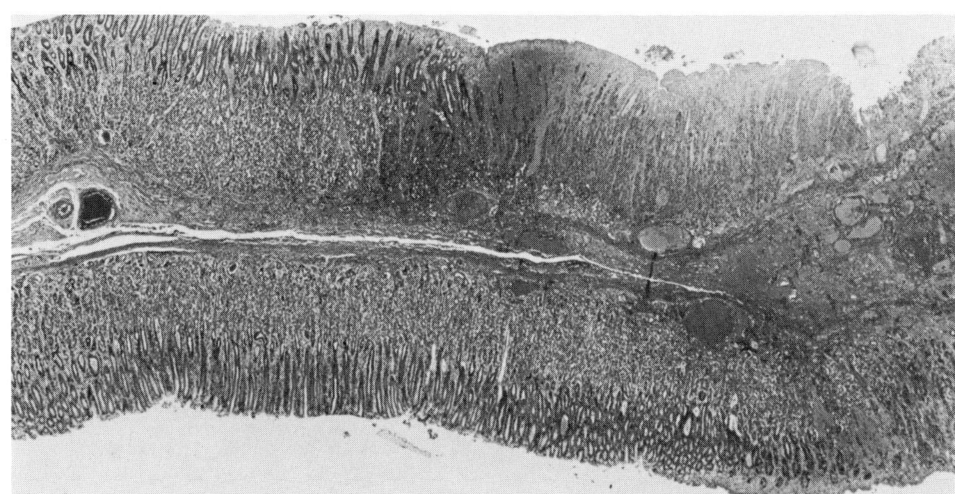

Figure 2–87. Area of coagulation necrosis in the abomasum of a calf caused by thrombosis due to invasion by fungal hyphae. The necrotic area is to the upper right and would be dark in color because of hemorrhage.

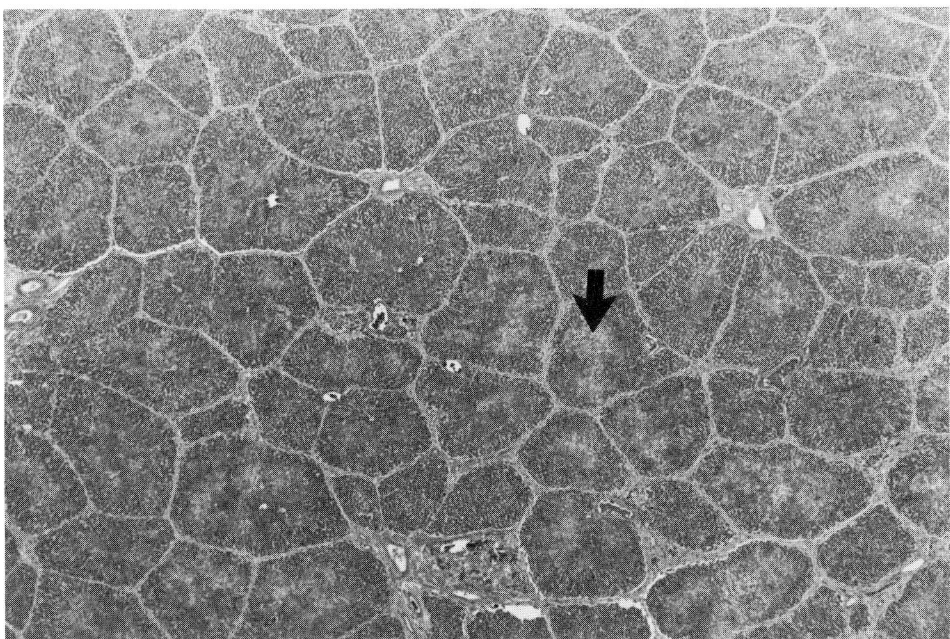

Figure 2–88. Acute anoxic hepatic necrosis in a centrilobular (arrow) or periacinar distribution. This type of lesion is usually related to acute circulatory failure.

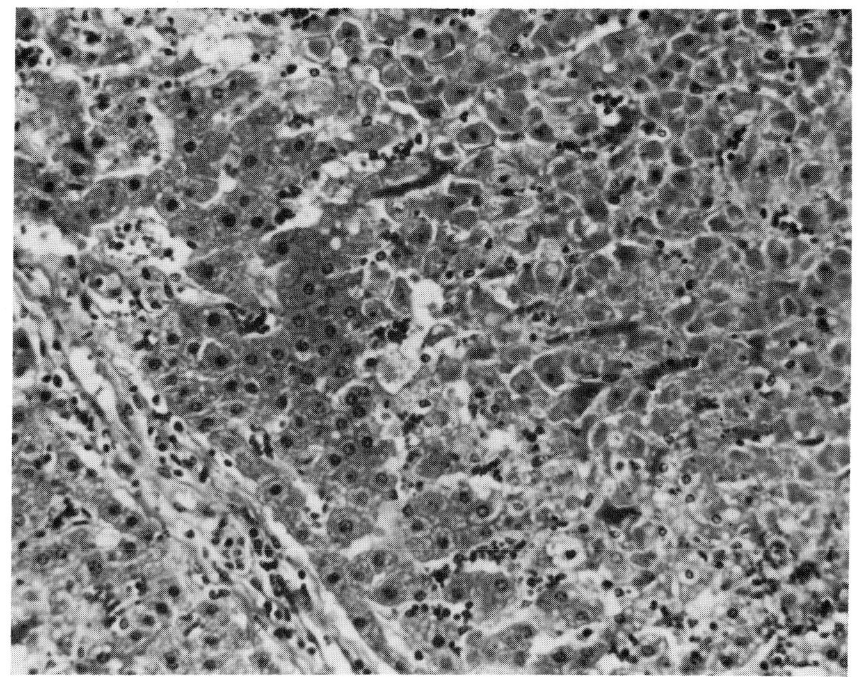

Figure 2–89. Higher magnification of a lesion similar to that in Figure 2–88. A portal area is to the left with viable cells near it, and necrosis of the cells is present near the central vein to the right.

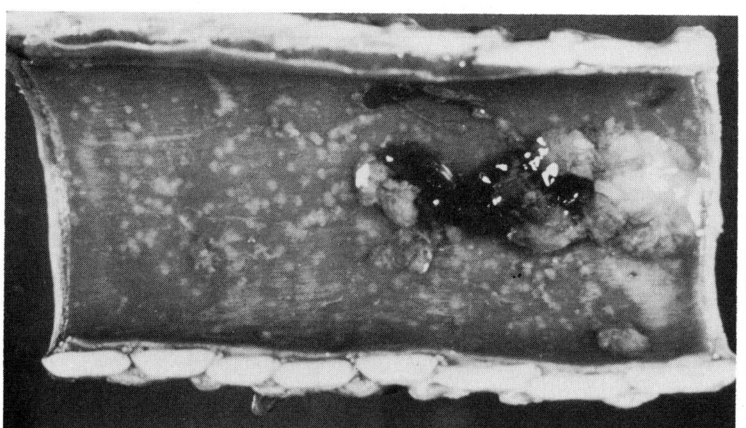

Figure 2–90. The white foci on the tracheal mucosa are areas of necrosis caused by infectious bovine rhinotracheitis virus. The mucosa is hyperemic and has inflammatory exudate on the surface to the right. The surface could become similar to that in Figure 2–94 as the lesion progresses.

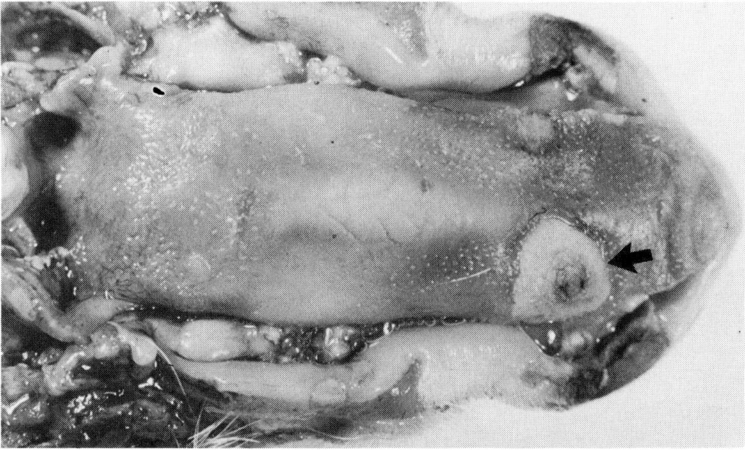

Figure 2–91. Caseous necrosis (arrow) of the tongue and buccal mucosa in a pig due to local injury and infection with *Fusiformis necrophorus*.

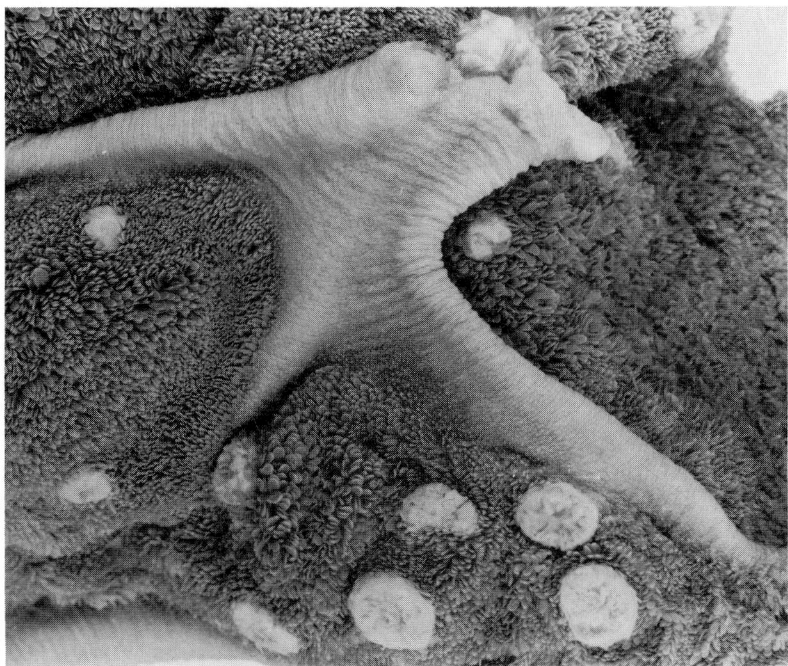

Figure 2–92. Areas of caseous necrosis in the rumen of a steer with similar pathogenesis to the lesion in Figure 2–10. These foci are the sites from which emboli spread to the liver to cause liver abscesses.

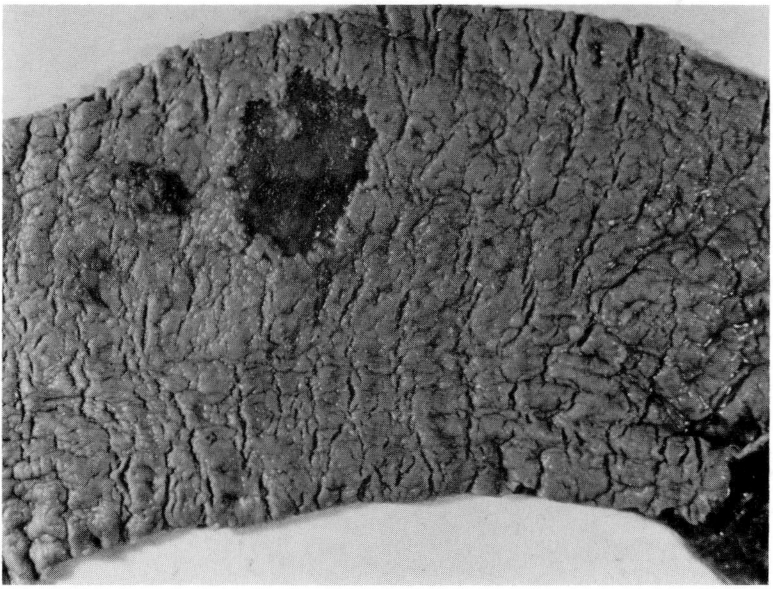

Figure 2–93. Caseous necrotic debris covering the intestinal mucosa in a pig. This type of lesion could be caused by *Salmonella choleraesuis*.

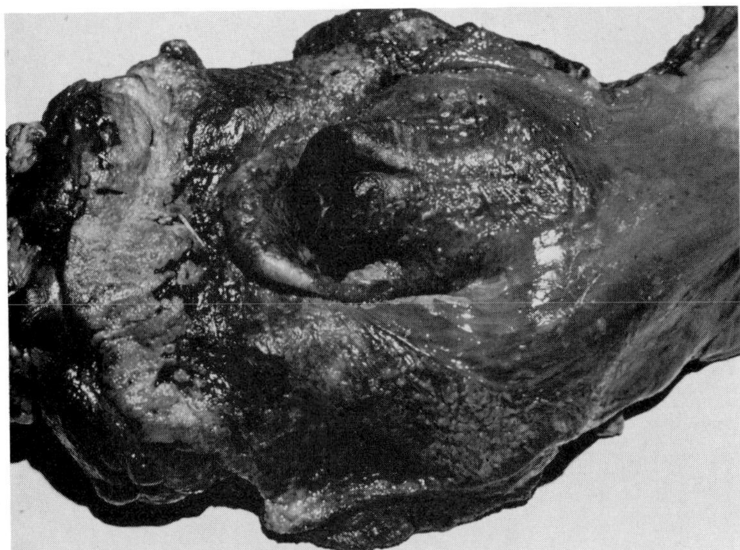

Figure 2–94. Extensive pale areas of surface necrosis of the pharynx and larynx in a steer probably caused by infectious bovine rhinotracheitis virus.

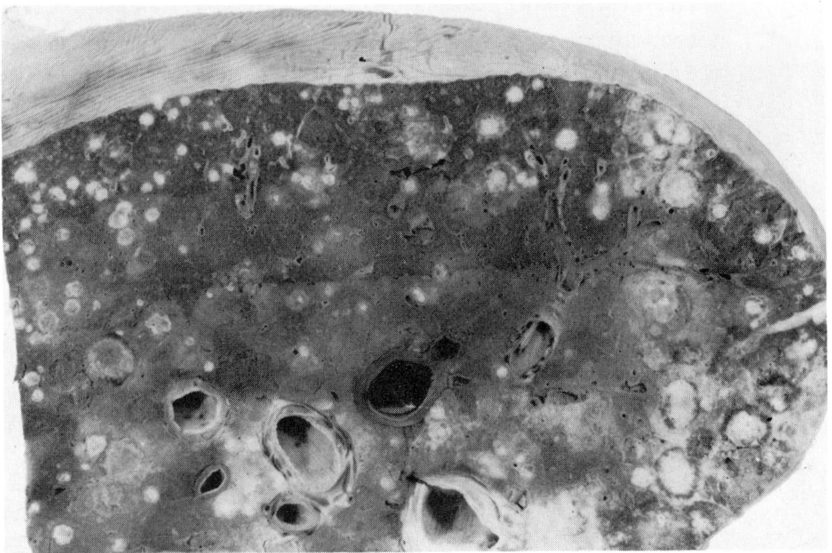

Figure 2–95. Pale areas of caseous necrosis due to fungal infection in the lung of a horse.

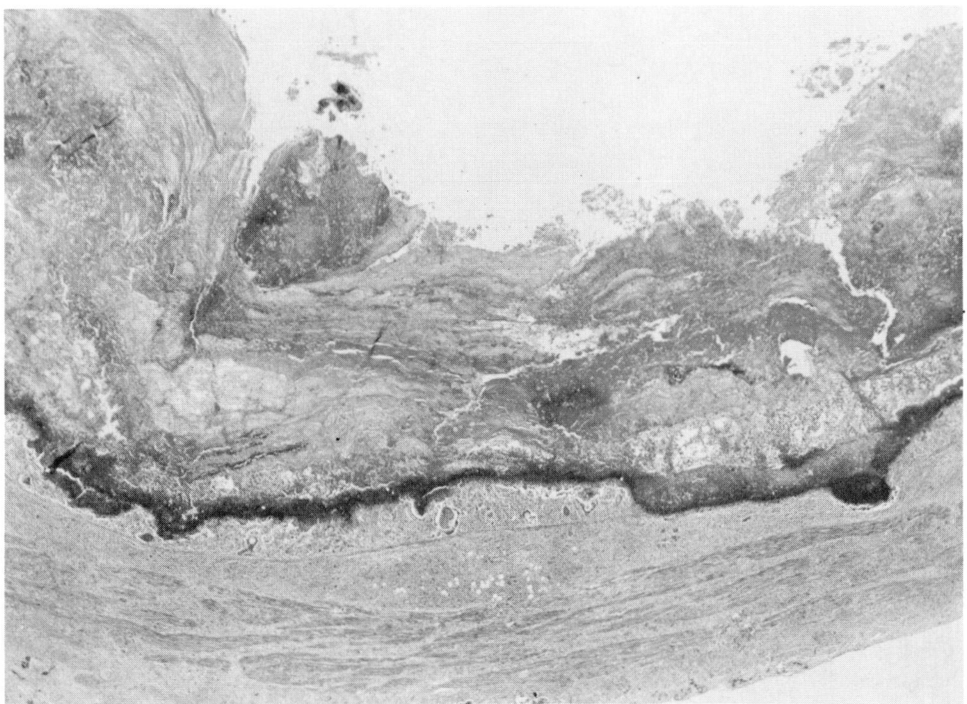

Figure 2–96. Caseous necrosis of the intestinal mucosa in a bird due to the protozoan infection histomoniasis. Note the line of demarcation at the junction of necrotic and viable tissue. This surface could have a gross appearance similar to that in Figure 2–93.

This is usually removed via lymphatic drainage with some help from macrophages. An abscess exhibits liquefaction necrosis composed of necrotic neutrophils.

Occasionally, other words or descriptive terms apply to necrotic lesions. The word ***malacia*** means softening and is used with reference to necrosis in nervous tissue. ***Focal necrosis*** implies numerous small white foci in random distribution in the liver or kidneys or other tissue. They may be pinpoint to 0.2 cm in size and indicate a microscopic caseous lesion probably caused by localization of a virus or bacteria (Figs. 2–97 through 2–101).

Reaction to Necrosis

Necrosis incites a reaction in surrounding viable tissue caused by substances released from the degenerate and necrotic tissue. The specifics of this reaction will be discussed in the chapter on inflammation. Tissue that is surgically removed, cooked and put into the peritoneal cavity does not induce a reaction, whereas an uncooked piece of tissue will. This point illustrates that it is the substances released from necrotic tissue that initiate the host's reaction to necrosis. Neutrophils and macrophages surround the area of necrosis and assist in lysing and liquefying the necrotic tissue for removal. The details of the methods of removal of necrotic tissue are not known. The general assumption would be that autolysis of necrotic cells is a major factor in removal, but this apparently is not so. If acute hepatic toxicity by carbon tetrachloride creates acute centrilobular necrosis, the Kupffer cells from the surviving areas repopulate the necrotic areas and contribute substantially to removing the necrotic cells, which is completed in about four days. If an inhibitor of enzyme synthesis is given with the carbon tetrachloride, the necrotic tissue remains intact without change for up to four days. Therefore, autolysis is not a significant factor and the tissue is not removed until the effect of the inhibitor declines to the level at which Kupffer cells enter the necrotic area and remove the necrotic tissue. This suggests that the removal process is primarily an extracellular enzymatic process carried out by cells attracted to the area for the task. This process occurs in a small

Text continued on page 72

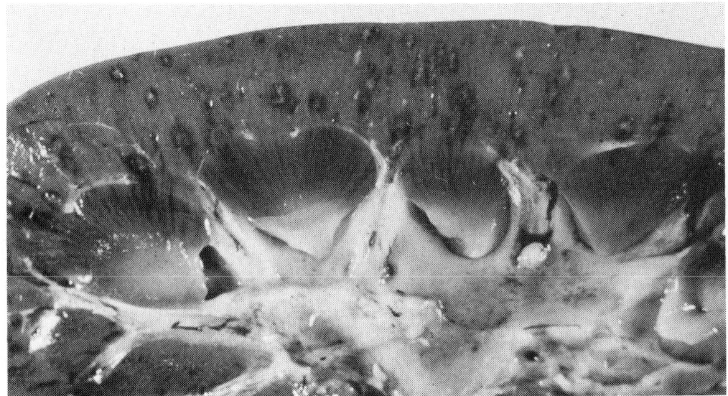

Figure 2–97. Focal areas of necrosis in a pig's kidney due to localized bacterial infection.

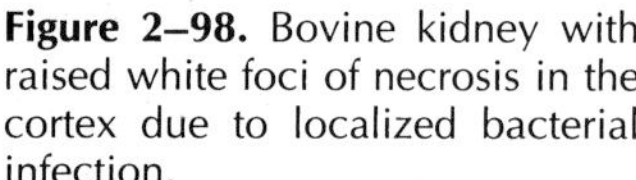

Figure 2–98. Bovine kidney with raised white foci of necrosis in the cortex due to localized bacterial infection.

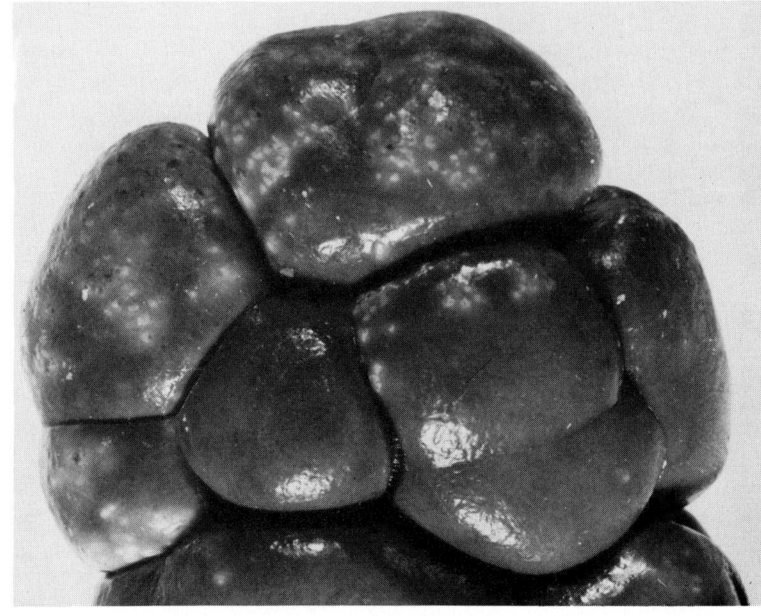

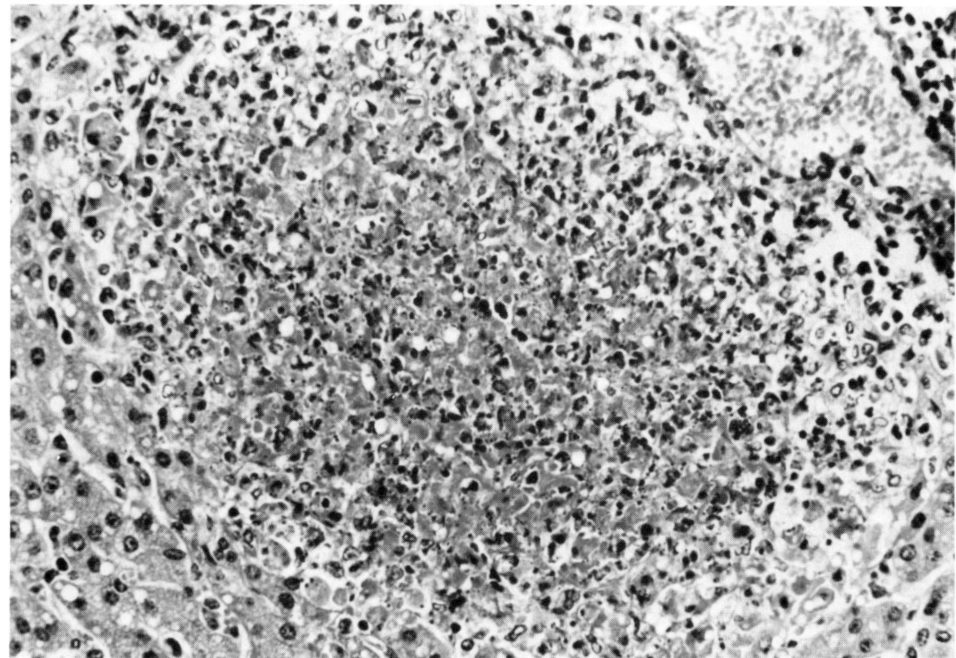

Figure 2–99. Focal caseous necrosis of the liver in infectious bovine rhinotracheitis virus infection in a bovine fetus. Note the loss of architecture and nuclear debris in the lesion. This lesion would appear as a pale focus in the gross specimen.

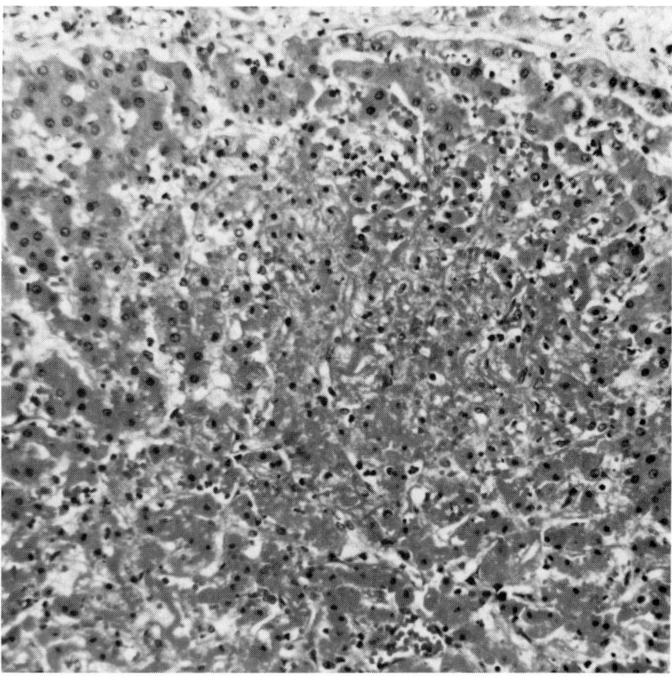

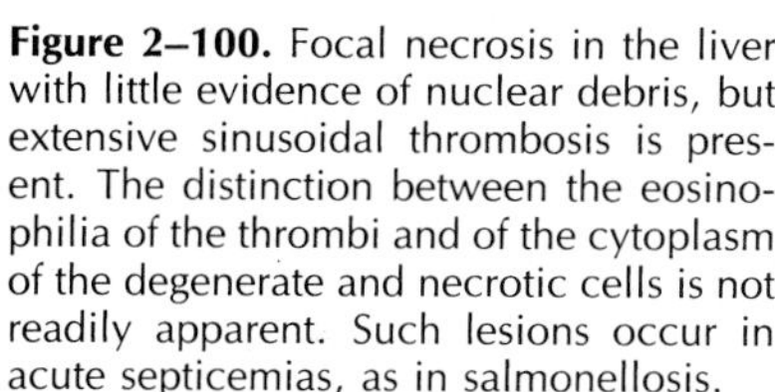

Figure 2–100. Focal necrosis in the liver with little evidence of nuclear debris, but extensive sinusoidal thrombosis is present. The distinction between the eosinophilia of the thrombi and of the cytoplasm of the degenerate and necrotic cells is not readily apparent. Such lesions occur in acute septicemias, as in salmonellosis.

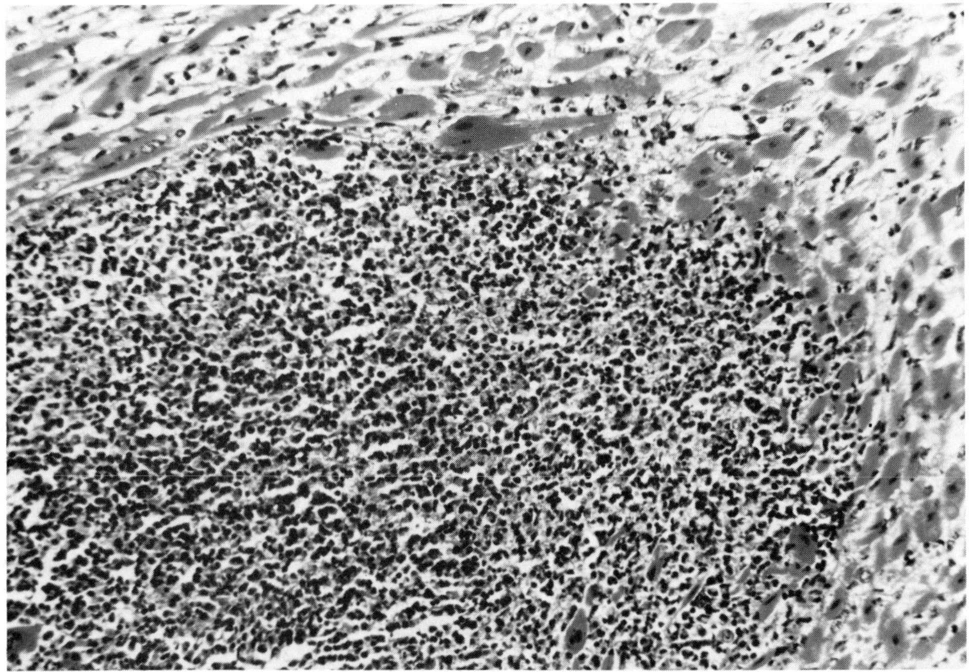

Figure 2–101. Destruction of muscle fibers in an area of caseous necrosis. This lesion would appear as a pale focus on gross examination. Compare with Figure 2–74, which is a similar lesion but more acute.

lesion in which regeneration is possible and will repair quickly. However, lesions in which a considerable area of tissue becomes necrotic, such as a sequestrum, will be lysed by macrophages and neutrophils and removed primarily in liquid form rather than primarily by phagocytosis. Eventually all the necrotic tissue will be lysed and removed. A scar formed of connective tissue may fill in the area where the necrosis occurred, or there may be partial regeneration and some scarring. The white ring of neutrophils, as well as hemorrhage in surrounding tissue, joined later by connective tissue, is of great assistance in gross recognition of necrosis. If a gross description refers to ***irregularly shaped and sized pale areas surrounded by a white line,*** the lesion is probably necrosis.

Necrosis on a surface has several names. An ***erosion*** is a shallow area of necrosis confined to epidermis that heals without scarring. An ***ulcer*** is an excavation of a surface produced by necrosis and sloughing of the necrotic debris and implies involvement of the tissue below the surface layer (Figs. 2–102 through 2–107). A ***slough*** is a piece of necrotic tissue in the process of separation from viable tissue and implies a process of shedding when used with reference to a surface. Examples would be sloughing of necrotic skin in swine erysipelas or a frozen gangrenous ear.

Degenerating and necrotic cells leak enzymes from the cytoplasm into the blood and can be measured in plasma. The different enzymes reflect particular locations and types of injuries. ***Alanine transaminase,*** previously known as serum glutamic-pyruvic transaminase (SGPT), is released from the cytoplasm of injured liver cells in moderate injury. ***Aspartate transaminase,*** formerly serum glutamic-oxalacetic transaminase (SGOT), is located in mitochondria and is released in more extensive injury. These are useful in determining the extent of damage in liver and muscle in particular and are of prognostic as well as diagnostic significance. Other enzymes used to evaluate tissue damage are ***lactic dehydrogenase*** (LDH), ***creatine kinase*** (CK) and ***alkaline phosphatase*** (AP). These are not really single enzymes, but each is a closely related family with several members called ***isoenzymes,*** each of which is able to catalyze similar reactions. Their presence in plasma is not a passive leakage but rather is due to specific types of injuries within cells. Most are removed from the plasma within a day or less. The half-life gives an indication of the persistence of injury over a period of time. The normal plasma levels of each

Text continued on page 76

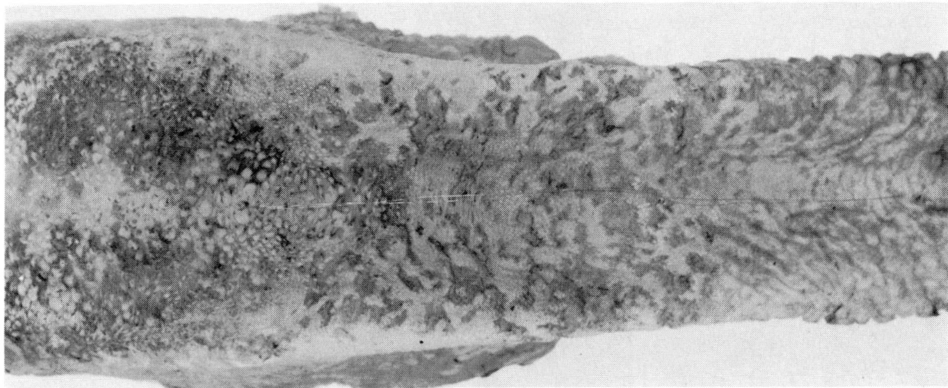

Figure 2–102. Erosion of epithelial surface of the tongue of a calf with bovine virus diarrhea. The pale tissue is normal. (Museum specimen.)

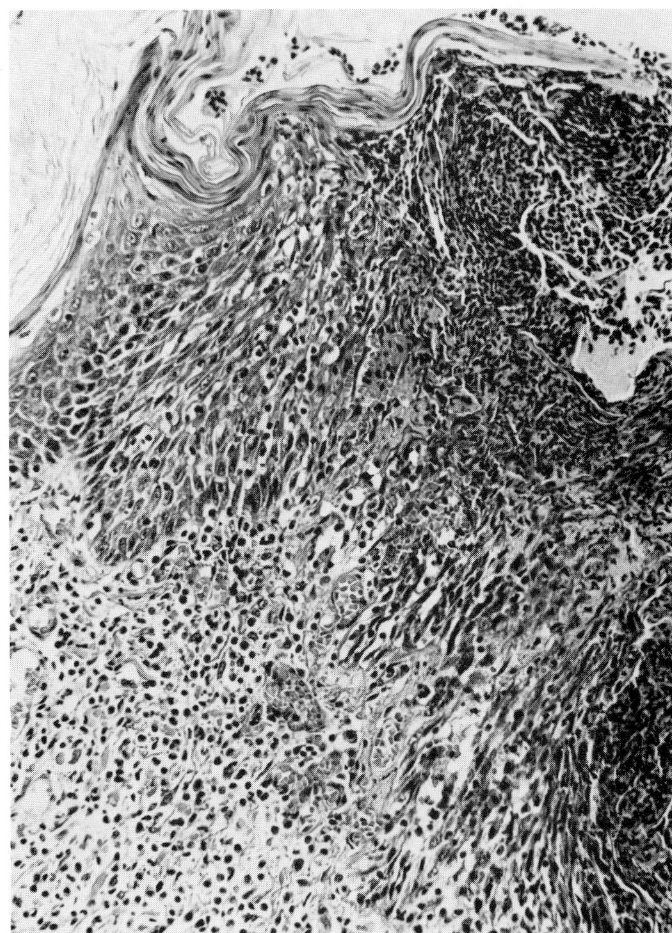

Figure 2–103. Skin surface at the top, normal to the left and extensive necrosis to the right. The necrosis, demonstrated by pyknotic nuclei and nuclear debris, extends into the dermis. From a dog with extensive dermatitis.

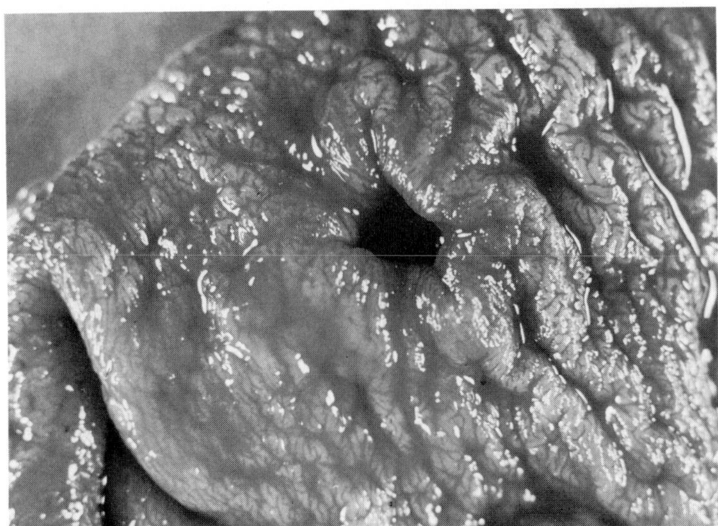

Figure 2–104. Gastric ulcer in a ringed seal. (Courtesy of J. R. Geraci.)

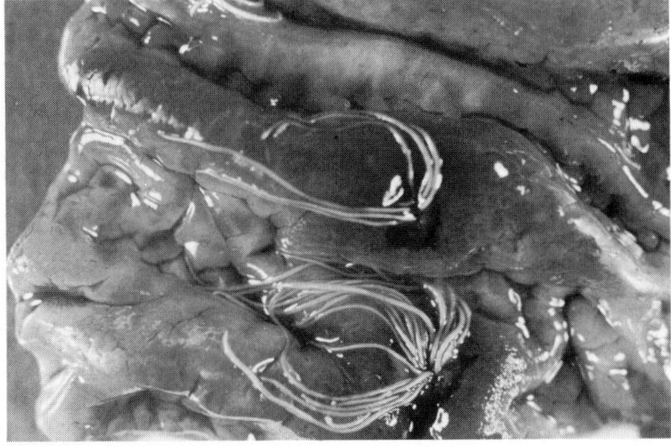

Figure 2–105. Gastric ulcer similar to the one in Figure 2–104, caused by parasites.

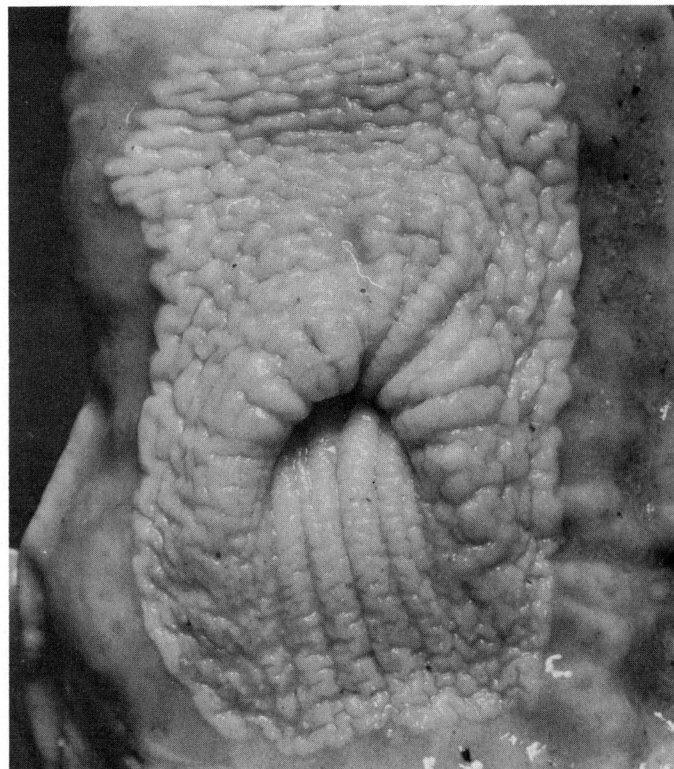

Figure 2–106. Normal squamous part of the gastric mucosa of a pig. The opening to the esophagus is in the center.

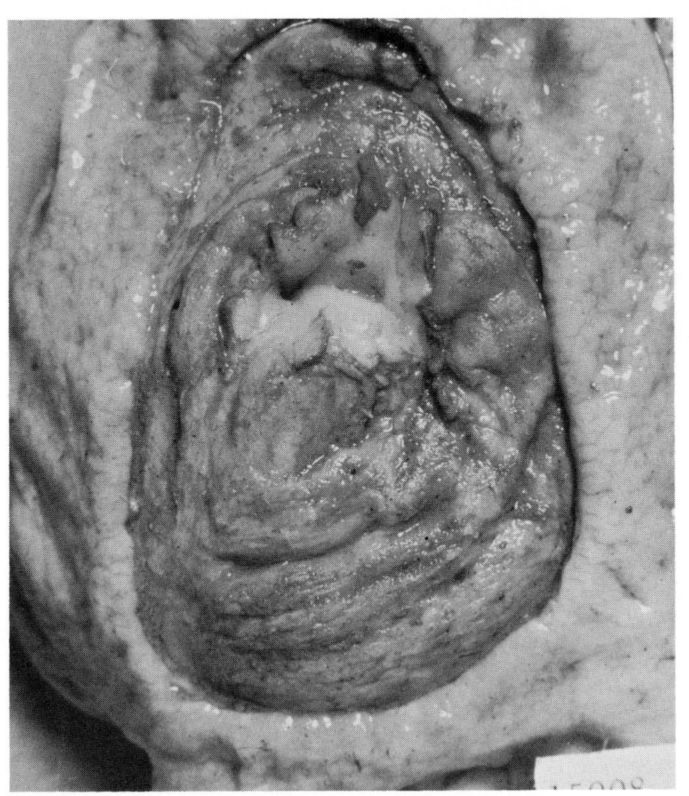

Figure 2–107. Complete ulceration of the squamous part of the gastric mucosa of a pig. The opening to the esophagus is to the center. This lesion is a common cause of death in pigs.

enzyme vary considerably among species, and the specificity for localization of lesions in particular tissues also varies with the species.

If an area of necrosis within an organ, particularly a large one, is surrounded by neutrophils and separated from viable tissue, it may remain as a solid mass for a long period as liquefaction proceeds from the outside. Internal liquefaction may be minimal. Such an isolated necrotic mass is called a ***sequestrum*** and the process is ***sequestration*** (Figs. 2–108 through 2–110). Examples occur in large infarcts, in skeletal muscle of downer cows and in acute mastitis. Sequestration is particularly significant if the sequestrum is bone tissue, because reabsorption and lysis become very difficult and the sequestrum remains as a chronic irritant. Mummification could possibly be used as a term to describe areas of coagulation necrosis. However, mummification usually refers to a fetus which died in utero, but in which the tissue dried out without putrefaction (Fig. 2–112). The various sequels to necrosis are indicated in Figure 2–113.

Necrosis of tissue is one of the most common and important lesions observed in disease. It may be part of other processes, such as cancer and inflammation, but is often a primary lesion.

Necrosis is the main lesion in infarction, which is common in the kidney and heart. Injection of irritating drugs causes necrosis of muscle tissue. Evidence of this necrosis is often found in slaughterhouses, at autopsy and even in cooked food on the dinner table. There are often multiple foci from repeated injections near the same site. Some types of mastitis often result in large areas of necrosis within the gland. Downer cows usually have varying degrees of necrosis in the hamstring muscles, and sometimes very large areas occur. Severe inflammation of the intestine results in a necrotic layer of exudate and tissue debris on the surface that has a dry or moist brown to pale color. The same may occur in the trachea or bronchi. Some bacteria such as ***Fusiformis necrophorus*** characteristically produce necrosis, as in liver abscesses and rumenitis in cattle, calf diphtheria and necrotic stomatitis in pigs.

The effects of necrosis on the host depend in large part on what types of cells are affected, where the affected cells are located, the number of cells affected and the rate at which they are affected.

Fat Necrosis

Fat necrosis is a distinctive type of necrosis and occurs in the abdominal cavity or under the skin. On cut surface, there are hard white gritty lumps (Fig. 2–114). The release of fat into connective tissue induces

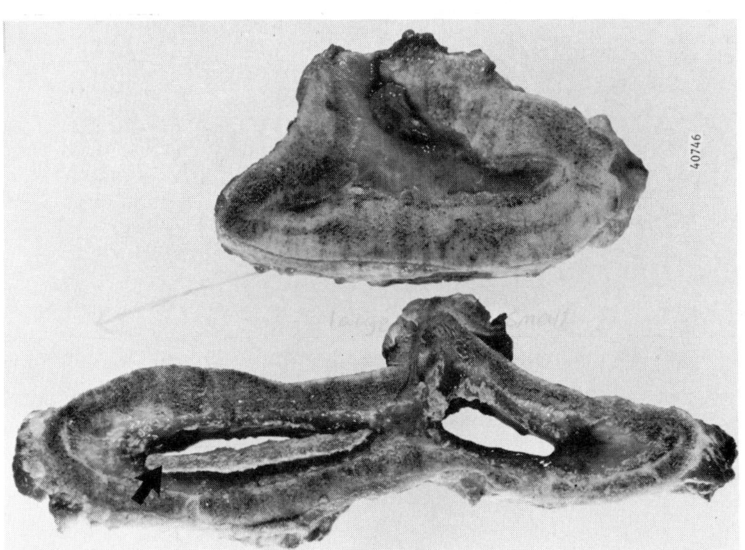

Figure 2–108. Two cross sections of the scapula of a horse with an infection from a penetrating wound. The lower specimen has a section of necrotic sequestered bone in a central space within the scapula (arrow).

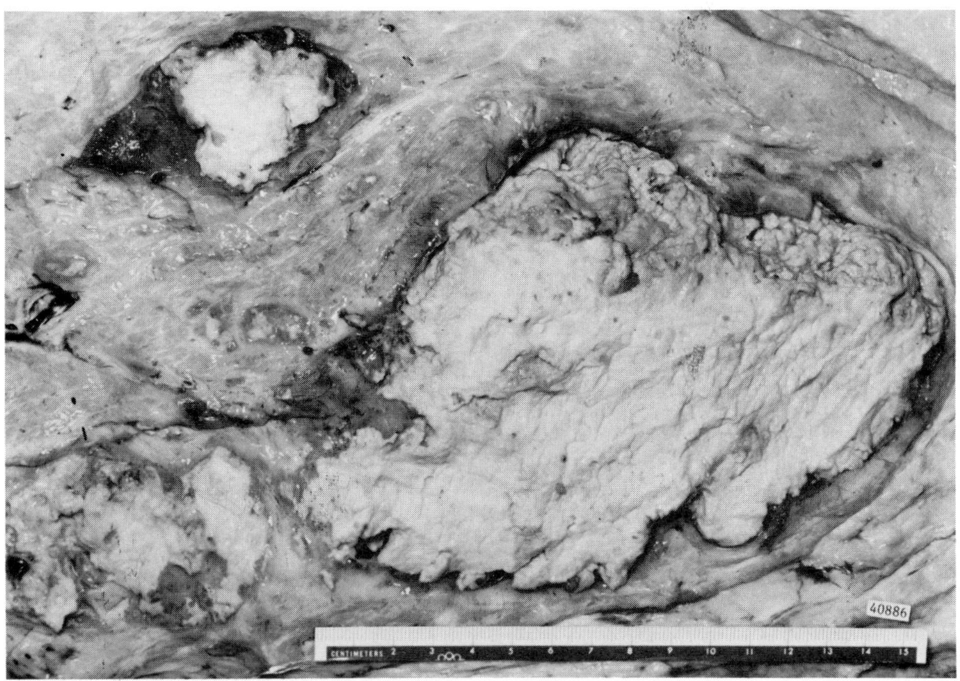

Figure 2–109

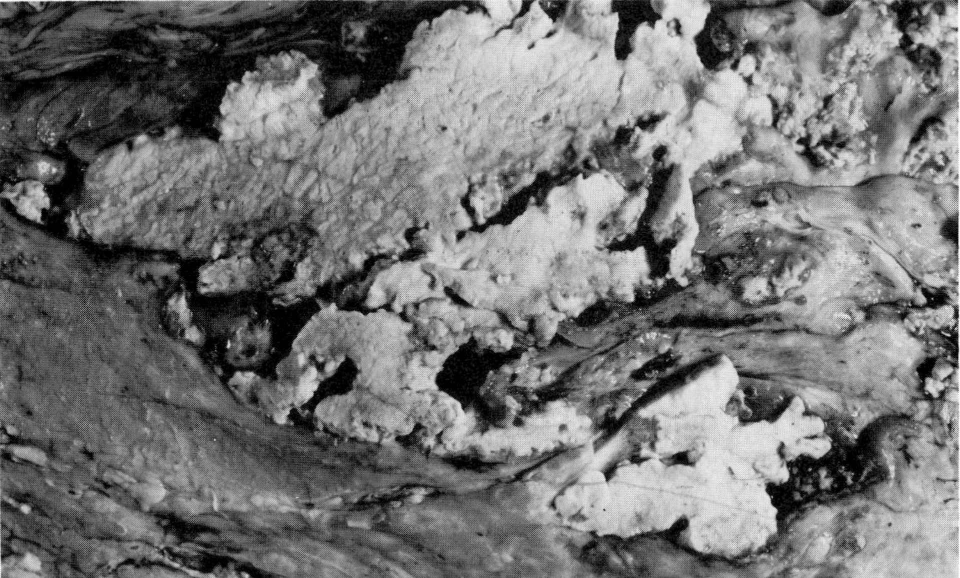

Figure 2–110

Figures 2–109 and 2–110. Areas of sequestration of necrotic tissue in the mammary gland of a cow. The pale necrotic tissue can be removed from the cut surface. The initial lesion was probably ischemic necrosis in an acute mastitis. The pale necrotic tissue often can be easily removed from the lesion because the separation from viable tissue is complete.

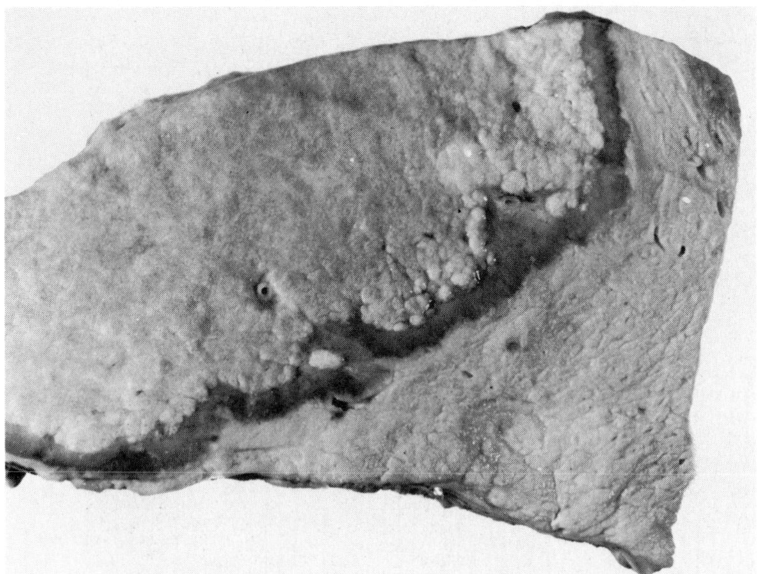

Figure 2–111. Another example of sequestered mammary tissue with a clear line of connective tissue separating the viable (to the right) and the necrotic tissue (to the left).

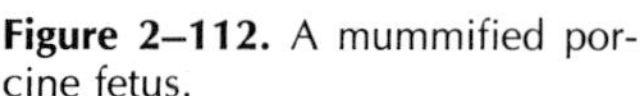

Figure 2–112. A mummified porcine fetus.

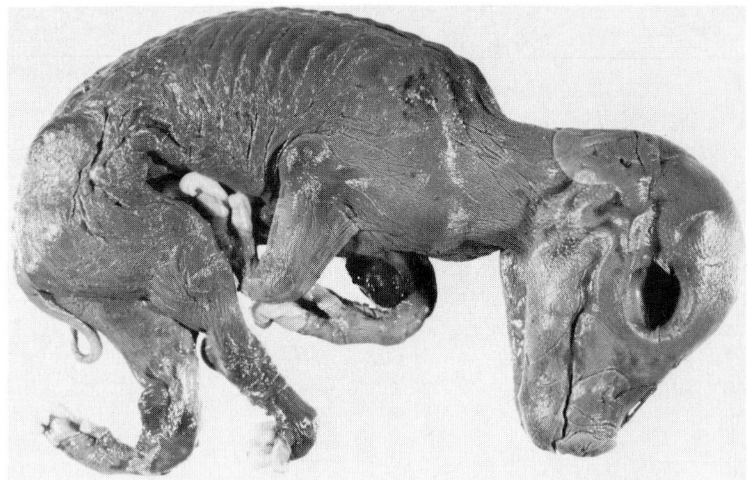

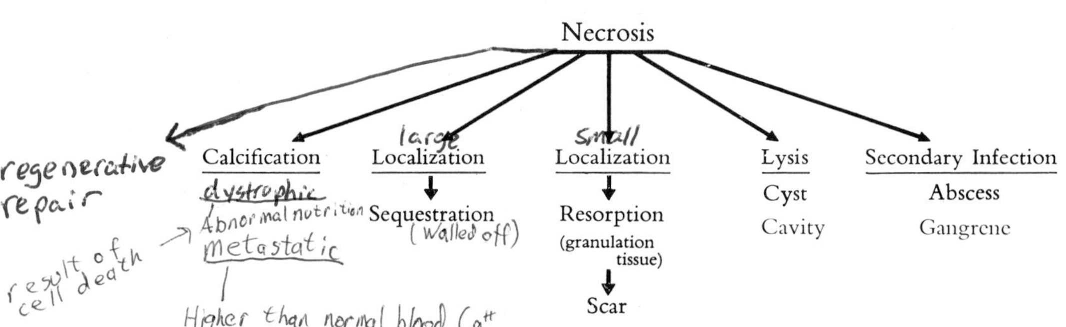

Figure 2–113. Sequelae of necrosis. (From Sandritter, W., and Wartman, W. B.: Color Atlas and Textbook of Tissue and Cellular Pathology. 3rd ed. Chicago, Year Book Medical Publishers, 1969. Reprinted by permission.)

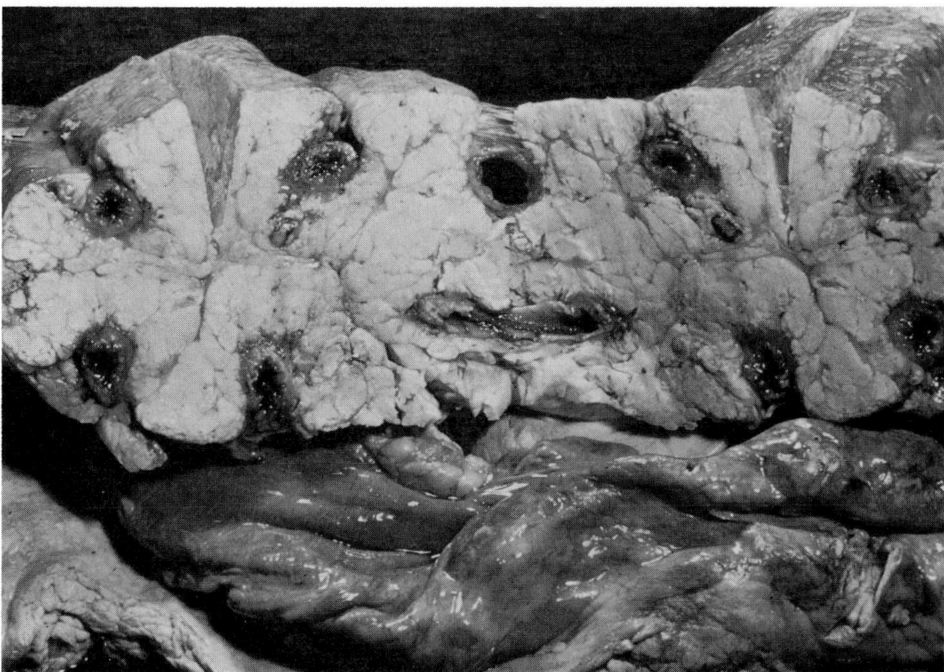

Figure 2–114. Extensive areas of fat necrosis around loops of intestine in a cow. The lesion is very hard and may lead to intestinal obstruction.

a ***marked inflammation and fibrosis,*** which contributes in large part to the firmness. Cholesterol clefts and calcification occur in the lesion, and giant cells and macrophages may be numerous. The lesion may be induced by trauma in several species and may be found in subcutaneous tissues or around the vagina after difficult parturition. In cattle, the lesion occurs as large, very hard lumps embedded in parts of large fat depots or may occur as hard flat plaques on the peritoneum. Evidence of this type of necrosis is usually found in slaughterhouse material. The explanation for large lesions in abdominal fat depots in fat animals is not clear, but there is a strong association between the lesion and eating forage containing fescue in the southeastern United States. Drainage from a lesion to nearby lymph nodes may cause lesions in the nodes as well. The large lesions may lead to obstruction of the intestine or ureter and result in death.

Inflammation in fat is called ***steatitis.*** There are several diseases in which necrosis of fat and steatitis are secondary effects. Necrosis of fat usually accompanies acute pancreatitis in dogs and may be the major component of the lesion in and around the pancreas. So-called "yellow fat disease" or ***steatitis*** of swine occurs primarily as a result of fish diets and is a quite mild inflammatory lesion. The fat becomes firm and is very yellow. Steatitis in cats, however, results in lumpy firm subcutaneous masses that are yellow to brown in color. Brown pigment is present in macrophages, and there are varying degrees of infiltration of neutrophils and macrophages, and later, fibrosis. Steatitis usually arises as a vitamin E deficiency. It does not produce the acute explosive lesion seen in pancreatitis.

Gangrene

Gangrene occurs when saphrophytic bacteria grow in necrotic tissue. The requirements are ***necrosis plus putrefaction.*** Gangrene is found in tissues that are easily accessible to saprophytes, such as the skin, lung, intestine and mammary gland. There are two types of gangrene, ***dry and wet;*** the only difference is the availability of fluid for rapid growth of the bacteria.

The ***dry type*** occurs in skin in which there is little fluid in the necrotic tissue because of evaporation and drainage but there are saprophytes. The cause of necrosis is usually ischemia, such as in freezing or vasoconstriction due to ergot poisoning or tight bandages and casts. There is a line of demarcation that usually progresses up the affected area between the viable and dark or black gangrenous tissue. The usual location is an extremity such as the tail, ears or limbs (Fig. 2–115). Animals seem to be able to walk on gangrenous limbs.

Wet gangrene is usually black in color, contains gas bubbles and has much hemorrhage and edema in and around the lesion (Fig. 2–116). It is often rapidly fatal because of systemic toxemia or rupture of the affected organ, such as the intestine. Gangrene in the lung is usually associated with acute aspiration pneumonia. The intestinal lesion is associated with twists or torsions that result in blockage of the vascular supply or compression of veins, which blocks venous drainage. It is common in colic in horses. The affected area of the intestine is black and is usually very distended with fluid prior to rupture. The necrosis together with the fluid and gas pressure soon lead to rupture.

Gangrenous mastitis usually starts out as acute coliform or staphylococcal mastitis in which necrosis of tissue occurs and the saprophytes gain access. The affected area is firm, cold, and blue to black, and gas bubbles can be palpated. The animal may be salvaged and the affected area will slough out. Castration by Burdizzo emasculator may result in gangrene if not carried out properly. Color alone or smell does not qualify a lesion as gangrenous. Gangrene usually has a distinctive odor, however, best exemplified by smelling the breath of a cow with gangrenous pneumonia.

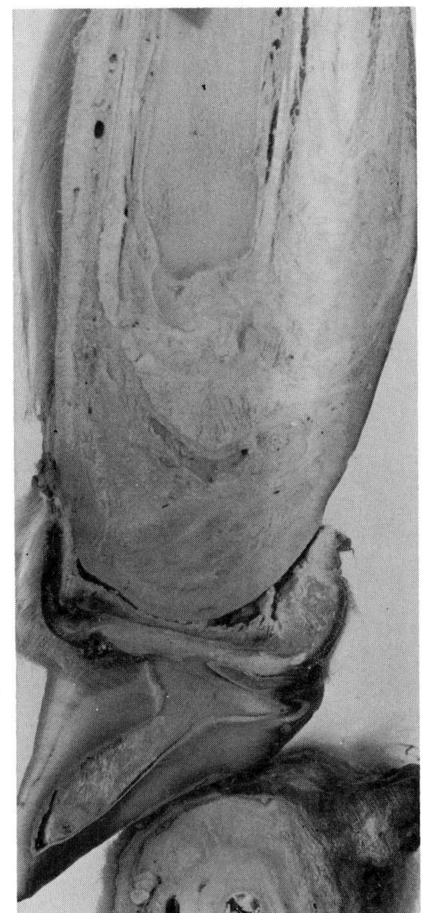

Figure 2–115. Dry gangrene of the limb of a calf. The hoof is necrotic and still attached but compressed owing to weight-bearing.

Tissues with acute circulatory problems such as a twisted loop of intestine or a prolapsed uterus are often very edematous, congested and relatively anoxic. Consequently, they are easily perforated during manipulations, but this alone does not necessarily indicate necrosis or gangrene. Sometimes a lesion is called gangrenous in error if the color is very black, as in extreme congestion of a twisted loop of gut. On the other hand, cytological features of necrosis may take up to six hours after actual death of the cells to be detectable by light microscopy. The precise nature or state of some lesions is difficult to define because clear-cut morphological features of specific processes may not be present or combinations of changes may be present. A firm background in physiology is essential to arrive at an understanding of the possible interpretations of such lesions, particularly those encountered during surgical procedures. Close consultation between the surgeon and pathologist is required for accurate interpretation.

Postmortem Changes

Some degree of postmortem change is present in most carcasses, particularly in

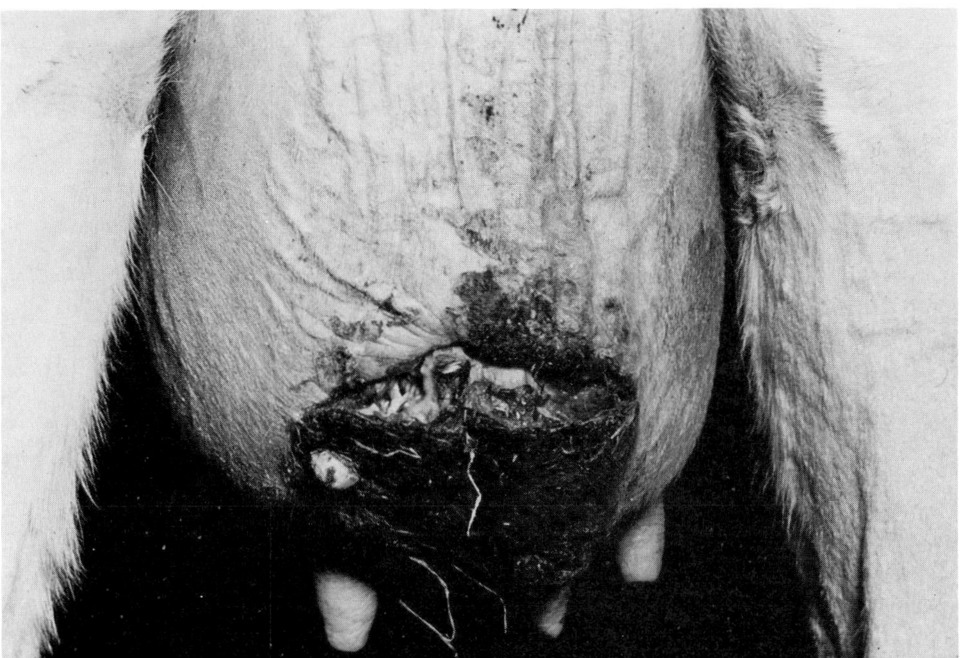

Figure 2–116. Wet gangrene in the mammary gland of a cow. Note the separation of the viable tissue from the necrotic tissue.

hot weather. These changes are evident on both gross and microscopic examination of tissue and ***must be differentiated from antemortem lesions.*** Considerable experience is required to make these distinctions, and much confusion arises in interpretations of findings until some confidence is gained. ***This point cannot be overstressed.*** It is embarrassing when all of the lesions described in a submission or shown to a client during an autopsy must be dismissed by the pathologist as postmortem changes. Therefore, it is important to specifically learn the range of postmortem change that may occur after death in each of the tissues and organs.

AUTOLYSIS

Autolysis means self-digestion by the tissues' enzymes that are present in, or released into, the cytoplasm of the cell after death. There is much variation among tissues in the content of proteolytic enzymes, which accounts for the variation in the degree of autolytic change among tissues. For example, liver, pancreas and kidney tissue change relatively quickly, whereas muscle tissue changes relatively little. Fixation stops the action of these enzymes. All of the nuclear and cytoplasmic changes described in coagulation necrosis occur in autolysis; however, the changes will probably be uniform in the tissue with no reaction such as occurs in necrosis.

A number of studies have been carried out to determine the progressive autolytic changes in cells at specific time periods and different temperatures.

Experimental evidence in rats indicates that a shift in weight and water levels of body organs occurs after death. At three hours after death, there was significant loss of weight from parts of the intestine and an ***increase in the heaviness of the lungs.*** If the lungs were severed from blood vessels and left in the thorax, the increase did not occur. This suggests that the reason for the increase was blood accumulation in the lungs. Other tissues that increased in weight were diaphragm, heart, abdominal muscle, ileum, cerebellum and kidney; the testicular weight decreased.

If the liver is removed from the body at the time of death and incubated in isotonic buffered saline, the features that normally occur in necrotic cells become visible rather rapidly. These changes are clumping of chromatin, lysis of chromatin and loss of differential staining. If the liver is left ***intact***

in the body, however, the changes occur much less quickly, even at the ultrastructural level. Functional activity remains for up to 24 hours. As mentioned earlier, cell death does not coincide with systemic death. There is a distinct difference in the rate of postmortem cell change during ***in vitro*** incubation and maintenance ***in vivo.*** Lysosomes remain in a relatively normal state for 24 hours after death ***in vivo.*** The release of lysosomal hydrolases may not contribute as much to necrosis or autolysis of hepatocytes as had once been thought. The nucleolus undergoes the most rapid changes and glycogen disappears from the cytoplasm quickly; endoplasmic reticulum dilates and mitochondria swell up, become round and lose their internal structure.

Some tissues are altered quickly after death and must be fixed rapidly to observe a lesion present at the time of death. The most sensitive are the retina, which becomes separated from the choroid; the seminiferous tubules, in which vacuolation in and between cells occurs; and the intestine, in which the epithelium over the villi falls off. The latter is important; the intestine is often examined because diarrhea is a common clinical problem resulting in death. Unless fresh and well fixed, minor lesions that may have great clinical significance will not be apparent. The brain softens into mush but is still worth fixing since cytological and structural details are surprisingly well preserved.

SPECIFIC TYPES OF POSTMORTEM CHANGES

In general, postmortem changes vary with the cause of death, air temperature, temperature of the body at the time of death, amount of time since death and presence of bacteria in the tissue.

Rigor mortis is the stiffening of all muscles after death and relates to contraction of muscle fibers as ATP decreases. ATP may be resynthesized from glycogen and thus delay rigor in well-fed animals with high muscle glycogen. Poorly nourished animals may develop rigor more quickly. Rigor classically begins in one to six hours and passes off in one or two days. It may be delayed or absent and is so variable in routine autopsy material as to have little value in interpretations. ***Algor mortis*** is the gradual cooling of the body after death.

Livor mortis is the gravitational settling of blood to the down side of the animal. It is most evident in the lung and skin as dark red coloration or in the kidney as a black zone of coloration in the cortex on one side, which has been called ***pseudomelanosis.***

Postmortem decomposition involves discoloration, softening, distention and displacement of tissues. ***Discoloration*** results from the breakdown of hemoglobin and the action of bacterial hydrogen sulfide on hemoglobin. The pretty shades of blue, green and purple are due to these changes. Discoloration also occurs because of lysis of erythrocytes with permeation of released hemoglobin into tissues, which turns them red; this is called ***imbibition.*** This change is evident on the inner surface of large arteries, as often observed in horses, and in most tissues, as often observed in aborted fetuses that died some time before abortion. Clear or reddish ***edema fluid,*** which appears to be a postmortem change, may be present beneath the skin but is difficult to explain. This is observed particularly in sheep. The diagnosis of black leg and malignant edema, which result in combinations of gas production, hemorrhage and edema, may be confused with postmortem changes. ***Softening*** is caused by autolysis with assistance from saprophytic bacteria or perhaps the normal bacterial flora of the tissue. This may be easily observed in livers and kidneys in animals that lay in the heat of a hot day prior to necropsy. The pancreas is very sensitive because of its enzymic content and softens rapidly, which is accentuated by handling. ***Distention*** occurs largely because of fermentation with gas production in the digestive tract. The gas distends all parts from the stomach down and extreme pressures may build in some organs. The stomach or diaphragm may rupture or the abdominal muscle may tear to produce hernias of various types. The problem of diagnosing bloat in ruminants is apparent.

Distention of the abdomen or intestines also causes ***pressure*** effects in other viscera. Large areas of the liver may be ***pale*** because the blood has been pushed out, or outlines of the loops of the intestine may be imprinted on the surface of the liver as a result of blood being pressed from one area of the liver into another. The myocardium may have large pale areas on the surface because of pressure, and these may be present within the muscle as well. Autolysis often gives the cut surface of the myocardium a mottled semicooked appearance that resembles degeneration and may be confusing. ***Gas bubbles*** are often present in the liver and kidney, usually in pale areas of autolysis and putrefaction, which are not uniformly spread through the tissues. These pale areas are often misinterpreted as areas of necrosis (Fig. 2–117). Bacteria in large numbers may be seen in autolytic tissue, especially the liver. Some species, such as horses, seem to have large numbers of such organisms in blood vessels in the brain, which appear often relatively shortly after death (Fig. 2–118).

Displacement may occur in the form of twists in the intestine, intussusception or herniations. If a tear or rupture occurs before death, there will be hemorrhage at the edges of the lesion, whereas ***no hemorrhage*** will be present in a postmortem tear. This is the main factor in differentiating an antemortem from a postmortem tear or rupture. Postmortem abdominal distention will push blood from the venous system in the abdomen to give pale viscera, but the hind limb muscles, lungs and neck region are very congested. A pig, horse or calf may die so quickly from shock with torsion of the entire root of the mesentery that there may be little color change in the intestines that might suggest a torsion. Unless the root of the mesentery is checked in animals with distended abdomens, this lesion will be missed. The mucosa of the rumen will peel off in large patches because of autolysis. The intestinal mucosa may have an accumulation of cells and mucus on the surface as a result of autolysis, and this change may be easily confused with an inflammation of the intestine. ***Bile*** will seep from the gallbladder into nearby tissues and stain them yellowish-brown. This is evident in any tissue in contact with the gallbladder and is often seen on the liver itself, stomach and mesenteric fat. Postmortem clots and chicken fat clots must be differentiated from thrombosis.

BACTERIAL FLORA OF TISSUES

It is becoming generally accepted that tissues in the body contain a ***normal bac-***

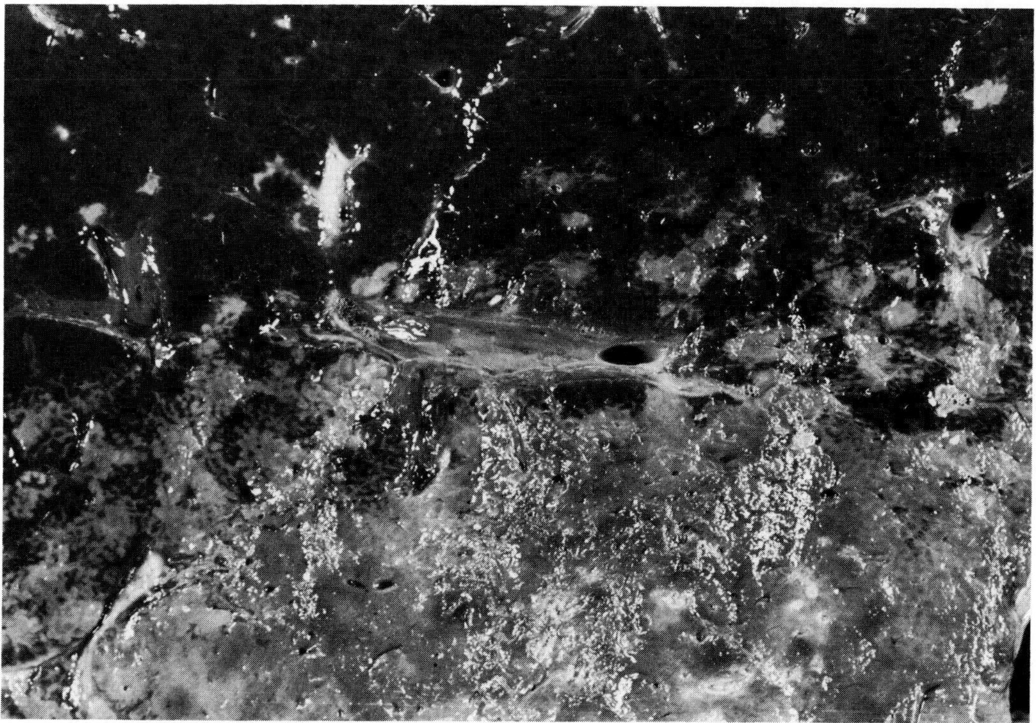

Figure 2–117. Bovine liver. The top dark area is relatively normal. The lower area is pale, and the middle area is a mixture of pale and dark areas. The pale areas are the result of autolysis, particularly related to growth of bacteria similar to that illustrated in Figure 2–118.

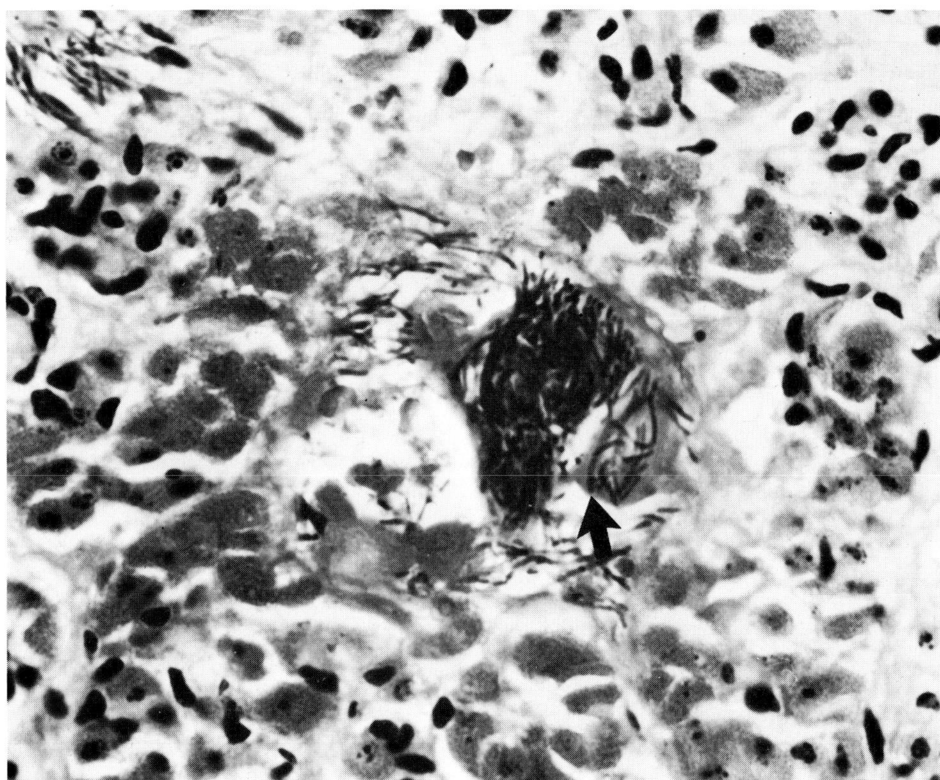

Figure 2–118. Pituitary gland of a horse with marked autolyses especially near colonies of bacteria (arrow). Such large rods in large colonies are often seen.

terial flora. This concept is well known in the digestive and respiratory tract, but there is difficulty in relating the idea of a normal bacterial flora to solid organs. There may well be normal viral flora as well, since viruses are found in tissue cultures of normal tissues. The normal bacterial flora is important here for two reasons. Firstly, if there is a flora, then it will contribute to autolysis and putrefaction if multiplication of organisms occurs after death. Secondly, if there is a normal flora in tissues, it must be considered in interpreting the results of bacterial culture of tissues from dead animals.

A number of studies have demonstrated normal bacterial flora in body tissues. This interest has arisen particularly as a result of storage of tissues or organs for transplantation purposes. These studies involved flora in biopsy specimens as well as the removal of tissues from dead bodies under strict sterile, surgical operating room technique at various time intervals after death. These studies have demonstrated that there is ***not*** an invasion of the body's organs by bacteria from the gut after death for at least 24 hours—so called postmortem invasion—if the tissues are kept cool. Bacteria found in tissues live there, and many are anaerobes. There is considerable variation in the flora among species and organs within species.

Two other points arise from these studies. ***There is a remarkable lack of correlation between culture results obtained from antemortem and postmortem samples from the same patients, and antibiotic therapy prior to death has little influence on culture results.*** The following quotations summarize some of the points. From Koneman and Davis (1974):

> We suggest the following model to explain the development of clinical infections in man. Viscera and tissues normally possess microflora, still of unknown nature, which vary in species from organ to organ, presumably through selective processes. In health their concentration is small, fewer than 10^5 organisms/Gm of tissue, possibly derived from intermittent seeding from

distant sites of contamination. At this low concentration, clinical disease rarely occurs; however, these organisms represent a potential source for the emergence of future infectious disease, either by mutation into more virulent strains, or through decline in local organ or generalized host resistance.

And from Koneman and colleagues (1971):

> The data suggest that neither the premortem clinical status of the patient nor the appearance of organs at autopsy is very useful in the prediction of the recovery of bacteria postmortem. Certainly when infection is suspected, bacteria usually are isolated (in about 90% of the cases) but they are also recovered from 70 to 80% of supposedly non-infected patients.
> It may be mistakenly believed by many that antibiotic therapy invalidates autopsy culture results. Carpenter and Wilkins, in their review of 2,033 autopsies, found no significant relationship between prior antibiotic therapy and the occurrence of positive heart blood and lung cultures. Wood and colleagues recovered bacteria from heart blood of substantial numbers of patients treated with antibiotics. Our data also substantiate the finding that the clinical use of antibiotics has little effect on the frequency with which bacteria can be cultured postmortem.

A series of papers by Gill and associates from New Zealand has shattered many traditional concepts about "postmortem invasion," bacteria in meat, meat spoilage by bacteria in stressed animals and the necessity to eviscerate carcasses soon after slaughter. They determined that, at 20°C, invasion of microorganisms does not occur in uneviscerated carcasses of healthy animals for 24 to 48 hours after death. They recognize a normal flora of clostridial organisms in some tissues. However, contamination of several tissues in carcasses by contaminated captive bolt pistols and sticking knives occurs quite easily between the time of "killing" and when the heart stops pumping blood.

PATHOLOGICAL PIGEMENTATIONS

Pigmentation or coloration is normal in some tissues, such as the corpus luteum, in which various shades of brown to yellow to orange are visible (over the life of the corpus luteum). The black color of the melanin in the iris of the eye and elsewhere is normal. There are examples, however, of ***lesions*** that characteristically have a color change associated with them, which may be visible grossly or microscopically. There is no particular connection or association between these groups of conditions, but they are examples of abnormalities in tissues or cells. Some are indications of degeneration and some are not, but they are all discussed together for convenience.

Pigmentations may be ***exogenous,*** that is, derived from outside the body, or ***endogenous,*** produced within the body.

Exogenous Pigmentation

PNEUMOCONIOSIS

Exogenous pigmentations are usually caused by inhalation of compounds in mineral or organic dust and become visible in the respiratory tract and draining lymph nodes. As a group, these occupational pathological pigmentations of the lung are called ***pneumoconiosis.*** They are of considerable concern in occupational health safety. They are not of concern to animals in industry since donkeys and mules are seldom used now in mines. Whether or not disease is caused depends on the concentration inhaled, the size and shape of particles, the chemical nature of the compound and the duration of exposure. Some of these chemicals induce chronic inflammation. Many occupational hazards known in humans, such as silicosis, anthracosis, siderosis, beryIliosis, calcicosis and asbestosis, are caused by chemical or dust inhalation while working in mining or quarry type environments. The compounds breathed in color the lung but may also induce chronic destructive lesions in the lung tissue, leading to respiratory insufficiency and sometimes cancer. They injure or kill macrophages during phagocytosis, releasing compounds that induce fibrosis.

ANTHRACOSIS

The only exogenous pigmentation of concern in animals is caused by ***anthracosis,*** which occurs as a result of inhalation of carbon compounds. It is found in urban dogs and in animals exposed to much dust. It is rarely of clinical significance but requires recognition and differentiation from other lesions. Grossly, the lungs may be gray or mottled in color. The bronchial nodes may be black, particularly the medullary regions where the particles are held in sinusoidal macrophages (Figs. 2–119 and 2–120). The microscopic lesion in the lung is centered around small bronchioles as collections of black granules in the wall of these structures. The precise location is difficult to assess and it may be found in macrophages or free in the tissue. The carbon that passes through the nasal passage and is deposited on the mucociliary apparatus will be cleared by ciliary action and then swallowed. What reaches the smaller airways may be phagocytized by alveolar macrophages and go up the same way or may be drained via the lymph as particles in fluid. The lymph drainage begins at about the junction of alveolar ducts with terminal bronchioles through openings into the interstitial tissue at that point. Macklin describes functional sumps as drains in this area. Particles may be drained with the fluid or some cells may pass out as well. Once in the lymph vessels, drainage of carbon to the nodes will occur, which accounts for their color. Some of the compounds do not drain completely, however, and remain in alveoli or in the tiny lymphatic vessels around the terminal bronchioles. If present in large quantities, chronic fibrosis may occur, but this is rare in animals. The normal drainage may be capable of removing all the pigment if the exposure is low, but an excess, as in some environments, may accumulate. Probably, inhalation of large quantities of tiny particles over a long period of time is required for a lesion that is visible grossly.

Endogenous Pigmentation

Most of the ***endogenous pigments*** may be divided into groups of those related to melanin or those derived from lipids, hemoglobin or porphyrins.

MELANIN

Melanin is a normal pigment made by melanoblasts and melanocytes and is present in cells that receive it from melanocytes. The melanin-producing cells are derived from neural crest tissue. The pigment is black grossly or microscopically, and very little is required in the tissue to induce a very black color. The granules are brown or black, depending on the concentration. Different species have melanin in different locations in addition to eyes and hair. The oral mucosa of dogs, sheep and other species may be partially pigmented; fish, amphibians and reptiles have considerable amounts in many internal organs. The lesions associated with melanin occur when the pigment is found in places or amounts

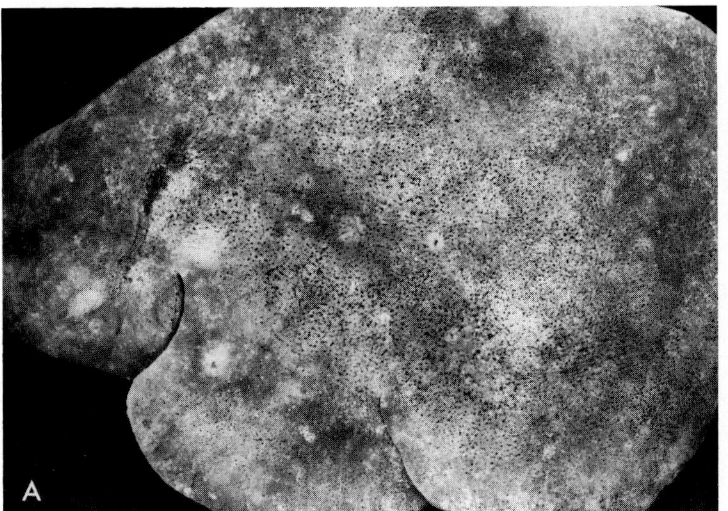

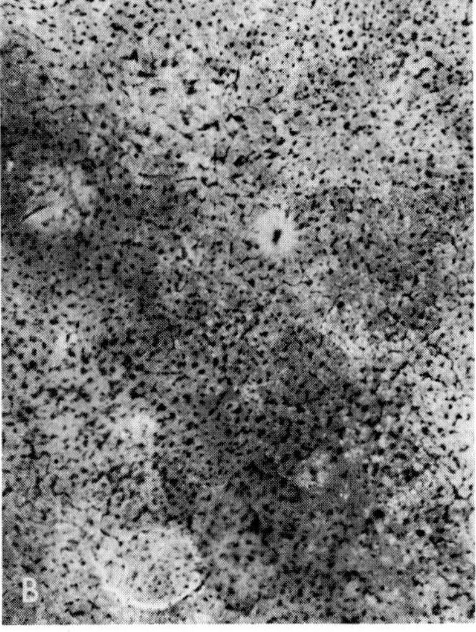

Figure 2–119. *A*, Lesion of anthracosis as visible on the pleural surface of a dog's lung. *B*, A close-up view of the same lesion. (Courtesy of B. Schiefer.)

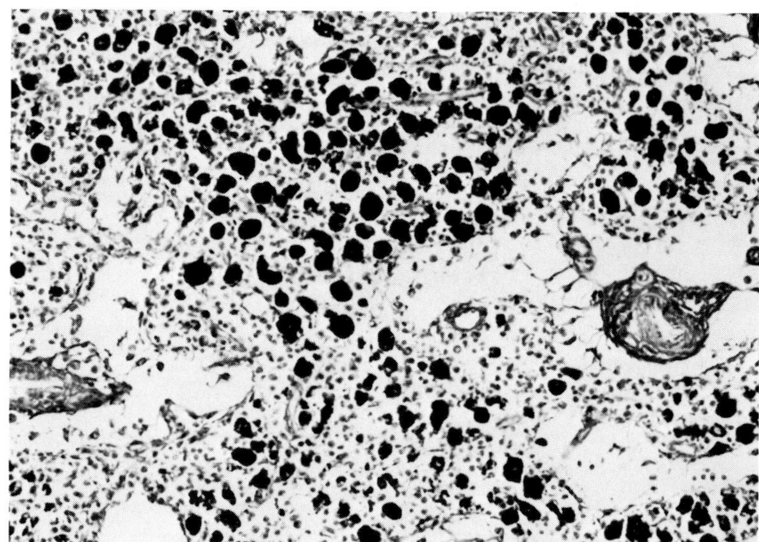

Figure 2–120. Anthracosis in a dog's bronchial lymph node. (Courtesy of B. Schiefer.)

that are not considered normal for the species concerned. An example is the nevus or mole in humans.

Melanosis is the presence of melanin in an abnormal location, such as on the pleura, meninges or heart, and is a congenital mislocation of melanocytes. Melanosis is not common and is found incidentally during autopsy or more commonly during inspection of carcasses in slaughterhouses. The organs are discarded at slaughter for aesthetic reasons. The lesion is found as irregularly sized and shaped black areas on the pleura, epicardium or meninges of sheep, cattle and pigs, as well as at other locations and in other species. Microscopically, there are scattered melanocytes mixed with fibroblasts. The lesion is usually on the surface of the organ but may occur in the interstitial tissue of the parenchyma. There is no functional lesion in the tissue (Figs. 2–121 through 2–123). Melanocytes can migrate into some types of inflammatory lesions (Fig. 2–124).

Tumors of melanoblasts and melanocytes are common and are called ***melanomas.*** They may be benign or malignant but usually have a poor prognosis. They can occur in many tissues but usually originate where precursor cells are numerous. They are found most often in the skin but may also occur in the oral cavity and eye of dogs as well as in horses and pigs. If the tumors contain melanin, they are easily identified grossly and microscopically by the black color (see Figs. 6–36 and 6–37). If little or no melanin is being produced because of lack of differentiation of the tumor cells, however, the cells may be very difficult to identify. Such a tumor is called an ***amelanotic melanoma.***

Melanin as used here is not one pigment. ***The chemical composition varies with the location in the body and with the species.*** All forms are oxidative derivatives of *l*-tyrosine bound to sulfur-containing proteins via several possible metabolic routes. Complete absence of melanin is a congenital defect and an affected individual is called an ***albino.*** The dihydroxyphenlalanine (dopa) test is used to identify the ***cells that have the capability to make melanin.*** Melanin is made from tyrosine. Dopa is a closely related chemical, dihydroxyphenylalanine, that, when placed on fresh tissue containing cells capable of producing melanin, forms a black granular precipitate. Macrophages that pick up granules of melanin are called ***melanophores*** and may be numerous in melanosis or melanomas, as they pick up pigment along with debris of dead melanin-producing cells.

LIPID PIGMENTS

Most of the pigments derived from lipids result from ***oxidation and polymerization of unsaturated lipids.*** The color and staining vary with the degree of oxidation and polymerization; thus, there is a great range of appearances that are all part of the same process. Traditionally, colored pigments

Text continued on page 90

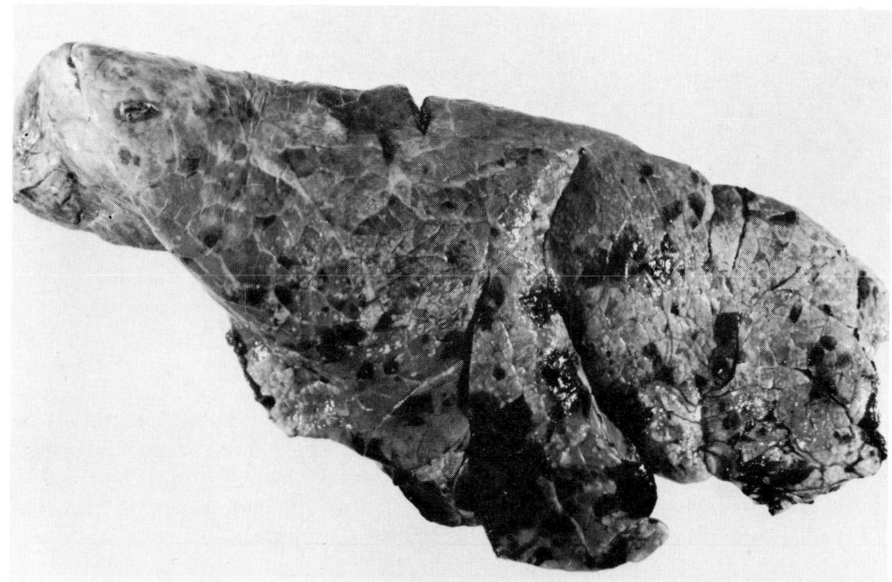

Figure 2–121

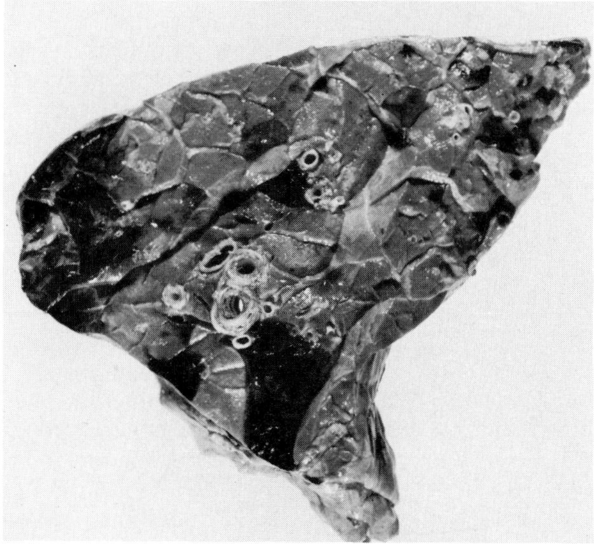

Figure 2–122

Figures 2–121 and 2–122. Congenital melanosis in a calfs' lung, showing external surface (Fig. 2–121) and cut surface (Fig. 2–122).

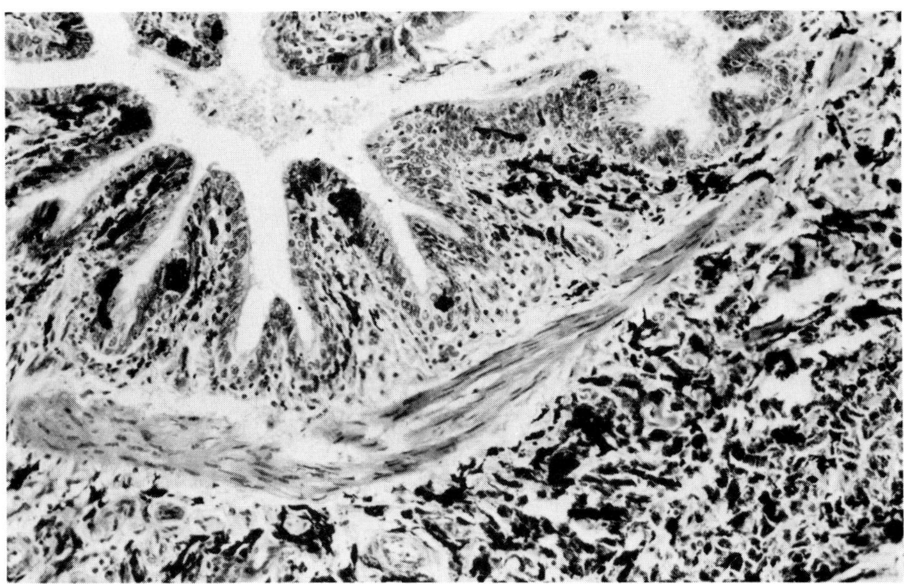

Figure 2–123. Melanosis in a calf's lung. The anatomical structure is normal, but there are melanocytes in the mucosa and outside the smooth muscle ring. This lung had melanocytes in the stroma of alveoli and interlobular tissue as well, but only in sporadic lobules.

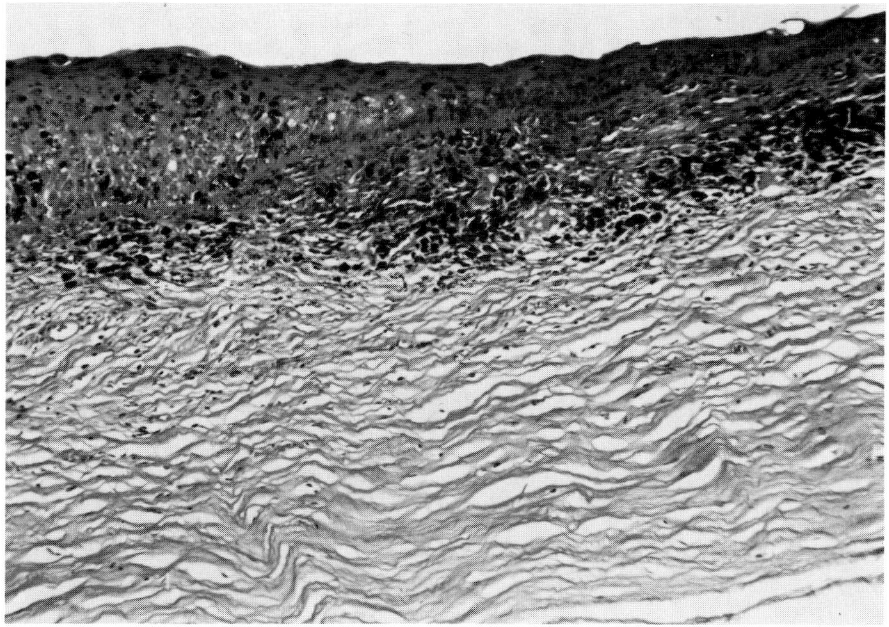

Figure 2–124. Pigmentary keratitis in a dog's cornea. The melanocytes have moved into the epithelium and cornea as part of the pathological response to injury.

have been named according to the particular situations and circumstances in which they occur and not by the composition of the compounds that give the color. Considerable confusion for the nonexpert exists in the classification of these pigments and is often based on differential reactions with a multitude of special stains. In general, the differences are quantitative rather than qualitative. The system used here to classify pigments is simplified into those found in macrophages and those found in the cells of parenchymal organs, although in both cases the pigment occurs in lysosomes.

Ceroid is found in macrophages following tissue damage or hemorrhage, or both, in which lipids have become free in the tissue. The pigment is generally brownish, granular and the product of partial breakdown of the lipids picked up by the macrophages. It is found in many types of lesions in which degeneration and necrosis have occurred and is common in mammary tumors of dogs (Fig. 2–125). It may occur with or resemble hemosiderin on hematoxylin-eosin stains but can be differentiated by special stains.

Lipofuscin is found as yellowish-brown granules in the cytoplasm of affected parenchymal cells. The pigment is a reflection of the content of autophagic vacuoles that contain partially metabolized lipid. It is caused either by an overload of work, by the formation of abnormal lipids, or by the inability to completely metabolize the lipids. Lipofuscin is often termed "wear and tear" pigment and tends to occur in mature or aged individuals.

These deposits are well known in neurons in dogs, in myocardial cells in cattle and in exhausted adrenal and thyroid glands in several species (Fig. 2–126). In the last, the glands are undergoing involution and atrophy. "Brown atrophy of the heart," sometimes called xanthosis, which is not unusual in Ayrshire cattle, is a lesion occurring in the heart of cattle and is found during meat inspection as an incidental lesion. It is not known to be clinically significant and is not really an atrophy. The dark brown color is very distinctive. ***Vitamin E deficiency*** may accentuate lipofuscin formation, and at times the pigment is called "vitamin E pigment." It occurs in smooth muscle in the intestine of vitamin E–deficient dogs and is visible enough grossly to be called "brown dog gut." The brown granules are very prominent in the cytoplasm of the smooth muscle cells often located around the poles of the nuclei. Some of the brown pigments found in hepatocytes are also lipofuscin. Some glandular epithelial cells such as in sweat, mammary or ceruminous glands contain brownish granules in the cytoplasm that are probably lipofuscin.

Jersey and Guernsey cattle have a yellow

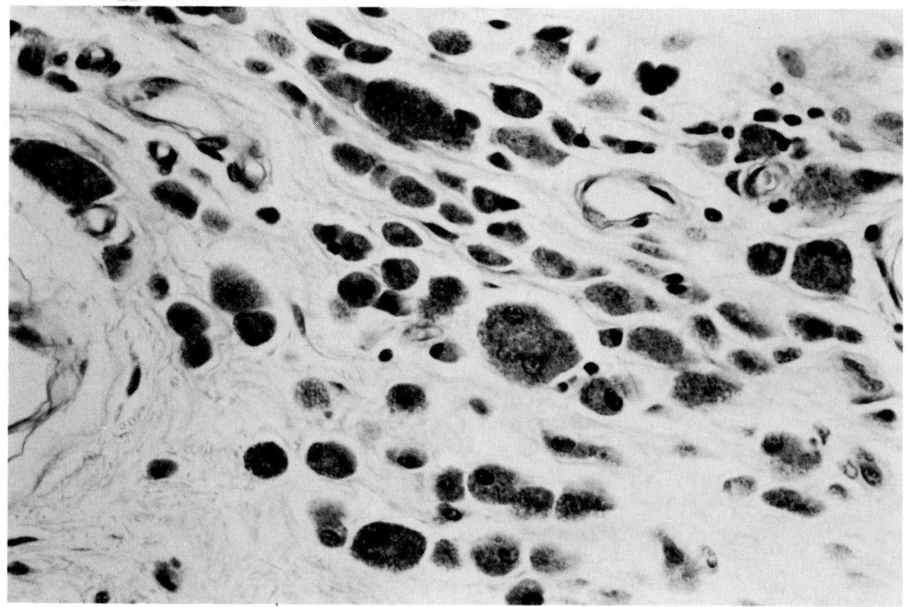

Figure 2–125. Ceroid pigment in macrophages in mesenchymal tissue in a mammary tumor of a dog.

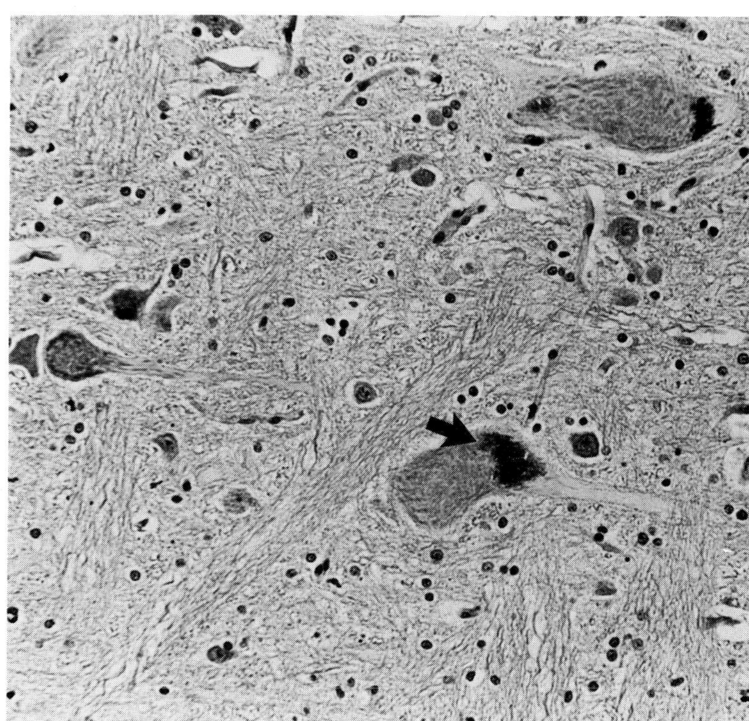

Figure 2–126. Neuronal lipofuscin in an old cat. The granules (arrow) are accentuated in this PAS stain. Individual granules are apparent but seem to become confluent as the concentration increases.

color to their fat and this is due to ***carotenoids,*** but these are not visible in routine tissue sections.

HEMOGLOBIN AND PORPHYRIN DERIVATIVES

The pigments derived from hemoglobin are hemosiderin, hematin and bilirubin.

1. Hemoglobin. ***Hemoglobin*** itself may be visible if released from red blood cells in large quantities. It will appear microscopically as a distinctive reddish-orange color in renal tubules if it crosses the glomerulus. The kidney is usually almost black in color when this occurs, and it is indicative of an acute hemolytic crisis. Chronic copper poisoning in sheep or cattle is a classic example.

2. Hemosiderin. ***Hemosiderin*** pigment is brown, contains iron and is usually present in macrophages of the reticuloendothelial system (Fig. 2–127). It is a common finding, and if quite prominent as a lesion, the term ***hemosiderosis*** is used. Iron is absorbed in the ferrous form and changes to the ferric form in the blood. There, it travels bound to transferrin, an iron-binding plasma protein. It is stored in reticuloendoethelial cells as ferritin, a protein (apoferritin)-iron complex, in many locations such as marrow and liver. Ferritin is diffuse in the cell and not visible, but if storage is concentrated in lysosomes, it is known as hemosiderin (insoluble ferritin aggregates), which is brown in hematoxylin-eosin-stained tissues (Fig. 2–128). Hemosiderin is 35 per cent iron by weight. It can be identified specifically with a Prussian blue stain in which the iron stains blue because it is loosely bound. The Prussian blue stain is often used on bone marrow to assess iron reserves.

If excess iron is absorbed or if much is released from red blood cells during hemolysis, the stores in macrophages will increase and considerable quantities may accumulate. The amount of hemosiderin may therefore be ***an indication of iron stores or of blood breakdown,*** depending on the circumstances that initiated the accumulation. The distribution in tissue may not be uniform, and hemosiderin seems to collect in clumps of macrophages, although their structure may be obscured by the pigment (Figs. 2–129 and 2–130). It may occur in renal epithelial cells if hemoglobin is passing the glomerulus and part is reabsorbed in the kidney. It may also occur in hepatocytes. In chronic left heart failure, red blood cells cross into the alveoli because of passive congestion and become phagocytized by

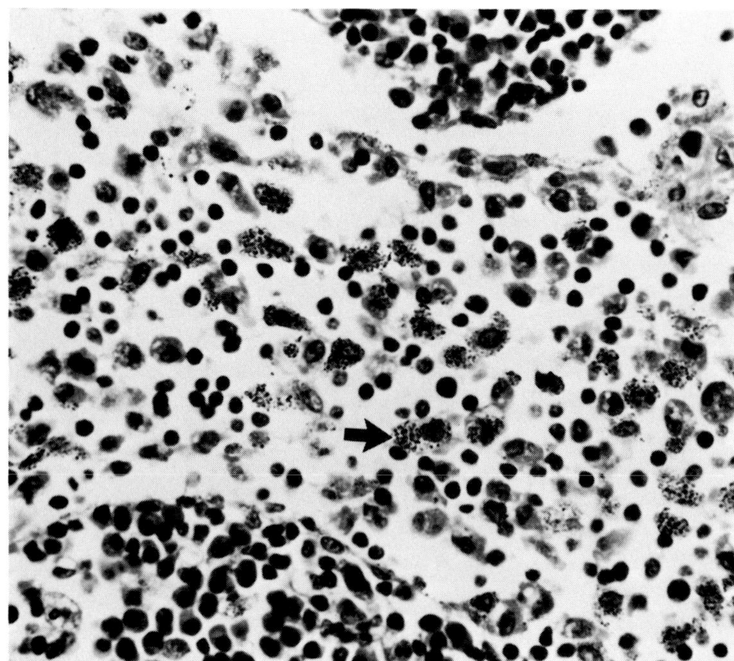

Figure 2–127. Hemosiderin granules in macrophages (arrow) in the medulla of a lymph node.

alveolar macrophages that gradually take on a brown color. These are so characteristic as to be called ***heart failure cells*** and are recognized because of the hemosiderin, which may grossly color the lung light brown (Fig. 2–131 and Fig. 3–17).

A pronounced concentration of hemosiderin in one area of a tissue is an indication of previous hemorrhage and may contribute to the color of a bruise. Old dogs often have brown, raised, granular lesions on the edge of the spleen. In section, these lesions contain iron, ceroid and hemosiderin, which create a very colorful appearance. They are called ***siderotic nodules*** and probably represent previous hemorrhage.

Xanthosis or xanthomatosis is a lesion in which the kidney becomes discolored black because of excess accumulation of non–iron staining brown pigment in renal tubular epithelium. There is a divergence of opinion as to whether the condition is a congenital metabolic defect or merely excess storage of a lipofuscin-type pigment. It occurs occasionally in cattle and is observed as very dark or black kidneys at slaughter. It is closely related to or similar to lipofuscin.

3. Hematin. ***Hematin*** results from the action of acid or alkali on hemoglobin. It is not a normal metabolite or precursor of hemoglobin but is formed in tissues when exposed to acid or alkali after death. Brown crystals are formed but are not intracellular. This feature helps differentiation from hemosiderin, the granules of which look similar to tissue sections. Hematin is used to identify blood in forensic laboratories and to identify the species from which the blood came.

Hematin is very common as "formalin pigment" when unbuffered formalin is used for fixation. It appears all through the tissue but mainly in blood vessels. It can be removed prior to routine staining. It does not stain blue with the Prussian blue stain because the iron is too tightly bound to react. Some parasites leave grossly visible brown pigments that resemble hematin in tissues in which they live or through which they migrate. These include malaria and some flukes and mites.

4. Bilirubin. ***Bilirubin*** is formed from the tetrapyrrole ring structure of hemoglobin when iron and protein have been removed. It is a normal by-product of hemoglobin breakdown but may occur at times in excess. Bilirubin may be formed in reticuloendothelial cells following phagocytosis and transported in the plasma to the liver by a protein carrier called haptoglobin. Bilirubin is normally present in serum at a low con-

PATHWAYS OF IRON UPTAKE AND DISTRIBUTION IN RETICULOENDOTHELIAL CELLS

Reference—Wixom, R. L., Prutkin, L., and Munro, H. N. (1980)
Int. Rev. Exp. Pathol. 22, 193–225

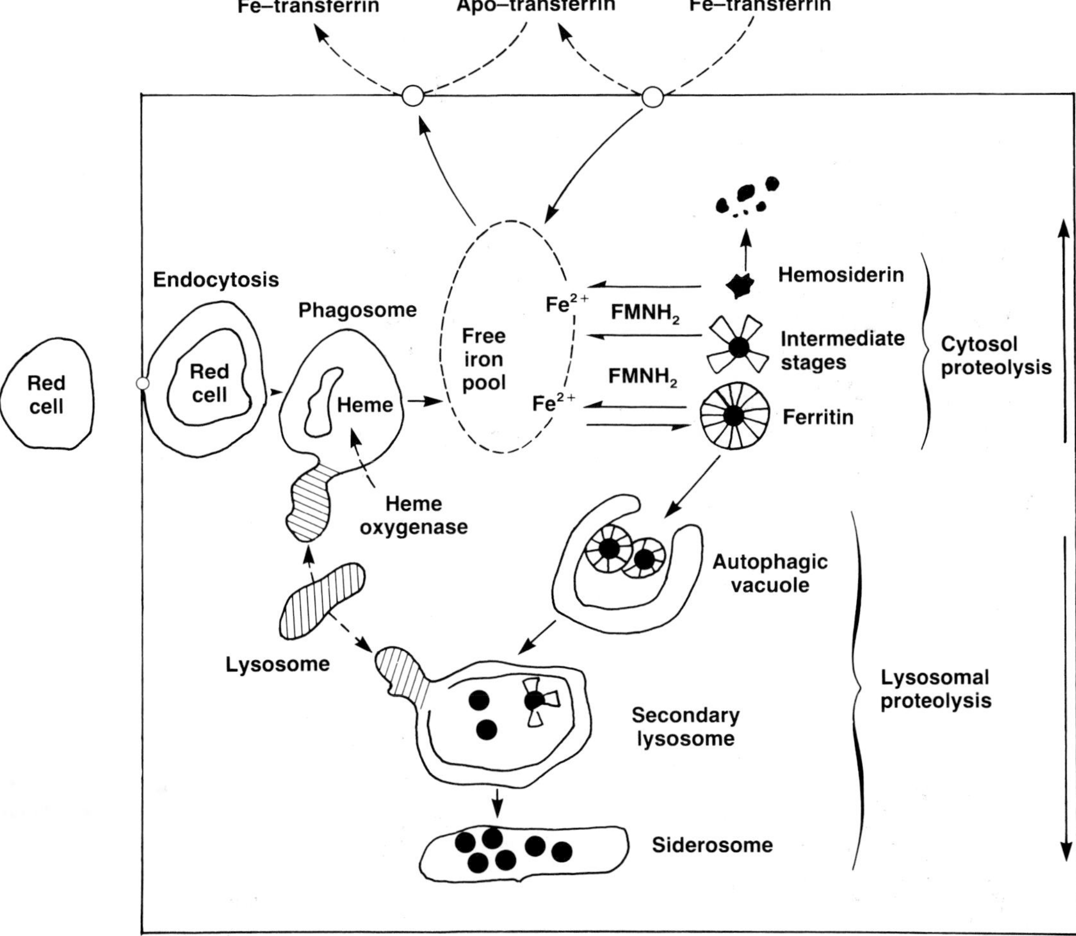

Figure 2–128. Diagram showing pathway of cellular uptake of iron from transferrin or in the form of effete red cells, and a proposed relationship to hemosiderin formation. The effete red cells are taken into cells of the reticuloendothelial system by endocytosis into sacs, which fuse with lysosomes to become phagosomes. This causes rapid digestion of the red cell protein, while heme oxygenase releases iron from the heme into a chelatable Fe^{2+} pool in the cytosol. This iron pool can also receive iron directly from transferrin, and also exchanges iron with ferritin by a mechanism in which the ferritin protein catalyzes the oxidation of Fe^{2+} to Fe^{3+} for storage within the ferritin, while reduced flavin nucleotides reduce the stored iron and return it to the cytosol at site marked by Fe^{2+}. Ferritin can be degraded by two mechanisms: (1) proteolytic enzymes in the cytosol degrade the protein shell; at some point in this process, ferritin ceases to be able to oxidize Fe^{2+} to Fe^{3+}, so that no more iron is laid down, but the stored iron continues to be reduced by $FMNH_2$ to Fe^{2+}, a process involving regeneration of $FMNH_2$ by mitochondria, not shown on the diagram. Consequently, this process completely mobilizes both the shell and core of the ferritin molecule and thus does not result in residual hemosiderin iron cores. (2) Ferritin is taken up by autophagic vacuoles that receive lysosomal enzymes, thus forming secondary lysosomes in which the protein shell is digested, but in which, unlike the cytosol, there is no reducing agent, so that the iron cores remain intact and become hemosiderin. (From Wixom, R. L., Prutkin, L., and Munro, H. N.: Hemosiderin: nature, formation and significance. Int. Rev. Exp. Pathol., *22*:193–225, 1980. Reprinted by permission.)

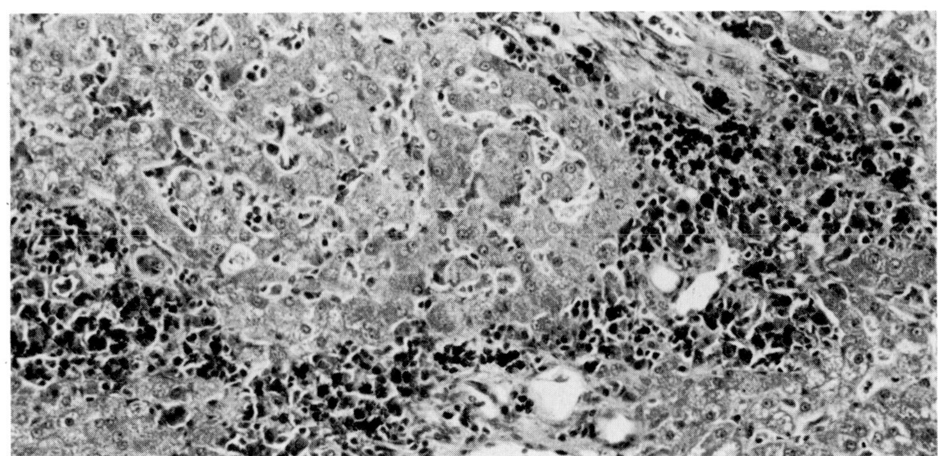

Figure 2–129. Collections of hemosiderin-laden macrophages in a dog's liver. Note the rather random distribution. The cause could be excess iron intake or excess destruction of erythrocytes.

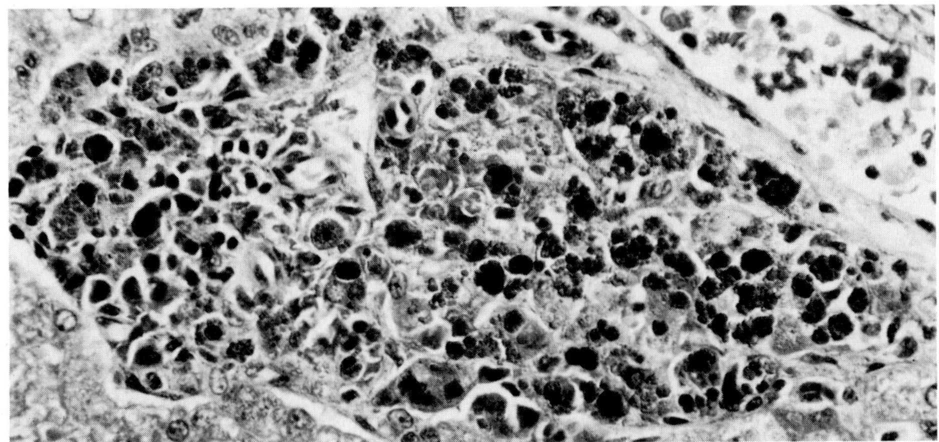

Figure 2–130. Closer view of a collection of cells with hemosiderin from the same liver as in Figure 2–129.

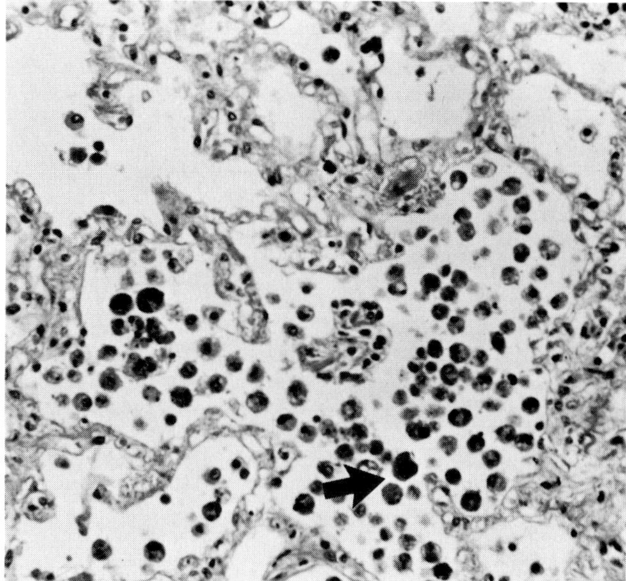

Figure 2–131. Numerous alveolar macrophages containing hemosiderin (arrow). Such macrophages are called heart failure cells when they occur diffusely throughout the lung in left heart failure.

centration. Hemoglobin in the plasma may be carried to the liver by haptoglobin or in the free state to be transformed into bilirubin within hepatocytes. Within hepatocytes, the bilirubin is conjugated with glucuronic acid and passed into the bile canaliculi to become part of bile. The bilirubin provides the normal brownish-orange color of bile. Occasionally, the brown color of bilirubin is observed within hepatocytes or in bile canaliculi. Bilirubin is acted on by the intestinal flora and is changed to ***urobilinogen,*** part of which is reabsorbed into the blood from the intestine. When feces are exposed to air following passage, further changes occur to form ***urobilin.*** Only conjugated bilirubin passes the glomerulus. Thus, although there are normally low levels of conjugated and nonconjugated bilirubin in the blood, only the conjugated form appears in the urine.

5. Jaundice. ***Jaundice,*** or ***icterus,*** occurs when bilirubin is present in the plasma in excess and all tissues are stained yellowish-brown. Jaundice is usually recognized first clinically on the sclera of the eye. The color of bilirubin is not evident on microscopic examination of tissues, but distention of canaliculi in the liver is usually visible (Fig. 2–132). Normally, bilirubin is not visible in canaliculi. If hemoglobin passes the glomerulus and is picked up by renal tubular

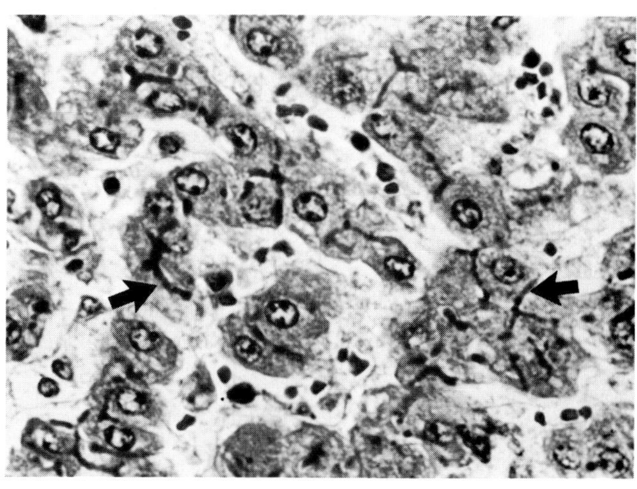

Figure 2–132. Hepatic canaliculi are distended with bilirubin (arrows), indicating excess formation or possible obstruction to outflow. An animal with this lesion would probably have jaundice.

epithelium, bilirubin may be formed in these renal cells and will be visible as brown granules. Biliverdin is the end product of hemoglobin breakdown in birds that do not form bilirubin.

Jaundice is of three types: prehepatic, hepatic and posthepatic. ***Prehepatic*** jaundice arises from acute hemolytic episodes that send bilirubin to the liver in larger quantities than can be processed, so it builds up in the blood as unconjugated bilirubin. Excess conjugated bilirubin will also appear in the blood, feces and urine from the overload. ***Hepatic*** jaundice occurs from direct damage to liver cells and release of conjugated and unconjugated bilirubin into the blood. In ***posthepatic*** jaundice, the bilirubin has passed through the liver cell but is blocked from entry into the intestine. As a result, the feces are pale. Blood levels of conjugated bilirubin rise because of reabsorption from the liver, and some will be present in the urine. The van den Bergh test will differentiate conjugated bilirubin from unconjugated bilirubin in serum. Therefore, by determining the levels of the two types of bilirubin in serum, measuring the conjugated bilirubin in urine and observing the color of the feces, in addition to assessing serum enzymes that indicate liver

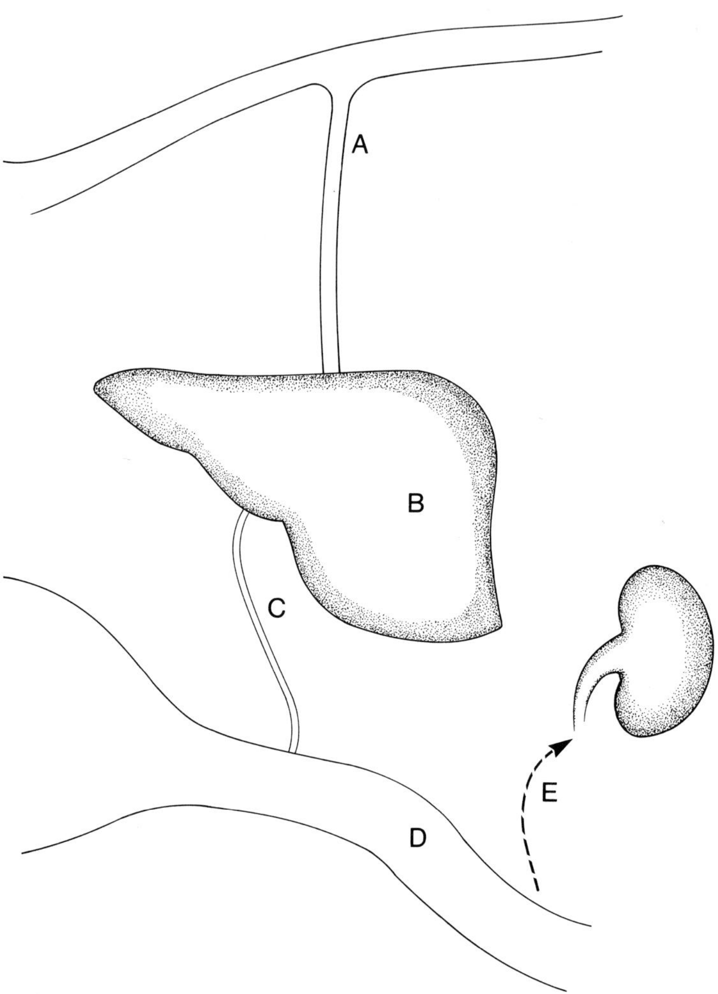

Figure 2–133. Diagrammatic representation of the pathogenesis of jaundice. *A,* The blood coming to the liver; *B,* the liver; *C,* the bile duct; *D,* the intestine; and *E,* reabsorption of urobilinogen and passage into the urine. Hemolysis or prehepatic jaundice would lead to excess unconjugated bilirubin in the intestine, resulting in darker feces and more reabsorption of urobilinogen, which would be detected in the urine. Obstruction to bile outflow or posthepatic jaundice would result in pale feces, no reabsorption to urobilinogen but much reabsorption of conjugated bilirubin into the blood from the liver. Destruction of hepatocytes or hepatic jaundice could give a mixture of these results, but analysis of serum enzymes would detect the damage to hepatocytes.

damage, diagnosis of the type of jaundice can be made (Fig. 2–133).

Jaundice is associated with photosensitization, acute hemolytic anemias (either intravascular as in copper poisoning or intraphagocytic as in autoimmune anemia) or blocked bile ducts caused, for example, by tumors or parasites. Acute toxic damage or viral infection of the liver may also manifest itself in jaundice. The interpretation of serum levels of bilirubin by using the test designed for human plasma is most accurate in the dog and less so in other species of animals.

6. Porphyrins. ***Porphyrins*** that accumulate in the blood may cause pigmentation of tissues along with jaundice and also photosensitization. The disease is called ***porphyria*** and may be congenital, hepatotoxic or primary. In the ***congenital*** type, there is a metabolic defect in the steps of breakdown of porphyrins. Some types accumulate and react with sunlight, resulting in edema and inflammation of nonpigmented areas of the body exposed to the light. The porphyrins collect in teeth and bones and result in so-called pink tooth of cattle. Also, the urine of affected cattle is quite dark. No harm comes to the animal unless it is exposed to sunlight. The ***hepatotoxic*** type arises from phylloerythrin, a metabolite of chlorophyll, that has photosensitizing properties. It accumulates when toxic damage to the liver impairs its normal degradation. The liver lesion is usually chronic and involves the bile duct system. Facial eczema of sheep caused by ingestion of the fungal toxin sporidesmin is a prime example. The ***primary*** type is caused by plants that contain compounds directly photosensitive by ingestion without hepatic injury. Examples are fagopyrism, which is poisoning by buckwheat, and hypericism, which is poisoning by a closely related species.

Pathological pigmentations are significant because they require differentiation from each other; some are more significant than others, and some have direct or indirect implications in the pathogenesis of a clinical disease. Their presence must be interpreted with accuracy and with care.

SUGGESTIONS FOR FURTHER READING

Degeneration

Allen, C. E., et al.: Biology of fat in meat animals. Madison, Wisconsin, North Central Regional Res. Publ. No. 234, University of Wisconsin, 1976.

Anderson, P. J., et al.: Hepatic injury: a histochemical study of intracytoplasmic globules occurring in liver injury. Arch. Pathol., *71*:89–95, 1961.

Arnold., J. P., and Weber, A. F.: Occurrence and fate of corpora amylacea in the bovine udder. Am. J. Vet. Res., *38*:879–881, 1977.

Boenig, H. V.: Free radicals and health: indicators for a unifying concept. J. Am. Geriatr. Soc., *14*:1211–1220, 1966.

Cheville, N. F.: Cell Pathology. 2nd ed. Ames, Iowa State University Press, 1983.

Danse, L. H. J. C., and Steenbergen-Botterweg, W. A.: Early changes of yellow fat disease in mink fed a vitamin E deficient diet supplemented with fresh or oxidised fish oil. Zentralbl. Veterinaermed. [A], *23*:645–660, 1976.

Glenner, G. G.: Amyloid deposits and amyloidosis. New Engl. J. Med., *302*:1283–1292, 1333–1343, 1980.

Hill, R. B., and La Via, M. F. (eds.): Principles of Pathobiology. 3rd ed. London, Oxford University Press, 1980.

Hruban, Z., et al.: Drug-induced and naturally occurring myeloid bodies. Lab. Invest., *27*:62–70, 1972.

Jellinek, H., et al.: Characteristics and fate of vascular fibrin deposition. Exp. Mol. Pathol., *26*:401–414, 1977.

Jennings, R. B., et al.: Ischemic tissue injury. Am. J. Pathol., *81*:179–194, 1975.

Jesaitis, A. J., and Cochrane, C. G.: Receptor-mediated endocytosis, host defense, and inflammation. Lab. Invest., *48*:117–119, 1983.

Johnson, H. A.: On the thermodynamics of cell injury: some insights into the molecular mechanisms. Am. J. Pathol., *75*:13–25, 1974.

Ladds, P. W., and Strafuss, A. C.: Eosinophilic cytoplasmic bodies in a bovine liver. Cornell Vet., *61*:486–489, 1971.

MacKnight, A. D. C., and Leaf, A.: Regulation of cellular volume. Physiol. Rev., *57*:510–573, 1977.

McConnell, E. E., and Talley, F. A.: Intracytoplasmic hyaline globules in the adrenal medulla of laboratory animals. Vet. Pathol., *14*:435–440, 1977.

McCord, J. M., and Fridovich, I.: The biology and pathology of oxygen radicals. Ann. Intern. Med., *88*:122–127, 1978.

Murray, M., et al.: Bovine renal amyloidosis: a clinicopathological study. Vet. Rec., *90*:210–216, 1972.

Osborne, C. A., et al.: Clinicopathologic progression of renal amyloidosis in a dog. J. Am. Vet. Med. Assoc., *157*:203–219, 1970.

Reid, I. M.: An ultrastructural and morphometric study of the liver of the lactating cow in starvation ketosis. Exp. Mol. Pathol., *18*:316–330, 1973.

Reid, I. M., and Collins, R. A.: The pathology of post-parturient fatty liver in high-yielding dairy cows. Invest. Cell Pathol., *3*:237–249, 1980.

Richter, G. W., et al.: Another look at lead inclusion bodies. Am. J. Pathol., *53*:189–217, 1968.

Rungger-Brandle, L., and Gabbiani, G.: The role of cytoskeletal and contractile elements in pathologic processes. Am. J. Pathol., *110*:361–392, 1983.

Slater, T. F.: Free radical mechanisms in tissue injury. *In* Bajusz, E., and Jasmin, G. (eds.): Methods and

Achievements in Experimental Pathology. Vol. 4. White Plains, New York, Albert J. Phiebig, 1969, pp. 30–53.

Sobel, H. J., et al.: Nonviral nuclear inclusions. 1. Cytoplasmic invaginations. Arch. Pathol., *87*:179–182, 1969.

Stenger, R. J.: Organelle pathology of the liver: the endoplasmic reticulum. Gastroenterology, *58*:554–574, 1970.

Suzuki, K.: Neuronal storage disease: a review. *In* Zimmerman, H. M. (eds.): Progress in Neuropathology. Vol. III. New York, Grune & Stratton, 1976, pp. 173–202.

Tamm, I.: Cell injury with viruses. Am. J. Pathol., *81*:237–250, 1975.

Tappel, A. J.: Lipid peroxidation and fluorescent molecular damage to membranes. *In* Trump, B. J., and Arstila, A. U. (eds.): Pathobiology of Cell Membranes. New York, Academic Press, 1975.

Thompson, S. W., et al.: Histochemical studies of acidophilic crystalline intranuclear inclusions in the liver and kidney of dogs. Am. J. Pathol., *35*:607–623, 1959.

Trump, B. F., and Arstila, A. U., (eds.): Pathobiology of Cell Membranes. Vol. 1. New York, Academic Press, 1975.

Trump, B. J., et al.: Cell death and the disease process. The role of calcium. *In* Bowen, I. D., and Lockshin, R. A. (eds.): Cell Death in Biology and Pathology. London, Chapman and Hall, 1981, pp. 209–242.

Van Vleet, J. F., et al.: Ultrastructural alterations in nutritional cardiomyopathy of selenium–vitamin E deficient swine. I. Fiber lesions. Lab. Invest., *37*:188–200, 1977.

Zmuda, M. J., and Quebbemann, A. J.: Localization of renal tubular uric acid transport defect in gouty chickens. Am. J. Physiol., *229*:820–825, 1975.

Necrosis

Anderson, J. F., and Werdin, R. E.: Ergotism manifested as agalactia and gangrene in sows. J. Am. Vet. Med. Assoc., *170*:1089–1091, 1977.

Caplan, E. S., and Kluge, R. M.: Gas gangrene: review of 34 cases. Arch. Intern. Med., *136*:788–791, 1976.

Dunnill, M. S.: A review of the pathology and pathogenesis of acute renal failure due to acute tubular necrosis. J. Clin. Pathol., *27*:2–13, 1974.

Farber, J. L., and El-Mofty, S. K.: The biochemical pathology of liver cell necrosis. Am. J. Pathol., *81*:163–177, 1975.

Farber, J. L., et al.: The pathogenesis of irreversible cell injury in ischemia. Am. J. Pathol., *102*:271–281, 1981.

Farber, J. I.: Membrane injury and calcium homeostasis in the pathogenesis of coagulative necrosis. Lab. Invest., *47*:114–123, 1982.

Frank, L., and Massaro, D.: Oxygen toxicity. Am. J. Med., *69*:117–126, 1980.

Freedland, R. A., and Kramer, J. W.: Use of serum enzymes as aids to diagnosis. Adv. Vet. Sci. Comp. Med., *14*:61–103, 1970.

Morison, R. S.: Death: process or event? Science, *173*:694–702, 1971.

Muller, H. K.: Mechanisms of clearing injured tissue. *In* Glynn, L. E. (ed.): Tissue Repair and Regeneration. Amsterdam, Elsevier-North Holland Biomedical Press, 1981, pp. 145–175.

Parry, E. W.: Studies on mobilization of Kupffer cells in mice. I. The effect of carbon tetrachloride induced liver necrosis. J. Comp. Pathol., *88*:481–487, 1978.

Parry, E. W.: Studies on mobilization of Kupffer cells in mice. II. Mobilization mediated by necrotic tissue injected intraperitoneally. J. Comp. Pathol., *88*:489–495, 1978.

Parry, E. W.: The mechanism of necrotic tissue removal in mouse liver following CCl_4-induced injury. J. Comp. Pathol., *89*:205–211, 1979.

Rappaport, A. M., and Hiraki, G. Y.: The anatomical pattern of lesions in the liver. Acta Anat., *32*:126–140, 1958.

Ribelin, W. E., and Deeds, F.: Fat necrosis in man and animals. J. Am. Vet. Med. Assoc., *136*:135–139, 1960.

Rumsey, T. S., et al.: Chemical composition of necrotic fat lesions in beef cows grazing fertilized "Kentucky-31" tall fescue. J. Anim. Sci., *48*:673–689, 1979.

Shier, W. T.: Cytolytic mechanisms—self destruction of mammalian cells by activation of endogenous hydrolytic enzymes. J. Toxicol. Toxin Rev., *1*:1–32, 1982.

Calcification and Pigmentation

Bagnara, J., et al.: Common origin of pigment cells. Science, *203*:410–415, 1979.

Bissell, D. M.: Formation and elimination of bilirubin. Gastroenterology, *69*:519–538, 1975.

Bonucci, E., and Sadun, R.: An electron microscope study on experimental calcification of skeletal muscle. Clin. Orthop., *88*:197–217, 1972.

Bradley, R., and Duffell, S. J.: The pathology of the skeletal and cardiac muscles of cattle with xanthosis. J. Comp. Pathol., *92*:85–97, 1982.

Capen, C. C., et al.: The pathology of hypervitaminosis D in cattle. Pathol. Vet., *3*:350–378, 1966.

Von Dirkesen, G., et al.: Uber eine enzootische "Kalzinose" beim Rind. Dtsch. Tieraerztl. Wochenschr., *77*:321–346, 1970.

Eggermann, J., and Kapanci, Y.: Experimental pulmonary calcinosis in the rat. Ultrastructural and morphometric studies. Lab. Invest., *24*:469–482, 1971.

Fox, D. L.: Pigment transactions between animals and plants. Biol. Rev., *54*:237–268, 1979.

Kajihara, H., et al.: Ultrastructure and morphogenesis of ceroid pigment. I. Phagocytosis and formation of lipid-containing lysosomes in Kupffer cells after intravenous injection of unsaturated lipids. Virchows Archiv. (Cell. Pathol.), *19*:221–237, 1975.

Lowenstine, L. J., and Petrak, M.: Iron pigment in livers of birds. *In* Montali, R. J., and Migaki, G. (eds.): Comparative Pathology of Zoo Animals. Washington, Smithsonian Institution Press, 1980, pp. 127–132.

Macklin, C. C.: Pulmonary sumps, dust accumulations, alveolar fluid and lymph vessels. Acta Anat., *23*:1–33, 1955.

Oberc, M. A., and Engel, W. K.: Ultrastructural localization of calcium in normal and abnormal skeletal muscle. Lab. Invest., *36*:566–577, 1977.

Riley, P. A.: Melanins and melanogenesis. Pathobiol. Annu., *10*:223–251, 1980.

Roberts, W. C.: Hepatic-cell pigment in congestive heart failure. Arch. Pathol., *82*:566–568, 1966.

Ross, M. A., et al.: Dystrophic calcification in the adrenal glands of monkeys, cats and dogs. Arch. Pathol., *60*:655–662, 1955.

Scott, D. W.: Dermatohistopathologic changes in bovine congenital porphyria. Cornell Vet., *69*:145–158, 1979.

Selye, H., and Berczi, I.: The present status of calciphylaxis and calcergy. Clin. Orthop., *69*:28–54, 1970.

Thompson, S. W.: Selected Histochemical and Histopathological Methods. Springfield, Ill., Charles C Thomas, 1974.

Whiteford, R., and Getty, R.: Distribution of lipofuscin in the canine and porcine brain as related to aging. J. Gerontol., *21*:31–44, 1966.

Wixom, R. L., et al.: Hemosiderin: nature, formation and significance. Int. Rev. Exp. Pathol., *22*:193–225, 1980.

Wolman, M.: Pigments in pathology. New York, Academic Press, 1969.

Wolman, M.: Lipid pigments (chromolipids): their origin, nature, and significance. Pathobiol. Annu., *10*:253–267, 1980.

Woodward, J. C.: A morphologic and biochemical study of nutritional nephrocalcinosis in female rats fed semipurified diets. Am. J. Pathol., *65*:253–264, 1971.

Zeman, W.: The neuronal ceroid-lipofuscinosis. *In* Zimmerman, H. M. (ed.): Progress in Neuropathology. Vol. III. New York, Grune & Stratton, 1976, pp. 203–223.

Postmortem Changes

Boyd, E. M., and Knight, L. M.: Postmorten shifts in the weight and water levels of body organs. Toxicol. Appl. Pharmacol., *5*:119–128, 1963.

deJongh, D. S., et al.: Postmortem bacteriology: a practical method for routine use. Am. J. Clin. Pathol., *49*:424–428, 1968.

Dillman, R. C., and Dennis, S. M.: Sequential sterile autolysis in the ovine fetus: macroscopic changes. Am. J. Vet. Res., *37*:403–407, 1976.

Gill, C. O., et al.: Tissue sterility in uneviscerated carcasses. Appl. Env. Microbiol., *36*:356–359, 1978.

Gill, C. O.: A review: intrinsic bacteria in meat. J. Appl. Bacteriol., *47*:367–378, 1979.

Gill, C. O., and Penney, N.: Microbiology of bruised meat. Appl. Environ. Microbiol., *38*:1184–1185, 1979.

Gill, C. O., and Penney, N.: Survival of bacteria in carcasses. Appl. Environ. Microbiol., *37*:667–669, 1979.

Gill, C. O., et al.: Survival of clostridial spores in animal tissues. Appl. Environ. Microbiol., *41*:90–92, 1981.

Koneman, E. W., et al.: Postmortem bacteriology. II. Selection of cases for culture. Am. J. Clin. Pathol., *55*:17–23, 1971.

Koneman, E. W., and Davis, M. A.: Postmortem bacteriology. III. Clinical significance of microorganisms recovered at autopsy. Am. J. Clin. Pathol., *61*:28–40, 1974.

Mackey, B. M., and Derrick, C. M.: Contamination of the deep tissues of carcasses by bacteria present on the slaughter instruments or in the gut. J. Appl. Microbiol., *46*:355–366, 1979.

McNaughton, A. F.: A histological study of postmortem changes in the skeletal muscle of the fowl *(Gallus domesticus)*. I. The muscle fibres. J. Anat., *125*:461–476, 1978. II. The cytoarchitecture. J. Anat., *126*:5–20, 1978.

Menckler, T. M., et al.: Microbiology experience in collection of human tissue. Am. J. Clin. Pathol., *45*:85–92, 1966.

Munger, L. L., and McGavin, M.D.: Sequential portmortem changes in chicken liver at 4, 20 or 37°C. Avian Dis., *16*:587–605, 1972.

Munger, L. L., and McGavin, M.D.: Sequential postmortem changes in chicken kidney at 4, 20 or 37°C. Avian Dis., *16*:606–621, 1972.

Nunley, W. C., et al.: Delayed, *in vivo* hepatic postmortem autolysis. Virchows Archiv. (Cell. Pathol.) *11*:289–302, 1972.

Pearson, G. R., and Logan, E. F.: Scanning electron microscopy of early postmortem artefacts in the small intestine of a neonatal calf. Br. J. Exp. Pathol., *59*:499–503, 1978.

Pearson, G. R., and Logan, E. F.: The rate of development of postmortem artefact in the small intestine of neonatal calves. Br. J. Exp. Pathol., *59*:178–182, 1978.

3

CIRCULATORY DISTURBANCES

In most instances, any type of lesion occurring in the body will involve or be influenced by the blood or blood vessels or both. Blood vessels are necessary for bringing nutriment in the blood to cells in the tissue and removing metabolic byproducts. Impairment of the function, composition or structure of the blood or blood vessels may have serious consequences for the tissues. This section deals with ***lesions related to blood vessels and blood that are common to all tissues in various kinds of tissue injury and that may be observed in the live or dead animal.*** These lesions are also involved in many major processes, such as inflammation and neoplasia, and in the special pathology of organ systems.

The circulatory changes common to many types of lesions may be summarized as follows (Fig. 3–1). Blood may leave the blood vessels and the lesion is termed ***hemorrhage.*** The lesion in which excess blood may be drawn into an area is ***hyperemia.*** Blood may passively accumulate in an area and this lesion is ***congestion.*** Excess fluid may accumulate in tissues and this lesion is ***edema.*** Blood may be kept from reaching an area of tissue; this process is named ***ischemia*** and the tissue is ***ischemic.*** If ischemia is complete, the tissue becomes necrotic; the affected area is an ***infarct*** and the process is an ***infarction.*** The blood may clot within blood vessels; this process is ***thrombosis*** and the solid clot is a ***thrombus.*** Solid structures may float in the blood vessels from one area to another. This process is ***embolism*** and the structure is an ***embolus.*** Generalized failure of peripheral circulation is known as ***shock.***

Each of these lesions will be discussed. The point should be stressed that these lesions are not specific disease entities but

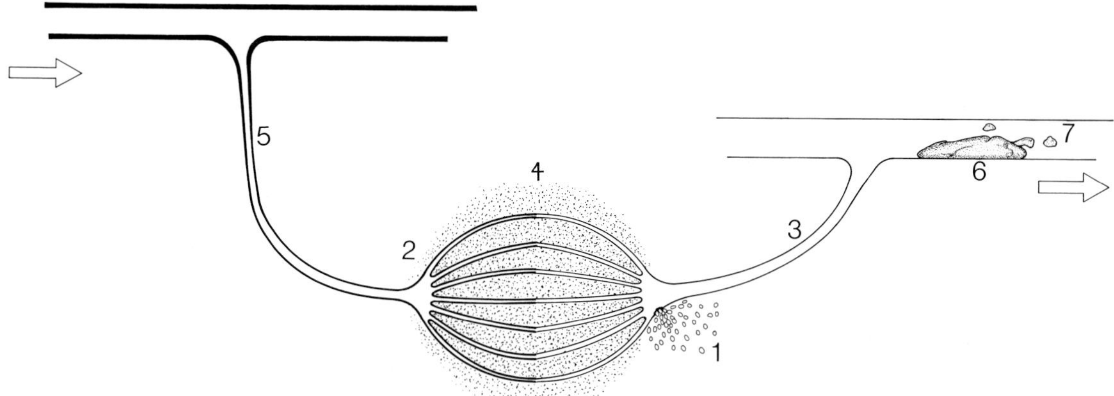

Figure 3–1. Diagrammatic representation of the circulation and of the main lesions common to the circulation in tissues. The arterial circulation is at the left, the venous circulation is at the right and the peripheral circulation is in the middle. Hemorrhage occurs when red blood cells escape from the vascular system (1). Hyperemia occurs if an increased amount of blood is actively drawn into a portion of the peripheral circulation (2). Congestion results when there is an impediment to the flow from a portion of the peripheral circulation (3). Edema is the accumulation of excess fluid in the connective tissue or stroma of a tissue (4). Ischemia results from the complete or partial impairment of blood flow to a tissue (5), and the peripheral area may be infarcted. Thrombosis occurs when blood clots inside the vascular system and forms a solid body, a thrombus (6). Embolism is the movement of a solid structure from one area to another, such as in the case of a piece of thrombus (7).

are general lesions and processes common to many tissues, organs and certain diseases. Attention will be drawn not just to the processes but also to their ***implications*** and ***complications.*** They may be primarily responsible for major disease or death of an organism, individually or collectively.

HEMOSTASIS

Several disease processes involve the coagulation system and hemostasis. Although these are encountered in studies of physiology, it is necessary to review some aspects here before proceeding with the specific circulatory lesions. These topics will arise again in the discussion of inflammation. An overall view of hemostasis is presented in Figure 3–2. A simplified version of the extrinsic and intrinsic systems is included in Figure 3–3. In the intrinsic clotting system, all the factors are present in plasma, whereas the extrinsic system is initiated by factors from outside the plasma. If both systems function, more fibrin is produced than when the intrinsic system operates alone.

It is sometimes difficult to envisage the presence or origin of the plasma factors involved in hemostasis. Most are normal constituents of the plasma proteins (Fig. 3–4). There is considerable species variation in the relative concentrations of albumin, globulin and fibrinogen in plasma of normal animals, and the levels are often altered in disease. Plasma levels of fibrinogen often increase in disease states, and this is particularly true in cattle diseases.

The factors involved in normal clotting are listed in Table 3–1. Thromboplastin is not a single substance but is best described as performing the function of catalyzing the conversion of prothrombin to thrombin. Substances with this activity occur in plasma, platelets and tissues. From the plasma come antihemophilic globulin (AHG), plasma thromboplastin component (PTC), Hageman factor, Stuart factor and factor V. From the platelets comes platelet thromboplastic factor, and from the tissues come thromboplastic precursors. These are both phospholipids and are synthesized by cells; active ingredients have not been specifically identified.

Prothrombin is a globulin circulating in plasma. Fibrinogen loses peptides under the influence of thrombin, a proteolytic enzyme, and repolymerizes to fibrin, which has a higher molecular weight than fibrinogen. Fibrin is stabilized by a factor in serum called FSF, fibrin stabilizing factor. Prothrombin, factor V and factor VII are made in the liver and require vitamin K for their production and activity.

Plasminogen or profibrinolysin is present

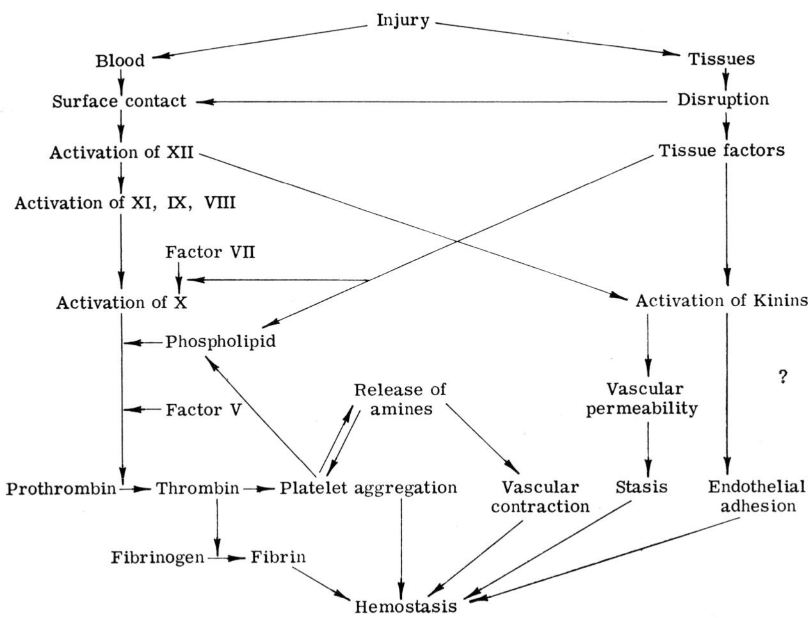

Figure 3–2. A comprehensive scheme of hemostasis. (From MacFarlane, R. G.: The hemostatis mechanism and its defects. Int. Rev. Exp. Pathol., 6:55–133, 1968. Reprinted by permission.)

in normal plasma. It becomes activated to form fibrinolysin or plasmin, which acts to break down fibrin. Numerous factors may activate plasminogen, including products of bacteria and granulation tissue. ***Thus, there are substances readily available in plasma and tissue to form a clot of fibrin and to remove the clot.*** Breakdown products of fibrinogen and fibrin may contribute to defective coagulation (Fig. 3–5).

The liver is the only source of fibrinogen, prothrombin and albumin, as well as most of the alpha and beta globulins, whereas gamma globulins are made by the lymphocytes and plasma cells. The plasma proteins have several important functions: maintaining osmotic pressure, acting as buffers, acting as a source of reserve body protein and serving as carriers of many substances, including hormones, lipids, vitamins and

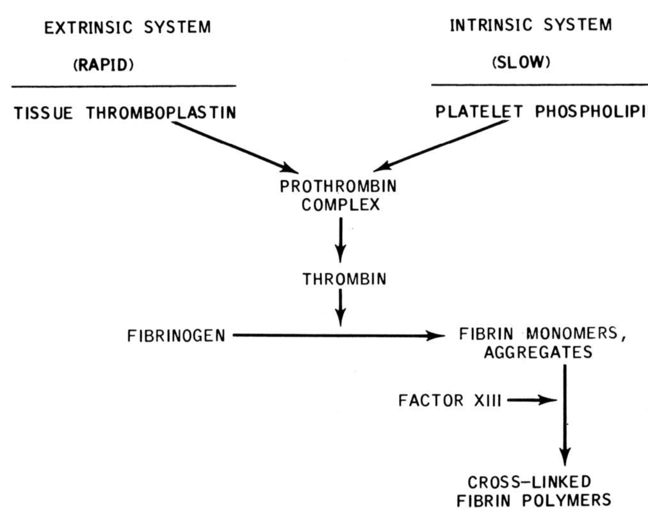

Figure 3–3. The major differences between and the major identities of the intrinsic and the extrinsic coagulation systems are summarized in this figure. Note that the extrinsic system of coagulation is more rapid, clotting plasma in seconds, and requires the action of tissue thromboplastin. The intrinsic system is slow, clotting plasma in minutes, and requires the action of platelet phospholipids. From the point at which prothrombin complexes are formed, both coagulation systems have a common route. (From Nalbandian, R. M., et al.: Consumption coagulopathy: practical principles of diagnosis and management. Mich. Med., *70*:794, 1971. Reprinted by permission.)

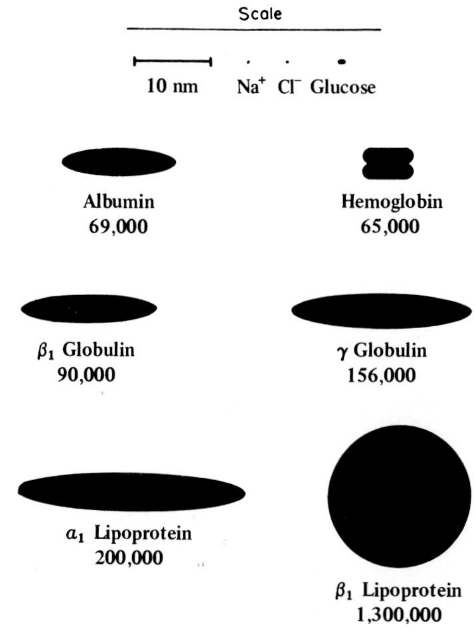

Figure 3–4. Relative dimensions and molecular weights of protein molecules in the blood. (From Harper, H. A.: Physiological Chemistry. 15th ed. Los Altos, California, Lange Medical Publications, 1975. Reprinted by permission.)

drugs. The components of the complement system are also normal plasma proteins.

HYPEREMIA

An understanding of hyperemia requires an appreciation of the anatomy and the physiological control of the terminal circulatory bed common to most tissues (Fig. 3–6). Under normal circumstances, blood may be flowing through a few of the capillaries in a tissue and may be shunted past many capillaries. Some organs vary in their function from time to time by having different areas take turns doing the work. Therefore, the amount of blood flow usually corresponds to the amount of work being carried out and so will vary in different areas at different times. These factors relate to the general concept of ***functional reserve.***

If, however, more blood is needed in an area, even beyond that needed for a heavy work load, then all the capillaries and shunts open, the vessels dilate and a much greater amount of blood is present. The tissue visibly becomes quite red because of the increased number of red blood cells present, and the blood present is arterial blood and therefore well oxygenated. This red area is ***hyperemic*** and the process is ***hyperemia,*** an ***active process*** whereby more blood is required in an area and is brought to it. Hyperemia most commonly occurs in inflammation, which is known for the bright red color it produces in tissues. In Figure 3–6, the blood either is being shunted past the entire capillary bed or is passing through only a few capillaries in the normal state. ***In hyperemia, all capillaries would be opened, dilated and filled with red blood cells.*** Hyperemia usually occurs in a ***localized area,*** because if it occurred all over the body, there would not be sufficient blood in the major vessels to maintain systemic blood pressure and shock would oc-

TABLE 3–1. BLOOD CLOTTING FACTORS AND SYNONYMS

International Classification*	Synonyms
Factor I	FIBRINOGEN
Factor II	PROTHROMBIN
Factor III	TISSUE THROMBOPLASTIN
Factor IV	CALCIUM
Factor V	PROACCELERIN Labile factor, Accelerator globulin (AcG)
Factor VII	PROCONVERTIN Serum prothrombin conversion accelerator (SLCA), Stable factor, Autoprothrombin I
Factor VIII	ANTIHEMOPHILIC FACTOR (AHF) Antihemophilic globulin (AHG), Platelet cofactor I, Plasma thromboplastic factor A
Factor IX	CHRISTMAS FACTOR Plasma thromboplastin component (PTC), Platelet cofactor II, Autoprothrombin II, Plasma thromboplastic factor B
Factor X	STUART FACTOR Stuart-Prower factor
Factor XI	PLASMA THROMBOPLASTIN ANTECEDENT (PTA)
Factor XII	HAGEMAN FACTOR
Factor XIII	FIBRIN STABILIZING FACTOR (FSF) Fibrinase, Laki-Lorand factor

*As recommended by the International Committee for the nomenclature of Blood Clotting Factors (1962). The most commonly used synonym is capitalized for each factor.

(Courtesy of Jean Dodds. Reprinted by permission.)

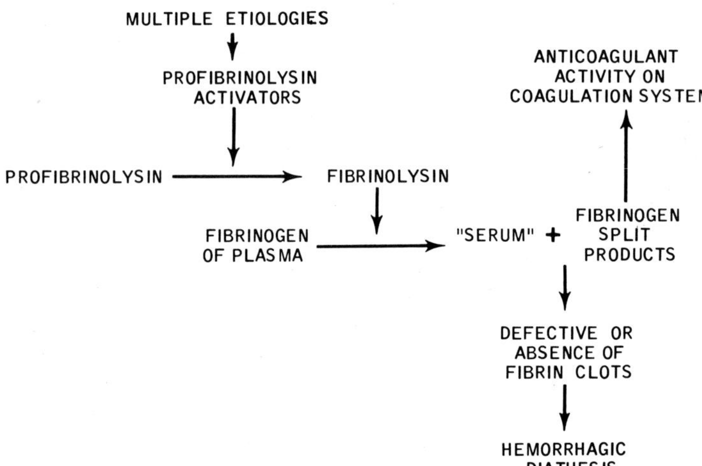

Figure 3–5. The important metabolic events in the primary activation of the fibrinolytic system are shown here. Note that profibrinolysin activators, rather than fibrinolysin, control the rate of activity on the substrate, the fibrinogen of plasma, and its conversion into fibrinogen split products. (From Nalbandian, R. M., et al.: Consumption coagulopathy: practical principles of diagnosis and management. Mich. Med., *70*:798, 1971. Reprinted by permission.)

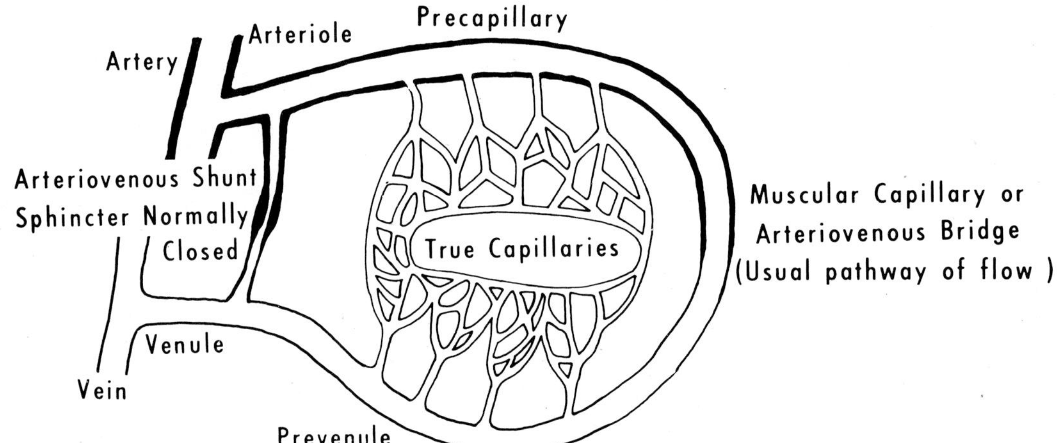

Figure 3–6. Diagrammatic representation of the microcirculation. (From Boyd, W.: A Textbook of Pathology. 8th ed. Philadelphia, Lea & Febiger, 1970. Reprinted by permission.)

cur. A blush is a well-known physiological hyperemia. Release of vasoactive substances, such as histamine and lactic acid, and nervous control of vessels play a role in initiating hyperemia. Since hyperemia is usually localized, the cause will be local as well.

VENOUS CONGESTION

Congestion implies that the flow of blood leaving an area is impeded and the blood therefore accumulates in the venous circulation (Figs. 3–7, 3–8 and 3–9). It is a ***passive*** process and results from impaired flow in veins. Congestion may be caused by physical obstruction of either small or large vessels or ***failure of forward flow,*** as in heart failure. Blood accumulates in dilated capillaries and venules, and the tissue appears blue because of the poorly oxygenated venous blood. Such a dark area is described as ***cyanotic.*** The microscopic appearance of congestion in Figure 3–7 is similar to that of hyperemia, and the circumstances (such as the presence of inflammatory cells) would have to be known in order to differentiate congestion from hyperemia.

Congestion may be either ***localized*** or ***generalized.*** An example of ***localized*** congestion is a strangulated piece of intestine in which the compression on the vessels is such that arterial blood still gets in through the muscular arteries but the pressure on the thinner-walled veins restricts the outflow and venous blood accumulates. Such a lesion may become almost black; the tissue will be anoxic but may not be necrotic—although necrosis will occur because of anoxia if the lesion persists. Localized congestion may develop rapidly or occur slowly (Figs. 3–10 through 3–13).

Generalized congestion involves the central circulation of the heart and major vessels (including the lung), since all the blood must flow through these organs. Congestion in this case may be caused by a number of factors: flow may be obstructed, the heart may be too weak to pump adequately or the blood may not be returned to the heart for repumping. These factors involve many aspects of heart disease dealt with in special pathology but a few points may be useful here for context. A defective valve will impair flow. A dilated thin-walled ventricle may not be strong enough to pump. There may be a chronic obstructive disease in the

Text continued on page 109

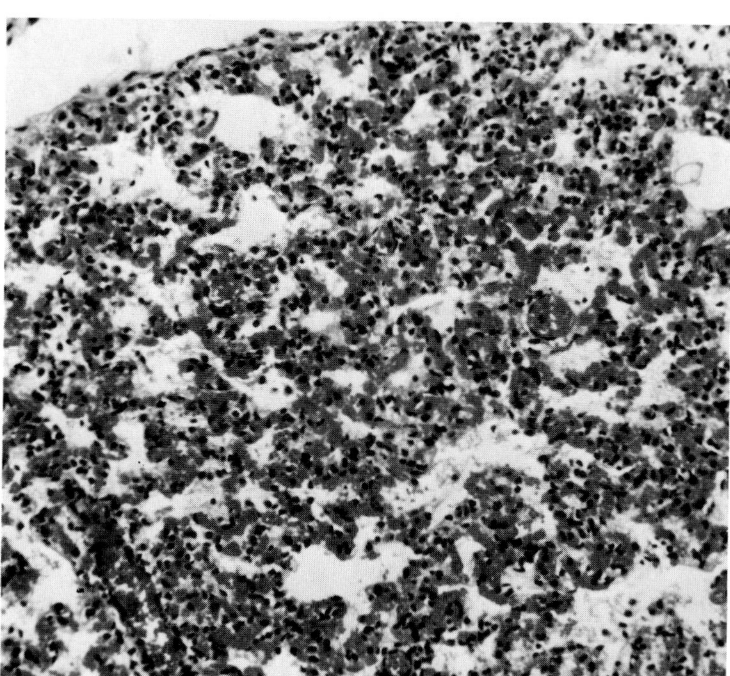

Figure 3–7. The alveolar capillaries in the lung are dilated and filled with red blood cells, and therefore the tissue is congested.

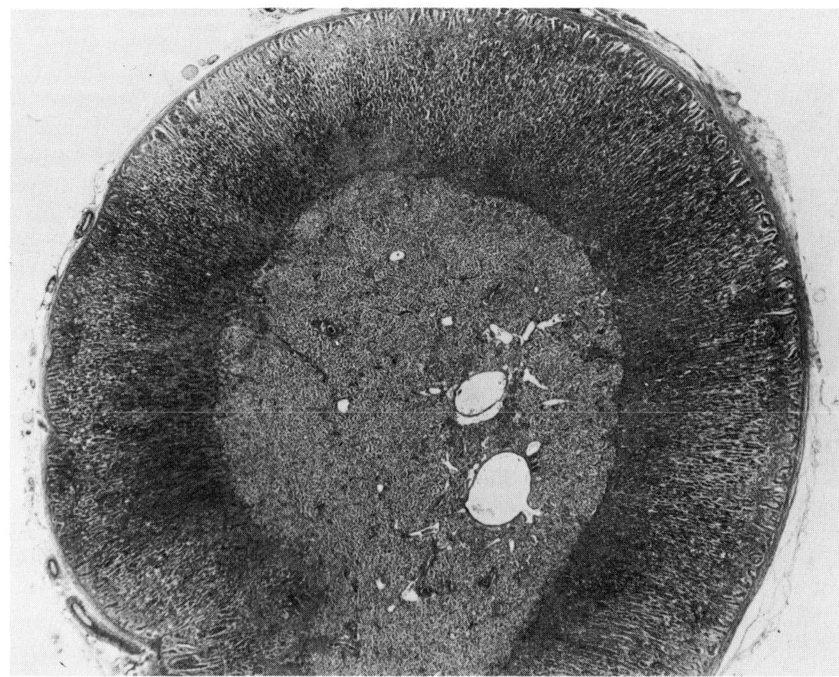

Figure 3–8

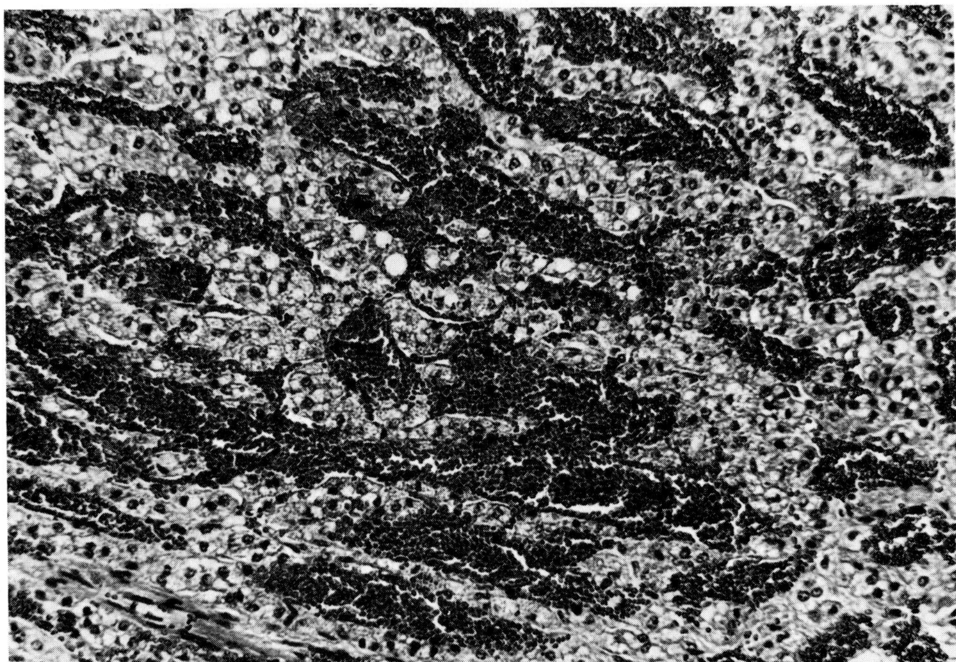

Figure 3–9

Figure 3–8. Congestion in the inner areas of the adrenal cortex of a horse with intestinal obstruction.
Figure 3–9. Microscopic view of a lesion similar to that seen in Figure 3–8, in which red blood cells fill the dilated sinusoids.

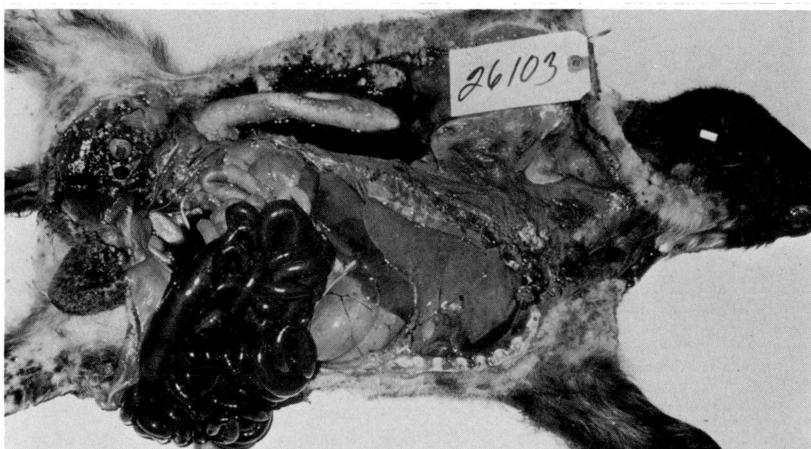

Figure 3–10. Lamb with extreme congestion of the section of intestine that has undergone complete volvulus (twist on a mesenteric axis).

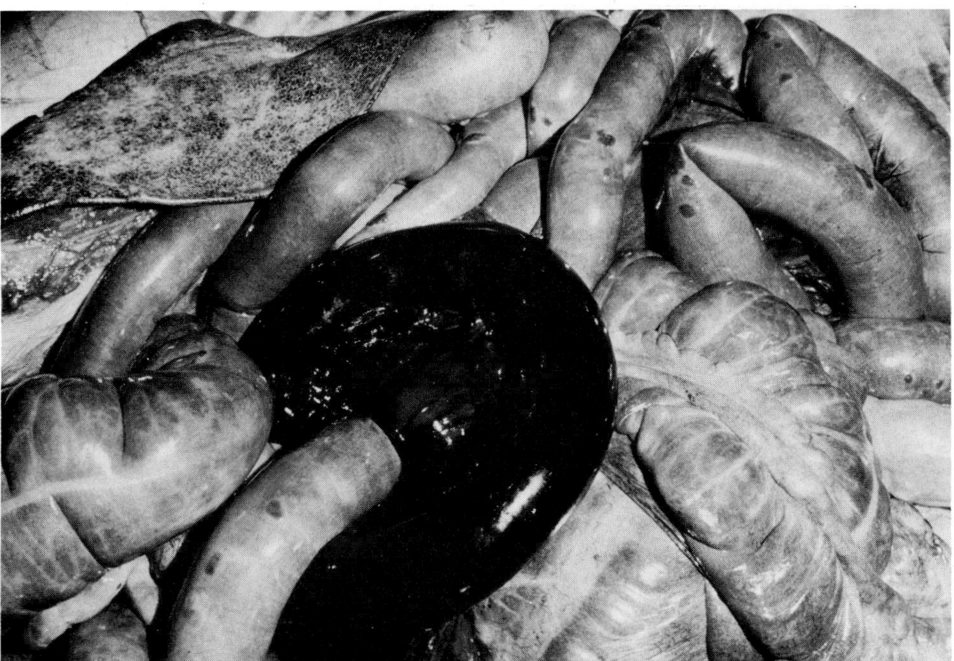

Figure 3–11. An extremely congested loop of intestine in a horse. This would indicate a localized obstruction to outflow of venous blood. The dark nodules on the serosal surface are areas of hemorrhage caused by migrating strongyle larvae and are sometimes called hemomelasma ilei because they often are black.

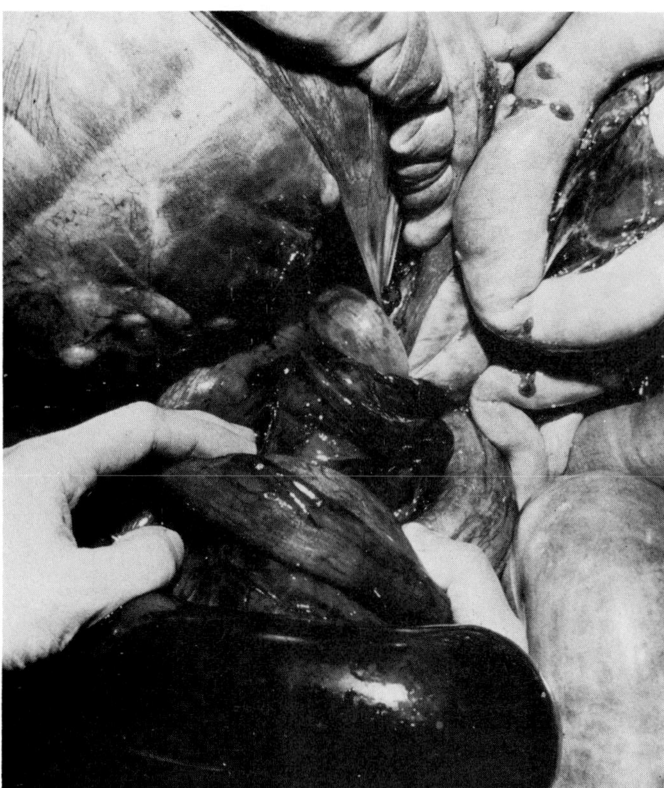

Figure 3–12. The cause of the congestion shown in Figure 3–11. A very tight volvulus is evident near the root of the mesentery.

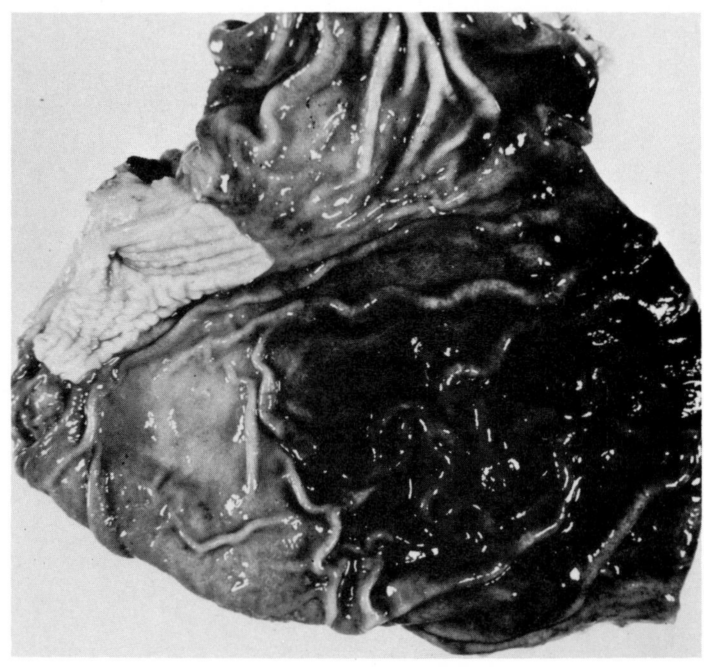

Figure 3–13. Dark fundic mucosa in a pig's stomach caused by congestion. This lesion seems to be a nonspecific indication of acute infections in pigs and is due to venous congestion with thrombosis. It is an indication of shock and sludging and is an important lesion to observe in pigs.

lung that impairs blood flow in general circulation. If the main impairment to flow is in the right side of the heart or the lungs, the blood will accumulate in the major veins and liver. If the problem is on the left side of the heart, blood will accumulate in the lungs. These problems are termed ***right-sided heart failure*** and ***left-sided heart failure,*** respectively (Fig. 3–14). Both may be either acute or chronic, but the chronic problem will be emphasized here because it has more obvious effects on other organs. Both may be fatal.

When blood accumulates in the systemic venous circulation in right-sided heart failure, fluid may accumulate in tissues. Increase in the hydrostatic pressure at the venous end of capillaries results in a counterbalancing of the positive action of the blood's osmotic pressure to draw tissue fluids into the vessels (see Edema, p. 119). The expression of this problem varies with species but usually results in fluid accumulation beneath the skin in the extremities and in the major body cavities. In the abdomen, the lesion is called ***ascites.***

The liver is particularly affected by increased hydrostatic pressure and slow flow. Hypoxia or anoxia, or a combination of the two, occurs around central veins in a periacinar distribution. If the anoxia persists and is severe, the hepatocytes may become necrotic. This may occur rather quickly, but the onset may be gradual, as in chronic heart failure. As the hepatocytes die and disappear, the red blood cells pool in the dilated sinusoids that remain and may eventually occupy much of the space formerly occupied by hepatocytes. These areas appear red or reddish-blue grossly and give the enlarged liver in chronic passive congestion its characteristic appearance (Figs. 3–15 and 3–16). The color pattern resembles that of the spice nutmeg, and the term ***nutmeg liver*** has become synonymous with ***chronic passive congestion*** of the liver (Fig. 3–17 *B* and *C*).

When the problem is on the left side of the heart, the accumulation of blood and increased hydrostatic pressure occur in the lungs. Fluid will collect in the lung and is characteristic of chronic left-sided heart failure. Also, red blood cells leak through the capillaries into alveoli and are picked up by alveolar macrophages. If the condition is chronic and severe, the breakdown products of the red blood cells appear in the alveolar macrophages in the form of hemosiderin. These are called ***heart failure cells*** because of their characteristic association with chronic left-sided heart failure (Fig. 3–17 *A*). The lungs are heavy and wet and dark in color.

HEMORRHAGE

Hemorrhage occurs when blood escapes from the blood vessels (Fig. 3–18). The vessel may be physically damaged so that

Text continued on page 112

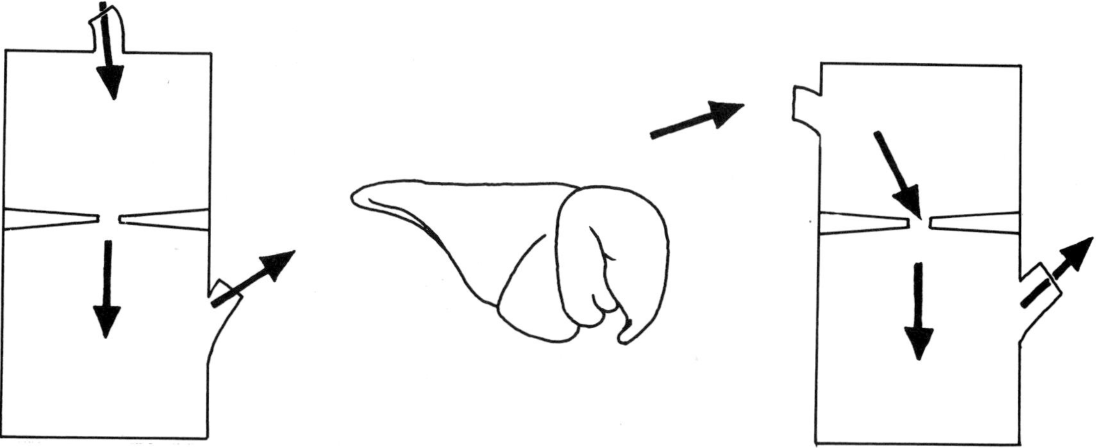

Figure 3–14. Diagrammatic representation of the central circulation with flow into the right heart, the lungs, and the left heart. Impediment to flow through the right heart or lungs will result in generalized venous congestion and right-sided heart failure. Impediment to flow from the left heart will cause venous congestion in the lung and, if prolonged, will extend to right-sided heart failure as well.

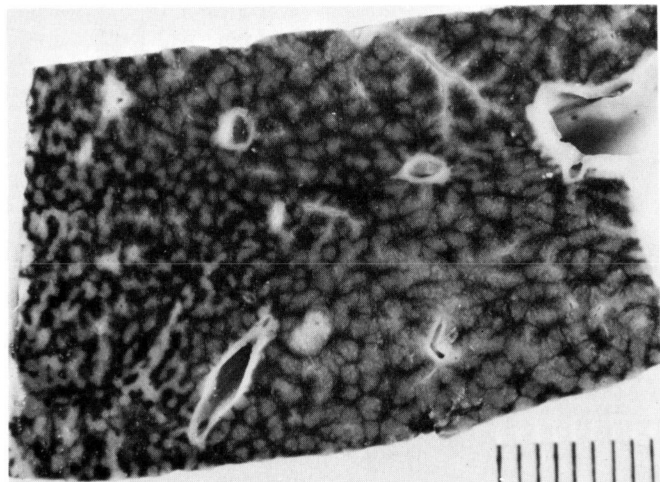

Figure 3–15. Chronic passive congestion in the liver. The dark areas are around central veins and the light areas are around portal triads.

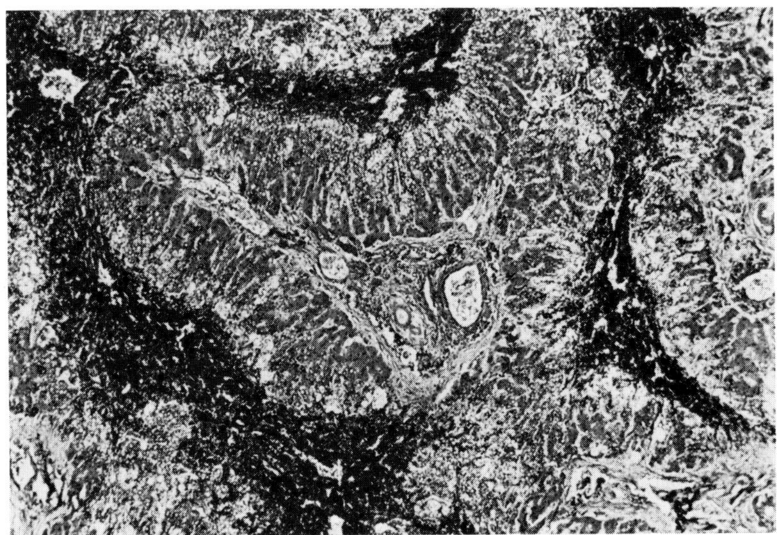

Figure 3–16. Chronic passive congestion of the liver. Hepatocytes in centrolobular areas have degenerated and died from anoxia, and erythrocytes now pool in these areas.

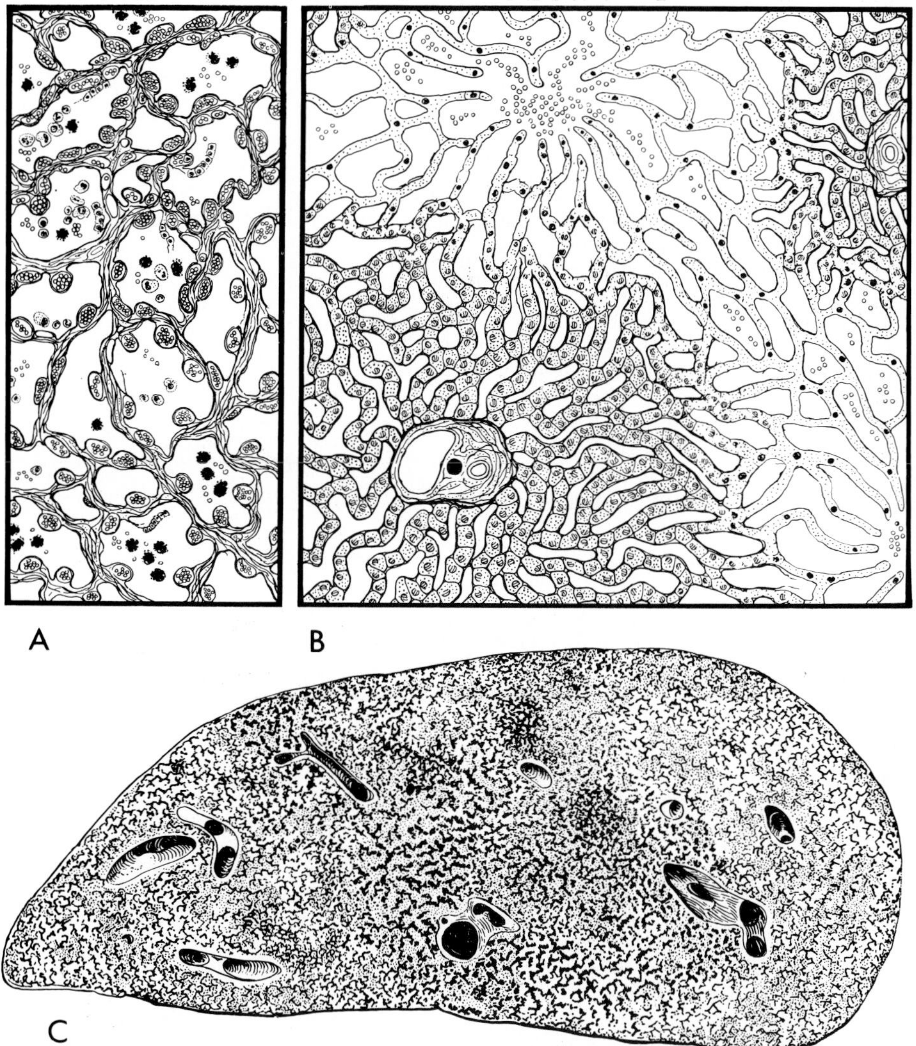

Figure 3–17. *A*, Chronic passive congestion of the lungs. Dilated capillaries bulge from the fibrotic alveolar septa. The alveolar lumina contain pigmented macrophages and chains of partly desquamated cuboidal alveolar epithelial cells. *B*, Chronic passive congestion of the liver. Note the dilated sinusoids and atrophic liver cells around the central vein in the upper center and the normal liver tissue around the portal tracts at the lower left and upper right. *C*, Chronic passive congestion of the liver. (From Fallis, B. D.: Textbook of Pathology. New York, McGraw-Hill, 1964. Reprinted by permission.)

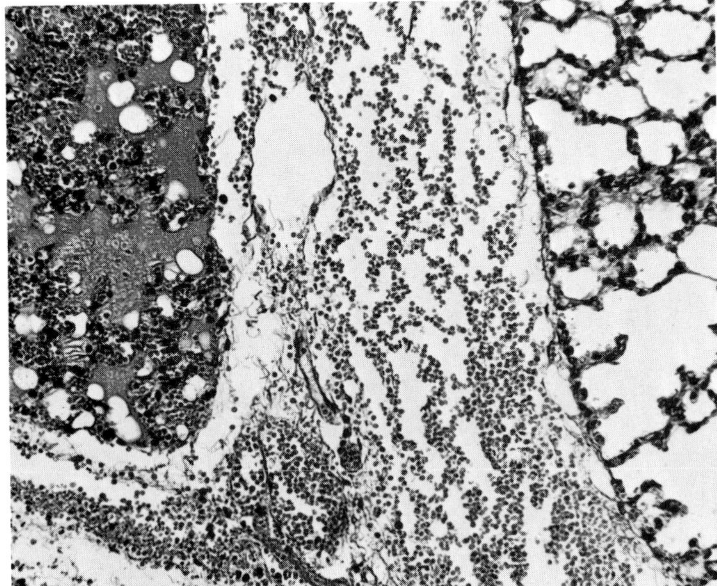

Figure 3–18. Hemorrhage between the lobules in a lung. Congestion edema and hemorrhage are present in the lobule to the left.

the cells simply flow out through a hole, or the cells may pass through an intact vascular wall by a process called ***diapedesis.*** Diapedesis occurs when there is increased venous hydrostatic pressure in vessels that are not visibly broken but perhaps somewhat anoxic and not functioning properly, or when the clotting mechanism is defective and the red cells seem to be able to pass through the wall very easily. Hemorrhage as a result of vascular damage may occur with ***inflammation, necrosis, trauma*** or ***neoplasia*** and is a very common lesion (Figs. 3–19, 3–20 and 3–21).

Specific adjectives are used to describe the gross appearance of hemorrhage. ***Petechial*** hemorrhage occurs as tiny, 1 to 2 mm foci. ***Ecchymotic*** hemorrhage occurs as larger areas up to 2 to 3 cm in size. ***Paintbrush*** type refers to extensive streaking

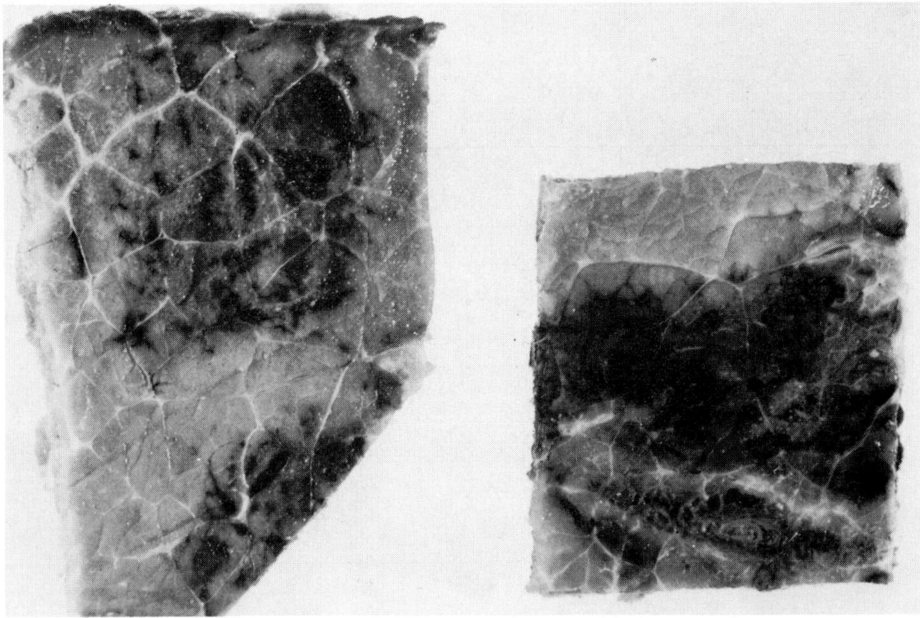

Figure 3–19. Hemorrhage in skeletal muscle of a calf caused by injection of an irritating drug.

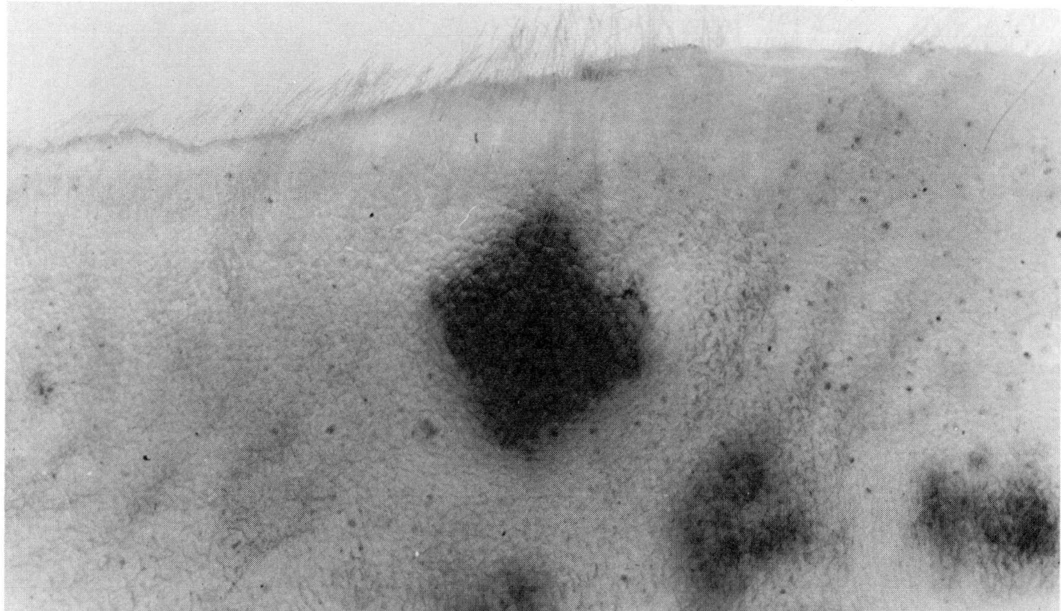

Figure 3–20. Congestion and hemorrhage in the skin of a pig with erysipelas—so-called diamond skin disease.

with hemorrhage, as if someone literally splashed red paint on the tissue. These three types usually occur on serosal or mucosal surfaces and are visible but cannot be palpated. When sufficient blood escapes and clots in one area to form a lump, the lesion is called a ***hematoma.*** It may vary in size from tiny to over a meter in diameter and is usually associated with trauma or a clotting defect (Figs. 3–22 through 3–30). Massive hemorrhage into a body cavity is called ***hemopericardium, hemothorax*** or ***hemoperitoneum,*** depending on the area affected.

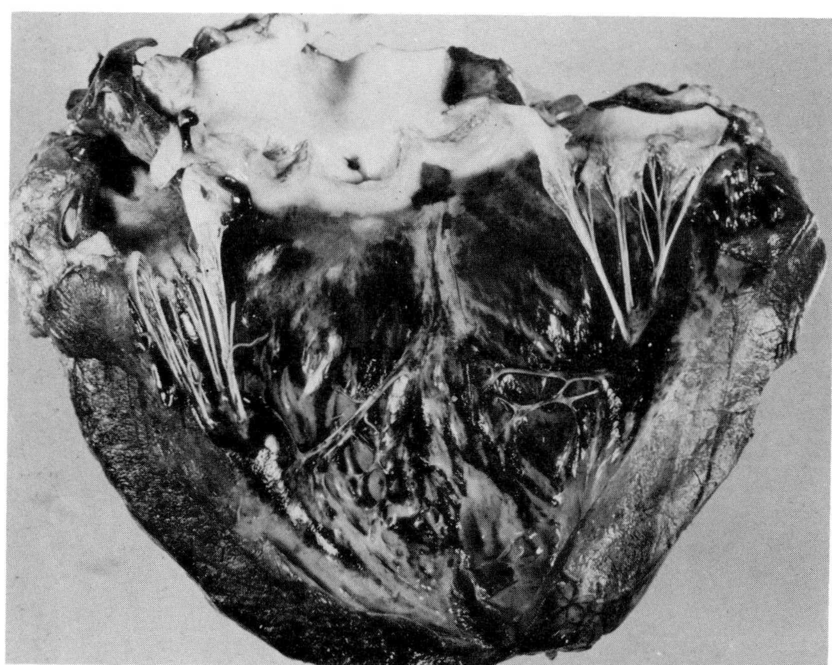

Figure 3–21. Paint-brush hemorrhage on the endocardium of a cow. These are usually agonal changes in cattle and horses and are very common.

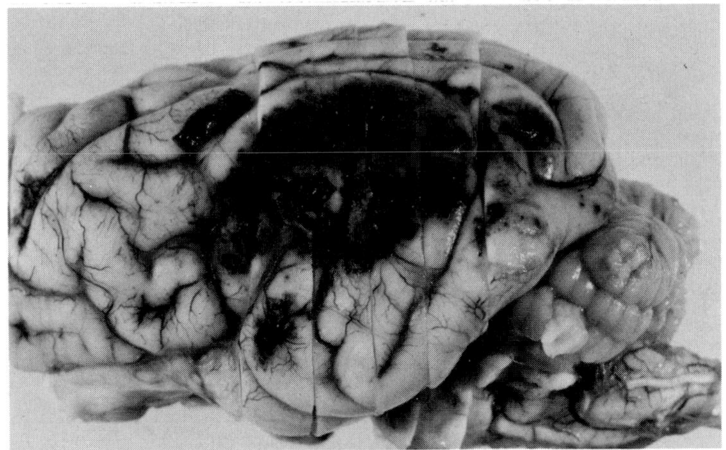

Figure 3–22

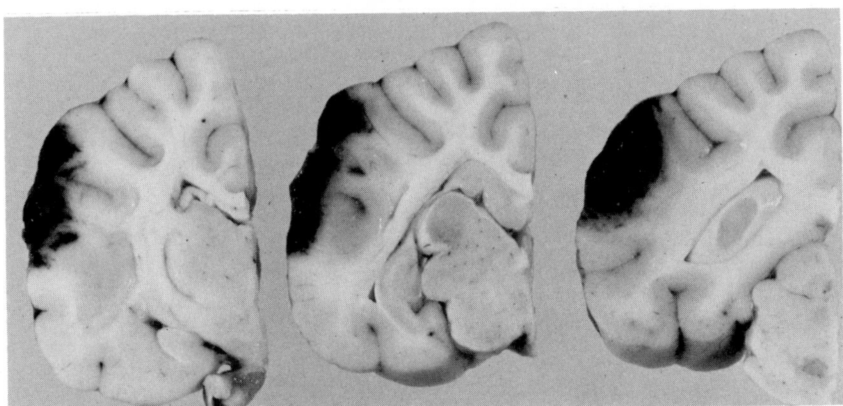

Figure 3–23

Figures 3–22 and 3–23. Hematoma in the cerebrum of a dog visible from the external surface (Fig. 3–22), as well as on the cut surface (Fig. 3–23).

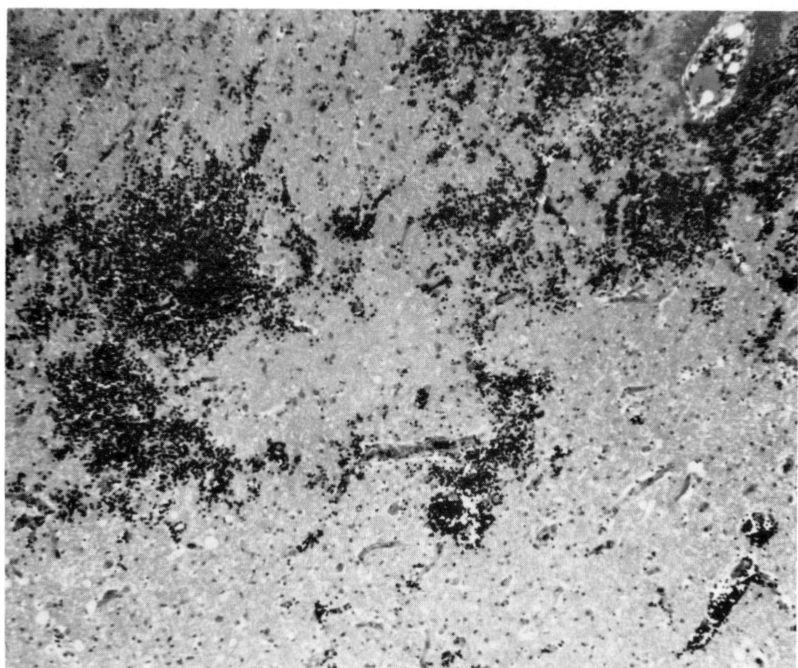

Figure 3–24. The microscopic appearance of the edge of the lesion seen in Figures 3–22 and 3–23.

Purpura is a clinical term applied to an animal that has extensive petechial and ecchymotic hemorrhages on serous and mucous surfaces (Fig. 3–31). It is a descriptive term and does not imply a specific disease. Purpura is characteristic of disease associated with platelets, including abnormal production, such as toxic depression or autoimmune depression. Platelets may be destroyed in excessive numbers as in autoimmune destruction or in disseminated intravascular coagulation, and these are loosely called consumptive "coagulopathies." Extensive and diffuse endothelial damage may also consume excessive numbers of platelets.

Ecchymotic and paint brush–type hemorrhages are often found at autopsy on the epicardial and endocardial surfaces of the heart in cattle and horses, as well as on the tracheal mucosa. These are often considered to be ***agonal,*** caused by labored breathing and terminal muscular activity in the process of dying. This lesion is often misinterpreted as being specifically associated with a septicemia (Fig. 3–21).

The ***color of hemorrhage*** depends on whether the blood was mainly arterial or venous, on the number of red cells in the lesion and on the amount of time elapsed since the hemorrhage occurred. Large collections of red cells are very dark in color because of the concentration and the anoxia. Microscopically, red cells are clearly visible in tissue outside of vessels and seem to be able to remain there intact for some days. They are disposed of by lysis or phagocytosis. Hemosiderin-laden macrophages and erythrophagocytosis are indications of former hemorrhage. A ***bruise*** is a result of hemorrhage, and the color arises from the color and number of red cells and their state of degeneration. Experimentally, muscle bruises at 8, 24 and 48 hours after injury in calves and lambs have characteristic features. Eight hour lesions have many red cells and many neutrophils but few macrophages. At 24 hours macrophages and neutrophils are present about equally, but by 48 hours macrophages far exceed neutrophils. Hemosiderin is present in macrophages by 48 hours. Fibroblasts and endothelial cells are greatly activated in the affected area. Gross examination reveals no differences in appearance until 48 hours, when a reddish-yellow color is evident in contrast to the reddish color of earlier lesions. Large numbers of macrophages of all shapes and sizes may be at work in a hematoma. Not all of the brown pigment

Text continued on page 119

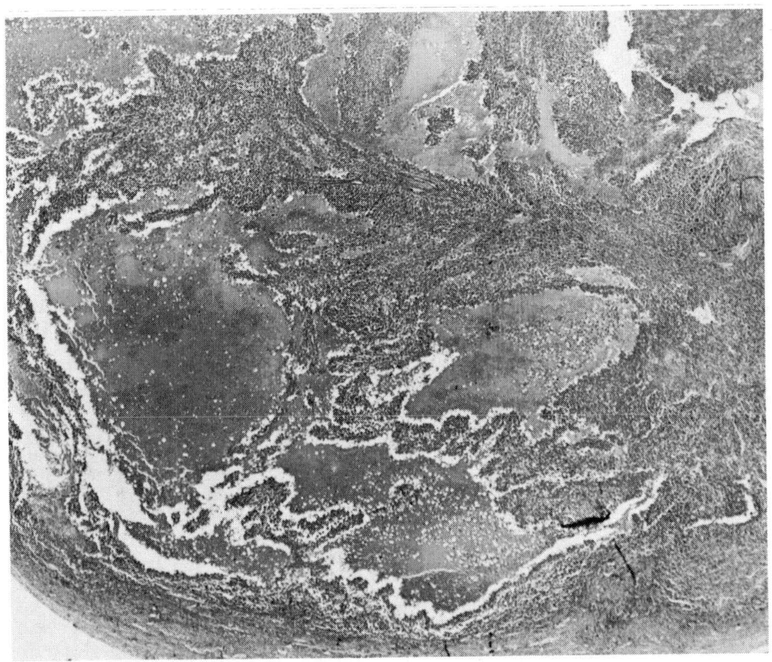

Figure 3–25

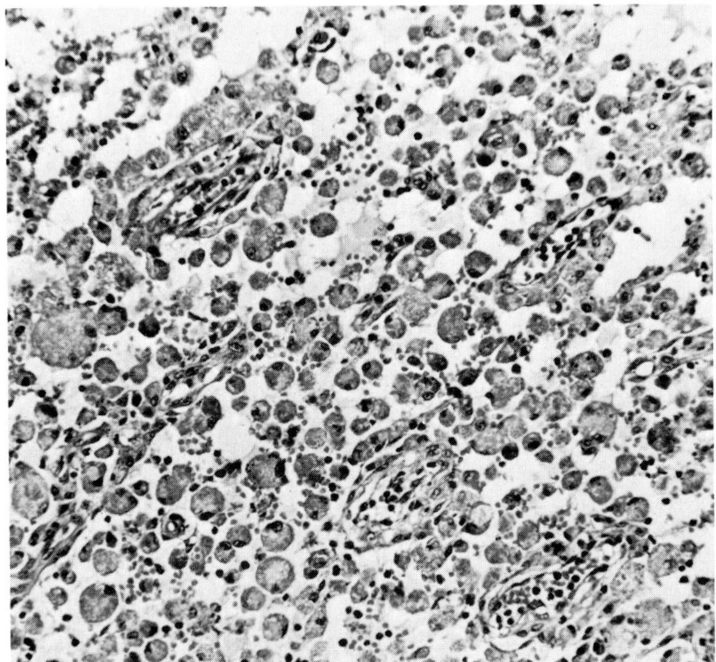

Figure 3–26

Figures 3–25, 3–26, and 3–27. A large subcutaneous hematoma containing islands of fluid and red blood cells surrounded by connective tissue stroma. Closer view is seen in Figure 3–26, with numerous macrophages ingesting free red cells. There are large numbers of variably sized macrophages (Fig. 3–27) that contain brown pigment (not visible in photo), some of which is hemosiderin and some of which is ceroid.

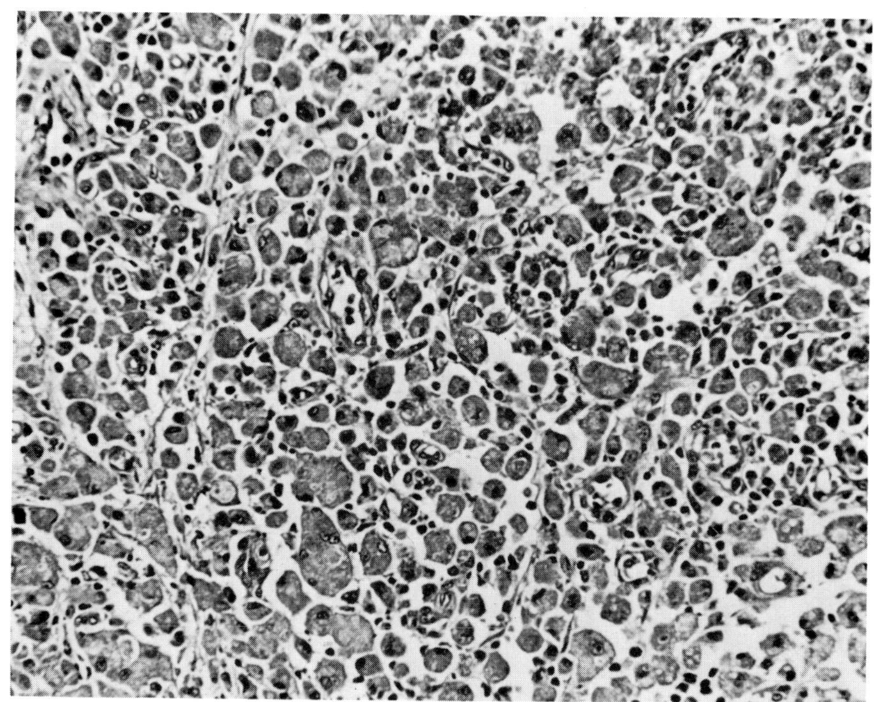

Figure 3–27. *See legend on the opposite page.*

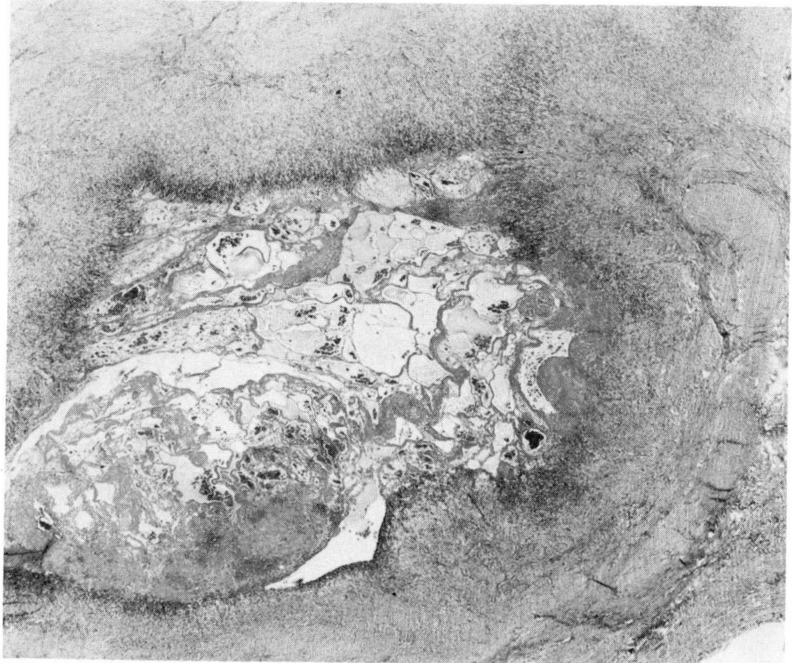

Figure 3–28. An old hematoma containing fibrin and fluid surrounded by a wall of connective tissue that is gradually filling in the space.

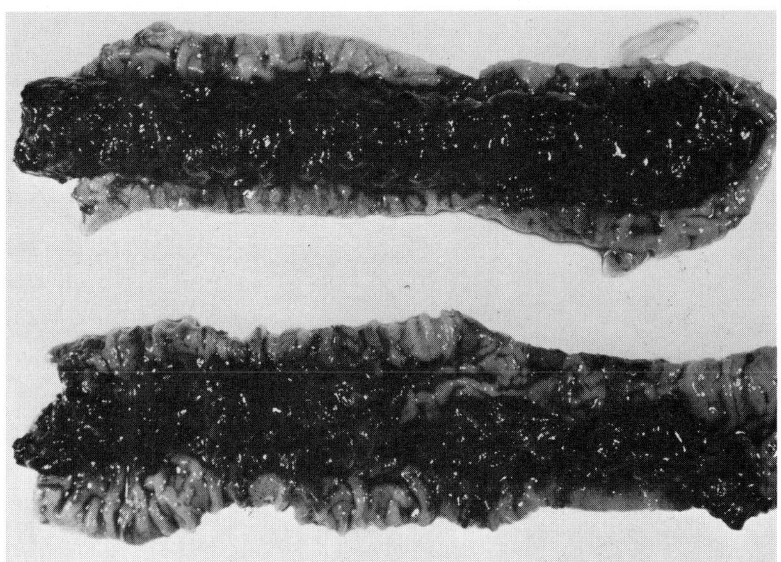

Figure 3–29. Hemorrhage into the intestinal lumen in a pig. Much of the blood has clotted. Such lesions occur in some acute bacterial infections such as those caused by *Campylobacter sputorum*.

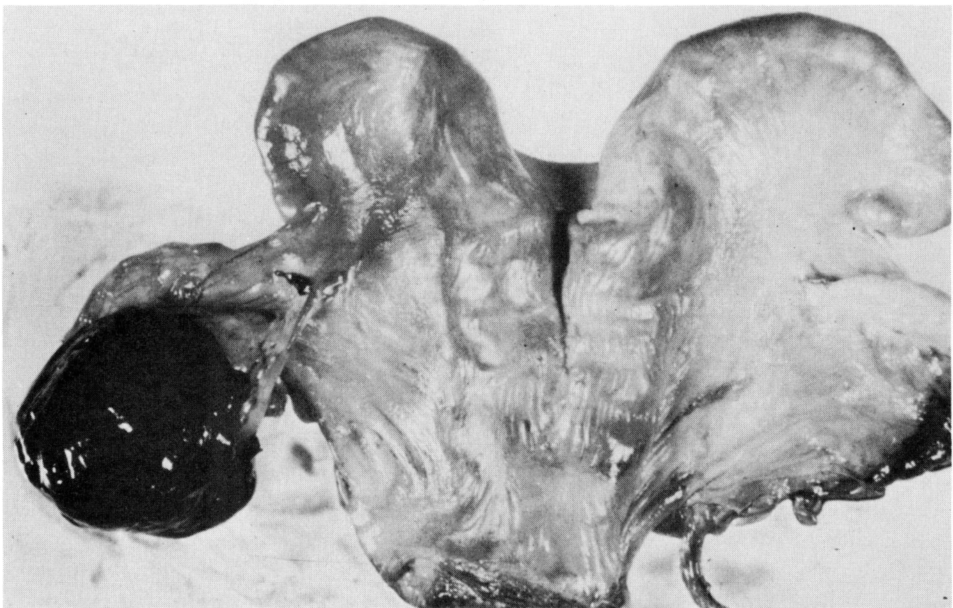

Figure 3–30. Hematoma in a cow's ovary due to trauma during rectal examination. It is not unusual for cows to bleed to death from such trauma.

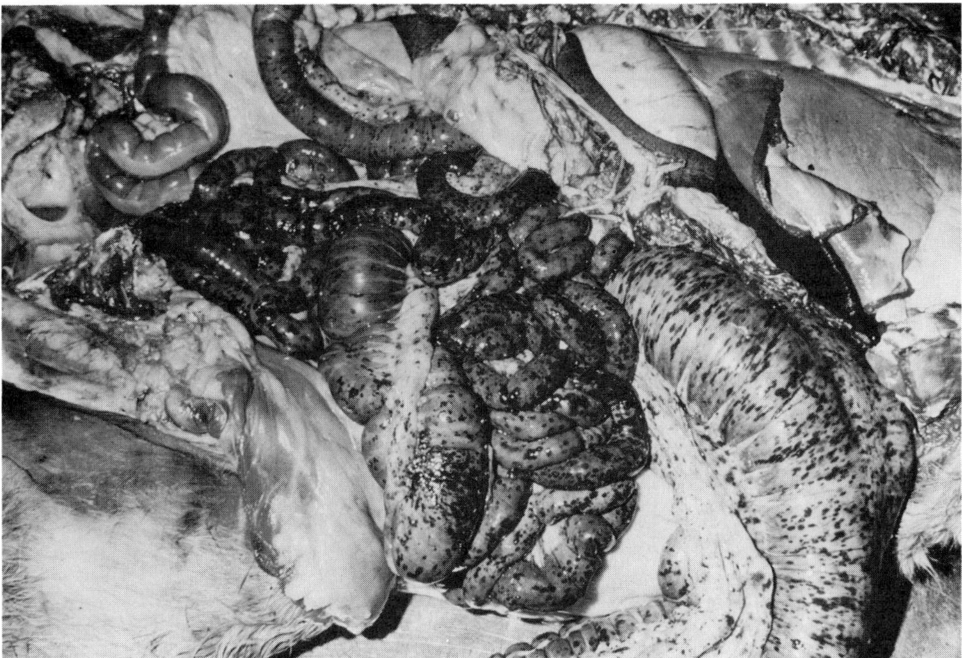

Figure 3–31. Petechial and ecchymotic hemorrhages and tiny hematomas on the serosal surfaces of the abdomen of a foal with purpura caused by an acute bacterial septicemia.

in the macrophages may be hemosiderin, since ceroid will probably be present—special stains will differentiate them.

Diseases that result in marked bleeding tendencies are named ***hemorrhagic diatheses.*** The basic problem usually is a clotting defect, either congenital or acquired. ***Congenital clotting defects*** are well known in humans and are being defined in animals with increasing frequency. Most steps in the clotting cascade may have defects to varying degrees, with the end result of each being a tendency to bleed after trauma (Table 3–2).

It should be clear that hemorrhage may occur in various circumstances from numerous etiological factors, many of which are not associated with inflammation. There is a tendency to consistently equate redness with inflammation and to refer to any redness as hemorrhagic. *This conclusion should never be taken for granted.* If the color of a tissue is abnormal because it is red, reddish-blue, blue or so dark as to be almost black, the color is due to red blood cells and either hyperemia, congestion, hemorrhage or some combination of the three. The problem is to decide, if possible, which it is and what its pathogenesis and significance are. *To call all such lesions hemorrhagic is to avoid making the real interpretation of the lesion.*

EDEMA

Edema is the abnormal accumulation of fluid ***in tissue spaces*** and is a ***lesion, not a specific disease.*** Causative factors in edema are as numerous as the many controls on volume and location of body fluids throughout the organism. In general, the etiology relates to hydrostatic pressure of blood, osmotic pressure of blood and tissue fluid, permeability of capillaries, lymphatic obstruction or any combination of these. Edema may be localized in a tissue or generalized in a large area or it may affect the whole body. The lesion may occur acutely, as in trauma or inflammation, or chronically, as in heart failure or renal disease. Edema can occur in any tissue, but some tissues have more space in which to accumulate fluid than others. If a tissue is literally filled with fluid, it will ooze through the surface. The lymphatic drainage takes care of normal fluid and will drain much

TABLE 3–2. SOME CAUSES OF HEMORRHAGE IN ANIMALS

Acquired Defect	Cause
Trauma	accident or surgical intervention
Poisoning	warfarin, moldy sweet clover, cottonseed meal, aspirin overdose
Vitamin deficiency	scurvy, absorptive failure, vitamin K deficiency
Liver disease	obstructive jaundice, infectious canine hepatitis, tumors, liver failure
Thrombocytopenia	idiopathic, virus, autoimmune disease, septicemia, splenomegaly, aplastic anemia
Intravascular coagulation and fibrinolysis syndrome	obstetrical complications, sepsis, malignancy, shock, liver disease, heart stroke, incompatible transfusions, heartworm disease
Platelet function defects	uremia, hyperestrogenism, allergies, drugs, chronic disease, malignancy
Drug-induced defects	aspirin, steroids, phenylbutazone (Butazolidin), live virus vaccines, nitrofurazones (Furacin), sulfonamides, antihistamines, local anesthetics, promazines, penicillins, phenothiazines, plasma expanders, anti-inflammatory drugs, estrogens
Hereditary Defect	**Cause**
Coagulation disorders	Hemophilias A and B, Factor VII deficiency, Factor X deficiency, Factor XI deficiency, von Willebrand's disease, hypoprothrombinemia, hypofibrinogenemia, afibrinogenemia
Platelet disorders	thrombasthenia, thrombocytopathy

(Courtesy of Jean Dodds.)

excess fluid, but it can be overloaded. The normal lymphatic drainage of tissues and organs for humans is described in Yoffee and Courtice (1970), and in general, drainage patterns are similar in animals.

Mechanisms of Edema Formation

Each of the ***main pathogenetic mechanisms*** of edema will be discussed. The normal control and relationships of tissue fluid must be clearly understood first (Fig. 3–32). The actual pressure values are included in Figure 3–33. The main ***filtration*** force that expels fluid from the vessel is the hydrostatic pressure at the arterial end of the capillary minus the osmotic pressure of the blood. The main ***absorption*** force that draws fluid into the vessel is the osmotic pressure of the blood minus the hydrostatic pressure at the venous end of the capillary.

HYDROSTATIC PRESSURE

Hydrostatic pressure of the blood is influenced mainly at the venous end of the capillary. Most important is an increase created by back pressure in the venous circulation. The increase in pressure pushing out counterbalances the osmotic pressure pulling in, and therefore the fluid ***fails to return*** to the vessel from the interstitial tissue. This mechanism predominates in chronic passive congestion (cardiac edema) and in any lesion in which the venous flow is obstructed (such as a twisted bowel).

OSMOTIC PRESSURE

Variations in osmotic pressure result from reduced plasma protein levels in blood and may occur from decreased formation or excessive loss of plasma from the blood. Albumin is most important in the maintenance of osmotic pressure and has four times the osmotic pressure of globulins. Failure to form plasma proteins results from malnutrition, usually in the form of emaciation, in which the building blocks for proteins are not available. Loss of protein may also occur through the intestine or kidney. Loss from the kidney is called the nephrotic syndrome; this syndrome may result from many causes, of which amyloidosis is one example. Defects in glomerular filtration mechanisms allow protein to be lost into the urine, and this is one of the reasons for checking urine for protein in routine clinical examination. A low osmotic pressure in the blood reduces the force to pull fluid in at the venous end of capillaries and also increases the pressure differential at the arterial end so that more fluid is pushed out.

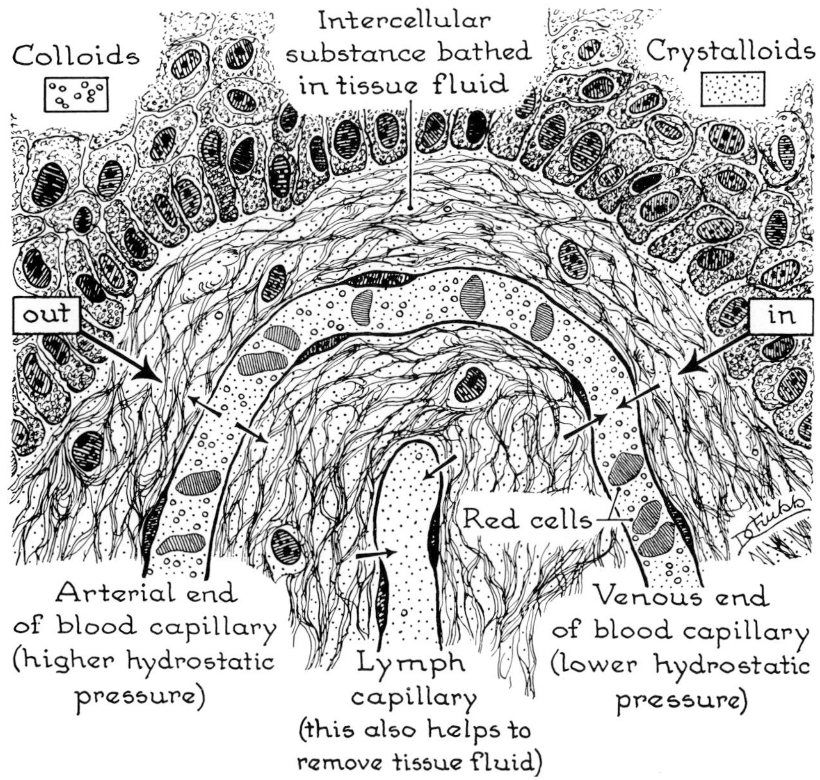

Figure 3–32. A diagram to show how tissue fluid is formed by capillaries and absorbed by capillaries and lymphatics. The colloids of the blood are represented as small circles and the crystalloids of blood and tissue fluid are represented as dots. Under normal conditions, only a very little colloid escapes from most capillaries, and the colloid that does escape is returned to the circulation by way of the lymphatics. (From Ham, A. W.: Histology. 6th ed. Philadelphia, J. B. Lippincott, 1969. Reprinted by permission.)

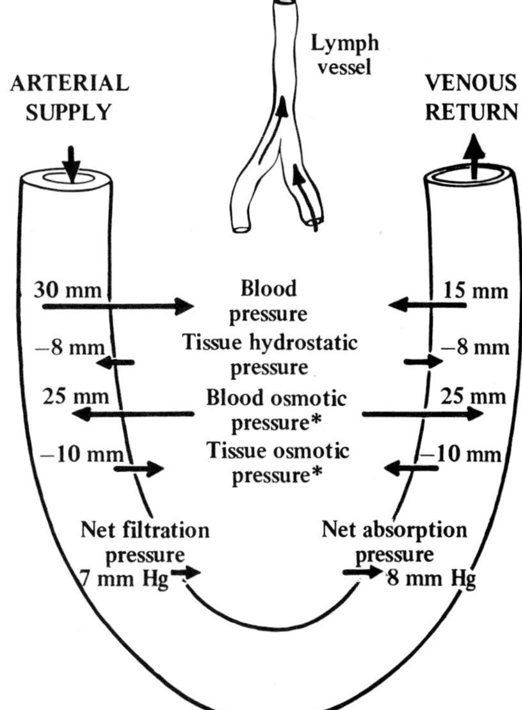

Figure 3–33. Capillary filtration and reabsorption ("Starling hypothesis"). The starred osmotic pressures are actually only due to the protein content of the respective fluids. They do not represent the total osmotic pressure. (From Harper, H. A.: Review of Physiological Chemistry. 15th ed. Los Altos, California, Lange Medical Publications, 1975. Reprinted by permission.)

This type of edema is sometimes called ***renal edema*** or ***debilitation edema.***

PERMEABILITY

Permeability changes result from ***direct damage,*** as in trauma or inflammation, and also from ***anoxia,*** as in heart failure. Endothelium is permeable to water and crystalloids, so the factors on either side of the endothelium may be more important than the endothelium itself. Injury to vessels and basement membrane allows plasma protein to leak into the tissue space, thus increasing the hydrostatic and osmotic pressures there, which in turn tends to hold fluid. Usually, this type of edema is localized and is called ***inflammatory edema.*** There is a variation in the structure of capillaries (Fig. 3–34), and edema may occur more easily from some than from others.

LYMPHATIC OBSTRUCTION

Lymphatic obstruction may occur when any lesion impedes normal lymphatic drainage by pressure or obstruction. Excess tissue fluid accumulates because normal amounts of lymph are still being formed. This type of edema is often associated with tumors that grow into and block lymphatics or with severe inflammation in which swelling impedes lymphatic flow.

The four pathogenetic mechanisms are summarized in Figures 3–35 through 3–38.

Recognition of Edema

Edema is recognized by ***excess clear fluid*** and is most easily visualized beneath the skin or between the layers of mucous membranes or the lobules in the lung, where there is space for accumulation to occur. The gray pattern of distended lymphatic vessels is visible in serosal surfaces such as the pleura or mesentery. Blood cells may be present in all proportions with the edema, depending on the etiological factors involved. Edema is more difficult to recognize grossly in a solid organ such as the kidney, which may be quite *swollen* although fluid is not visible. Sometimes the edema fluid will have a ***yellowish tinge,*** which indicates that the damage to vessels has allowed much plasma protein to escape from the tissue.

Microscopically, the appearance of edema is variable. If little or no protein is present in the fluid, it will be invisible and may only be detected by recognizing ***dilation of lymphatics*** in the tissue. They can dilate to amazing proportions. If protein is present, the dilated lymphatics will contain light ***pink***-staining fluid on hemotoxylin-eosin preparation that will become increasingly red with the increased percentage of protein in the fluid. The color variation may be an indication of the ***extent of vascular damage*** in an inflammatory lesion. In some edematous lesions, dilated lymphatics do not stand out and excess protein is not visible but there is a general spreading out of tissue components. This type may be difficult to recognize (Figs. 3–39 through 3–45). Large amounts of fluid will exude from the cut surface of an edematous organ such as the lung, if left in a tray. Edematous organs are wet and heavy (Figs. 3–46 through 3–48). If edema persists for a long time, it will induce the formation of ***connective tissue*** and cause permanent thickening in the tissue. Extreme edema in the entire body, as occurs in some aborted fetuses, is called ***anasarca.*** Special fixatives, such as Bouin's, will retain edema fluid better than formalin.

Pulmonary edema is a common lesion and is often the immediate cause of death in many different disease conditions, even though the specific etiology may not be clear. Edema is such a characteristic lesion in some specific diseases that it is incorporated into the name of the disease, e.g., "gut edema" caused by ***Escherichia coli*** in pigs and "malignant edema" caused by ***Clostridium septicum*** in several species. The "bottle jaw" of sheep with haemonchosis is subcutaneous edema, as is "stalking up" in the limbs of horses.

Edema is easily overlooked and underestimated both grossly and microscopically. Look for it carefully.

Fluid in Body Cavities

Excess fluid ***in a body cavity*** may be called hydrothorax, hydropericardium, hy-

Text continued on page 131

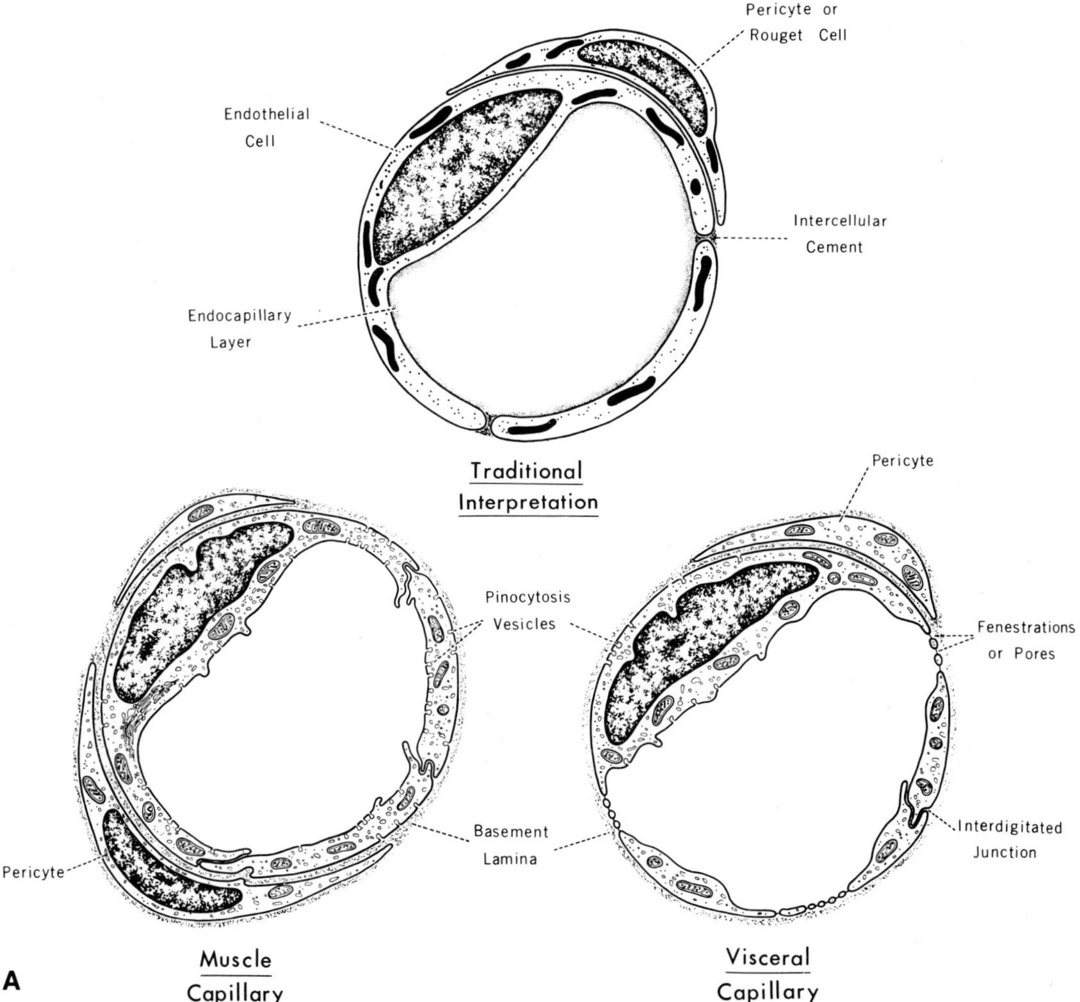

Figure 3–34. *A*, The top drawing illustrates capillary structure as visualized when only the light microscope was available. Endothelial cells were supposed to be joined edge to edge by an appreciable amount of intercellular cement, and their inner surfaces were thought to be coated with absorbed protein. The nature of the pericapillary cell was not established, and the existence of a basement membrane, the pinocytotic vesicles, and the fenestrations in visceral capillaries, which are seen with the electron microscope and shown in the lower drawings, was not known. (From Bloom, W., and Fawcett, D. W.: A Textbook of Histology. 9th ed. Philadelphia, W. B. Saunders Company, 1968.)

(Illustration continued on following page)

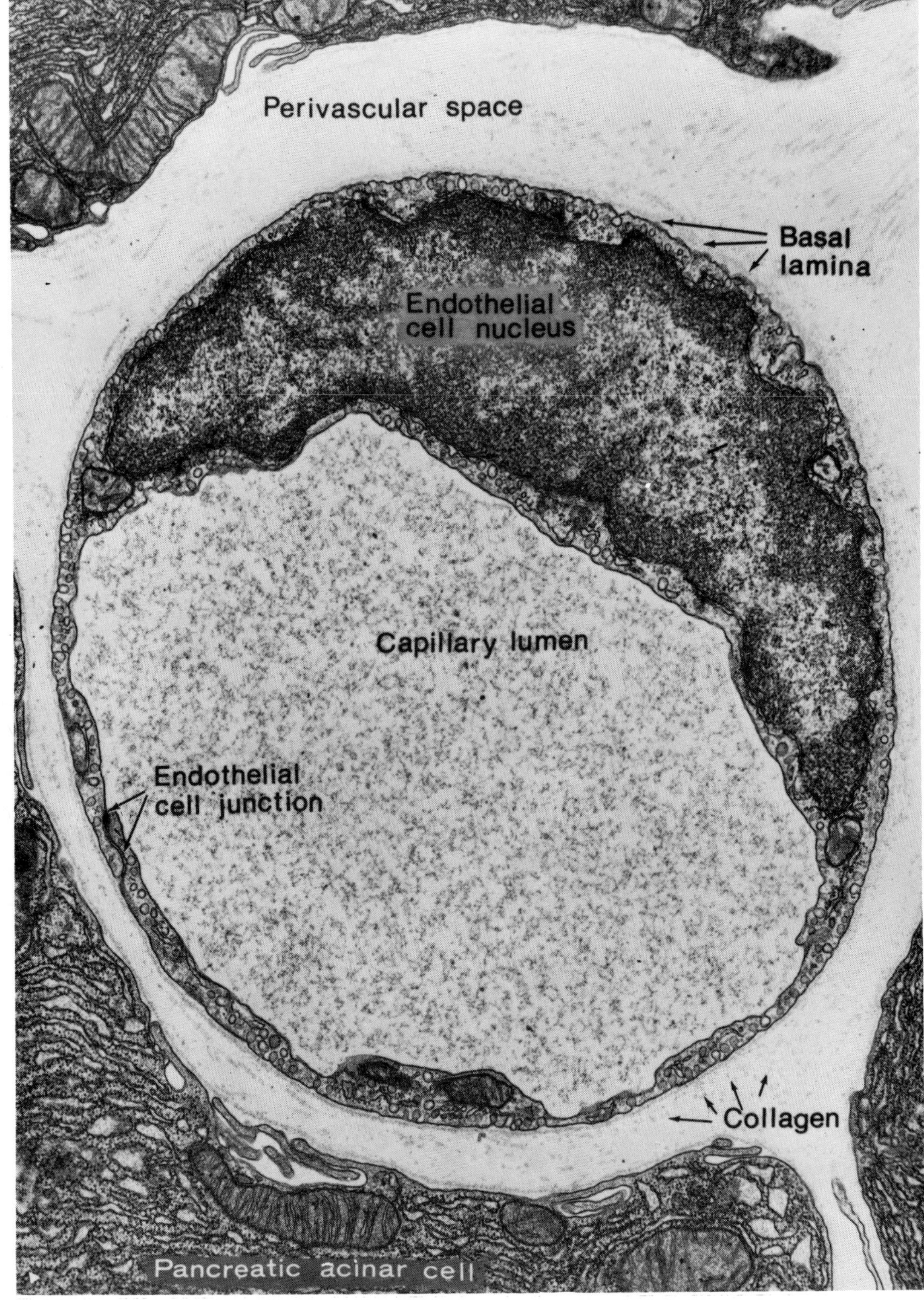

B

Figure 3–34 *Continued. B,* Ultrastructure of a capillary. (Courtesy of R. Bodender.)

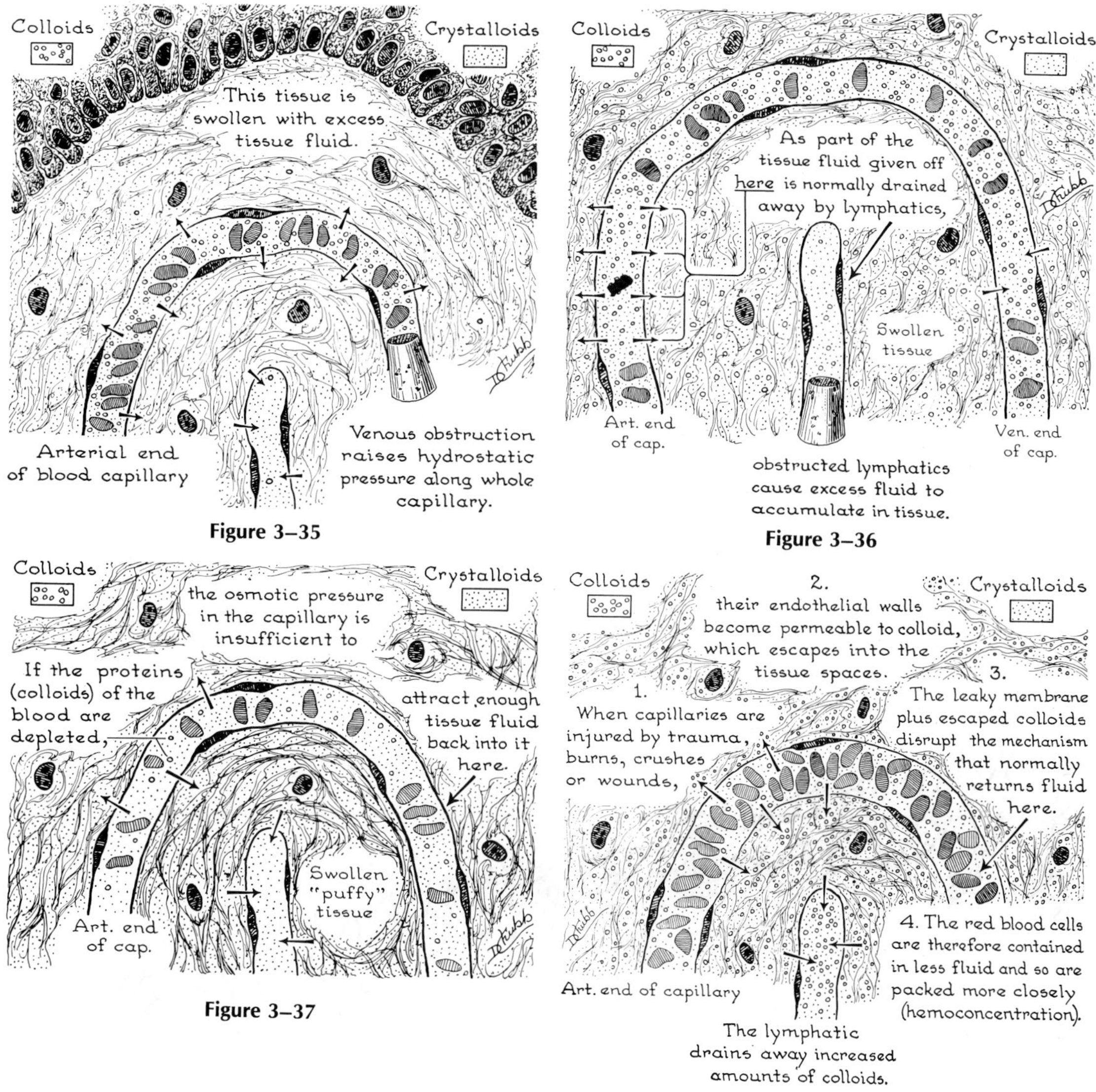

Figure 3–35. Diagram showing how an obstruction to the outflow of blood from the capillaries (back pressure on veins) can cause an increased amount of tissue fluid to form from the capillaries and also interfere with its absorption.

Figure 3–36. Diagram showing how the obstruction of lymphatics may cause an increased amount of tissue fluid to be present in the tissues they normally drain. It should also be observed that the amount of colloid in the tissue fluid increases when lymphatics are obstructed, because such colloid as normally escapes from the capillaries is normally drained away by the lymphatics.

Figure 3–37. Diagram showing how a lack of colloid in the blood increases the amount of tissue fluid.

Figure 3–38. Diagram showing how plasma escapes when the endothelial walls of capillaries are injured by burns, crushes, nearby wounds, or other means. Notice that as plasma leaks away from the capillary, the number of red blood cells in relation to plasma increases. This is called hemoconcentration. Observe also how, under conditions of this sort, increased amounts of colloid are drained away by the lymphatic capillaries. (From Ham, A. W.: Histology. 6th ed. Philadelphia, J. B. Lippincott, 1969. Courtesy of D. W. Fawcett. Reprinted by permission.)

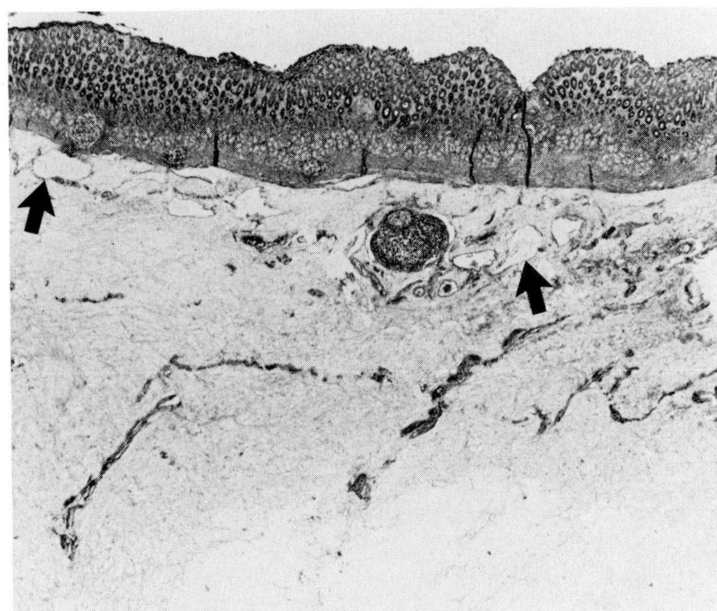

Figure 3–39. Submucosal gastric edema in a pig with gut edema. Note the separation of submucosal stroma and dilated lymphatic vessels (arrows).

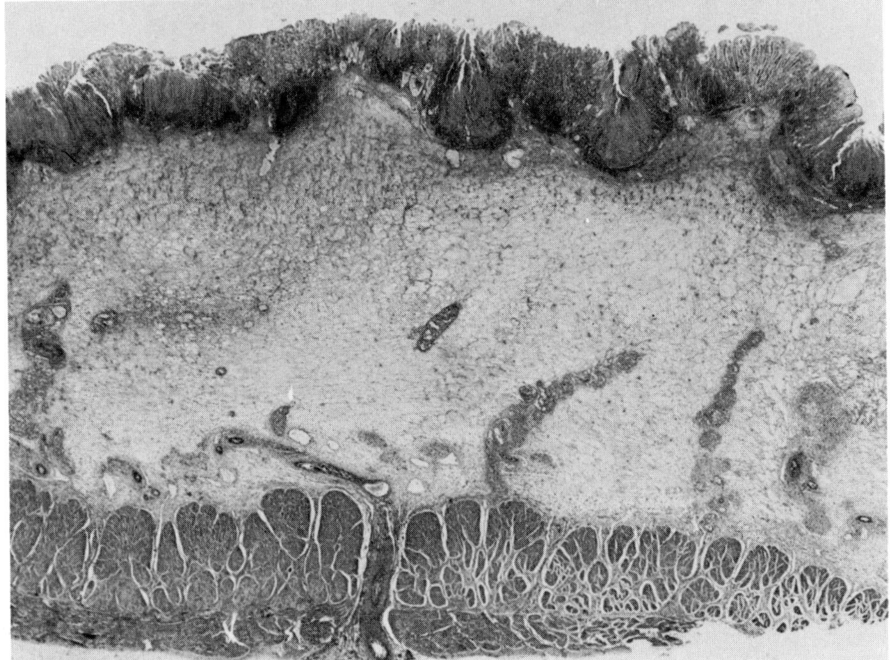

Figure 3–40. Submucosal edema in the abomasum of a calf. Mucosa is at top, and muscle layers are at bottom. Note the thickness of the entire wall.

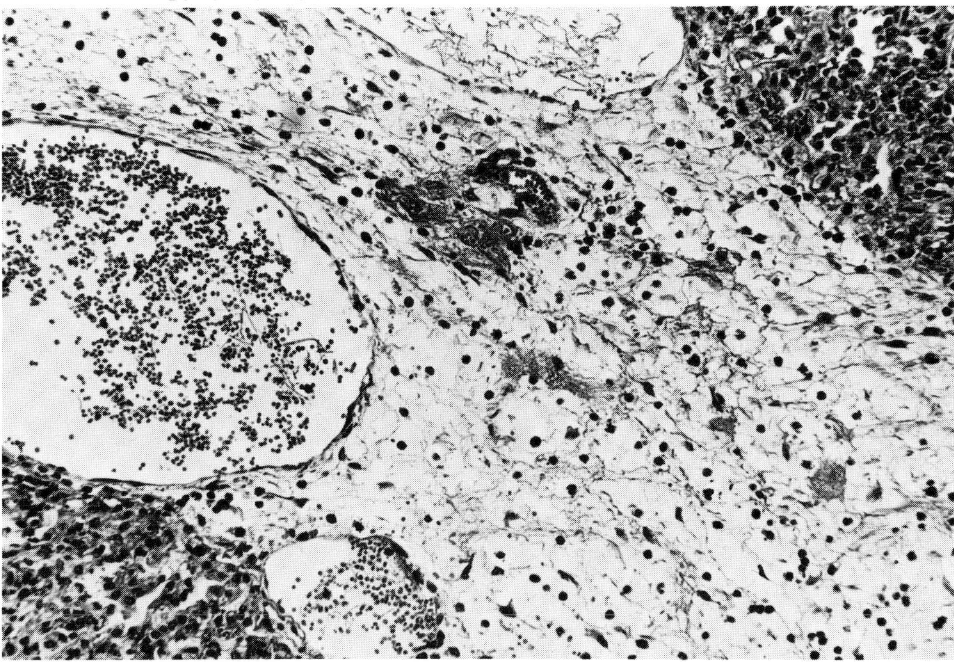

Figure 3–41. Pulmonary edema with dilated interlobular lymphatic vessels containing red cells and bits of fibrin. There is diffuse accumulation of fluid that has spread all of the components in the interlobular septum.

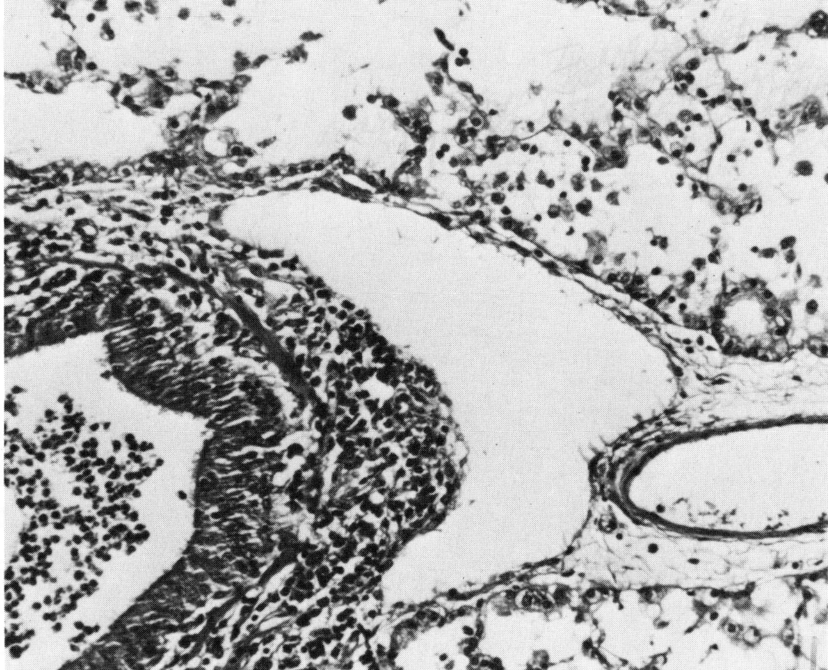

Figure 3–42. Lung of a pig. From left to right, a bronchiole, a dilated lymphatic vessel, and a vein. The dilated lymphatic vessel is filled with fluid that contains very little protein and therefore does not stain.

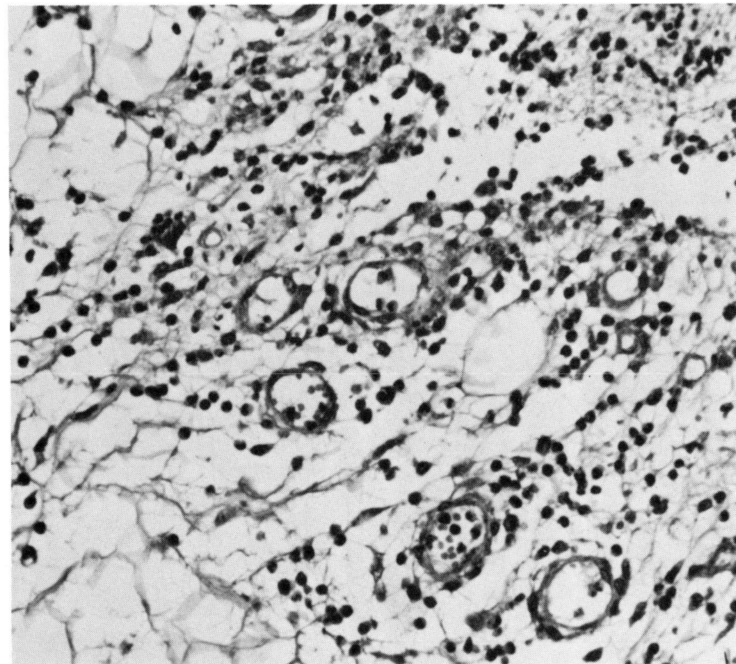

Figure 3–43. Loose areolar tissue around a synovial membrane spread out and separated by edema in an early inflammation of the joint. This type of lesion is not often easily recognized and may be overlooked.

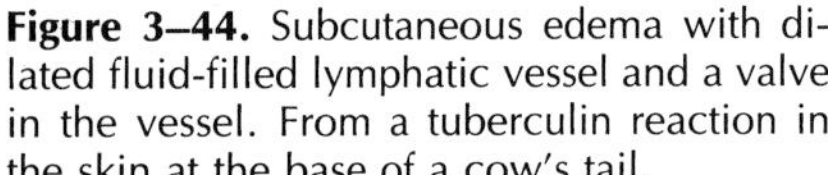

Figure 3–44. Subcutaneous edema with dilated fluid-filled lymphatic vessel and a valve in the vessel. From a tuberculin reaction in the skin at the base of a cow's tail.

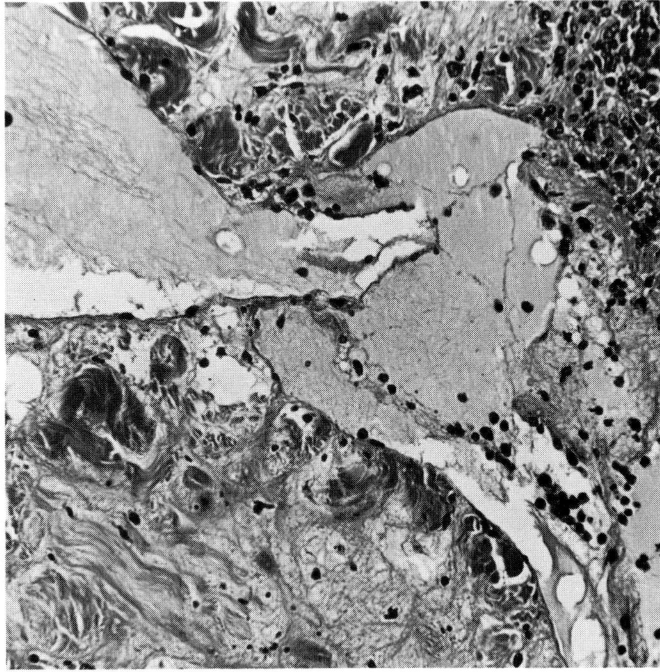

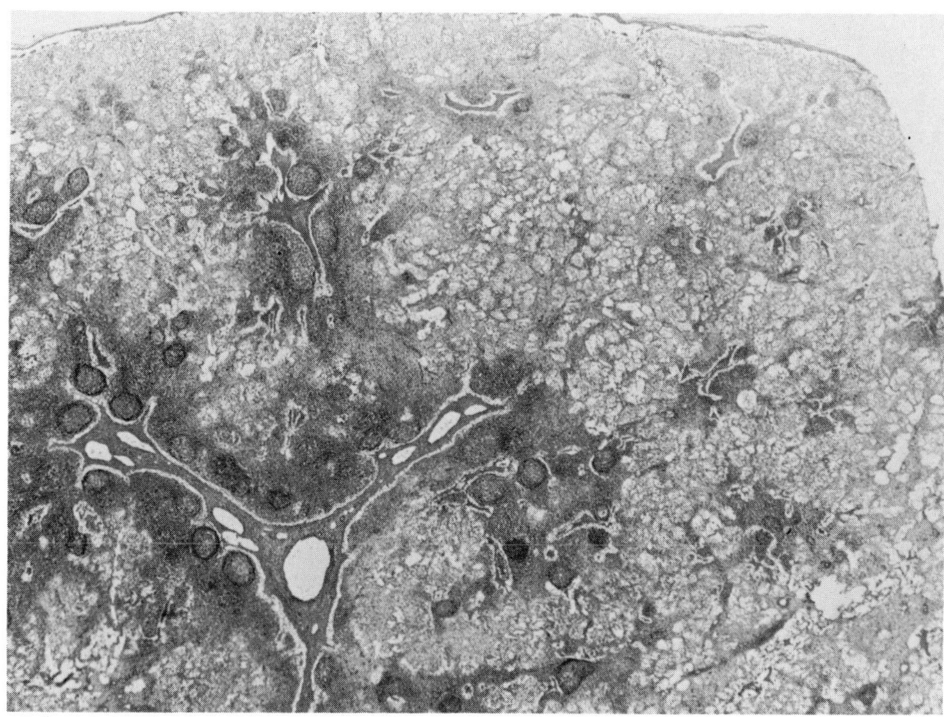

Figure 3–45. Edematous lymph node in a pig. Note the expansion of the medullary regions. Grossly, this node would be large and wet.

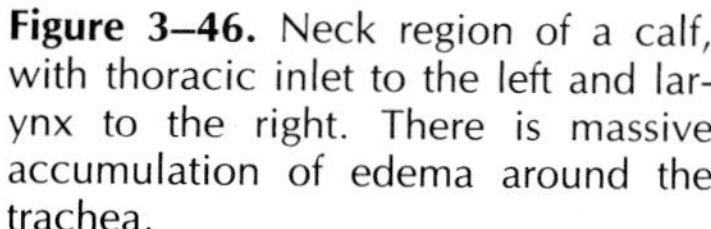

Figure 3–46. Neck region of a calf, with thoracic inlet to the left and larynx to the right. There is massive accumulation of edema around the trachea.

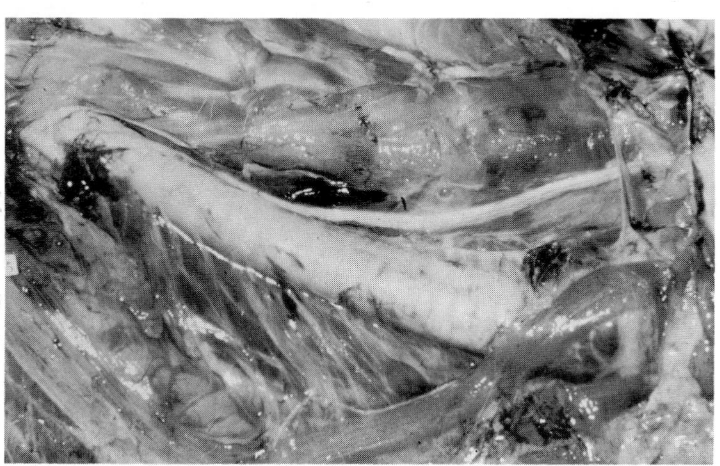

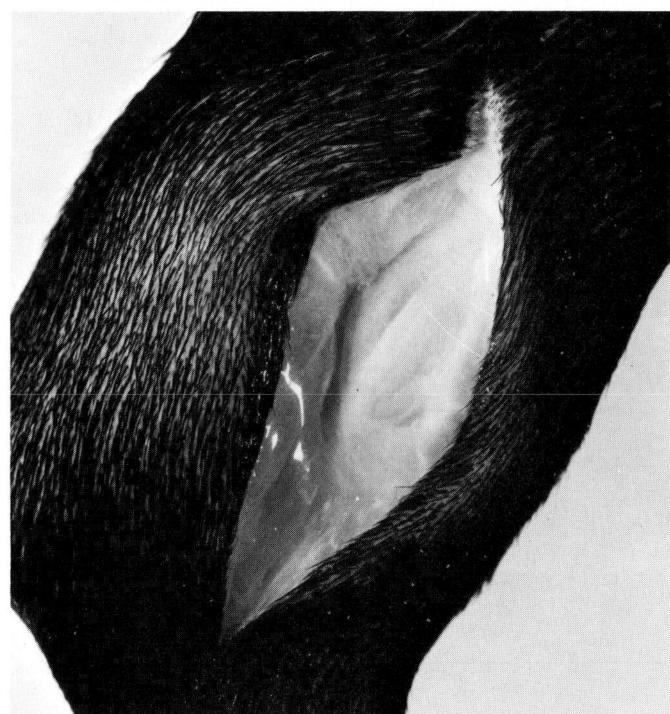

Figure 3–47. A dog's leg with very extensive subcutaneous edema.

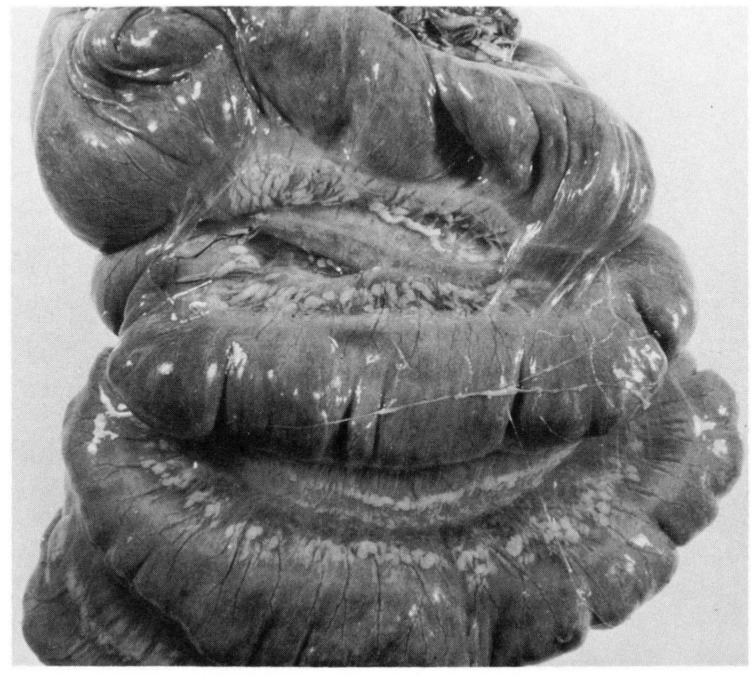

Figure 3–48. Subserosal edema in the mesentery of a pig and strands of fibrin on a shiny serosal surface. Similar strands of fibrin are often found on serosal surfaces at postmortem examination and are associated with edema of the organ concerned. Edema in this area is common in cases of gut edema of pigs.

drocele or ascites. If considerable protein is present in these fluids, some degree of coagulation may occur, especially on exposure to air, resulting in a yellow to white colored coagulum in the fluid. ***Hydrothorax*** arises from leakage of surface pleural lymphatic vessels in very edematous lungs. This is often prominent in left-sided heart failure. ***Hydropericardium*** arises from excess flow of lymph from within the myocardium, usually as a result of vascular damage or degeneration in the myocardium. It is a characteristic lesion of mulberry heart disease in pigs (Fig. 3–49).

Ascites occurs by several means. (1) Chronic passive congestion or right heart failure consistently causes ascites through increased venous hydrostatic pressure in abdominal organs, particularly in the liver. Most of the fluid leaks through the capsule of the liver into the abdomen. Obstruction to flow in the vena cava by a lesion such as a liver abscess results in a situation within the abdomen that is similar to right-sided heart failure. Chronic liver disease, particularly fibrosing obstructive lesions and chronic congestion, may also be a cause of ascites. In such cases, the portal venous flow will not pass through the liver easily, and there is increased venous hydrostatic pressure in the portal system. Edema occurs in the intestines, in the mesentery and in the abdominal cavity. (2) In chronic renal disease, the flow of blood in the kidney may be reduced, which activates the renin system and eventually raises the blood volume and the intravascular hydrostatic pressure. (3) Hypoproteinemia results in generalized edema and ascites because the fluid remains in tissues. (4) Some tumors that are implanted in the abdominal cavity spread or are carried to the lymphatic vessels in the ventral diaphragm, through which lymph normally flows into the thorax. The tumor cells grow into these lymphatic vessels, blocking them and thus preventing drainage of abdominal fluid. This occurs in some ovarian and some intestinal tumors. The points at which lymphatic or venous obstruction may occur and thus induce ascites are shown in Figures 3–50 and 3–51.

THROMBOSIS, ISCHEMIA AND INFARCTION

The clotting system is designed to operate when blood is removed or escapes from a blood vessel, usually because of injury. The process of ***hemostasis*** consists of the key processes of vasoconstriction, clumping of platelets and formation of fibrin. Strictly speaking, ***coagulation*** refers only to the formation of fibrin.

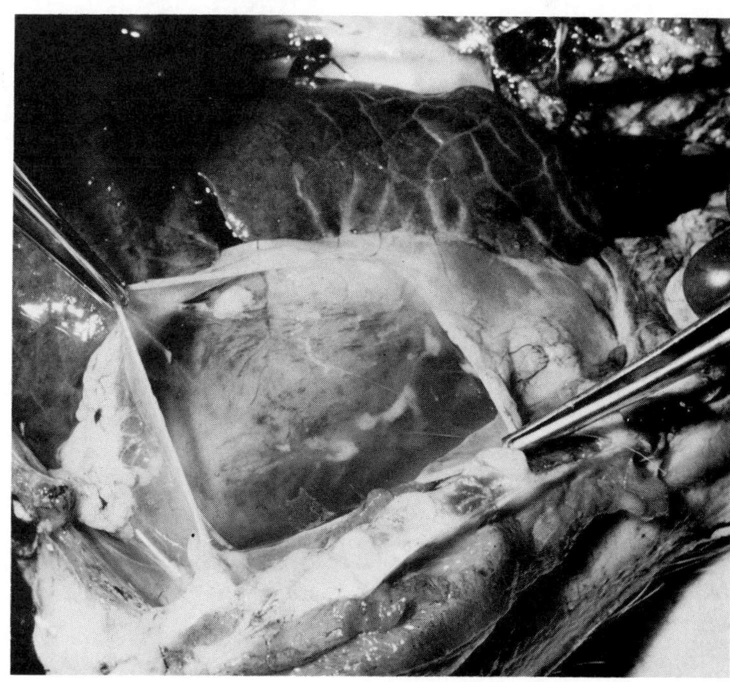

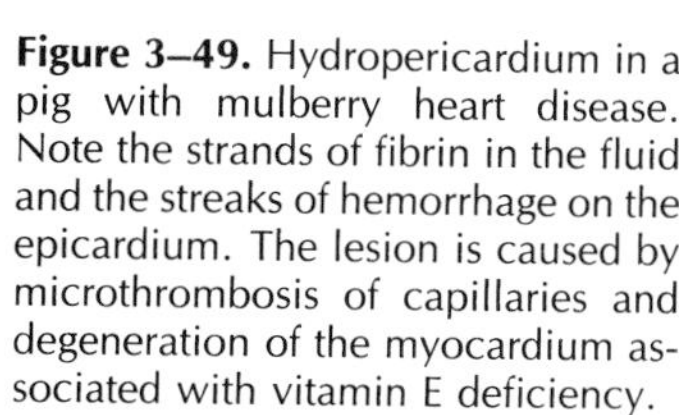

Figure 3–49. Hydropericardium in a pig with mulberry heart disease. Note the strands of fibrin in the fluid and the streaks of hemorrhage on the epicardium. The lesion is caused by microthrombosis of capillaries and degeneration of the myocardium associated with vitamin E deficiency.

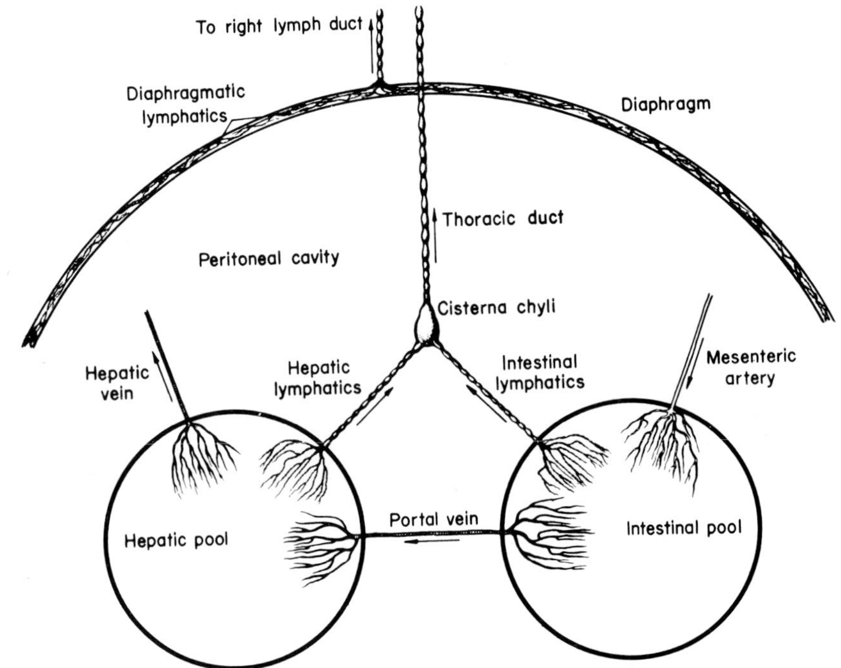

Figure 3–50. Diagrammatic representation of tissue fluid pools and their lymphatic drainage, implicated in the formation of ascites. (From Yoffey, J. M., and Courtice, F. C.: Lymphatics, Lymph and the Lymphomyeloid Complex. New York, Academic Press, 1970. Reprinted by permission.)

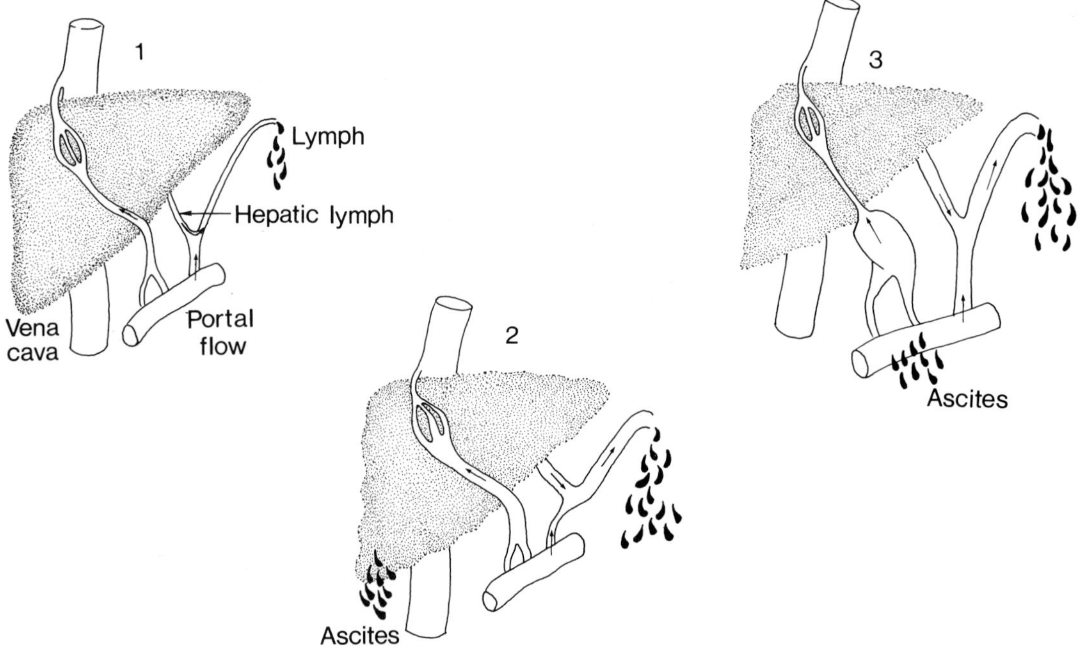

Figure 3–51. Formation of ascites. *1,* Normal flow. *2,* Outflow impediment due to physical obstruction, such as an abscess or increased venous hydrostatic pressure as in right-sided heart failure. The result is increased flow of lymph from the liver and leakage through the capsule to form ascitic fluid. *3,* Chronic obstructive lesion in the liver, such as fibrosis. The result is leakage of fluid from the intestinal serosa due to increased venous hydrostatic pressure to form ascitic fluid and increased lymphatic drainage from the abdomen. (Modified from Yoffey, J. M., and Courtice, F. C.: Lymphatics, Lymph and the Lymphomyeloid Complex. New York, Academic Press, 1970. Reprinted by permission.)

A ***thrombus*** is a solid structure formed ***in*** the blood stream ***from*** the normal constituents of the blood, and the process by which it forms is called ***thrombosis.*** Thrombi are different from extravascular and postmortem clots. They are composed of platelets, fibrin and red and white blood cells in varying proportions, depending on local circumstances.

Thrombosis usually begins with platelets becoming sticky and adhering to each other and to the endothelium. They may separate or degenerate and lyse in clumps, depending on the nature of the etiology. Clumping may be induced by contact with bacteria, collagen, basement membrane or injured endothelial cells, possibly as the result of an injury to a blood vessel. The clumped platelets attempt to plug up any defect that might allow blood to leave the vessel. Clumped or degenerate platelets release thromboplastin, which activates the formation of thrombin, which in turn activates the formation of fibrin from fibrinogen (see Fig. 3–2). The formation of thrombin may occur by way of either the intrinsic or the extrinsic clotting system. The ***intrinsic*** system involves activation of the stepwise series of enzyme reactions to form thrombin. The ***extrinsic*** system involves contact of blood with lipoproteins from tissue debris, which are called ***thromboplastin*** (see Fig. 3–3). Many of the components of hemostasis and thrombosis are the same. Normal hemostasis is designed to stop bleeding by plugging a hole inward from the outside, and then just to the edge of the hole. Thrombosis fills the hole from the inside and by doing so creates a physical mass, the thrombus, in the lumen. Before considering the fate of the mass, attention will be given to how it is built.

Causes of Thrombosis

The main factors influencing the formation of a thrombus are the rate of blood flow and flow patterns, the blood vessel wall and the composition of blood itself.

RATE OF FLOW AND TURBULENCE

Mechanical factors relate primarily to the ***rate of flow*** and the ***turbulence*** of blood. In arterial blood, the platelets travel midstream and do not easily reach the endothelial surface unless the rate of flow reduces, turbulence occurs or there is a major injury to the endothelial surface. Any platelets that do attach to the surface are easily swept off by flow and pulsation. If injury to the endocardium or endothelium of large arteries does occur, any thrombus that forms will initially be composed of mostly platelets and fibrin because the rate of flow usually sweeps red and white cells away, although white cells stick more easily than red cells do. Once a mound forms, turbulence becomes a factor and more blood cells may be caught up in the fibrin, partly because fibrin is chemotactic for neutrophils. ***The fibrin, platelets and white cells account for the white color of arterial thrombi.***

In veins, the slower flow allows the whole process to occur more quickly. These thrombi are more loosely arranged and often contain more red cells than arterial thrombi do. Also venous thrombi tend to be larger and extend as a tail downstream from the original site as the flow is further reduced and the turbulence occurs below the site of origin. Venous thrombi tend to begin near valves and venous plexuses, both of which involve turbulence in a slow flow pattern (Fig. 3–52). In both instances, bits may break off and travel either to an end artery or back to the lungs via veins. Formation of red venous thrombi often results from predisposing factors, such as shock or heart failure that slow blood flow, and possibly from local injury.

INJURY TO THE VESSEL WALL

Injury of any type to the vessel wall may induce thrombosis, with the degree and acuteness of injury being proportional to the degree of thrombosis (Fig. 3–53). Beneath the endothelium lies any one or a combination of the following: basement membrane, subendothelial microfibrils or elastin. ***Each of these may react with components of the blood by different biochemical processes in the induction of a thrombus.*** Outside of these lie collagen fibers that react with blood in still a different manner. Venous, but not arterial, endothelium can release thromboplastin, which takes part in fibrinolytic activity. ***Platelets adhere primarily to subendothelial structures*** (Fig. 3–54). Histamine from platelets contracts

Text continued on page 137

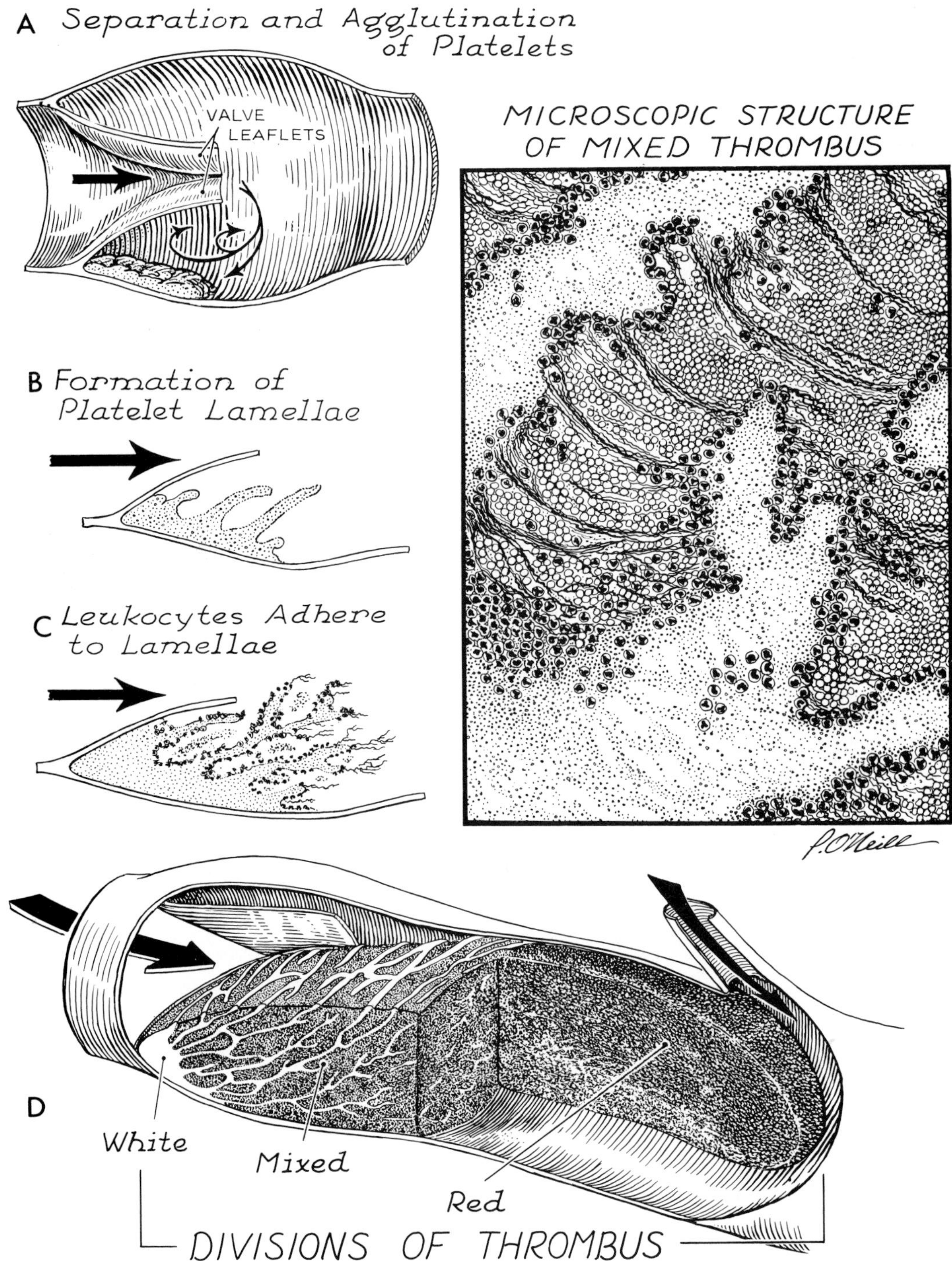

Figure 3–52. Thrombosis. *A* through *D* show the formation of a thrombus, beginning in the valve pocket of a vein. Note the lines of Zahn in *D*. In the microscopic view, note the granular masses of platelets with marginated leukocytes and the interposed erythrocytes and fibrin strands. (From Fallis, B. D.: Textbook of Pathology. New York, McGraw-Hill, 1964. Reprinted by permission.)

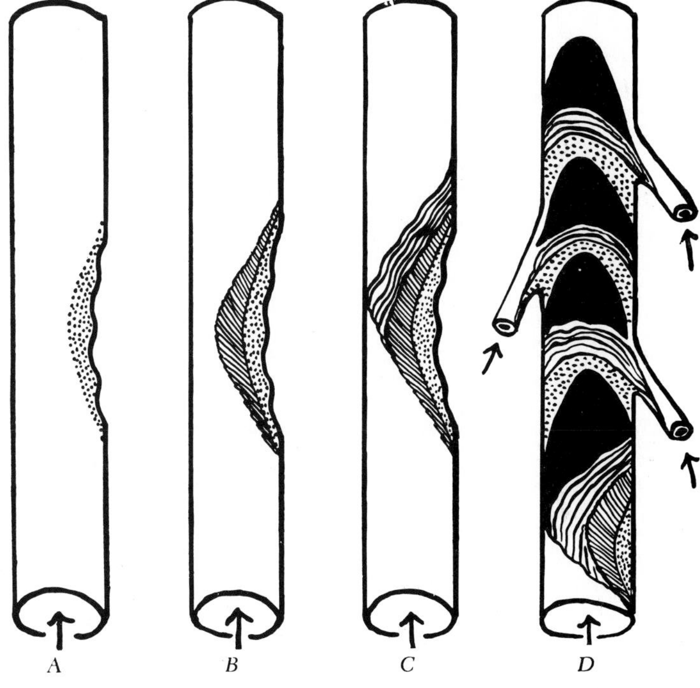

Figure 3–53. Injury to vessel wall. *A,* Platelet thrombus; *B,* addition of white blood cells; *C,* fibrin; *D,* the effects of turbulence and flow patterns are evident, as well as the dark areas of clotting that tail downstream once the lumen is occluded. (From Boyd, W.: Textbook of Pathology. Philadelphia, Lea & Febiger, 1970. Reprinted by permission.)

1. Adhesion

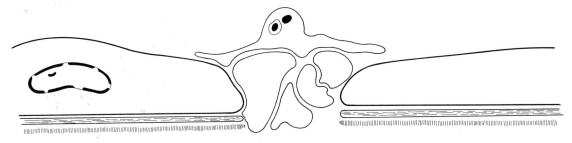

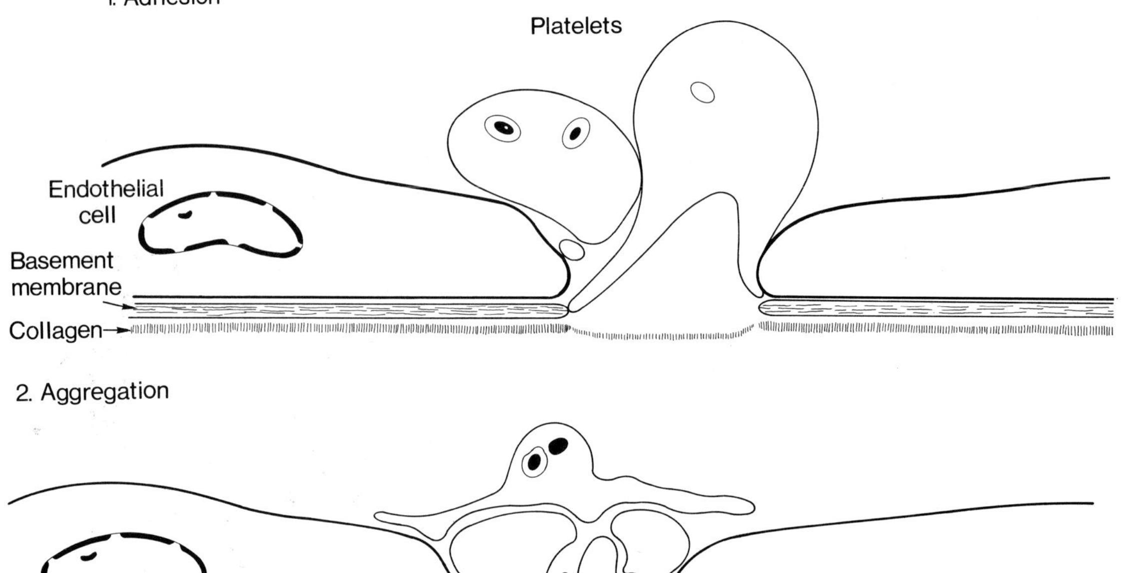

3. Consolidation

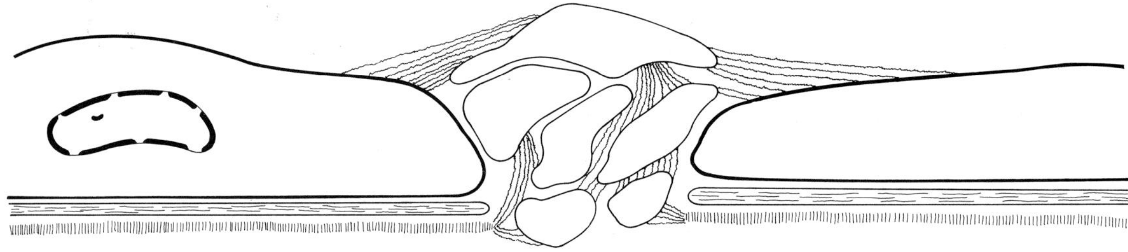

Figure 3–54. Stages in platelet aggregation and deposition of fibrin. (Modified from Cheville, N. F.: Cell Pathology. Ames, Iowa State Press, 1976. Reprinted by permission.)

endothelial cells and thus exposes interendothelial gaps. The essential feature of the process is the formation of the thrombotic hemostatic plug composed of platelets, whereas fibrin is of less significance at the earliest stages. Later fibrin stabilizes the plug. Complex control systems confine the thrombus to the site of injury and maintain the kinin, complement and fibrinolytic systems to acceptable levels of activity. Once the plug is stable, factors are released from platelets, which are chemotactic to neutrophils, which are themselves chemotactic, and macrophages are attracted to remove debris and fibrin. Simultaneously repair is under way and appropriate endothelial cells, collagen and fibroblasts are induced to participate. ***Thus, the process of thrombosis induces inflammation and repair*** (see Chapter 4). Whether the injury occurs on heart valves or in arteries or veins, many of the factors mentioned in connection with turbulence are involved. Common injuries include trauma, damage by localization of bacteria on a vascular surface, viral infection of endothelial cells, migration of parasites in or through vessel walls and factors that change flow patterns, such as outside pressure from an abscess or tumor. Repeated puncture of the jugular vein is a common cause of the serious or fatal consequences of thrombosis.

CHANGES IN THE BLOOD

Changes in the blood may be a primary or a predisposing factor in thrombosis. Certain systemic conditions, such as shock or toxemia, may activate Hageman factor or cause the platelets to release thromboplastin, and these cause the blood to become sticky. This may compound a slow flow problem or be compounded by injured or anoxic capillary endothelium in a toxemia. Thrombi may occur in large vessels, such as the pulmonary arteries, or in capillaries and venules in certain organs. This general mechanism will be discussed again with shock and disseminated intravascular coagulation.

Results of Thrombosis

The ***results of thrombosis*** may be as follows. ***Lysis*** and complete removal occur in a minor vascular injury through resorption of the fibrin by fibrinolysis and neutrophils. The fibrinolytic system counterbalances the coagulation system, and the compound plasmin lyses fibrin. ***Plasmin*** is formed from a β globulin called plasminogen, a normal component of plasma, and is activated during stress, infection or shock, as well as being released from injured tissue. ***Contraction*** of a thrombus will occur if it remains on a surface. Connective tissue and capillaries will grow into it and form a permanent new layer on the inside of the vessel. The ***organized thrombus*** will be covered by endothelium and, if in an artery, may develop a new elastica. If the thrombus fills the lumen of a vessel, organization may involve the formation of new canals in the thrombus and allow some reflow to occur in the ***recanalized thrombus.*** Fibrin thrombi in capillaries are called ***hyaline thrombi.*** Examples of thrombi or their effects are shown in Figures 3–55 through 3–73.

The vasa vasorum, the collateral circulation or both may take over the function of a thrombosed vessel temporarily or permanently. Thrombosis is particularly significant in organs with minimal collateral circulation, such as the heart, kidney and brain. In some organs, such as the lung, thrombosis may be extensive without serious effect.

Thrombi may form rapidly or slowly or by periodic episodes. They may be ***red, white*** or ***laminated,*** depending on the arrangement of components, and ***septic*** or ***nonseptic,*** depending on whether or not they are infected with virulent bacteria. They may be ***valvular*** if on the valves of the heart or ***mural*** if on the wall of a vessel, completely obstructive or partially so, or they may be shaped like a ***saddle*** at a bifurcation point. Thrombi may also be ***arterial, venous, capillary*** or ***lymphatic.*** They must be distinguished from postmortem clots and chicken fat clots, which are smooth with a shiny surface and are not attached to an endothelial surface. Distinction between the two is not always easy, particularly when postmortem clots are tangled around the chordae tendineae of the valves or located in the indentations of the auricles.

A further point necessary for correlation of clinical and pathological findings is that ***thrombi may undergo dissolution in a short time,*** either ***in vivo*** or during the first few hours ***post mortem.*** Experimental evidence

Text continued on page 148

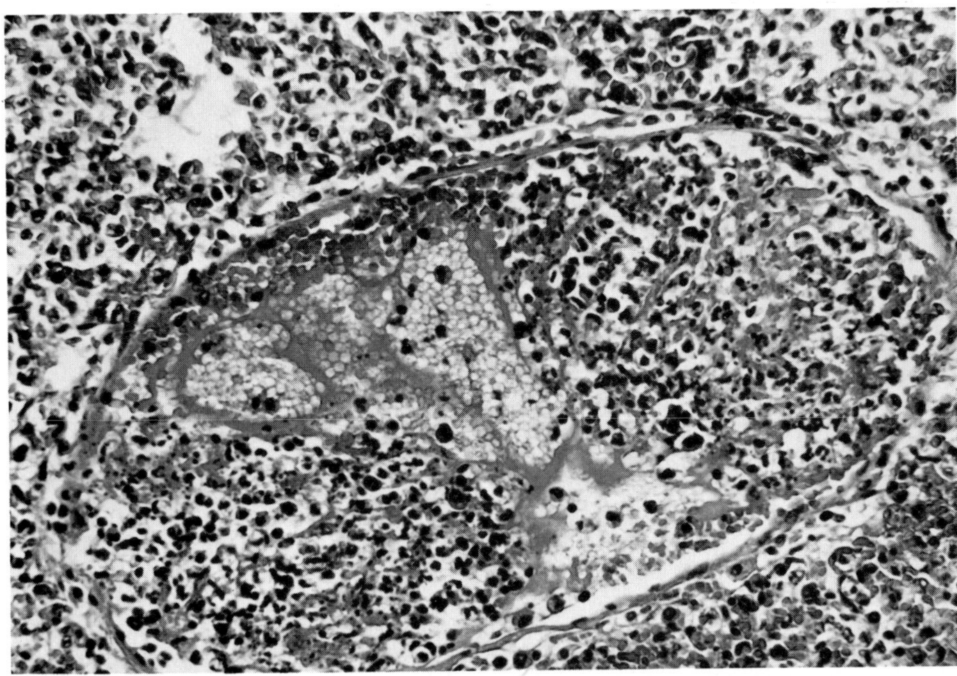

Figure 3–55. Early mixed thrombus in a vein in a lung of a mouse with acute septicemia. Note the strands of fibrin and large numbers of cells in the thrombus. Many of the nuclei of the cells are becoming fragmented.

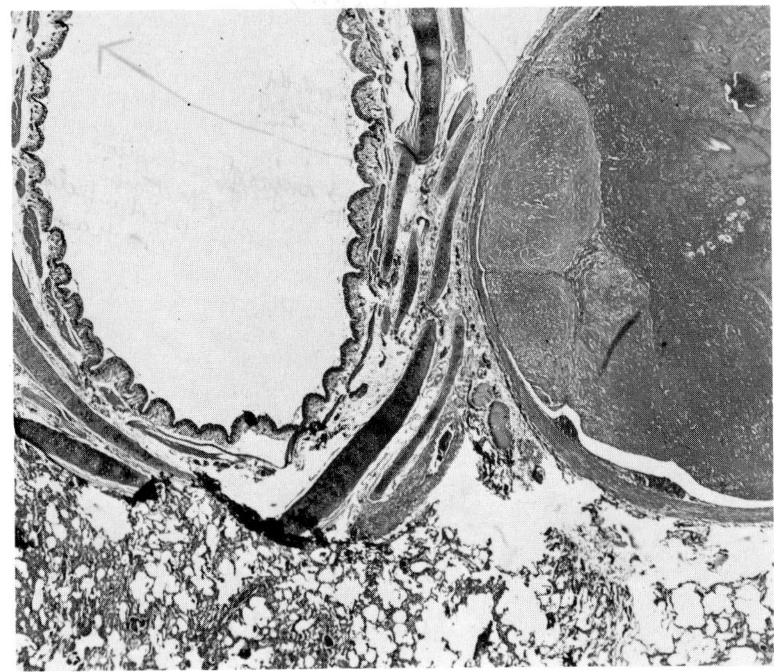

Figure 3–56. Well-formed thrombus in a pulmonary vein. The separation from the vessel wall is a shrinkage artifact of fixation.

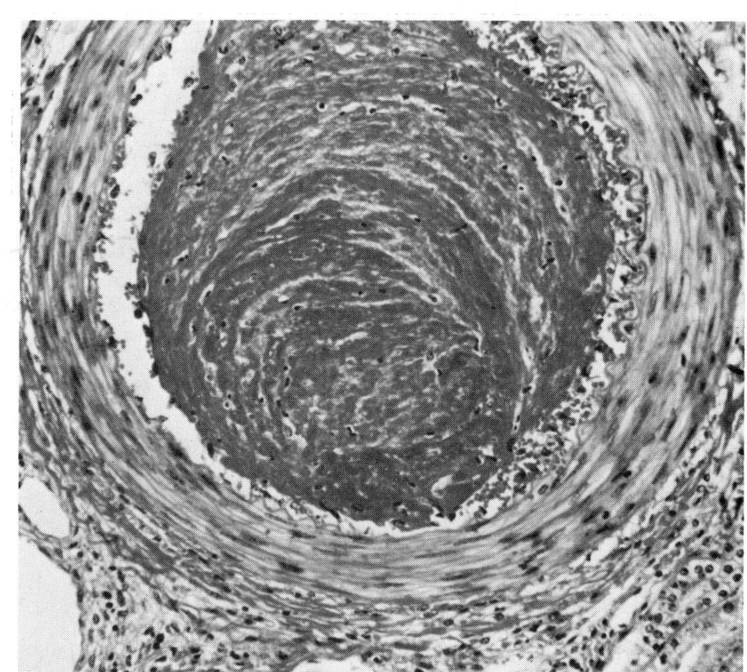

Figure 3–57. Early thrombus in a renal artery.

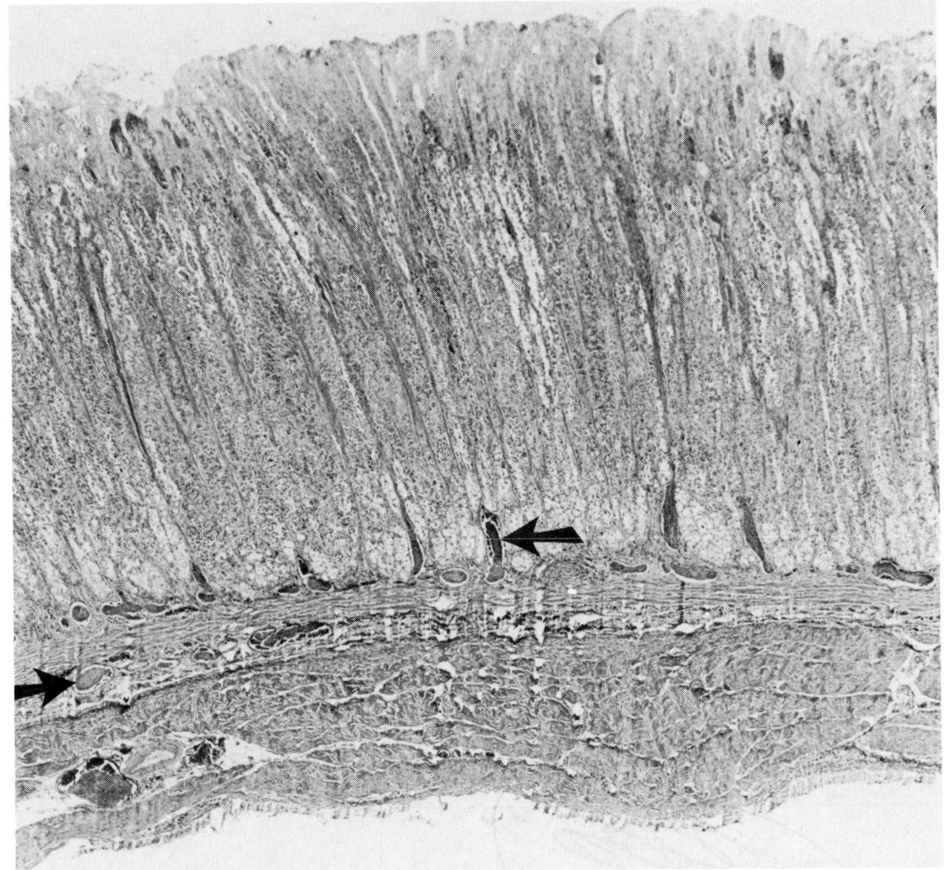

Figure 3–58

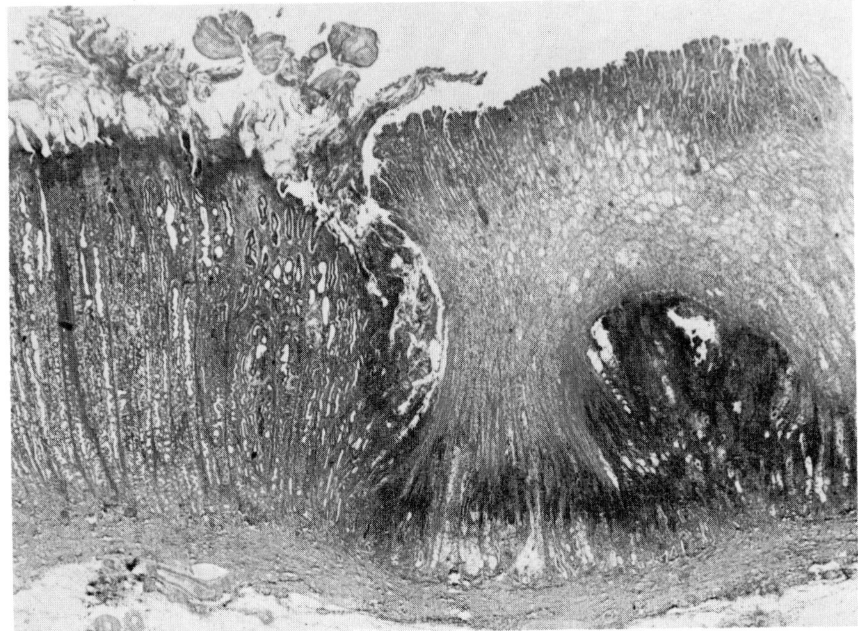

Figure 3–59

Figures 3–58 and 3–59. Thrombi in veins at the mucosal-submucosal junction and extending into the mucosa of a pig's stomach (arrows). These thrombi often lead to venous infarction of the gastric mucosa in pigs and are a common lesion, probably indicative of acute circulatory failure in severe infections (Fig. 3–59). The area to the upper right is necrotic. The gastric mucosa will be dark red grossly (see Fig. 3–13), and the necrotic surface may slough off if the pig survives the acute episode.

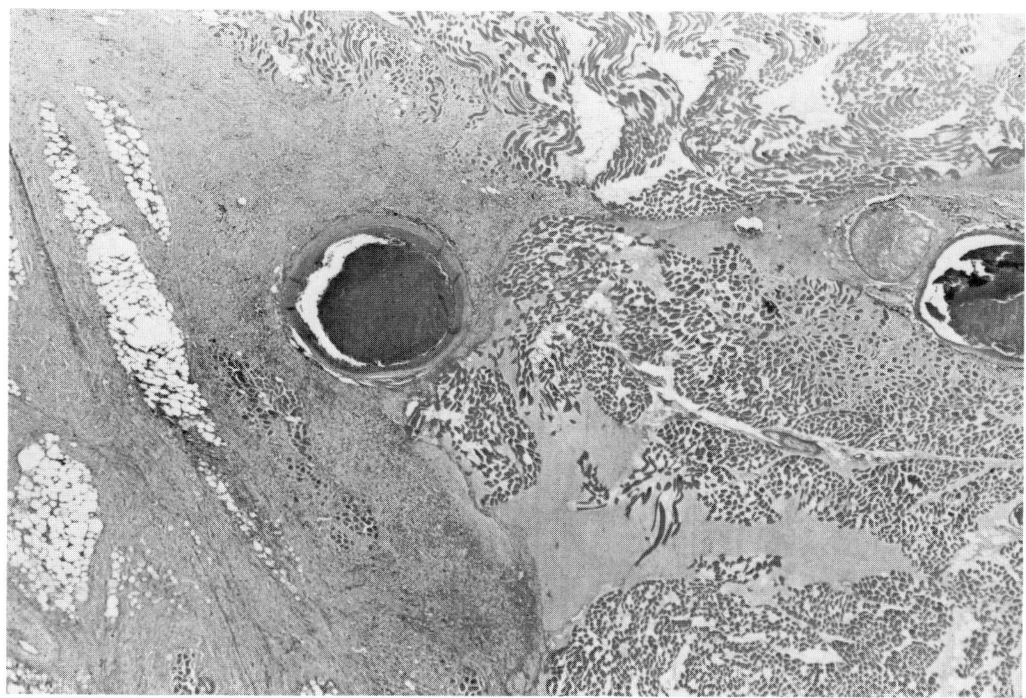

Figure 3–60. Thrombus in the thigh muscles of a downer cow that is probably related to the acute ischemic necrosis observed in many of these cases (see Fig. 2–76).

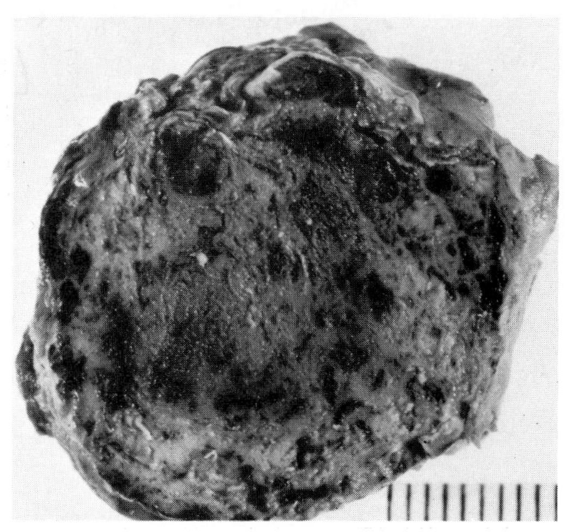

Figure 3–61. Gross appearance of a cross section of a thrombus.

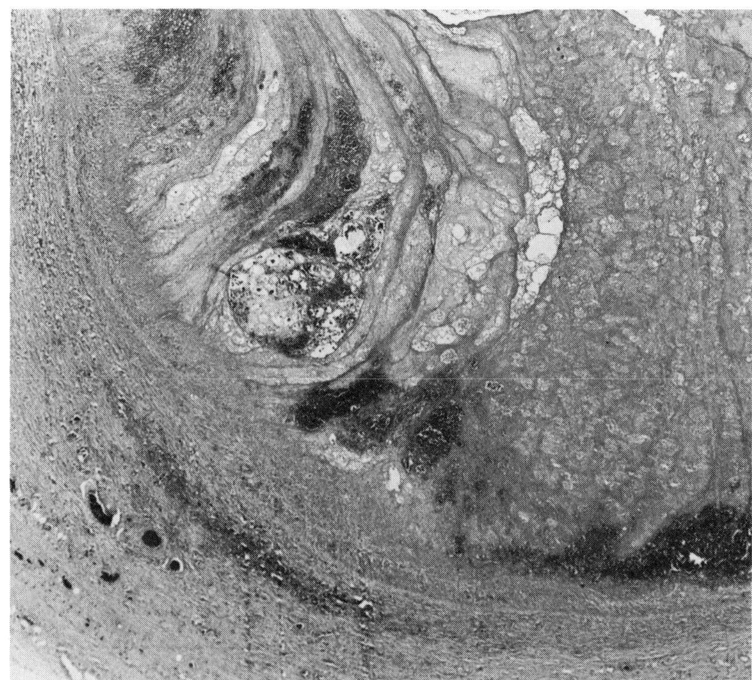

Figure 3–62. Connective tissue is beginning to grow into and replace the thrombus. Note the lamination of the fibrin with plasma and platelets between the laminae. Pockets of erythrocytes are also present in the dark areas.

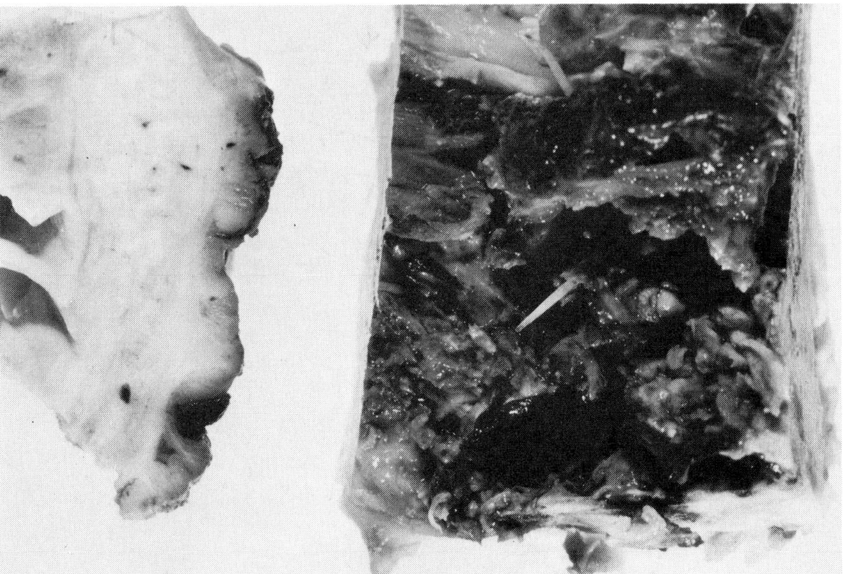

Figure 3–63. Parasitic thrombosis due to Strongylus vulgaris in the mesenteric arteries of a horse. A cross section of thickened arterial wall is on the left and the luminal surface is on the right. Note the parasite protruding from the thrombus. In the cross section, the marked thickening of the vessel wall is evident. This type of lesion often leads to colic in horses from ischemia either due directly to the thrombus or due to embolism into smaller vessels.

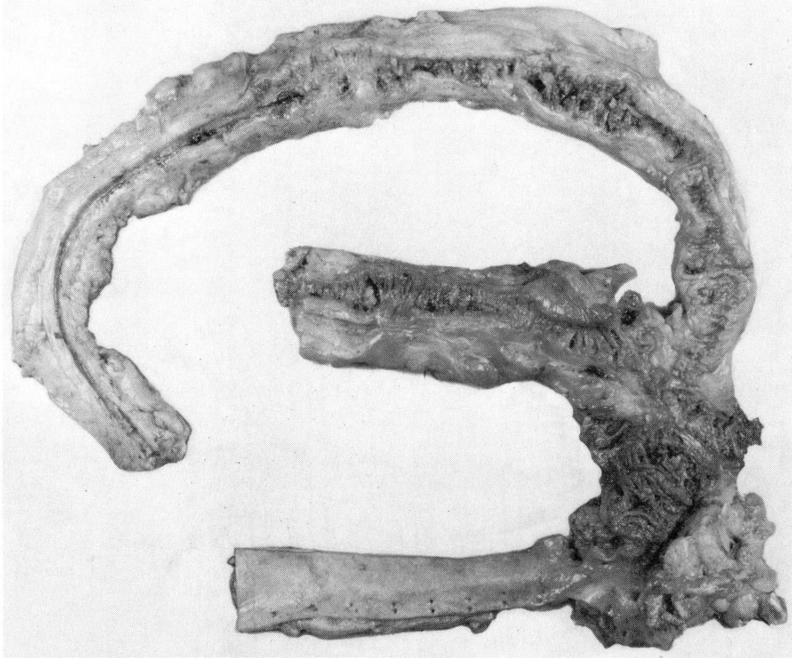

Figure 3–64. Dissected mesenteric arteries from a foal with experimentally induced Strongylus vulgaris infection. Note the luminal surfaces of the arteries, which have a very corrugated luminal surface caused by organized ridges of former thrombi and which also are probably associated with an inflammatory reaction caused by the parasites. Such lesions are very common in natural infections in horses. (Courtesy of B. M. McCraw.)

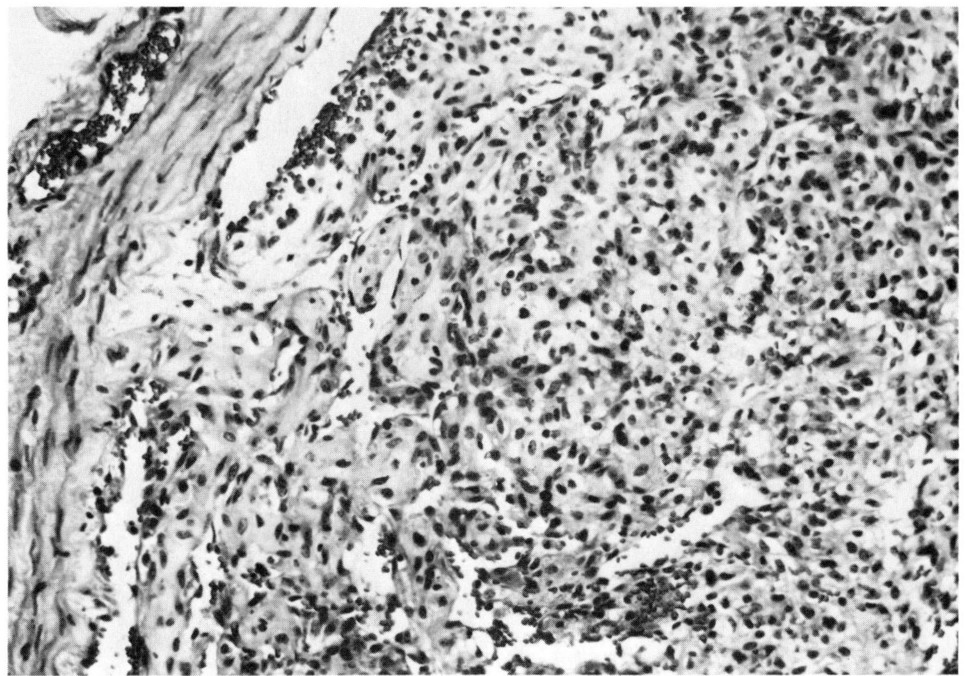

Figure 3–65. An organizing thrombus with possible recanalization and a point of attachment to the vessel wall on the left.

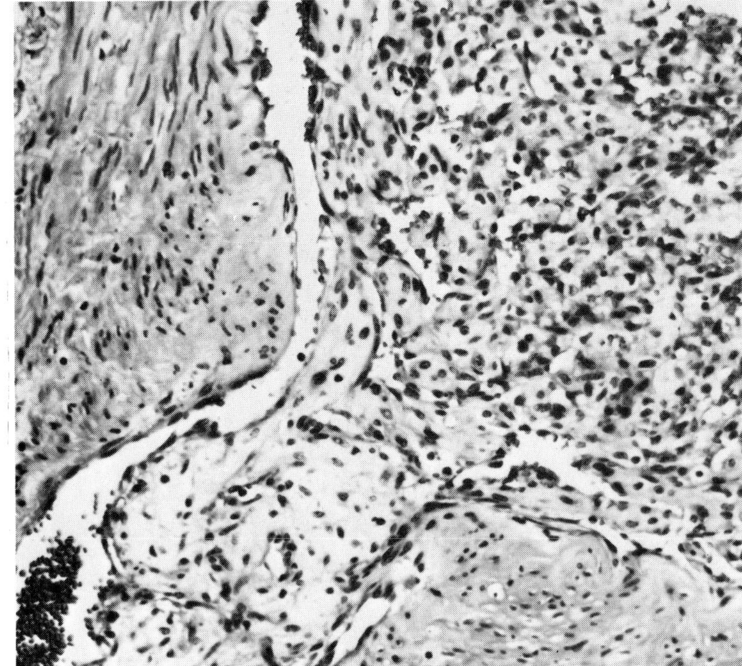

Figure 3–66. The same lesion as seen in Figure 3–65 at the junction with a branch of the artery.

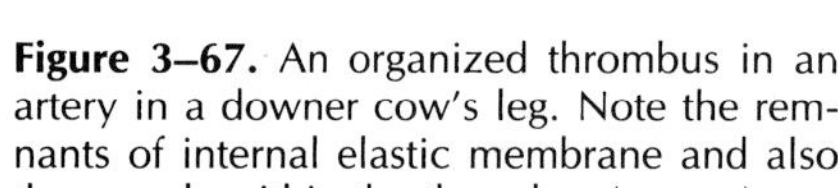

Figure 3–67. An organized thrombus in an artery in a downer cow's leg. Note the remnants of internal elastic membrane and also the vessels within the thrombus (arrows).

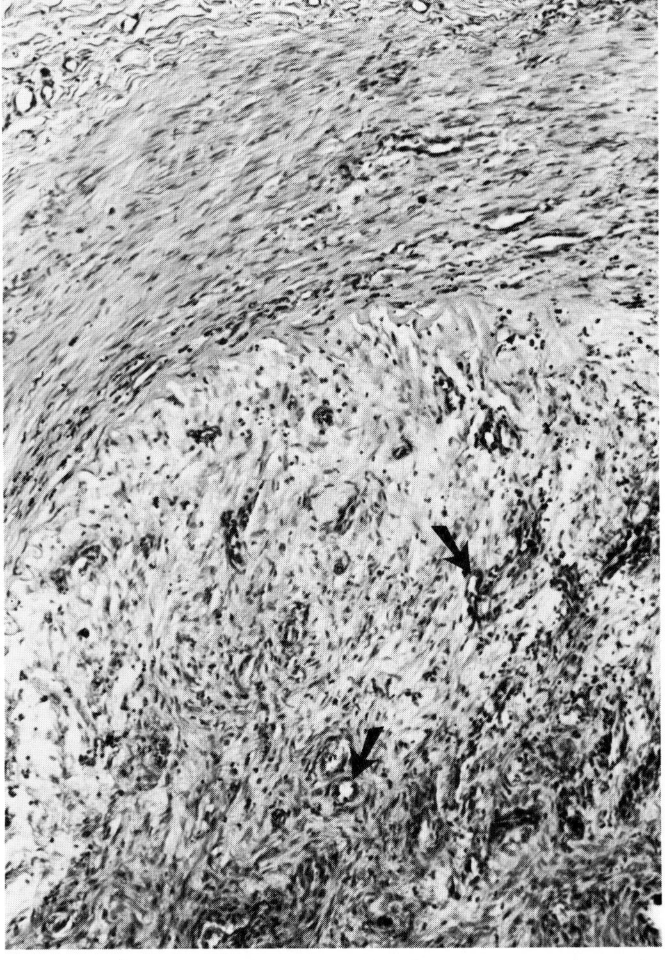

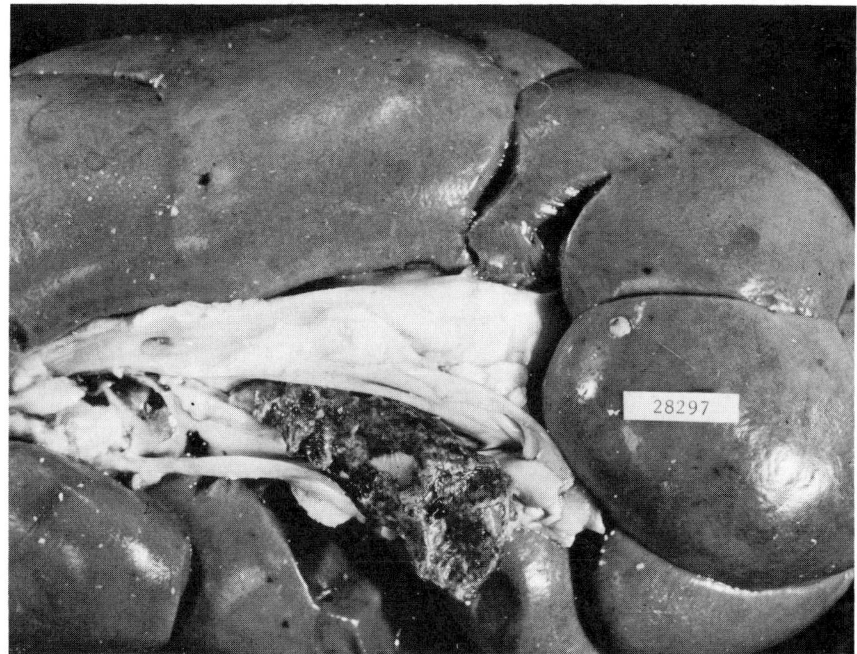

Figure 3–68. A large mixed thrombus in a cow's renal vein.

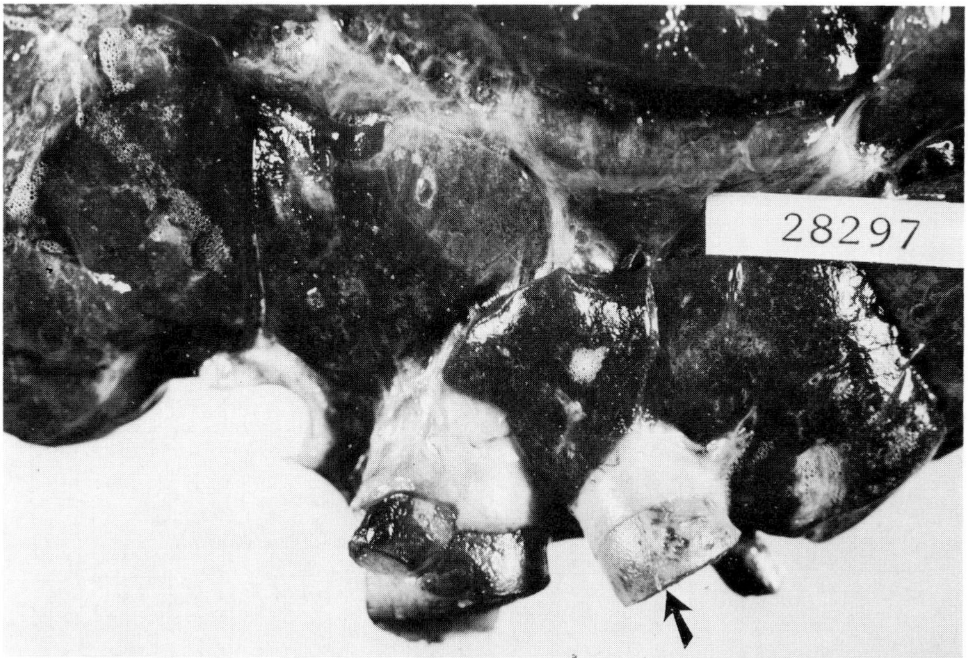

Figure 3–69. Thrombi protruding from the cut surface of pulmonary arteries in the lung of a cow (arrow). Note the congestion and edema with froth in the lung.

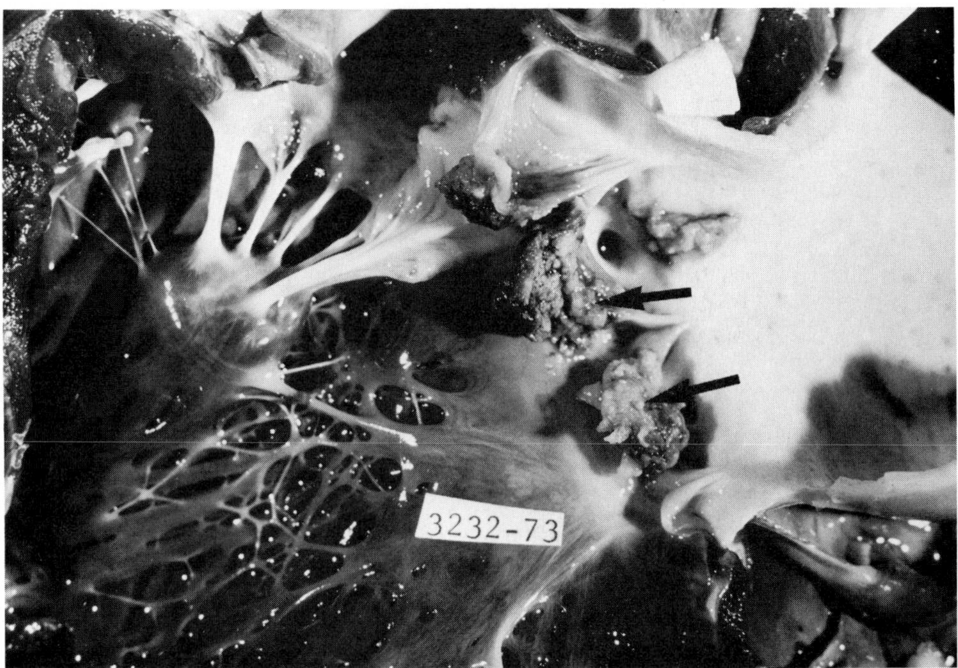

Figure 3–70. Thrombosis of heart valves in a cow (arrows). Embolism is common from such a lesion.

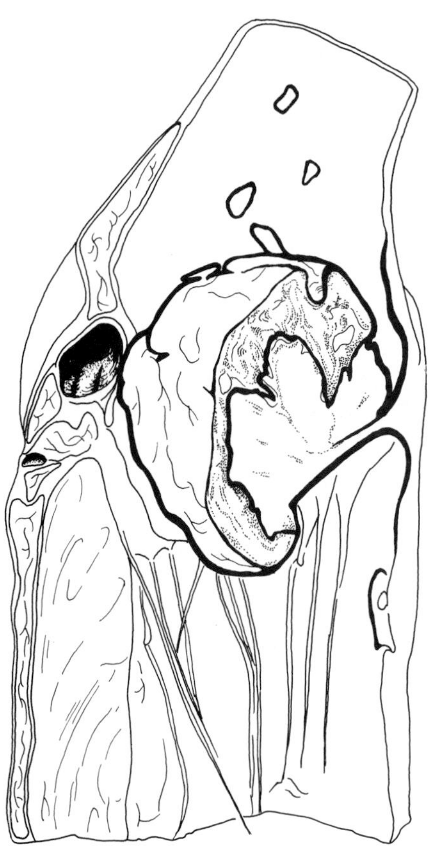

Figure 3–71. Chronic infection on the heart valves of a horse. *Inflammation* and *thrombosis* are mixed in the outer layers of the lesion, and *organization* is occurring from the base of the valve. Thus, three major processes are occurring at the same time in this lesion. Also note embolism.

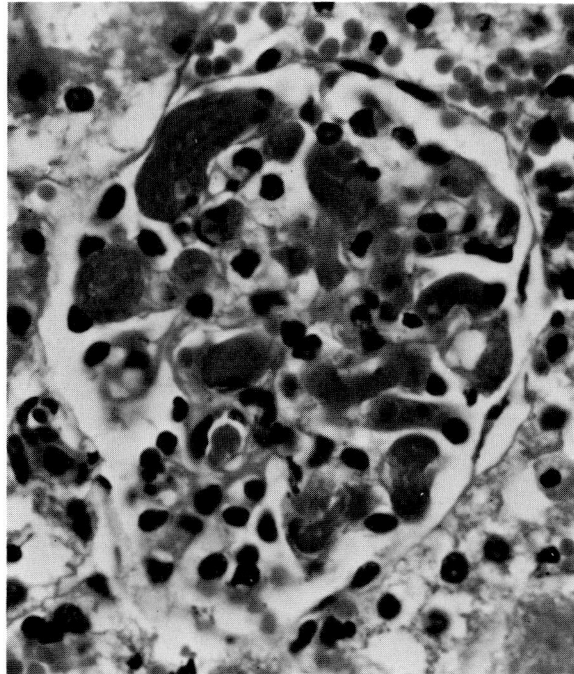

Figure 3–72

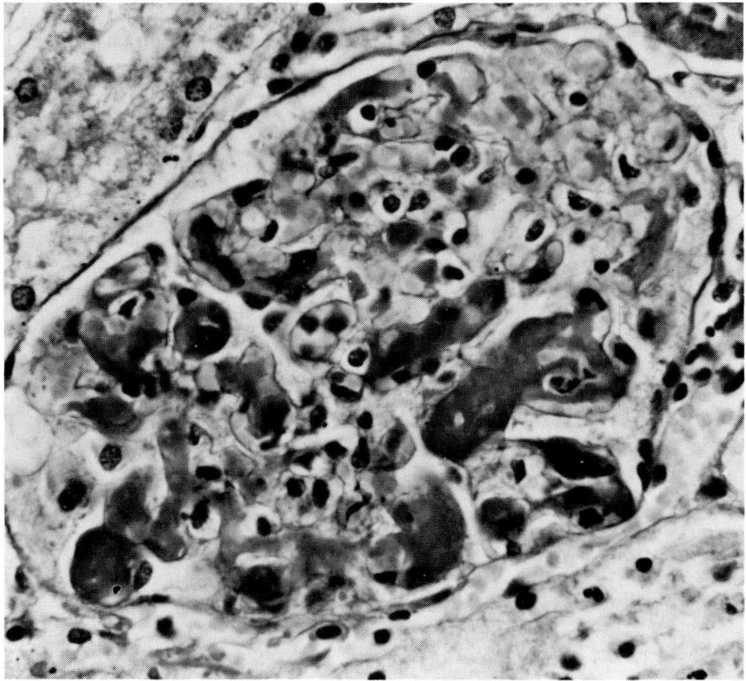

Figure 3–73

Figures 3–72 and 3–73. Hyaline thrombi in glomerular capillaries in intravascular coagulation. This lesion may be induced by severe shock or acute septicemias.

indicates that thrombi formed acutely may have dissolved to a great extent by three hours post mortem, and most autopsies are not conducted during that interval under normal circumstances. The disappearance of thrombi occurs particularly after shock and disseminated intravascular coagulation. This mechanism of dissolution is considered to be the fibrinolytic system. Discrepancies may occur between the extent of thromboembolism observed in gross and microscopic examinations and the cardiopulmonary consequences observed prior to death by the clinician.

Ischemia

Ischemia is a local reduction in flow of blood to an area and usually refers to the flow of arterial blood. The reduction may occur rapidly or slowly. ***The result is dependent on the organ, the size of the vessel, the degree of occlusion and the degree of collateral circulation.*** If ischemia occurs in an end artery, as in the brain, heart or kidney, the result is likely to be acute necrosis of the tissue supplied by that vessel. If the obstruction is gradual, atrophy may occur. The cause is usually a thrombus or an embolus, but functional ischemia may be due to vasoconstriction, as in diabetes or ergot poisoning.

Ischemia may be partial and result in ***anoxia*** or hypoxia rather than necrosis. Four types of anoxia occur in tissue: ***stagnant,*** resulting from reduced flow of oxygenated blood, as in shock or heart failure; ***anoxic,*** resulting from insufficient oxygenation of blood, as in a severe pneumonia; ***anemic,*** caused by low hemoglobin or reduced capacity to carry hemoglobin; ***histotoxic,*** resulting from the inability of cells to use oxygen, as in toxic damage to cells.

Infarction

Acute ischemic coagulation necrosis of an area of tissue is called ***infarction,*** and the area of necrosis is called an ***infarct.*** The shape and size of the infarct will be dependent on the area served by the blocked vessel. A classic example is the triangular area of the renal cortex served by an arcuate artery (Figs. 3–74 and 3–75). Typically, the tissue is pale and surrounded on all sides by a red line of hemorrhage that is due to leakage from necrotic vessels at the junction of the viable tissue, possible attempts at reflow, and an ***inflammatory*** reaction. A white line of neutrophils develops inside the red line in two or three days and is part of the inflammatory response to the necrotic tissue. The necrotic tissue undergoes liquefaction by autolysis with the assistance of the liquefactive action of the neutrophils. Connective tissue forms outside the line of neutrophils and fills in the space as resorption of the liquefying tissue occurs, mainly via lymphatics (Fig. 3–76). Resorption may take two or three weeks or longer. The area ends up as a depressed pale scar.

Not all infarcts are pale; some are red or a mixture of red and pale. The capsular blood supply may remain intact, and if it does, a narrow rim of viable tissue remains at the surface. Dilation of these vessels and hemorrhage give a red color to the surface. Some infarcts form slowly and ischemia is gradual, which might result in great dilation of vessels within the infarct while it is forming, causing it to be red in color. If a thrombus forms in a vein, the area of necrosis may be filled with blood and the edge will not be distinctly demarcated initially. Usually, red infarcts become pale as red cells lyse in the necrotic tissue.

It is common to think of infarcts primarily as being related only to arteries, but ***venous infarction*** does occur, as in the small venules in the stomach of a pig in shock. Venous thrombosis causes necrosis in the hind legs of downer cows. It is not unusual to find renal infarcts of various ages, sizes, shapes and colors in the same kidney. Sometimes venous or capillary infarcts occur, but thrombi are not found in the lesion. The reason for this is that the ***thrombi may be lysed by fibrinolysis*** after or during the process of necrosis, and only a series of examinations of similar lesions at different time periods reveals the thrombi. It has been demonstrated experimentally that resorption of thrombi can occur in a brief period, as mentioned previously.

Pulmonary infarcts are always red and swollen. Usually, either the pulmonary or the bronchial circulation is already compromised and some incident causes a thrombus in the other. Collateral circulation is impaired and anoxia and necrosis are gradual. The collateral circulation is active for a while and pumps blood in for as long as possible,

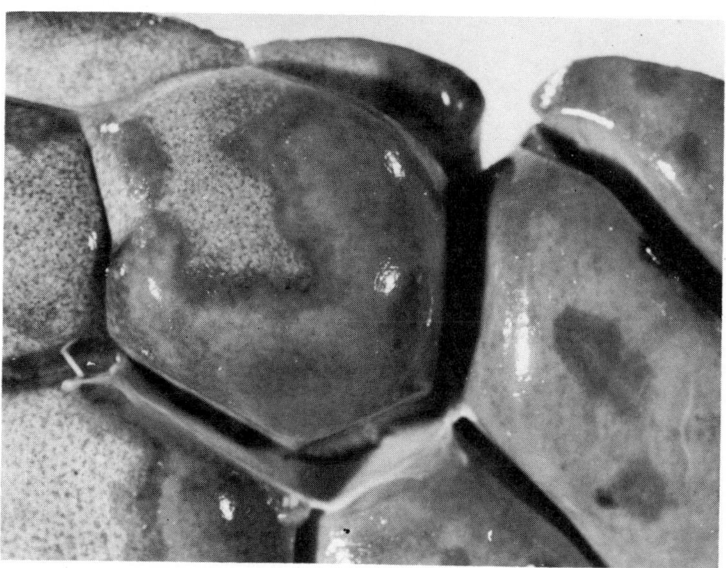

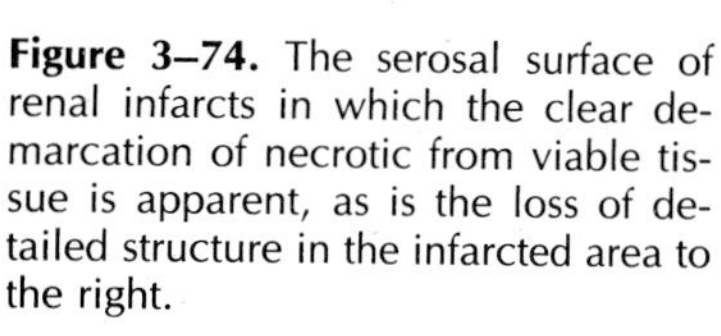

Figure 3–74. The serosal surface of renal infarcts in which the clear demarcation of necrotic from viable tissue is apparent, as is the loss of detailed structure in the infarcted area to the right.

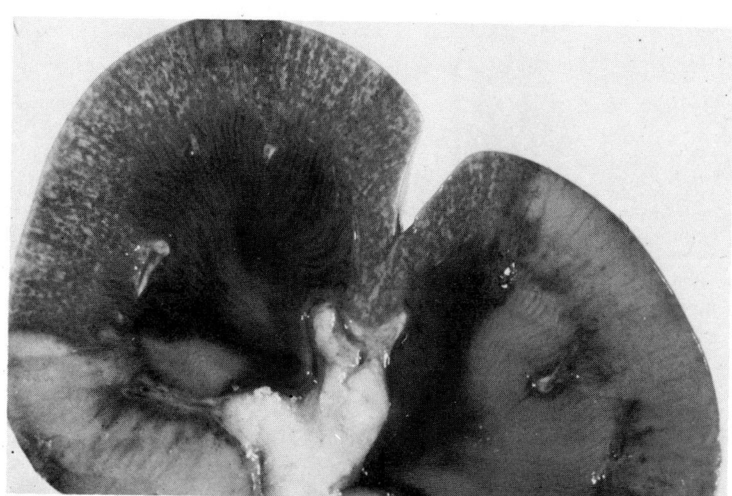

Figure 3–75. Cut surface of the same lesion as seen in Figure 3–74. Note the pale color of the degenerate and necrotic tissue.

Acute Infarction ⟶ 8-10 hrs ⟶ pale discrete Area ⟶ 2-4 days ⟶ pg 149 ⟶ 3-5 days ⟶ sequence below

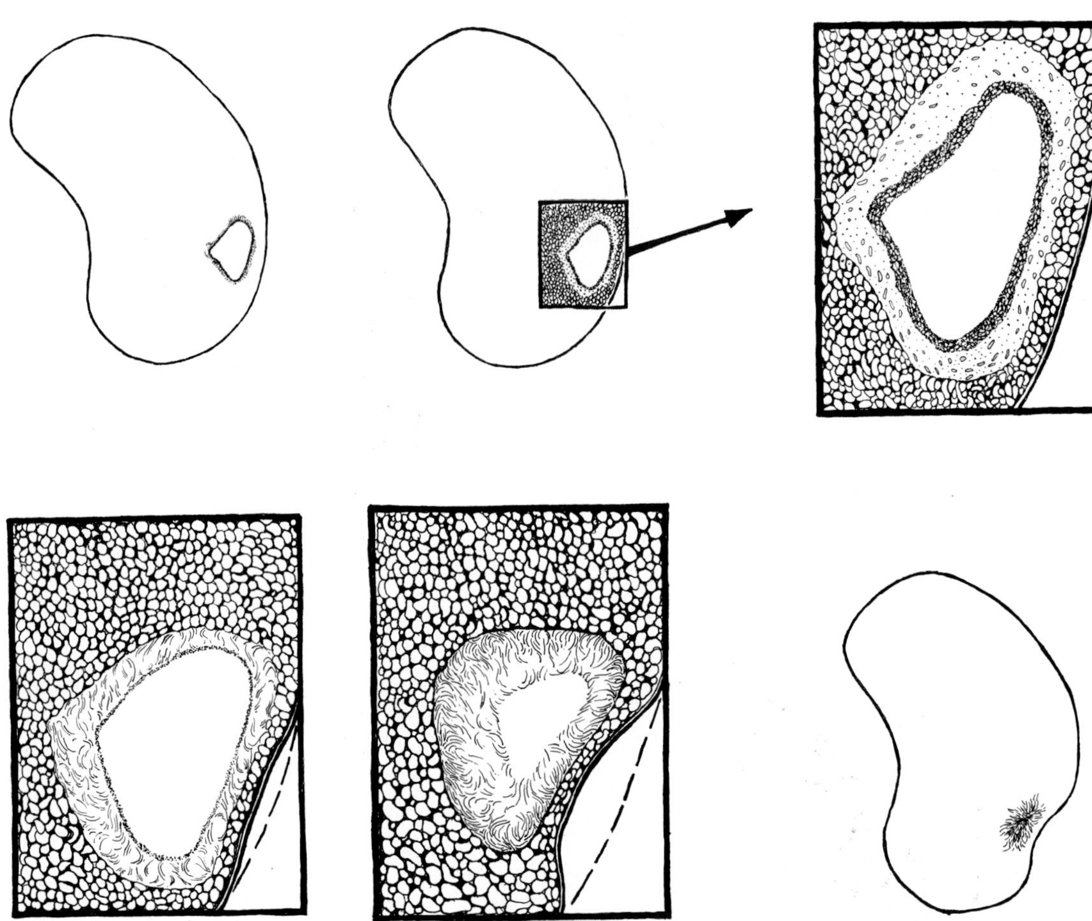

Figure 3–76. Diagrammatic representation of the resorption of an infarct. *Top left,* Discrete pale area surrounded by a white line. *Top center and right,* Necrotic tissue in the middle, with zone of neutrophils around the edge and connective tissue nearest the renal tissue. *Lower left,* Necrotic tissue is resorbed as the connective tissue increases. Note depression from the surface. *Lower center,* Further growth of connective tissue, resorption of necrotic tissue, and depression of the lesion below the surface. *Lower right,* A healed depressed scar.

occurs the same regardless of location (scar tissue)

which accounts for the red swollen appearance of the infarct.

The classic infarct is not difficult to recognize if it is present for two or three days. ***Acute infarction may be very difficult to recognize,*** however. This problem has been studied in detail in human coronary disease. As mentioned previously, a few hours are required from the time of necrosis until morphological evidence is apparent. Slight color changes are difficult to interpret. The problem of recognizing degrees of ischemia is particularly important in intestinal accidents such as volvulus or incarceration. It is most difficult to determine whether or not normal function will return following surgery or whether there has been sufficient anoxia to lead to necrosis, rupture or gangrene. The texture and color of the affected portion of intestine even one hour after surgery gives little indication of the prognosis. Loss of motility, progressive edema and darkening of color may take two to three hours in cases that appear initially to have returned to normal. The prognosis also relates to the extent of sloughing of villous epithelium during the initial anoxic stage and to the progressive subsequent microvascular thrombosis which follows.

EMBOLISM

An ***embolus*** is a solid abnormal mass transported from one part of the body to another in the circulatory system, and the blocking of a vessel by such transported fragments is ***embolism.*** Emboli usually end up caught in a vessel that has a lumen smaller than the embolus. If the vessel is an end artery, the embolus may cause an infarct. ***Embolism is a common cause of infarction.*** If the vessel is a vein, the embolus will probably eventually lodge in the pulmonary circulation. Emboli may be groups of tumor cells, colonies of bacteria or foreign bodies injected into the blood or pieces of a thrombus that have broken off from a primary site.

Embolic dissemination is an important means of spreading disease within the body. A classic example is a septic thrombus either on a left heart valve and showering septic emboli throughout the body or on a right heart valve and showering septic emboli into the lung (Fig. 3–70). Venipuncture often produces emboli of pieces of skin or hair. Injection of air during venipuncture may cause air embolism and occlusion of cerebral vessels and has been used in some species as a means of euthanasia. Fungal hyphae have an affinity for blood vessels and may spread as emboli; mycotic rumenitis in cattle is a good example. A common cause of clinical illness and death in horses is colic caused by migration of ***Strongylus vulgaris*** larvae in the walls of the celiac and anterior mesenteric arteries. The results are thrombosis in these vessels and showers of emboli to the intestine, which cause anoxia, possibly infarction and abnormal motility of the gut that results in colic (Figs. 3–77 and 3–78). Pulmonary and cerebral fat embolism from fractures is a significant cause of death in humans after serious car accidents. Liver abscesses in cattle may be located near the vena cava, into which they eventually rupture with massive septic embolism to the lungs. Some bacterial species seem to travel in colonies and lodge in capillaries to cause necrosis or acute inflammation—for example, ***Actinobacillus equuli*** in the kidneys of horses and ***Hemophilus somnus*** in the brains of cattle. Embolism from thrombi in deep veins of the leg is a serious concern in phlebitis in humans. Partial occlusion of coronary arteries by chronic atherosclerosis may lead to anoxia and ischemia of myocardium in humans. Rupture of an atheromatous plaque into the lumen of an artery will probably lead to thrombosis and embolism by fragments of the plaque.

NONSPECIFIC CIRCULATORY CHANGES

Correlation of clinical with pathological findings is desirable, and in many cases, the correlation is satisfying to both the pathologist and the clinician. Sometimes, however, the lack of correlation is disturbing to one or both. This situation leads to theorizing about what probably happened and sometimes overinterpretation as well as underinterpretation of certain changes. Among the changes that may be difficult to interpret at postmortem examination in terms of significance to the cause of death are shock, dehydration, acidosis and alkalosis. These are somewhat nonspecific factors, in part related to circulatory changes. Some discussion of the evaluation and possible significance

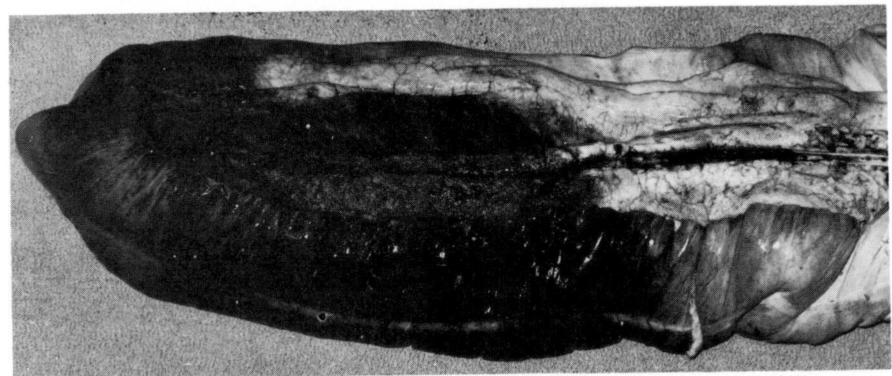

Figure 3–77

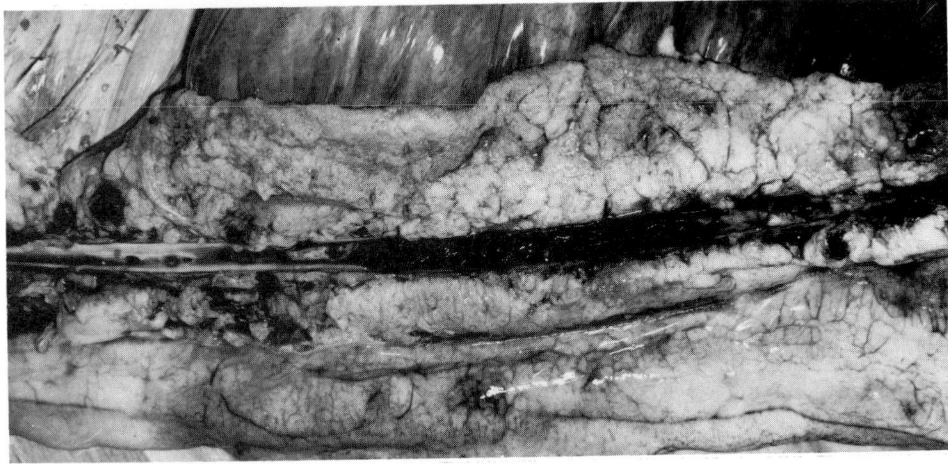

Figure 3–78

Figures 3–77 and 3–78. Colon of a horse that is very dark due to severe congestion. One of the thrombi causing the lesion is shown in Figure 3–78.

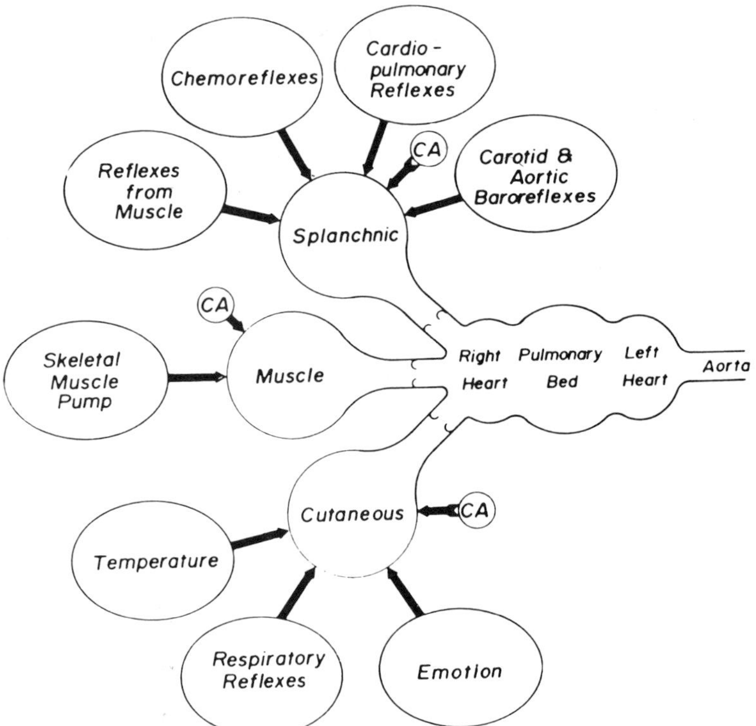

Figure 3–79. Mechanisms involved in regulation of capacity of splanchnic, muscle and cutaneous venous beds. CA, circulatory catecholamines. (From Shepherd, J. T., and Vanhoutte, P. M.: Role of the venous system in circulatory control. Mayo Clin. Proc., *53*:247–255, 1978. Reprinted by permission.)

of these is appropriate. These factors may relate much more to abnormal physiology than morphology and are perhaps more readily assessed in the living animal.

Shock

Shock is a clinical term that means ***peripheral circulatory failure with pooling of the blood in the terminal circulatory bed in small vessels, mainly capillaries and venules.*** If all capillary beds were to open up, there would not be enough blood to fill the major vessels. This is the problem in shock: insufficient blood is returned to the heart, blood pressure falls and flow is decreased. The result is usually a ***redistribution*** of blood in the circulation, although loss of blood will have a similar effect. The mechanisms involved in regulation of blood volume in various parts of the circulatory system are illustrated in Figures 3–79 and 3–80. The venous system is of great importance because it normally holds 70 to 80 per cent of the blood and must return that blood to the central circulation efficiently.

Clinically, the patient becomes inactive, weak and pale and has cool skin, rapid respiratory and heart rates, reduced urine formation and hypotension. Tissues are not oxygenated normally, lactic acidosis develops and the sequence becomes self-perpetuating.

The causes of shock may be classified as septic, hypovolemic, cardiogenic and neurogenic, all of which are largely self-explanatory. ***Hypovolemic*** shock is associated with hemorrhage, trauma, loss of fluid in burns, and major surgery. ***Cardiogenic*** shock refers to diminution of output of the central pump. ***Septic*** shock implies septicemia or extreme localized infection, usually with gram-negative organisms, which in turn implies endotoxemia. The main problem is intravascular coagulation. ***Neurogenic*** shock usually results from pain or severe emotional upset, but fainting is not really a primary form of shock. ***Shock may be a major contributing factor or perhaps the main cause of death.***

LESIONS INDICATIVE OF SHOCK

1. Congestive Atelectasis. There are lesions found post mortem that may be very suggestive, or in some cases diagnostic, of severe shock. Pulmonary edema may result from numerous causes and may occur with congestion, a mild interstitial pneumonia and some collapse of alveoli. The term ***congestive atelectasis*** is appropriate for these changes, which are also called shock lung (Fig. 3–81). An example of the pathogenesis for each cause of this lesion—trauma, intestinal obstruction, infection and blood loss—is illustrated in Figure 3–82. Each has a final common pathway leading to peripheral circulatory failure. This sequence is compounded by a nonspecific reflex hypertension within the lung as a result of anoxia. The hypertension would be an advantage in some situations but may compound a problem in others. In many animals, these lung lesions are observed but are considered mild and often overlooked as being insignificant. The lesions are sufficient to be the immediate cause of death, although specific etiology may be impossible to determine.

2. Visceral Pooling. In cattle that die with a failing circulation, considerable fluid may be present in the intestine, and the fluid contains so many red cells that the fluid looks like blood. There are no blood clots, however, and the color is very dark. This lesion is the result of diapedesis from dilated anoxic capillaries in villi. The lesion is called ***visceral pooling*** but unfortunately is often mistaken for inflammation and called hemorrhagic enteritis.

3. Acute Renal Tubular Necrosis. A fall in blood pressure causes reflex renal ***vasoconstriction,*** which sets off the following chain of events. The reduced flow causes the release of renin from the juxtaglomerular apparatus. Renin acts on the liver to activate angiotensinogen, a globulin produced by the liver, and splits off angiotensin I to form angiotensin II, which raises the systemic blood pressure. Angiotensin II also acts on the adrenal cortex, releasing aldosterone to cause sodium and water retention and therefore increasing the blood volume. This whole sequence is beneficial if blood loss is the problem, but sometimes increased blood volume may be detrimental, as in heart failure. The renal lesions associated with shock arise from ***excessive vasoconstriction*** in the initial stages of the sequence, to the point that ***acute ischemic degeneration and necrosis*** occur randomly throughout the kidney. The random distribution is the result of the normal pattern of

Text continued on page 156

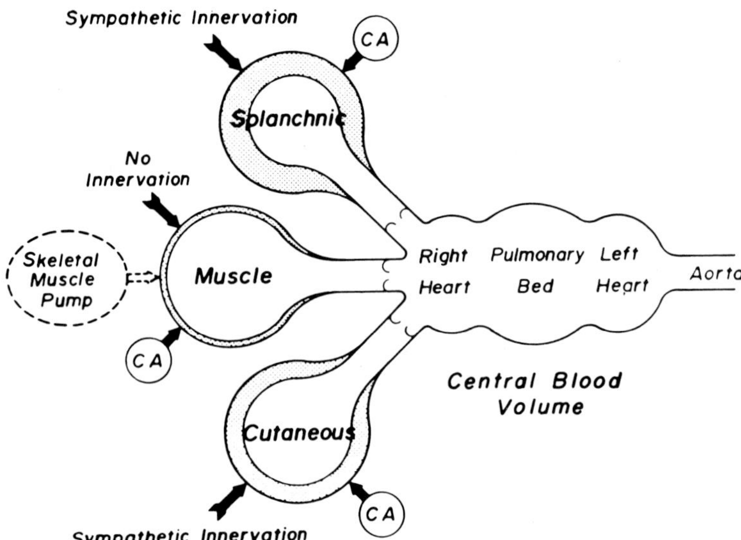

Figure 3–80. Regulation of central blood volume and cardiac filling pressure by major components of systemic venous system—splanchnic, muscle and cutaneous veins. Active changes in venous capacity are caused by contraction or relaxation of smooth muscle in venous walls. Whereas splanchnic and cutaneous veins have an abundance of smooth muscle (shaded areas) and a rich sympathetic innervation, muscle veins have little smooth muscle and few, if any, sympathetic nerves. The skeletal muscle pump has a major role in reducing capacity of muscle veins. CA, Circulatory catecholamines. From Shepherd, J. T., and Vanhoutte, P. M.: Role of the venous system in circulatory control. Mayo Clin. Proc., *53*:247–255, 1978. Reprinted by permission.)

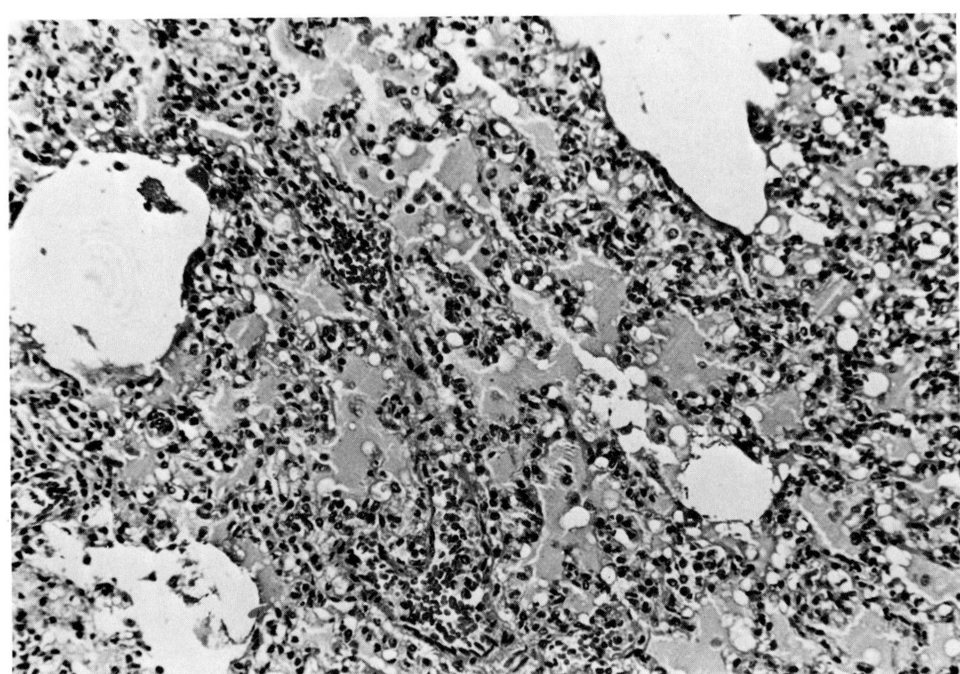

Figure 3–81. Congestive atelectasis. There is collapse, edema, and thickening of alveolar walls. The lesion might be called a diffuse interstitial pneumonia.

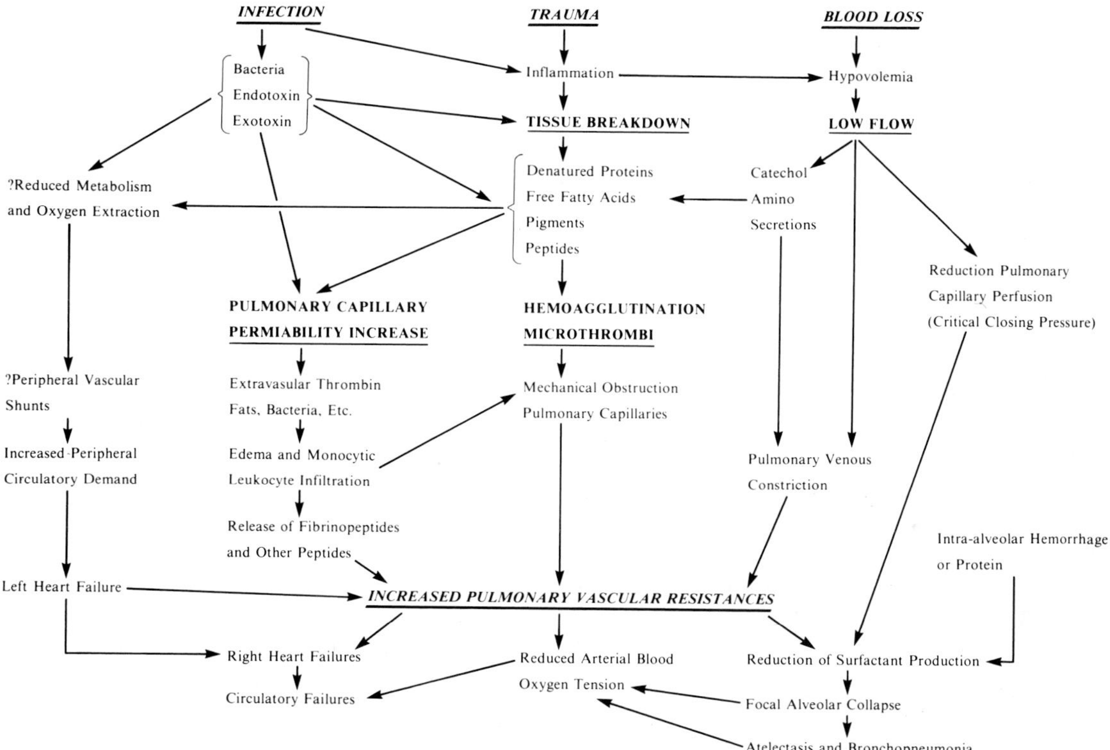

Figure 3–82. Schematic diagram of the concept of a final common path of circulatory failure for many types of lesions and diseases. Study this diagram carefully. Note that most of the factors toward the top lead to reduced perfusion of the lung, partly due to thrombosis and sludging but also due to reflex hypertension in the lung due to anoxia. (From Clowes, G., et al.: The nonspecific inflammation reaction leading to respiratory failure after shock, gangrene and repair. J. Trauma, *8*:899, 1968. Reprinted by permission. Improved from the original by Gary Cody.)

variation in the degree of function in different areas at different times as part of functional reserve.

The lesion is called ***acute tubular necrosis.*** Epithelial cells degenerate, die and fall into the tubular lumen, edema occurs in the interstitium, and if the basement membrane of the tubule is disrupted, the irritating contents of the tubule are released into the interstitium and may cause inflammation. Grossly, the kidney may be mottled in color, or if the lesion has been present for some time, pale, irregularly sized and shaped areas of degeneration and necrosis will be present. Oliver called this lesion tubulorrhexis and was instrumental in helping others appreciate the significance of the lesion with various etiological factors, such as trauma and poisoning. ***This lesion is very useful for interpreting the significance of shock.***

Congestive atelectasis and acute tubular necrosis are indications of the cause of death in many instances of death after trauma. The classic crush syndrome results in renal failure and pneumonia by the mechanisms mentioned previously.

4. Sludging. Sludging refers to slowing down of the circulation, settling out of red cells from plasma and increased stickiness of blood. A chicken fat clot results from sludging (Figs. 3–83 and 3–84). The significance of sludging was well demonstrated by Knisely (1961), who developed a system by which he could observe the settling out, slow flow and venous thrombi in the posterior vena cava. He infected monkeys heavily with ***Plasmodium knowlesi*** and found that sludging was very prominent as the illness progressed to death (Fig. 3–85). In similarly infected animals given heparin, clinical signs were markedly diminished, indicating that the main effect of the parasite was increased ***stickiness*** of the blood, which led to illness and death through activation of components of the clotting system. Sludging is common in shock.

5. Disseminated Intravascular Coagulation. Disseminated intravascular coagulation (DIC) refers to widespread, or at times localized, formation of microthrombi in capillaries, arterioles and venules. The condition is a complication of many disease states, including some cases of shock. DIC is ***intravascular coagulation*** and can arise by way of the extrinsic or intrinsic systems or by stasis of flow. There may be defective clearing of activated clotting factors or defective fibrinolysis. DIC often affects the entire peripheral circulatory vasculature but tends to affect particular organs. The effect will vary with the species and the etiology. Hyaline thrombi may be evident in the pulmonary capillaries, glomeruli or myocardial capillaries. Loose thrombi may occur in the sinusoids of the liver or adrenal cortex. The extent of thrombosis varies with the amount and speed of formation of thrombin. ***Congestion and hemorrhage*** are probable in a severely affected area, and on occasion, it is assumed that the thrombi were present but have been lysed, perhaps after death. ***Necrosis*** may also occur in these severe lesions.

These lesions of DIC are common in the acute gram-negative septicemias in animals. They are the bases of the venous infarcts of the fundic mucosa of the stomach in pigs in several acute infectious diseases. The blue color of the ears of pigs with *Salmonella* septicemia is caused by venous thrombi of DIC.

DIC may be caused by antigen-antibody complexes, tissue damage, intravascular hemolysis, endotoxin and systemic hypersensitivity or by extensive diffuse endothelial damage. Neoplastic cells may also initiate the process. The generalized Shwartzman reaction induces DIC. Viruses that replicate in endothelial cells may initiate the conditions. An example of DIC is infectious canine hepatitis, in which viral replication in endothelial cells leads to destruction of these cells and release of tissue thromboplastin into the blood stream, which activates the intrinsic system, causes platelets to adhere to the site of injury and activates plasmin formation. Purpura often occurs because of loss of platelets.

DIC is a very important nonspecific process that may contribute substantially to the cause of death. DIC can produce shock and shock can produce DIC. In short, the problems are the formation of fibrin and the clumping of platelets in flowing blood as well as the consumption of platelets that may lead to purpuric hemorrhage.

Microthrombosis is common in various forms of tissue injury including mechanical, chemical, and radiation trauma, and there is often a common reaction of the vasculature and surrounding tissue to such injury. An example of lesions associated with burns is illustrated in Figure 3–86; the explanation

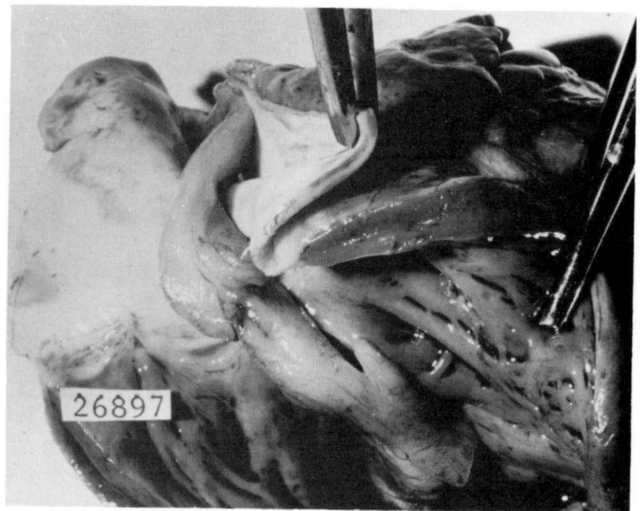

Figure 3–83

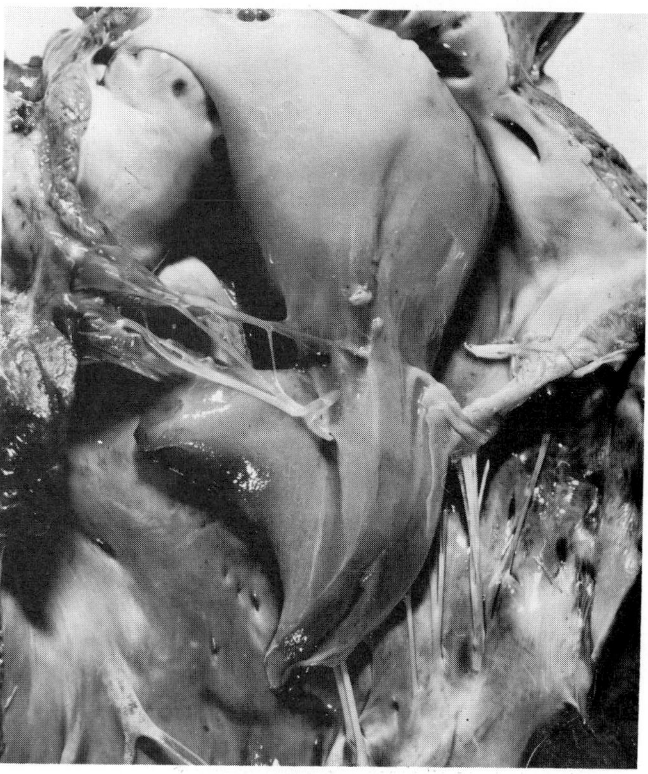

Figure 3–84

Figures 3–83 and 3–84. Chicken fat clot in a calf's heart (Fig. 3–83) and a close-up of another (Fig. 3–84). Note how the latter is caught in the chordae tendineae and auricular wall because it was fluid prior to death and coagulated later.

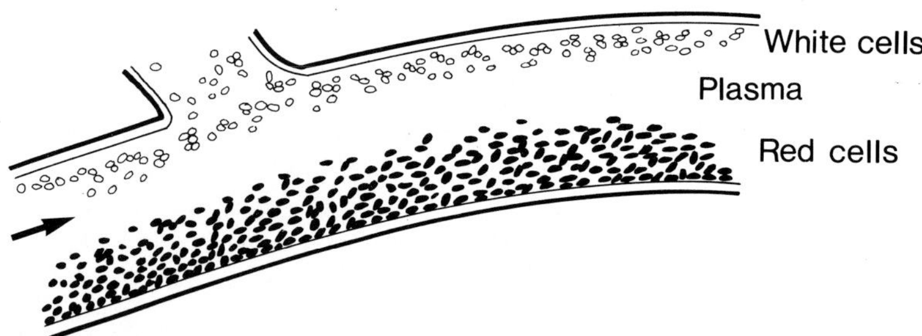

Figure 3–85. Diagrammatic representation of sludging in a vein. The plasma, most of the white cells, and the top layers of the red cells are moving, but the red cells are settling out, slowing down, and clumping together to form a sludge. (Drawn from Knisely, M. H., Warner, L., and Harding, F.: Ante-mortem settling. Microscopic observations and analyses of the settling of agglutinated blood-cell masses to the lower sides of vessels during life: a contribution to the biophysics of disease. Angiology, *11*:535, 1960. Reprinted by permission.)

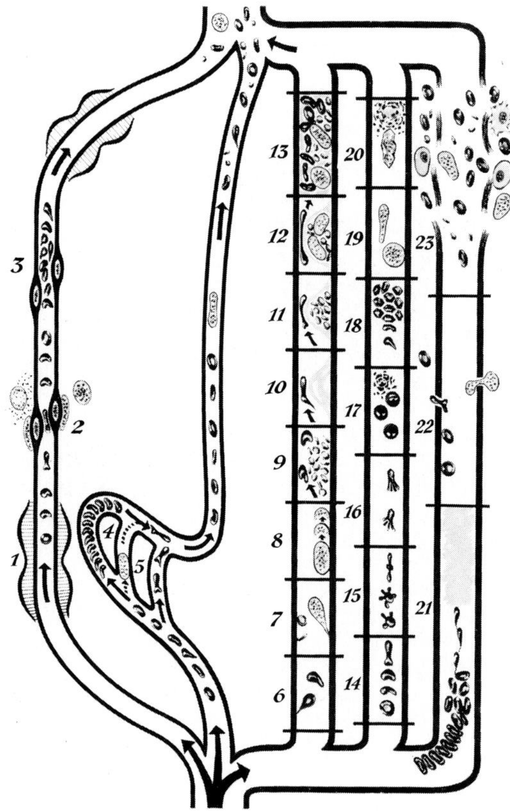

Figure 3–86. Pathophysiology of burned tissue. See text for explanation. (From Branemark, P. I., Breine, U., Joshi, M., et al.: Microvascular pathophysiology of burned tissue. Ann. N.Y. Acad. Sci., *150*:474–494, 1968. Reprinted by permission.)

of the pathogenetic mechanisms involved related to the numbers 1 to 23 in this illustration is as follows.

Arteriolar constriction is a common phenomenon (1). Sometimes arteriolar dilatation occurs, or even an alternation of constricted and dilated arteriolar segments. In the true capillaries the endothelial cells may swell (2), thereby reducing the capillary lumen and impairing nutritive flow of blood. This phenomenon is structurally and functionally connected with changes in the periendothelial granular cells and pericytes. Even adjacent tissue mast cells may play a role in this mechanism by disrupting and liberating the content of their granules into the ground substance, the extracellular space and the perivascular space.

Dilatation of venules and venular stasis (3) is an early and important phenomenon in tissue injury. Microvascular architecture differs in various tissues. If capillary shunts or arteriolar-venular shunts exist (4), blood may be short-circuited and thereby bypass the nutritive part of the capillary bed. Granulocytes are often rigid and may block the nutritive capillaries temporarily or even permanently (5). Wall-adhering erythrocytes (6), granulocytes (6) and platelets (7) are characteristic phenomena in tissue injury. Increased numbers of granulocytes, which adhere to and roll along the endothelium (8), are a constant finding.

Microthrombi are formed and may consist of platelets (9), fibrin (10) or a combination of fibrin and platelets (11), and may even include red cells and white cells, thereby forming a classic microthrombus (12). These wall-adhering thrombi often allow single blood cells to pass (9–12). They may, however, also completely block the lumen (13), temporarily or permanently. The erythrocytes (14) may change in shape to crenated cells (acanthocytes) (15), which, however, often maintain a great deal of the plasticity of the normal red cell (16). Sometimes the red cells turn into spherocytes (17), which may be disrupted, causing hemolysis. When spherocytes are compressed into in a vessel, they change into characteristic hexagonal bodies (18). The white cells may exhibit different degrees of plasticity (19), but may also turn into rigid corpuscles (20). Disruption of granulocytes with liberation of their granules into the lumen has been established as an in vivo phenomenon (20), which appears to be significant in the development of tissue injury. An aggregation of red cells may, to some extent, influence nutritive flow of blood (21). Often, however, the aggregates are plastic and deformable enough to pass even narrow nutritive capillaries, and when the flow rate is increased, the cells move as solitary bodies. The noncorpuscular plasma constituents of blood may change appreciably in composition, accompanied by disturbances in microvascular rheology. Thus, significant abnormalities occur, for example, in plasma proteins, lipoproteins and lipids.

The endothelial wall becomes disrupted functionally with leakage of plasma, resulting in edema and the passage of single blood cells (22), or structurally, resulting in bleeding into the tissue and more or less complete breakdown of the microcirculation (23). This is then followed by derangement and necrosis of the tissue.

Acidosis and Alkalosis

The normal blood pH is maintained between 7.35 and 7.45 by several buffer systems, the main one being bicarbonate and carbonic acid. Excess of bicarbonate, or a deficiency of carbonic acid, leads to severe ***alkalosis*** at a blood pH of about 7.8. A deficiency of bicarbonate or, conversely, an excess of carbonic acid leads to ***acidosis*** at a pH of about 7.0. Values beyond these points are seldom tolerated, since they are usually lethal. The ratio of carbonate to carbonic acid is more important than the total amounts.

Metabolic disturbances affect mainly bicarbonate, and respiratory problems affect carbonic acid or more particularly, carbon dioxide. The most common of these is ***metabolic acidosis.*** It occurs in diarrhea as a result of loss of sodium and bicarbonate from the body, in renal insufficiency as a result of retention of acidic metabolites and in ketosis of diabetes or starvation. Horses with severe colic develop metabolic acidosis because shock reduces oxygen availability, and general anaerobic metabolism increases to compenstate. This produces much lactic acid, the level of which is closely related to the prognosis. ***Metabolic alkalosis*** occurs following prolonged vomiting with loss of acid. It is also important in stressed cattle when adrenal steroids cause sodium retention and subsequent loss of hydrogen and potassium through the kidney as acidic urine. This is a frequent postsurgical problem in cattle and may account for the clinical signs in a slow response after surgery. ***Respiratory acidosis*** occurs in pneumonia, in which exchange of carbon dioxide is impaired. ***Respiratory alkalosis*** results from excess loss of carbon dioxide during rapid respiration.

The clinician must establish the extent of acidosis or alkalosis and then must decide on the cause in order to determine whether the problem is metabolic or respiratory. Acidosis and alkalosis may contribute significantly to clinical illness and death.

Dehydration

Dehydration is expressed clinically as sunken eyes and loss of elasticity in the skin. A loss of 15 per cent of the body weight as fluid will cause death. ***Dehydration leads to circulatory failure, hypovolemic shock and renal failure.*** Postsurgical electrolyte imbalance associated with dehydration may also slow recovery and lead to complications. It is most significant in peracute neonatal diarrhea because the turnover of electrolytes is more rapid in the young and deficiencies are more acutely expressed. The intestinal mucosa has a normal net absorptive function because absorption exceeds secretion. Villous cells digest and absorb whereas crypt cells secrete. Diarrhea results if secretion exceeds absorption. This could be caused by a viral disease such as transmissible gastroenteritis in pigs, destroying villous epithelium, or by hypersecretion of crypt cells, as in enterotoxic colibacillosis. Malabsorption, digestive failure and excess fermentation of undigested food increase the osmotic pressure in the intestine, causing more fluid to be in the lumen, and also contributes to diarrhea (see Figure 7–1). Increased pore size between epithelial cells and vascular injury may allow plasma proteins such as fibrin into the intestinal lumen. If hemorrhage occurs, as in a severe enteritis, there has been a 10,000-fold increase in permeability. By comparison, hypermotility, if it occurs, is apparently of little significance in diarrhea. A calf with scours may die of metabolic acidosis and dehydration with no or minimal visible gross or light microscopic lesions in the intestine. A normal newborn calf has the following volumes of fluids as percentages of body weight: 5 per cent blood plasma, 25 per cent interstitial and 40 per cent intracellular. A three-week-old calf has corresponding amounts of 5 per cent, 15 per cent and 50 per cent. The vulnerability of the newborn to fluid loss is apparent. A 1000 pound cow has 5 gallons of blood plasma and 15 gallons of interstitial fluid. A moderately dehydrated cow (4 to 6 per cent) requires 25 ml of fluid per pound of body weight to become rehydrated and 50 ml if it is severely dehydrated (over 6 per cent). These figures emphasize the signficance of dehydration. The relationships of plasma electrolytes to each other, as well as their absolute amounts, are also quite significant, in addition to the volume of fluid mentioned previously.

As stated earlier, the group of nonspecific circulatory changes may be highly significant individually or in combination as contributions to illness and death. The lesions may be subtle, difficult to interpret or overlooked. An awareness of their significance as factors leading to illness and death will increase the ability of the pathologist and clinician to recognize and evaluate them.

SUGGESTIONS FOR FURTHER READING

General

Attar, S., et al.: Alterations in coagulation and fibrinolytic mechanisms in acute trauma. J. Trauma, *9*:939–965, 1969.

Baker, P. L., et al.: Experimental fat embolism in dogs. J. Trauma, *9*:577–586, 1969.

Bennett, B.: Coagulation pathways: interrelationships and control mechanisms. Semin. Heamtol., *14*:301–318, 1977.

Bleyl, U., and Rossner, J. A.: Globular hyaline microthrombi—their nature and morphogenesis. Virchows Arch. (Pathol. Anat.), *370*:113–128, 1976.

Borner, H., and Klinkmann, H.: Pathogenesis of acute noninflammatory renal failure. Nephron, *25*:261–266, 1980.

Casley-Smith, J. R., et al.: Tissue changes in chronic experimental lymphoedema in dogs. Lymphology, *13*:130–141, 1980.

Clark, D. R.: Circulatory shock: etiology and pathophysiology. J. Am. Vet. Med. Assoc., *175*:78–81, 1979.

Coe, N. P., and Salzman, E. W.: Thrombosis and intravascular coagulation. Surg. Clin. North Am., *56*:875–890, 1976.

Davenport, D. J.: Platelet disorders in the dog and cat. Part 1. Physiology and pathogenesis. Comp. Cont. Ed., *4*:762–776, 1982.

Gill, J. R.: Edema. Ann. Rev. Med., *21*:269–280, 1970.

Harvey, H. J.: Fatal air embolization associated with cryosurgery in two dogs. J. Am. Vet. Med. Assoc., *173*:175–176, 1978.

Hayes, M. A., et al.: Acute necrotizing myelopathy from nucleus pulposus embolism in dogs with intervertebral disk degeneration. J. Am. Vet. Med. Assoc., *173*:289–295, 1978.

Henschen, A., et al. (eds.): Fibrinogen—Recent Biomedical and Medical Aspects. International Symposium on Fibrinogen, New York, 1981. Walter De Gruyter (Hawthorn), 1982.

Hermans, J., and McDonagh, J.: Fibrin: structure and interactions. Semin. Thromb. Hemost., *8*:11–24, 1982.

Herndon, J. H., et al.: Fat embolism: a review of current concepts. J. Trauma, *11*:673–680, 1971.

Hulland, T. J.: Arteriosclerotic changes in the visceral arteries of sheep. Can. Vet. J., *1*:195–205, 1960.

Jacobs, R. R., et al.: Fat embolism: a microscopic and ultrastructure evaluation of two animal models. J. Trauma, *13*:980–993, 1973.

Jennings,, R. B., et al.: Ischemic tissue injury. Am. J. Pathol., *81*:179–198, 1975.

Jesaitis, A. J., and Cochrane, C. G.: Receptor-mediated endocytosis, host defense and inflammation. Lab. Invest., *48*:117–119, 1983.

Kaley, G., and Altura, B. M.: Microcirculation. Vol. 1. Baltimore, University Park Press, 1977.

Kitchens, C.S.: The anatomic basis of purpura. *In* Spaet, T. H. (ed.): Progress in Hemostasis and Thrombosis. Vol. 5. New York, Grune & Stratton, 1980, pp. 211–244.

Lalonde, J.-M. A., and Ghadially, F. N.: Ultrastructure of experimentally produced subcutaneous haematomas in the rabbit. Virchows Archiv. (Cell Pathol.), *25*:221–232, 1977.

Losowsky, M. S., and Scott, B. B.: Ascites and oedema in liver disease. Br. Med. J., *3*:336–338, 1973.

Mason, R. G., and Saba, H. I.: Normal and abnormal hemostasis. An integrated view. Am. J. Pathol., *92*:775–811, 1978.

McCausland, I. P., and Dougherty, R.: Histological ageing of bruises in lambs and calves. Aust. Vet. J., *54*:525–527, 1978.

Mckay, D. G., et al.: Mechanisms of thrombosis of the microcirculation. Am. J. Pathol., *63*:231–241, 1971.

Modell, J. H.: The pathophysiology and treatment of drowning. Acta Anaesthesiol. Scand. (Suppl.), *29*:263–279, 1968.

Moser, K. M., et al.: In vivo and post mortem dissolution rates of pulmonary emboli and venous thrombi in the dog. Circulation, *48*:170–178, 1973.

Mustard, J. F.: Factors influencing thrombus formation in vivo. Am. J. Med., *33*:621–647, 1962.

Mustard, J. F., and Packham, M. A.: Thromboembolism—a manifestation of the response of blood to injury. Circulation, *42*:1–21, 1970.

Mustard, J. F., and Packham, M. A.: The reaction of the blood to injury. *In* Movat, H. Z. (ed.): Inflammation, Immunity and Hypersensitivity. New York, Harper & Row, 1971.

Robin, E. D., et al.: Pulmonary edema. N. Engl. J. Med., *288*:239–246, 299–304, 1973.

Shepherd, J. T., and Vanhoutte, P. M.: Role of the venous system in circulatory control. Mayo Clinic Proc., *53*:247–255, 1978.

Sixma, J. J., and Webster, J.: The hemostatic plug. Semin. Hematol., *14*:265–299, 1977.

Skjorten, F.: On the nature of hyaline microthrombi. A light microscopical, immunofluorescent and ultrastructural study. Acta Pathol. Microbiol. Scand., *73*:489–501, 1968.

Skorecki, K. L., and Brenner, B. M.: Body fluid homeostasis in man. A contemporary overview. Am. J. Med., *70*:77–88, 1981.

Thomas, A. N., and Stephens, B. G.: Air embolism: a cause of morbidity and death after penetrating chest trauma. J. Trauma, *14*:633–638, 1974.

Van Vleet, J. F., et al.: Ultrastructural alterations in nutritional cardiomyopathy of selenium–vitamin E deficient swine. II. Vascular lesions. Lab. Invest., *37*:201–211, 1977.

Van Vleet, J. F.: Ultrastructure of hyaline microthrombi in myocardial capillaries of pigs with spontaneous "mulberry heart disease." Am. J. Vet. Res., *38*:2077–2080, 1977.

Van Vleet, J. F., et al.: Pathologic alterations in hypertrophic and congestive cardiomyopathy of cats. Am. J. Vet. Res., *41*:2037–2048, 1980.

Van Vleet, J. F., et al.: Pathologic alterations in congestive cardiomyopathy of dogs. Am. J. Vet. Res., *42*:416–424, 1981.

White, N. A., Moore, J. N., and Trim, C. M.: Mucosal alterations in experimentally induced small intestinal strangulation obstruction in ponies. Am. J. Vet. Res., *41*:193–198, 1980.

Yoffee, J. M., and Courtice, F. C.: Lymphatics, Lymph, and the Lymphomyeloid Complex. New York, Academic Press, 1970.

Circulatory Failure

Balis, J. U., et al.: Glucocorticoid and antibiotic effects on hepatic microcirculation and associated host responses in lethal gram-negative bacteremia. Lab. Invest., *40*:55–65, 1979.

Brinkhous, K. M., and Scarborough, D. E.: Some mechanisms of thrombus formation and hemorrhage following trauma. J. Trauma, *9*:684–691, 1969.

Clowes, G. H. A., et al.: The nonspecific pulmonary inflammatory reactions leading to respiratory failure after shock, gangrene and sepsis. J. Trauma, *8*:899–914, 1968.

Collan, Y., et al.: Ultrastructural changes in the gastric mucosa following hemorrhagic shock in pigs. Circ. Shock, *4*:13–25, 1977.

Day, S. B. (ed): Trauma: Clinical and Biological Aspects. New York, Plenum Publishing Corporation, 1975.

Greene, C. E., et al.: Disseminated intravascular coagulation complicating aflatoxicosis in dogs. Cornell Vet., *67*:29–49, 1977.

Hardaway, R. M., III: The problem of acute severe trauma and shock. *In* Day, S. B. (ed.): Trauma: Clinical and Biological Aspects. New York, Plenum Publishing Corporation, 1975.

Hardaway, R. M.: Cellular and metabolic effects of shock. J. Am. Vet. Med. Assoc., *175*:81–86, 1979.

Haskins, S. C.: An overview of acid-base physiology. J. Am. Vet. Med. Assoc., *170*:423–428, 1977.

Jacobson, M. E.: Endocrine aspects of trauma. *In* Day, S. B. (ed.): Trauma: Clinical and Biological Aspects. New York, Plenum Publishing Corporation, 1975.

Kannel, W. B., et al.: Role of blood pressure in the development of congestive heart failure—the Framingham study. New Engl. J. Med., *287*:781–787, 1972.

Kirk, J. E.: Premortal clinical biochemical changes. Adv. Clin. Chem., *11*:175–212, 1968.

Knisely, M. H.: The settling of sludge during life. Acta Anat. (Basel) (Supp. 41), *44*:1–64, 1961.

Knisely, M. H., et al.: Ante-mortem settling. Angiology, *11*:535–588, 1960.

Krum, S. H., and Osborne, C. A.: Heatstroke in the dog: a polysystemic disorder. J. Am. Vet. Med. Assoc., *170*:531–535, 1977.

Lord, P. F.: Neurogenic pulmonary edema in the dog. J. Am. Anim. Hosp. Assoc., *11*:778–783, 1975.

McGovern, V. J.: The pathology of shock. Pathol. Annu., *6*:279–298, 1976.

Moon, H. W.: Mechanisms in the pathogenesis of diarrhea: A review. J. Am. Vet. Med. Assoc., *172*:443–448, 1978.

Moore, J. N., et al.: Clinical evaluation of blood lactate levels in equine colic. Equine Vet. J., *8*:49–54, 1976.

Moss, G., et al.: Cerebral etiology of the "shock lung syndrome." J. Trauma, *12*:885–890, 1972.

Oliver, J., et al.: The pathogenesis of acute renal failure associated with traumatic and toxic injury. Renal ischemia, nephrotoxic damage and the ischemuric episode. J. Clin. Invest., *30*:1307–1440, 1951.

Saldeen, T.: Blood coagulation and shock. Pathol. Res. Pract., *165*:221–252, 1979.

Schiefer, B., and Searcy, G.: Disseminated intravascular coagulation and consumption coagulopathy. Can. Vet. J., *16*:151–159, 1975.

Schramel, R., et al.: Congestive atelectasis. J. Trauma, *8*:821–826, 1968.

Teplitz, C.: The ultrastructural basis for pulmonary pathophysiology following trauma. J. Trauma, *8*:700–712, 1968.

Wigton, D. H., et al.: Infectious canine hepatitis: animal model for viral-induced disseminated intravascular coagulation. Blood, *47*:287–296, 1976.

4

INFLAMMATION AND REPAIR

Inflammation is a fascinating subject. As the host's main defense mechanism against all forms of injury, it is a cornerstone of biology and a marvel of evolutionary complexity. The many interactions of the inflammatory process with other biological processes and the checks and balances through feedback systems are impressive. By definition, ***inflammation is the vascular and cellular responses of living tissue to injury,*** a simple but all-encompassing definition. Injury results in chemical changes in the injured cells or tissue that call forth the inflammatory reaction. The process is generally manifested as redness, heat, swelling and pain. These cardinal signs of inflammation have been known and recognized for many centuries and are exemplified in Figure 4–1. Celsus usually receives credit for defining and recording the signs as rubor (for redness), tumor (for swelling), dolor (for pain) and calor (for heat). A fifth cardinal sign, loss of function, was added later and refers to the tendency to avoid using the part that hurts. ***Any inflammatory lesion carries the suffix "itis,"*** which is quite specific; for example nephritis and hepatitis. If a lesion is not inflammatory, it should not be called an "itis."

FUNCTION OF THE INFLAMMATORY RESPONSE

The purpose of the inflammatory process is to minimize the effect of an irritant to the particular injured tissue. The main response to injury is the accumulation of ***fluids*** and ***cells*** in the injured area. The overall plan for these fluids and cells is to ***dilute, local-***

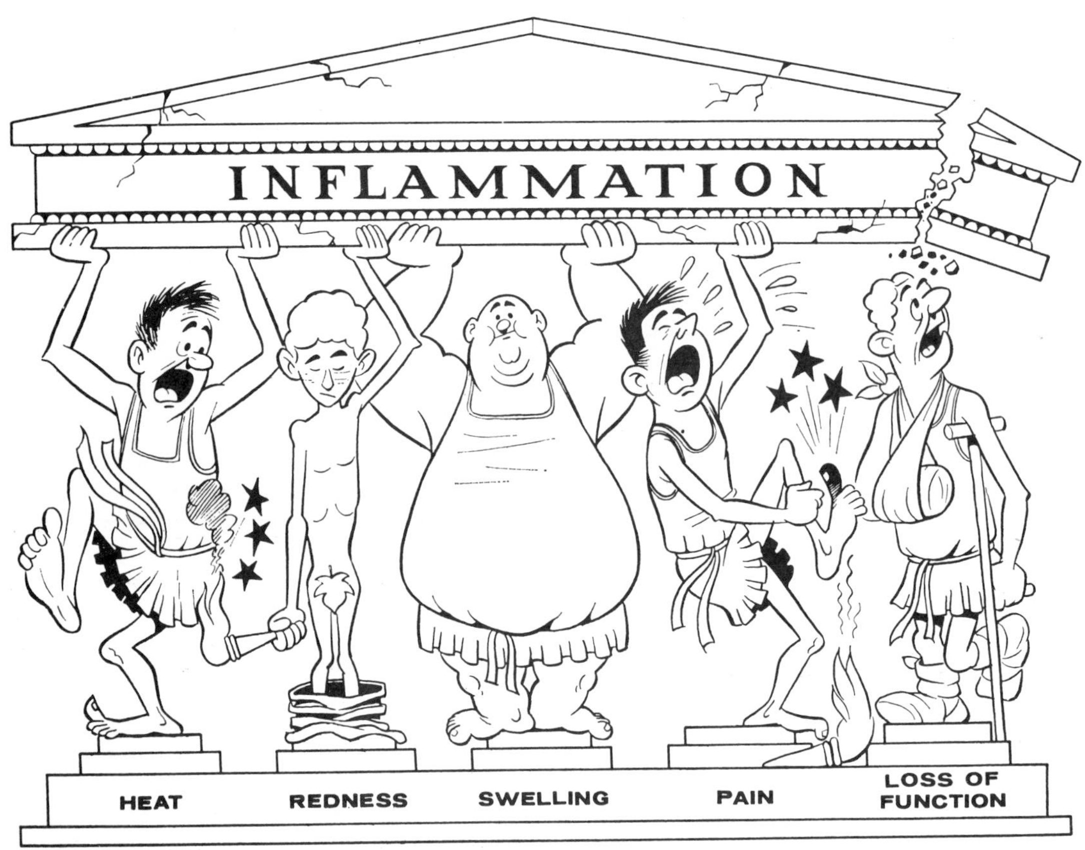

Figure 4–1. The cardinal signs of inflammation. (From Forscher, B. K. [ed.]: Chemical Biology of inflammation. New York, Pergamon Press, 1968. Reprinted by permission.)

ize, destroy and ***remove*** the irritant and to induce ***replacement*** of any injured tissue. The fluids and cells together are referred to as ***exudate,*** which means that they have ***entered the tissue from the blood in an active process.*** They are the means for recognizing the inflammatory process in tissues. The process is complex and involves many biochemical reactions that lead to functional and morphological alterations. ***The immune system and the hemostatic functions of the body are often closely involved in the process, and this adds to the complexity of interactions.***

Inflammation is caused by living and nonliving agents that have the capacity to injure living tissue. The living forms include microorganisms, such as bacteria, viruses, fungi and protozoa, as well as larger parasitic organisms. The nonliving agents include physical and chemical injuries such as those resulting from trauma, irradiation, heat, cold and toxins. Actually, the living agents cause their damage through physical and chemical means by killing cells directly or by secreting substances that are injurious to cells or that cause a harmful host reaction. The concept of ***the host's reaction causing injury*** is quite significant and will come up repeatedly, especially in connection with immune mechanisms of injury.

Table 4–1 provides an overview of the effort to dilute, localize, destroy and remove irritants and lists the components of blood that participate in exudation and healing. Exudates occur ***into*** tissues and ***onto*** serosal, mucosal and integumentary surfaces. They vary in type and composition depending on the tissue, the species of animal and the causative factor. ***Exudates are often mixed with degenerative and necrotic components of tissue, components of the hemostatic system, products of the immune response and repair mechanisms.***

Considerable effort is required to mentally visualize and to actually recognize these interactions in tissues on gross and microscopic examination. The integration of information from Chapters 2 and 3 into this chapter will be essential.

Many nonspecific biochemical factors in serum aid in the destruction of etiological agents. The outpouring of fluid, which is really edema, dilutes the effect of the agent. Fibrin acts as a physical barrier to spreading and confines the irritant. Destruction or confinement by antibody refers to the effect on tissues and on microorganisms, both of which may serve as recognizable foreign antigens. Phagocytosis aids in removal and destruction. The immune system is also involved in the form of antibodies, lymphocytes and macrophages, all of which participate in the lysis of cells and microorganisms. Replacement involves new growth of connective tissue cells resident in the tissues or a degree of regeneration, or both.

One could look at inflammation as a game with an offense, the etiological agent, and a defense, the host. The relative strength, strategy and reserve capacity of each will influence the outcome. If the offense is too strong, the host is quickly eliminated and the agent must find a new team to play against. If the defense is too strong, the agent must plan carefully and avoid a confrontation on the host's terms. The offense can win by using sudden short bursts of ***strength*** and ***surprise*** and by striking ***a weak point*** in the defense. The defense requires time to mobilize reserves in the form of white blood cells and tissue response and will probably be able to sustain prolonged attack if it has ***time*** and ***normal production facilities*** for white blood cells. The defense has many intricate formations to throw at the offense. The initial fibrin barrier, manned by neutrophils, will be aided by the heavy artillery of the macrophages. Sometimes, there is no winner or loser, but the battle may be very close, prolonged and destructive for the agent and the host. Thus, the inflammatory process is essential for body defense but may end up killing the host by committing too many of the body's resources to defense or by allowing the battle to get out of hand in a location vital to the host's survival.

TABLE 4–1. FUNCTIONS OF INFLAMMATORY EXUDATE

Exudate		Function	Method
Fluid	serum plasma	dilute	edema
		localize	fibrin
		destroy	antibody phagocytosis cellular immunity lysis
Cells	neutrophils eosinophils basophils lymphocytes –plasma cell monocytes –macrophage –epithelioid cell –giant cell	remove	lysis phagocytosis
		replace	fibrosis regeneration

There is a tendency to equate inflammation with infection, but this is quite misleading. Not all infections result in inflammation, and inflammation occurs without infection. Some agents are harmful to one species or age group of animals and are not harmful to others. Some parasitic agents live in symbiosis with the host; others survive well and injure the host only moderately. Injury results when there is a degree of incompatibility between the host and the agent, and this usually takes place at the biochemical level of interaction between the proteins or other antigens of one and those of the other. These factors involve the basics of the host–parasite relationship (Chapter 7).

Some agents cause the host to react in a characteristic and consistent manner and, in a manner of speaking, leave their fingerprints. The individual attempting to make a diagnosis will learn from such observations and will begin to make deductions based on species, age, circumstances, lesions present and the type and location of exudate. These observations can assist in identifying an agent's activities, just as learning the habits of a particular thief helps a detective. Such observations are valuable but must be checked out by laboratory tests, since other agents may mimic a particular response or new agents may appear.

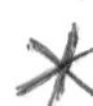

Inflammation is a large subject, and it is necessary to maintain some perspective as the story progresses. The approach here will be somewhat chronological, that is, the acute response first, then the chronic responses and then repair. Each involves both vascular and cellular responses and these will be divided for purposes of convenience, but the fact that they occur together should be kept in mind. Essentially, the individual parts of the process will be discussed separately, and then the process will be assembled. The interactions of the hemostatic and immune systems will be superimposed. The appearance, pathogenesis and significance of different kinds of exudates will be discussed. Repair mechanisms will come later in the discussion but actually begin soon after the inflammatory process begins.

There is a tendency to learn the theory or facts of inflammation while losing sight of its characteristic appearance in tissues, how it can be identified and what is actually occurring in terms of functional processes in the tissues. These must all be combined. The point should be stressed again that *overall perspective* is essential. Keep the view of the forest separated from that of the trees and the other way around but be able to focus back and forth between the two. Some will study inflammation for the theory and some will study it for the art and to practice recognition, diagnosis and prescription of therapy. These are two different missions, but both require understanding of the processes.

COMPONENTS OF THE INFLAMMATORY RESPONSE

The Vascular Response

The exudation of cells and fluids occurs from small venules and capillaries. Most of the exudation occurs from the venules.

What causes these components to leave the vessels and how do they get out? The *pattern of flow changes* in the vessels, they ***dilate,*** their walls become ***permeable*** to some of the contents of the blood that normally do not pass the vessel wall and fluids and cells cross from the blood into the tissue spaces.

The dilated arterioles and capillaries cause hyperemia, and, since the venules also become ***dilated,*** a degree of congestion also occurs; these components will vary in proportion in different lesions. Exudation requires flowing blood, however. There is more blood flowing into the injured area and the flow is slow. As the vessels become ***leaky,*** the viscosity of the blood increases, leading to sludging and increased hydrostatic pressure. The flow pattern is altered and laminar patterns are disturbed, so that white cells, red cells and platelets may ***touch each other and the endothelial surfaces.*** Endothelial injury may activate components of the coagulation system.

These events are controlled and influenced by ***chemical mediators*** (Fig. 4–2). Details of actions of these mediators are indicated at the appropriate points in this chapter. The mediators are usually present in an inactive form that is activated by the injury. Once activated, some factors are self-perpetuating and some activate others. Many have functions in common; their effects may be additive or they may set off or contribute to other functions. Some are activated inside the blood vessel in the area of inflammation, some are released in the tissue after they leave the vessel and some are activated from the tissue. ***Primarily, these chemicals dilate vessels and alter permeability, but some attract white blood cells into the tissues.*** They alter the junctions of endothelial cells with other endothelial cells and with the basement membrane, and this allows fluid to leave. The basement membrane is also biochemically altered with the result that it becomes leaky. The extent of injury will influence the degree of release of chemical mediators, the extent of leakage and the size of the compounds that come out. Of the plasma proteins, albumin will be released first; more damage will allow the escape of fibrinogen.

The chemical mediators are amines, proteases and polypeptides and include histamine, serotonin, kinins, plasmin, complement, anaphylotoxins, prostaglandins, lysosomal esterases and lymphocytic and macrophage products. There are new com-

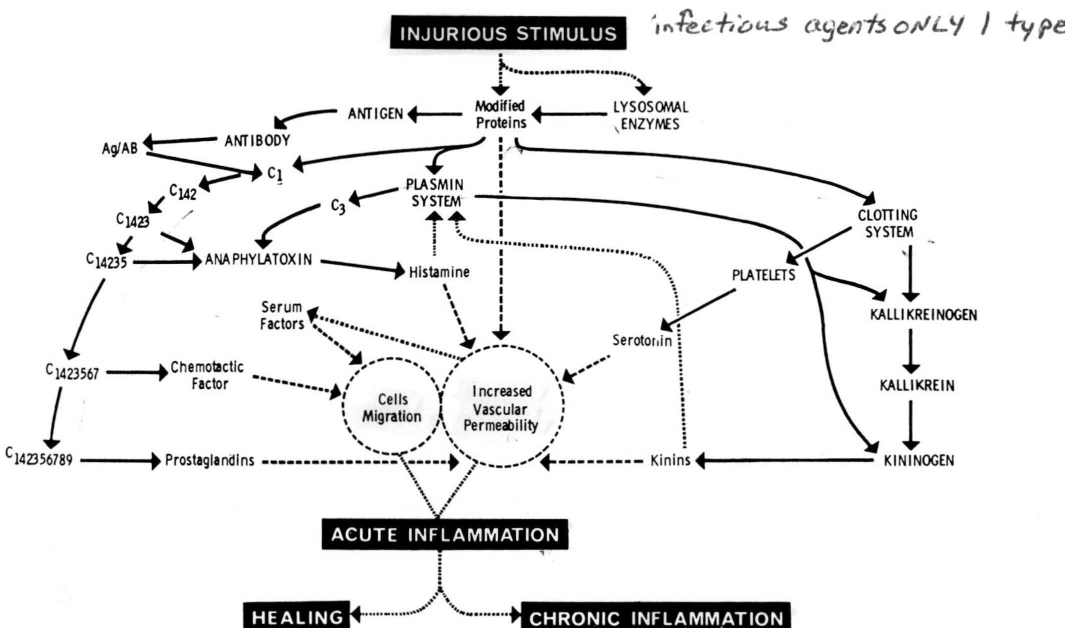

Figure 4–2. Events in inflammation mediated by chemical mediators. This figure should be examined periodically during the study of the remainder of the chapter in order to integrate the aspects of coagulation, chemical mediators and immunologically induced influences. (From Forscher, B. K., and Houck, J. C.: Immunopathology of Inflammation. Amsterdam, Excerpta Medica, 1971. Reprinted by permission.)

pounds being discovered and unknown compounds being purified regularly, as indicated by the voluminous literature on their structure and function (Table 4–2). (See Ryan and Majno, 1977.)

Histamine is contained in and released from mast cells that are present in most tissues, and especially near very small blood vessels, but it is also released from platelets and basophils (Figs. 4–3 and 4–4). Histamine is released from membrane-bound granules within the mast cells and induces dilation of arterioles and increased permeability of capillaries and venules. The action is ***relatively brief***; sustained action comes from other mediators. In some species, serotonin has actions similar to those of histamine. ***Anaphylotoxins*** are effectors of histamine release. ***Prostaglandins*** stimulate the release of histamine and thus act very early in the inflammatory process. Prostaglandins contribute to the genesis of fever, pain, vasodilation and increased permeability. Bradykinin stimulates prostaglandin release from cells. There is increasing evidence that mast cells are not fixed in tissues but may move into the epithelium of mucosal surfaces, and thus closer to surface stimuli. They may proliferate in tissues in some forms of inflammation.

Kinins are present in plasma alpha-2-globulins in an inactive form as ***kininogens*** and are the most potent mediators. They act in vasodilation by increasing vascular permeability and enhancing migration of leukocytes, and they may cause pain. Kinins are activated by plasma enzymes called ***kallikreins*** and are inactivated by ***kininases,*** which are carboxypeptidases found in plasma and tissues (Fig. 4–5). Kallikrein is a plasma enzyme system present in and released from neutrophils, and it generates the formation of kinins. ***Bradykinin,*** the best known kinin, increases vascular permeability, contracts smooth muscle, dilates vessels and induces pain.

Plasmin causes liberation of kinins and ***complement,*** which influence permeability and also lyse fibrin. Hageman factor may be influential in activation of plasmin (Fig. 4–6). These mediators essentially influence permeability, but some are also active in attracting neutrophils outside the vessel and in stimulating degranulation and release of compounds from cells that maintain the inflammatory process.

Cholinergic and adrenergic stimulation affect the immunological release of mediators. β ***adrenergic stimuli*** suppress and ***cholinergic stimuli*** enhance the release of me-

TABLE 4–2. CLASSIFICATION OF ENDOGENOUS MEDIATORS OF INFLAMMATION

Origin	Major groups	Major mediators
Plasma	Kinin system	Bradykinin Kallikrein Plasminogen activator
	Complement system	C3 fragments C5 fragments C567 complex C kinin
	Clotting system	Fibrinopeptides Fibrin degradation products
Tissues	Vasoactive amines	Histamine 5-hydroxytryptamine
	Acidic lipids	Slow-reacting substance of anaphylaxis Prostaglandins
	Lysosomal components	Cationic proteins Acid proteases Neutral proteases
	Lymphocyte products	Migration inhibitory factor Chemotactic factors Lymphotoxin Skin reactive factors Mitogenic factor Lymph node permeability factor
	Others	Endogenous pyrogens Leukocytosis factors Substance P Neurotensin Cyclic AMP

From Ryan, G. B., and Majno, G.: Acute inflammation. Am. J. Pathol., *86*:184–276, 1977.

MAST CELL OR BASOPHIL

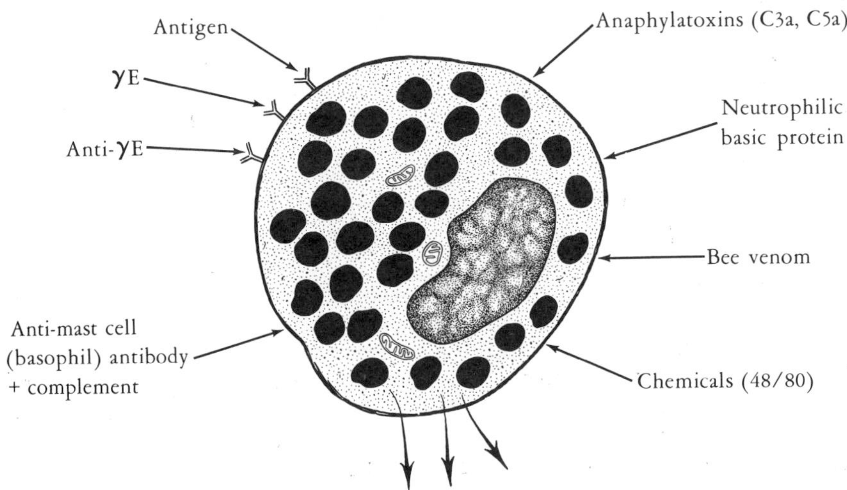

RELEASE OF VASOACTIVE AMINES

Figure 4–3. Stimuli that can induce release of vasoactive amines from mast cells or basophils. (From Bellanti, J. A.: Immunology II. Philadelphia, W. B. Saunders Company, 1978.)

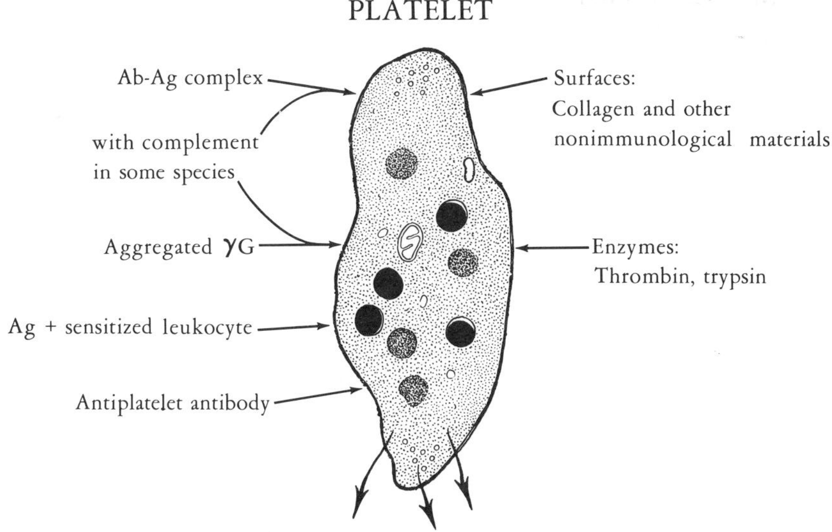

Figure 4–4. Some stimuli that can induce release of vasoactive amines from platelets. (From Bellanti, J. A.: Immunology II. Philadelphia, W. B. Saunders Company, 1978.)

diators. These actions are regulated by ***cyclic AMP,*** which is increased by β adrenergic stimuli and decreased by cholinergic stimuli. The stimuli enhance or suppress activation of adenyl cyclase, which in turn controls the production of cyclic AMP. This mechanism is considered to be a factor in asthma, in which cholinergic stimuli add to the release of mediators induced by exposure to antigen.

As illustrated by Figures 4–5 and 4–6, it seems that bradykinin, C3a and C5a are most important in increasing vascular permeability and C5a in chemotaxis. Plasmin generates kinins, cleaves C3 and lyses fibrin. Factor XII initiates the clotting, fibrinolytic and kinin systems. In addition, strong amplification is provided by the further results of kallikrein activation of Factor XII.

The Cellular Response

The migration of cells occurs primarily from venules soon after the vascular changes are set in motion. ***Neutrophils*** are usually first to leave and gain exit by moving to the edge of the endothelium, sticking to the endothelium and actively seeking a space between the endothelial cells. They push pseudopodia into the space and bulge through, and the rest of the cell follows. They seem to pass through the basement

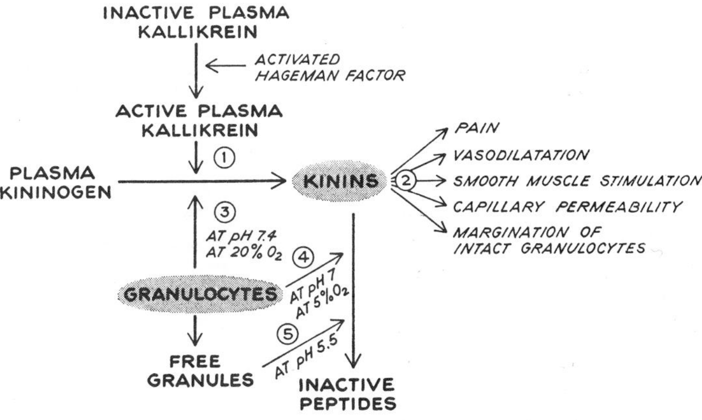

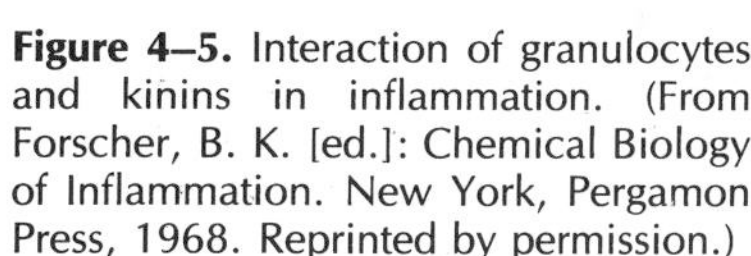

Figure 4–5. Interaction of granulocytes and kinins in inflammation. (From Forscher, B. K. [ed.]: Chemical Biology of Inflammation. New York, Pergamon Press, 1968. Reprinted by permission.)

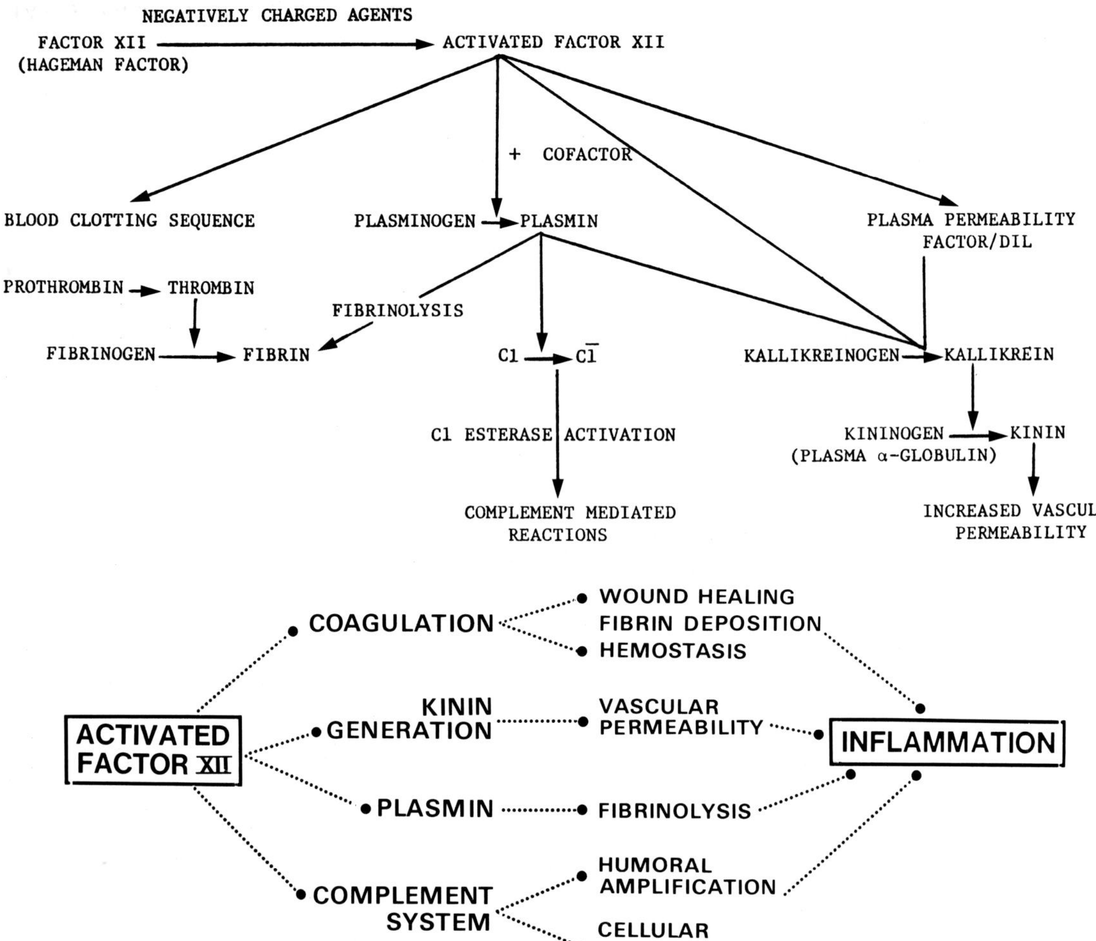

Figure 4–6. Involvement of Hageman factor in the interrelations of inflammatory and clotting mechanisms. Activation of the first component of the blood clotting mechanism, Hageman factor, also results in the activation of other biological reactions, including plasmin, complement and kinin systems. Plasmin induces fibrinolysis, complement activation, local inflammation and cell lysis; kinin, a biologically active polypeptide fragment that is split off plasma α-globulin, enhances vascular permeability and causes dilation of small vessels. Reaction of an individual to a variety of inciting events sets off an interrelated series of responses, both immune and nonimmune, leading to blood clotting, clot lysis, inflammation and cell lysis. (Courtesy of D. Slausen.) The Inflammatory Process. D. O. Slausen, 27th Annual Mtg. of the American College of Veterinary Pathologists on "Mechanisms of Inflammation," Miami, Florida, December 1976.

membrane as though it did not exist and crawl over other elements, such as fibrin or tissue cells, toward their destination. Eosinophils and neutrophils have ameboid capabilities, but red cells do not; lymphocytes have considerably less ability to move actively than neutrophils have. Monocytes actively contribute to their own exiting and soon become macrophages. Some animals, such as poultry, fish and reptiles, have cells named ***heterophils*** that perform functions similar to neutrophils. Neutrophils do not normally stick to endothelium or to each other, so there must be biochemical and surface charge alterations on their surfaces and perhaps those of endothelial cells to contribute to the mutual stickiness. The specific details of the mechanism have not been clarified.

In acute inflammation, neutrophilic exudation is soon followed by monocytic exudation. ***The monocytes quickly mature into macrophages that are also called histiocytes since they patrol within tissues.*** Distinction will not be made here between macrophages derived from monocytes and those derived from tissue histiocytes, but in an inflammatory lesion most are derived from monocytes. If the skin is scraped until it bleeds and a coverslip is taped to the lesion, it is possible to study the time sequence of exudation of cells by removing the coverslip for staining and examination at specific intervals. This is called the ***Rebuck skin window technique.*** Neutrophils predominate by four to six hours, by 12 hours macrophages are numerous and the two are about equal by 24 hours, when lymphocytes begin to appear. This is an experimental model and the responses will vary somewhat depending on the etiological factors.

Neutrophils that come into the exudate seem to travel toward a place in the tissue as though they were being drawn there by some force. The process by which the attracting site determines the migration route is called ***chemotaxis,*** and the biochemical substances responsible for the attractive influence are called ***chemotactic factors.*** There are two main functions for neutrophils once they enter the tissue and collect in groups. One function is ***phagocytosis,*** and the other is the ***release of lysosomal enzymes***, which lyse cells and tissue in the area. Both of these processes are themselves chemotactic. Several factors have chemotactic attraction for neutrophils: some viruses, some bacteria, kinins, fibrin, antigen-antibody complexes, complement, lymphocyte secretions (called lymphokines) and collagen degradation products. The process becomes self-perpetuating, and the tissue damage caused by neutrophils adds to the vascular permeability and exudation of cells. Other factors add further to chemotaxis: ***substances released from necrotic cells, coagulation products and fibrinolysin.*** Some chemotactic factors attract neutrophils, monocytes and eosinophils equally, and some have preferential attraction for one specific cell or combination of cells. More specifically, the two most important chemotactic factors are soluble products produced by bacteria and the products of the complement system. For neutrophils, C3 and C5, as well as closely related factors, and $C\overline{567}$ are the main active components of the complement system. The activity of the C3 and C5 components is induced by both immunological reactions and by bacterial proteases and proteolytic enzymes in plasma and tissue, such as plasmin and other tissue proteases. The chemotactic factors influence contractile proteins of the phagocytes. Monocytic chemotactic substances include C3 and C5 fragments, factors formed in antigen-antibody interactions, bacterial factors, neutrophil products and factors liberated from sensitized neutrophils.

If the original inciting agent persists and multiplies in spite of the defense, much tissue damage may occur, and the process will continue as long as the agent persists. Macrophages, lymphocytes, plasma cells and fibroblasts may soon appear in considerable numbers to assist with the battle, and these are usually an indication of a subacute or chronic lesion.

Complement is influential in several aspects of inflammation, but mainly in chemotaxis. This compound is normally found in plasma and is really a complex system of enzymes that may be activated and that has strong biological functions. The "classical" system comprises nine components that, if activated in sequence, cause lysis of cells. The key step is activation of the third component, and this can also be accomplished by the "alternate" pathway, through which C3 is activated directly without need for C1 and C2. Some components of the system are active in phagocytosis, in increasing permeability of vessels and in chemotaxis. The lysosomal enzymes from neutrophils may activate complement components, as may plasmin, thrombin, some bacterial enzymes and, in particular, antigen-antibody complexes (Fig. 4–7). More specifically C3a increases vascular permeability and is chemotactic for neutrophils. C5a induces increased vascular permeability and is chemotactic for neutrophils and macrophages; $C\overline{567}$ is also chemotactic. C3a and C5a, often called anaphylotoxins, induce the release of histamine from platelets and mast cells. Necrotic tissue, such as infarcted myocardium, contains an enzyme that is able to split a chemotactic factor from C3.

There is a tendency to think of all inflammatory reactions in textbook fashion, which is usually only an experimentally determined sequence. Different etiological agents will cause different circumstances to exist in the tissue, and the reactions may vary considerably in cell type and time sequence, even in acute lesions. Therefore, the textbook picture is seldom observed in natural disease states in which neither the time of initiation nor the etiological agent is known at the time of observation. It is the knowledge gained from experimental findings, however, that allows extrapolations and interpretations to be made in naturally occurring lesions.

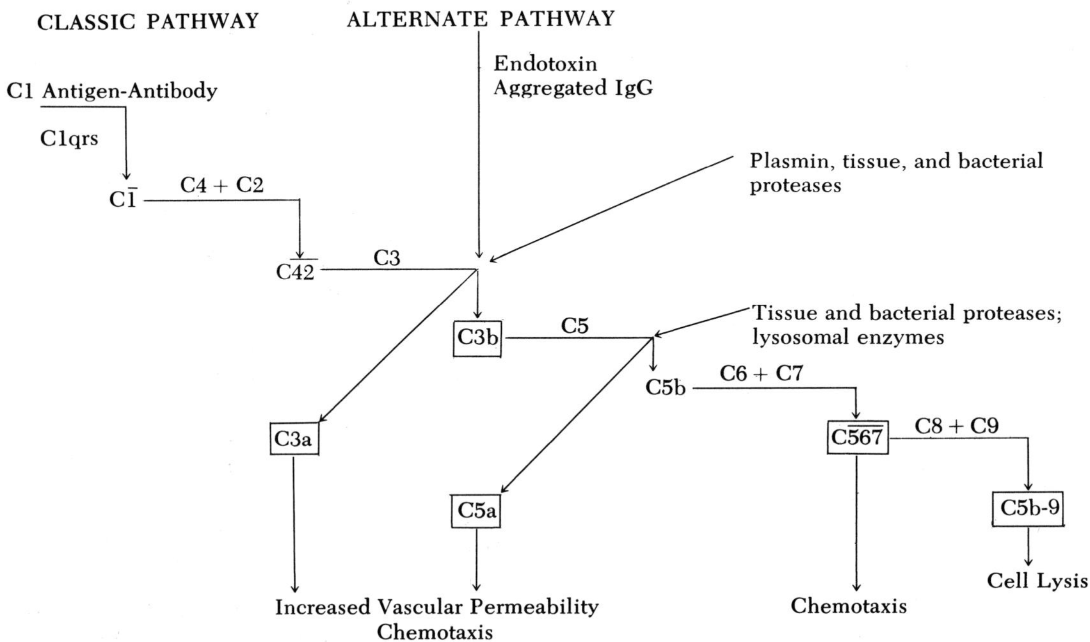

Figure 4–7. The complement system. (From Robbins, S. L., and Cotran, R. S.: Pathologic Basis of Disease. 2nd ed. Philadelphia, W. B. Saunders Co., 1979.

This point is important for perspective and aids in increasing one's appreciation for experimental pathology.

The paper by Rebuck and Crowley (1955) contains a review of inflammation that begins with the year 1828 and deals in particular with the role of white blood cells. The paper by Ryan and Majno (1977) provides an extensive review of the acute inflammatory response and includes over 550 references.

Each of the cell types involved in the inflammatory exudate (Fig. 4–8) will now be discussed.

GRANULOCYTIC SERIES

This series refers to ***neutrophils, eosinophils*** and ***basophils,*** the neutrophils being the most numerous. Neutrophils function within the blood or tissues primarily to ***phagocytize*** and often to release their lysosomal enzymes to ***lyse*** debris. They contain abundant lysosomes that have a large number of different types of enzymes and seem to be armed for any occasion. The process of ***phagocytosis*** is illustrated in Figure 4–9. Particles such as microorganisms are taken into the cell and are digested to bits of debris that may be expelled from the cell. The ***phagosome*** fuses with the ***lysosome*** to become a ***phagolysosome*** in which the ingested particle is exposed to the lysosomal enzymes. Some of the enzymes kill microorganisms, and others digest the remnants. Some organisms are more easily phagocytized than others, and if ***opsonic antibodies*** are produced by the antibody-forming cells, the work of uptake is facilitated. To be phagocytized is not necessarily to be killed. Some agents are quite resistant to digestion, may remain inside the phagocyte (particularly macrophages) for prolonged periods and are protected from the defense mechanisms of antibody and lymphocytes. In some instances, when phagocytosis of bacteria occurs, the process seems paralyzed in terms of internal digestion. Some viral infections in macrophages create these circumstances. The process of phagocytosis often results in the release of lysosomal enzymes from the cells, and these may influence the clotting mechanisms as well as acting as pyrogens.

1. Neutrophils. ***Neutrophils*** are present in most, if not all, inflammatory exudates, but their numbers may vary, depending on the agent and the host's reaction to the

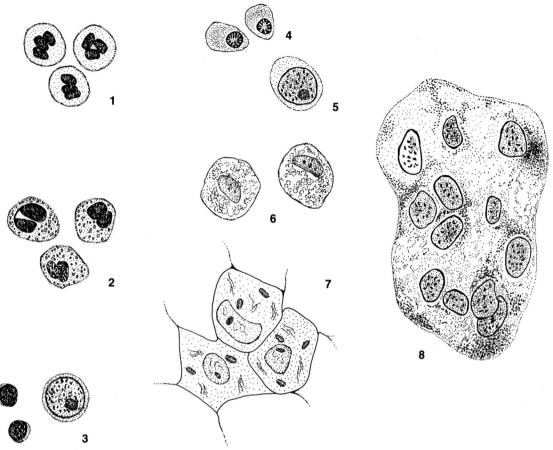

Figure 4–8. Some of the cells involved in inflammatory exudate: (1) neutrophils, (2) eosinophils, (3) small and large lymphocytes, (4) plasma cell, (5) cell in transition between a lymphocyte and a plasma cell, (6) macrophage, (7) epithelioid cell, (8) giant cell.

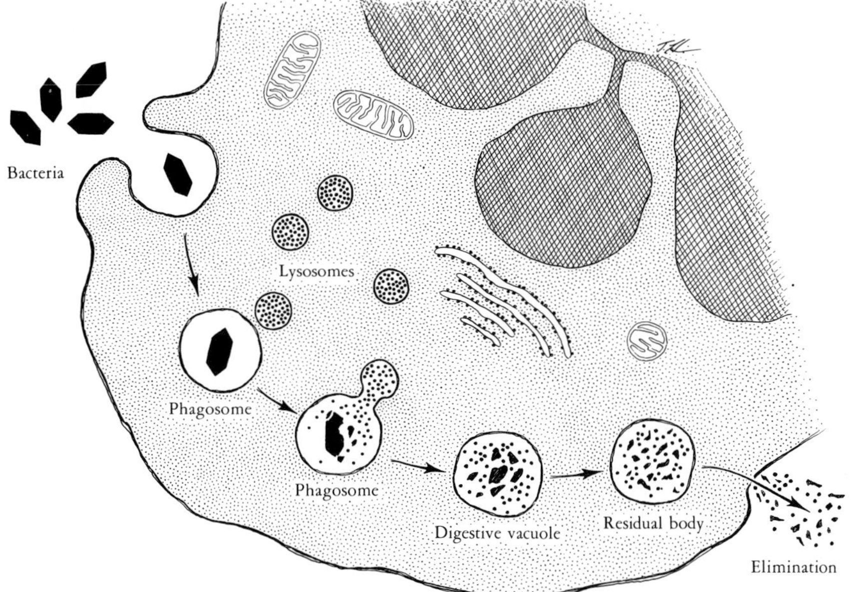

Figure 4–9. Schematic representation of phagocytosis, showing the ingestion process and intracellular digestion. (From Bellanti, J. A.: Immunology II. Philadelphia, W. B. Saunders Company, 1978.)

agent (Figs. 4–10, 4–11 and 4–12). Masses of dead and dying neutrophils are the chief constituents of ***pus.*** The fluid nature of pus occurs because of the digestive lysosomal enzymes released from the neutrophils that act on other neutrophils and nearby tissue. They have ameboid activity and can crawl on fibrils such as fibrin. They do not swim well in fluid but do respond to chemotaxis. They occur in pus as the predominant cell in an inflammatory exudate in response to infection by pyogenic bacteria; ***they respond by chemotaxis to necrotic tissue*** and quickly surround it to begin liquefaction. They also respond dramatically to ***antigen-antibody reactions that fix complement.*** Neutrophil products include cationic proteins, acid proteases and neutral proteases. The cationic proteins increase vascular permeability by releasing histamine from mast cells, are chemotactic for monocytes and may inhibit movement of neutrophils and eosinophils. Acid proteases act primarily within phagosomes. Neutral proteases degrade extracellular components such as collagen, basement membrane, fibrin, elastin and cartilage and are thus responsible for the tissue destruction associated with collections of neutrophils in tissue. They can also induce the release of kinins and initiate chemotactic activity from C3 and C5 fragments.

In tissue sections, their cytoplasm stains variably and may not be apparent, but the nucleus is the identifiable feature. As they degenerate, the nucleus becomes pyknotic and breaks up. The nucleus is usually identifiable for some time after the death of the cell.

The phagocytic processes in neutrophils and macrophages have many similarities. Most particles which become phagocytosed are first coated by opsonic serum factors, usually IgG or opsonic fragments of C3. Both cell types have Fc receptors for IgG opsonins and a C3 receptor. Often leakage of lysosomal enzymes from the cell occurs during the phagocytic process as degranulation occurs within the phagocyte. Phagocytes require energy for their defense functions. The oxygen-dependent bactericidal mechanisms use hydrogen peroxide and superoxide ions to kill the phagocytosed bacteria. ***Myeloperoxidase,*** contained in neutrophil granules, markedly increases the efficiency of hydrogen peroxide particularly in the presence of a halide ion—thus the name hydrogen peroxide–myeloperoxidase-halide system. The latter system is of greater significance than the superoxide system. Hydrogen ion production in the phagocytes reduces the pH, and thus bacterial growth. Lysozyme contained within the phagocyte attacks bacterial cell walls.

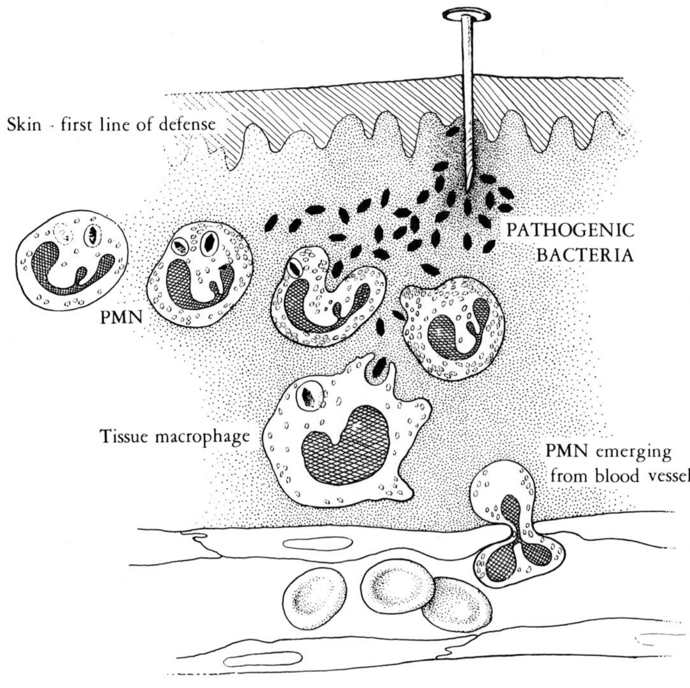

Figure 4–10. Schematic representation of phagocytosis by polymorphonuclear leukocytes (PMN) and tissue macrophages after penetration of the skin and introduction of pathogenic bacteria into deeper tissues. The PMN's are more efficient in phagocytosis than the macrophages. Note the PMN's are mobilized into tissues from blood vessels during the inflammatory response. (From Bellanti, J. A.: Immunology II. Philadelphia, W. B. Saunders Company, 1978.)

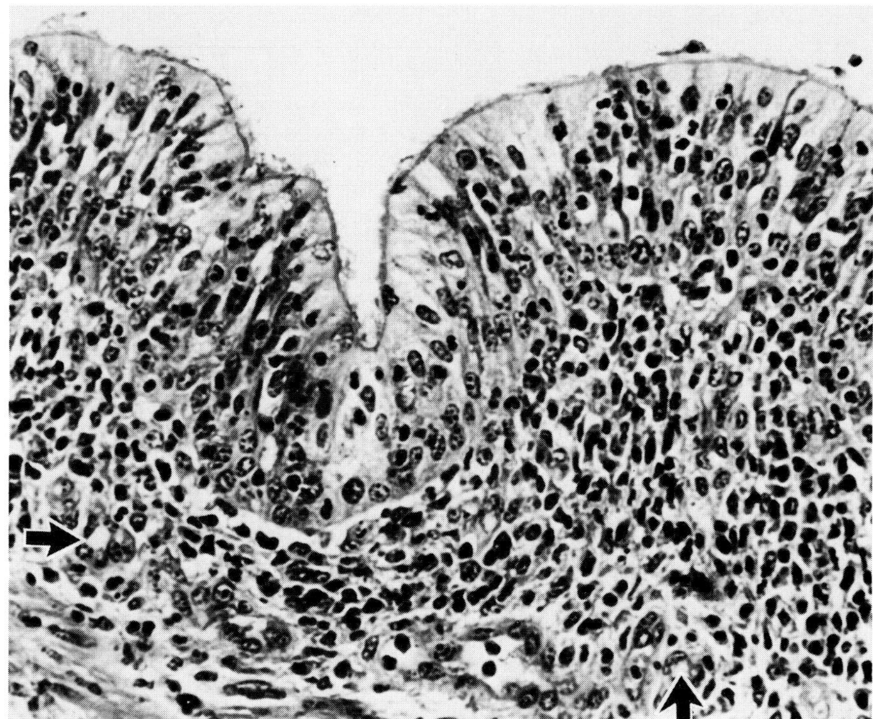

Figure 4–11. Neutrophils are present in the epithelial layer and are passing into the lumen of a bronchus. They have come from small vessels in the lamina propria (arrows) but this is difficult to visualize among the mononuclear cells in that area. It is surprisingly difficult to clearly visualize cells in the process of exudation from vessels in tissue sections.

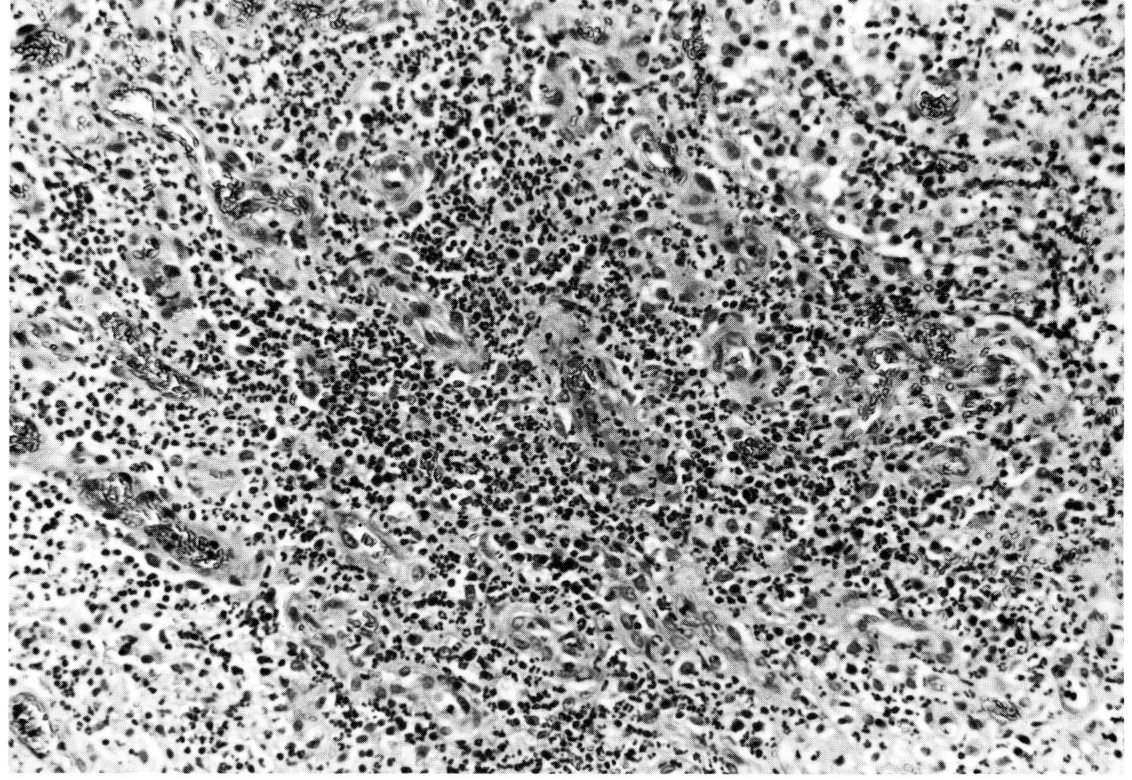

Figure 4–12. Neutrophils in an acute inflammation of soft tissue. Note the shape of their nuclei. It is the means by which they are identified in tissues.

The bone marrow may be examined to determine the state of regeneration if large numbers of neutrophils have been used and more are needed. The percentage and, more importantly, the absolute number in the circulating blood can be established from a ***total and a differential white cell count.*** The ability of the marrow to respond may be partially interpreted from this information. A ***regenerative shift*** in the differential count indicates that more neutrophils are being made, as indicated by the numbers of cells circulating and by the immature forms present. A ***degenerative shift*** implies that the marrow is not producing cells quickly enough, as indicated by the low or normal total number of cells and the higher percentage of band forms than of cells with segmented nuclei. If the offense wipes out the reserves before an adequate marrow response can occur, the game will be over. If the defense cannot produce new recruits because of debility or overcommitment to other functions, the game will also end—but more slowly.

Species vary in their normal total and differential white blood cell counts. Each must be learned or a small data card should be carried for ready access to the information. The book by Schalm and co-workers (1975) should be consulted for detailed information. The ***neutrophil to lymphocyte ratio*** is 3.5:1 in dogs, 1.8:1 in cats, 1.1:1 in horses and 0.5:1 in cattle. Corticosteroids induce ***leukopenia, lymphopenia*** and ***neutrophilia*** in animals with a high proportion of lymphocytes. Those species with high proportions of neutrophils respond to steroids with ***leukocytosis,*** neutrophilia and lymphopenia.

The marrow activity for generation of cells is controlled by ***chalones.*** The specific generation time for each of the cell types in various species has not been determined, but information is available for some. Thus, only generalizations can be mentioned here. Neutrophils have a generation time of about seven days and a half-life in circulating blood of about six hours. Therefore, the entire pool is replaced about four times every day. They leave the blood to go into tissue and do not return. ***Apparently, most are lost on the mucosal surfaces of the urinary, digestive and respiratory tracts.*** The total pool comprises those neutrophils that are circulating and those that are in the vessels but marginated temporarily in reserve. Species vary in the numbers available for quick release from the marrow; for example, a dog responds quickly if the circulating reserves are used up suddenly, whereas a calf remains leukopenic for a few days, during which its defenses are reduced. The marrow usually contains a larger number of cells in reserve or in the final stages of development, but, as was mentioned previously, the ability to respond quickly varies.

Congenital and inherited deficient functions of neutrophils occur; one example is the ***Chédiak-Higashi syndrome,*** in which large abnormal granules are formed. This syndrome has been identified in several species. The cyclic neutropenia of collie dogs is a periodic depression of bone marrow production of neutrophils. In both instances, affected individuals are very prone to infection.

2. Eosinophils. *Eosinophils* generally react to stimuli similar to those for neutrophils but have specific chemotactic responses. Their red granules on hematoxylin and eosin staining distinguish them from neutrophils, but they may be confused with globule leukocytes in tissue sections of mucous membranes. Eosinophils are usually prominent in certain stages of the reaction to ***parasitic migration*** in tissue and in so-called ***allergic reactions,*** but this latter point is so general and nonspecific as to be of little use in microscopic interpretation. It is difficult to make a specific association with the presence of eosinophils in any diseases other than parasitic ones. They are numerous in the acute Arthus reaction, in some granulomas, in the exudate in the meninges of pigs with salt poisoning and in eosinophilic myositis or chloroma in cattle but may occur in any inflammatory lesion. They are phagocytic and produce pus if present in sufficient numbers. The source, generation time and life span of eosinophils is similar to that of neutrophils.

3. Basophils. *Basophils* are the least numerous of the granulocytes and in many respects are similar in form and function to the mast cells, although some of their granules resemble those of neutrophils. They are not specifically associated with lesions in common diseases of animals as a main component of exudate. Some consider basophils to be immature circulating mast cells. Basophils have a life span of 10 to 12 days and are made in the marrow.

MONONUCLEAR CELLS

The mononuclear series includes monocytes, lymphocytes, plasma cells, macrophages, epithelioid cells and giant cells.

1. Lymphocytes. *Lymphocytes* are smaller than macrophages, are not phagocytic and are primarily associated with the host's immune response. They, too, are very versatile. They are less mobile than macrophages and probably respond to chemotaxis. ***It is not possible to determine from observing lymphocytes in routine tissue sections where they came from or precisely what their function may be*** (Figs. 4–13, 4–14, and 4–15). Techniques are being developed, however, to make such interpretations in experimental situations. Again, it is only as a result of experimental work that possible interpretations can be rendered on the significance of lymphocytes in lesions of naturally occurring diseases. For purposes of this discussion, it is necessary to digress at this point to put the ***source*** and ***functions*** of lymphocytes into perspective. There is some evidence that lymphocytes may become macrophages.

The discussion may seem unduly complicated, but a perspective is necessary to relate to possible interpretations of the function of lymphocytes in lesions or to evaluate the host response in tissue sections of lymph nodes and follicles.

Lymphocytes are produced in the lymph nodes, bone marrow, spleen and thymus and in the lymph follicles on many mucous membranes (the most prominent being Peyer's patches of the intestine) and the tonsils (Fig. 4–16). ***They migrate from, between and among these locations, in and out of the blood and lymph and from lymph nodes and nodules.*** Figure 4–17 illustrates the traffic into and out of a lymph node.

Two main functional groups of lymphocytes exist: one that results in the production of all types of ***antibody for humoral immunity*** and one that produces lymphocytes to function in the various aspects of ***cellular immunity.*** They are the mobile instructional apparatus for the immune system. The first are called ***B lymphocytes*** and the second are called ***T lymphocytes.*** The T cells are derived from lymphocytes that at some point passed through and were influenced by the thymus gland to respond in cellular immune reactions. The name "B cells" is derived from the bursa of Fabricius in chickens, where this distinction in lymphocyte function was first demonstrated (Fig. 4–18). Both T and B cells occur in lymphoid tissues and are made in the spleen and lymph nodes. B cells are made in lymph follicles and T cells are made in the area just peripheral to lymph follicles. The various stages of development of lymph follicles indicate stages in production or stimulation of production of B cells. A large area of activity and proliferation of lymphocytes around a follicle indicates T cell production. The situation becomes

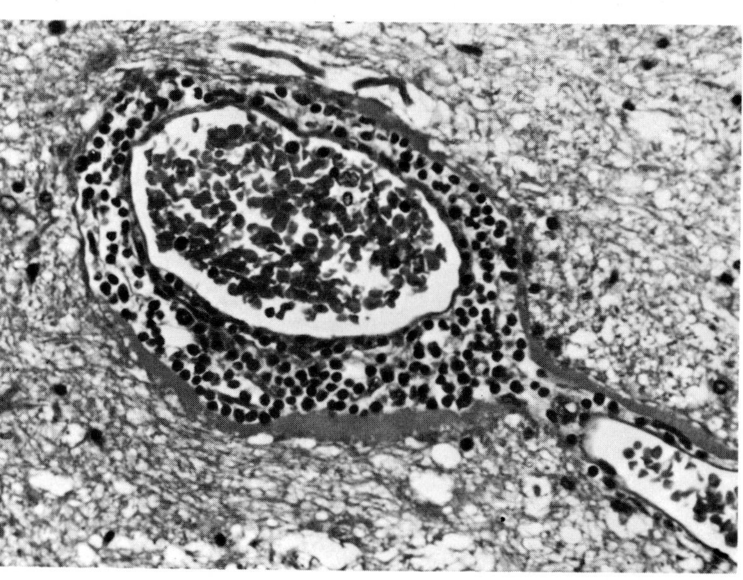

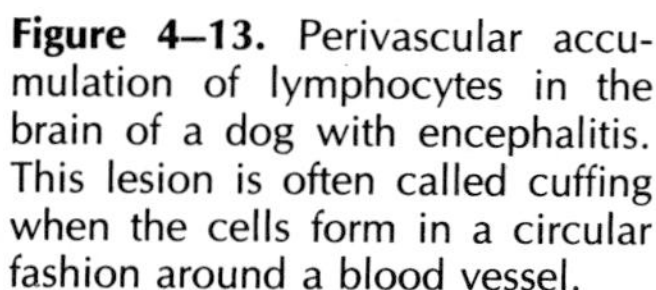

Figure 4–13. Perivascular accumulation of lymphocytes in the brain of a dog with encephalitis. This lesion is often called cuffing when the cells form in a circular fashion around a blood vessel.

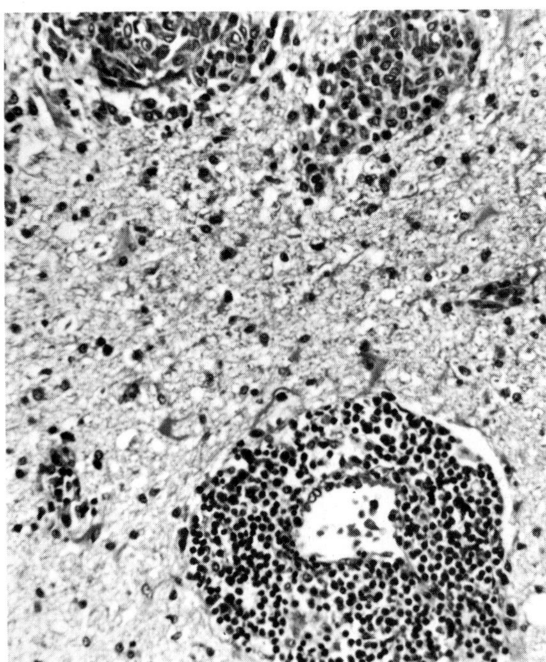

Figure 4–14. Same type of lesion as seen in Figure 4–13 (bottom). Note the collection of macrophages around nearby vessels (top).

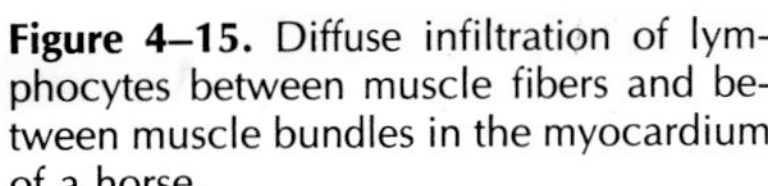

Figure 4–15. Diffuse infiltration of lymphocytes between muscle fibers and between muscle bundles in the myocardium of a horse.

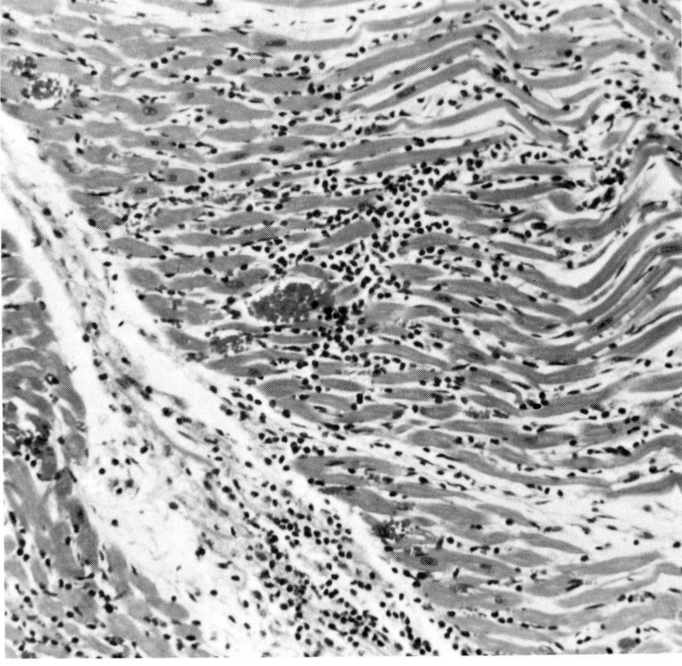

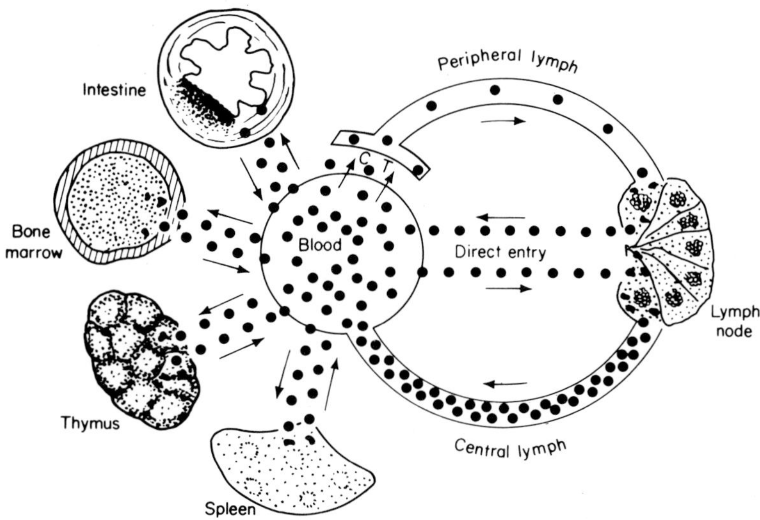

Figure 4–16. Illustration of some of the main cellular migration streams in the lymphomyeloid complex. This diagram was originally devised to illustrate lymphocytic migration streams. It is now known that there also is extensive migration of macrophages and macrophage precursors and of immature plasma cells; these are not illustrated in the diagram. Cells reach the blood stream either by obtaining access to the lymph stream (indirect entry) or by passing through the walls of blood vessels (direct entry). Lymphocytes from bone marrow and spleen reach the blood by direct entry. Lymphocytes leaving lymph nodes and thymus use both the direct and the indirect entry, in varying proportions. The connective tissue migration stream (CT) includes the serous cavities, such as the peritoneum. (From Yoffee, J. M., and Courtice, F. C.: Lymphatics, Lymph and the Lymphomyeloid Complex. New York, Academic Press, 1971. Reprinted by permission.)

more complex because some T cells also act as cofactors in the production of antibody by B cells. T cells produce their effects by directly contacting cells and killing them or by secreting substances called ***lymphokines*** that act on antigens or other cells. Lymphokines mediate the inflammatory process primarily via the T lymphocytes and their products, which are chemotactic for macrophages, neutrophils and basophils. They can also inhibit macrophage migration. It is important to note that lymphocytes may be present, even in large numbers, in lesions that are not immunologically induced. Reference will be made to the functions of lymphocytes in the discussion of immunologically mediated lesions. Lymphocytes are often present in lesions around small blood vessels and tend to form a cuff around the vessel. NK (natural killer) lymphocytes have recently been recognized to have many functions, including direct cytotoxicity against target cells such as tumour cells, production of interferon and general surveillance functions.

Lymphocytes are found both within and outside the blood stream, as mentioned previously. There seem to be two populations of lymphocytes based on life span: one whose life span is 2 to 4 days and one with a life span of 100 to 200 days. Some human lymphocytes have been found that

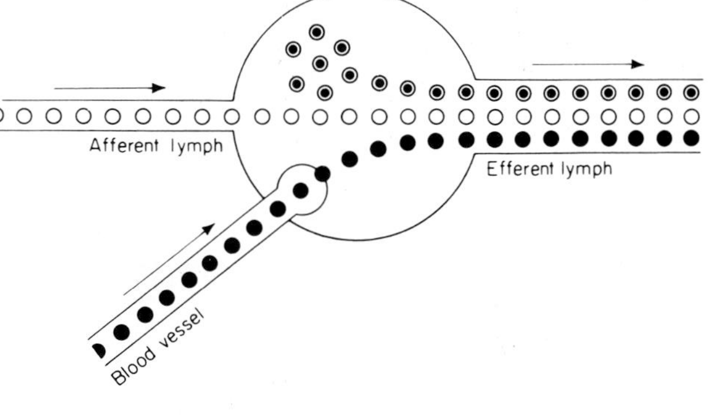

Figure 4–17. The origin of lymph-borne (indirect entry) lymphocytes in the efferent lymph of a lymph node. These cells may be derived from (1) lymphocytes reaching the node through the afferent lymphatic vessel, (2) lymphocytes in the blood stream that enter the node by passing through the walls of blood vessels, especially the postcapillary veins and (3) lymphocytes formed in the node. (From Yoffee, J. M., and Courtice, F. C.: Lymphatics, Lymph and the Lymphomyeloid Complex. New York, Academic Press, 1971. Reprinted by permission.)

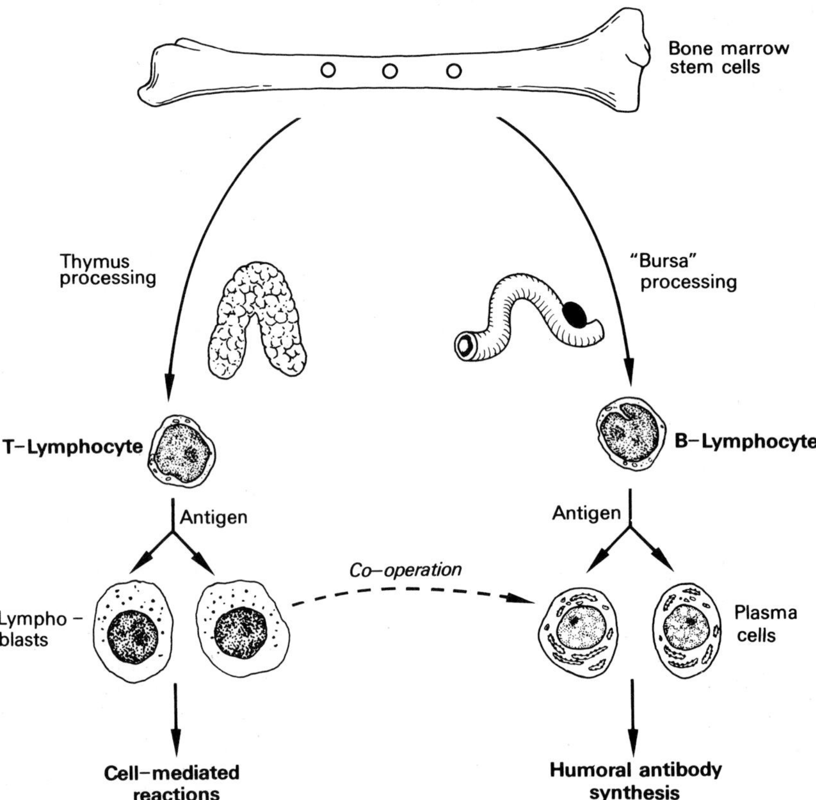

Figure 4–18. Processing of bone marrow cells by thymus and by gut-associated central lymphoid tissue to become immunocompetent T- and B-lymphocytes, respectively. Proliferation and transformation to cells of the lymphoblast and plasma cell series occur on antigenic stimulation. (From Roitt, I.: Essentials of immunology. Philadelphia, F. A. Davis Co. [Blackwell Scientific Publications], 1971. Reprinted by permission.)

lived from 3 to 20 years. In calves, two hundred million cells per minute enter the blood by the thoracic duct; 10 per cent of these cells are new and the remainder are recirculating. There does not seem to be a correlation between the number of lymphocytes in the total circulation and the number in the blood, so the blood counts may not reflect total numbers available. The sizes of the organs that produce lymphocytes are not necessarily a reflection of the numbers in the blood. A functional pool is available that can quickly add to the circulation if required.

2. Plasma Cells. ***Plasma cells*** form by a process of maturation or conversion from B lymphocytes. Their function is to make and store ***antibody.*** Usually, the lymphocyte is directed to make the antibody and during the process of production becomes a plasma cell. Thus, plasma cells in tissue indicate that there has been a ***humoral immune response*** to an antigen of some type, perhaps from a microorganism, but it does not mean that the antibody produced is protective against that organism or agent. It is not possible to tell by looking at a plasma cell what type of antibody is being made (Fig. 4–19), but this can be determined by specific antiglobulin staining with fluorescent antibody labeling. The host may make several different kinds of antibodies in response to different ***antigens*** of an organism. These antibodies may be detected and measured by several different serological methods indicating a response by the host to the organism. Even though there has been a detectable response, however, none of the various kinds of antibody are an indication of ***protection*** of the host from the agent. They only indicate ***exposure*** to the agent. Fortunately, however, many antigens induce antibody that neutralizes, kills or inactivates the agent and its products or causes them to be phagocytized. The specific aspects of response and protection must be determined for each agent and each host species in order to determine the ***precise mechanism of protection,*** and that is not a simple matter.

Plasma cells are usually present along with lymphocytes in tissue. They are numerous along the sinusoidal linings of the medullae of lymph nodes and the red pulp of the spleen after antigenic stimulation. Assuming that an antigen came by way of the lymph to a lymph node from a site of infection upstream from the node and that a lymphocyte begins to make antibody in the node, how does the antibody get back to where it is needed? Apparently, the lymphocyte may leave the node soon after it begins antibody production and go to the site the long way via the blood stream, or it may make its way around the perilymphatic vessels of the tissues upstream from the node to the site. How it knows where to go is not known, but it will probably arrive as a lymphocyte and become a plasma cell to finish the task of production and secretion. Plasma cells are rarely seen in circulating blood. If a lymphocyte is at the site and is available for initiation of antibody production, the entire task can be completed at the site. ***Transition forms between lymphocytes and plasma cells are often seen in tissue.*** Plasma cells are not common in clean healing wounds because there is little foreign antigenic material.

The formation of mature plasma cells from lymphocytes requires four or five days. Heavy and light chain immunoglobulins are made separately on polyribosomes and are released into the cisternae of the rough endoplasmic reticulum, where they are formed into molecules with different ratios of heavy and light chains. These molecules are passed to the Golgi apparatus, where carbohydrate is added prior to secretion.

3. Macrophages. ***Macrophages*** in tissue are functionally and morphologically the same as tissue ***histiocytes*** and are derived from blood monocytes made in the bone marrow. Their function is primarily phagocytosis for purposes of disposal, or at least partial breakdown, of the phagocytized material. Specific receptors are present on macrophages that assist phagocytosis. One receptor recognizes particles coated by IgG; another recognizes particles coated with complement; and another recognizes particles that have altered or denatured membranes. A population of macrophages ex-

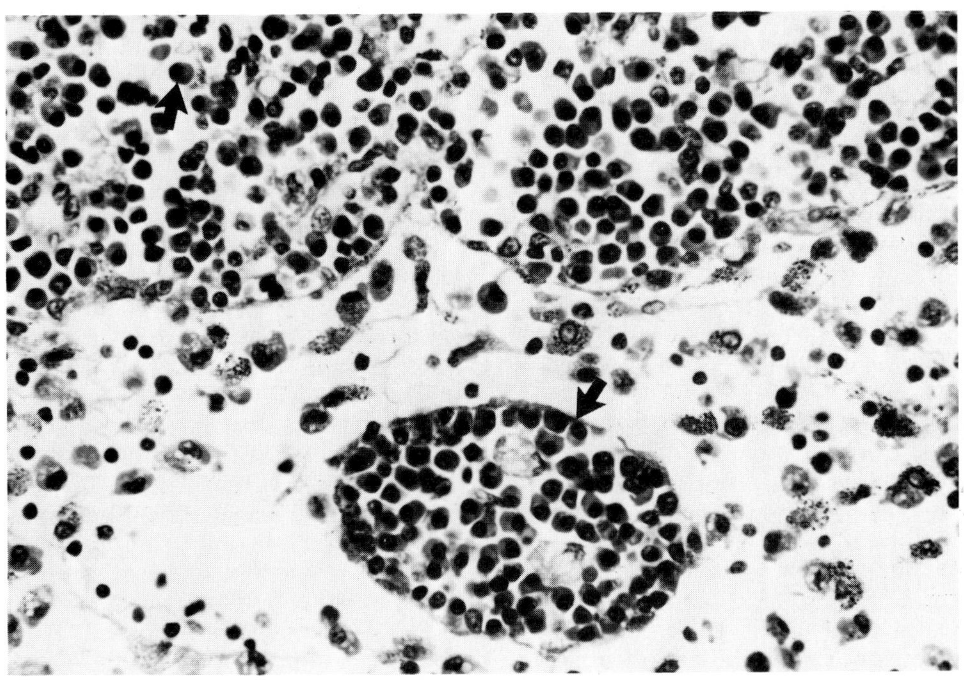

Figure 4–19. Plasma cells (arrows) in the medullary region of a lymph node. Note the density of the cytoplasm and the location of the nuclei. Hemosiderin is present in macrophages in sinusoids.

hibits marked functional heterogeneity. This may be due to differences in maturity or origin or actual subclasses of cells. They usually kill microorganisms by the same methods as neutrophils, and they dispose of debris in a similar fashion. They apparently process many antigens before handing them over to the lymphocytes to make antibody. If the antigens are broken down readily, the macrophages do not persist; but if much antigen accumulates in their cytoplasm and is not broken down to any extent, the presence of these cells persists in the lesion.

Activated macrophages are prepared to contribute to many defense mechanisms. Activation occurs through secretions of sensitized T cells, by contact with immune complexes and by cleavage products (C3a and C3b) from C3. In chronic inflammation the most significant function of activated macrophages are (1) secreting neutral proteases that can cleave C3, degrading collagen and elastin and activating plasminogen; (2) releasing complement activators chemotactic for other macrophages; (3) killing tumor cells; (4) killing or controlling intracellular organisms; (5) producing interferon; (6) secreting endogenous pyrogen; (7) forming tissue thromboplastin; (8) secreting plasminogen activator; (9) synthesizing prostaglandin; (10) stimulating fibroblast proliferation and collagen synthesis.

Thus, chronic inflammatory exudate persists if antigen persists.

Macrophages have difficulty with some components of bacterial cell wall, components of mycobacteria and some plant products. They may have difficulty disposing of these antigens for four reasons: coating with host antigen, being held on the cell membrane, being held in an area of the cytoplasm away from lysosomes and inadequacy of lysosomal enzymes to break them down.

Macrophages respond to chemotaxis, especially as directed by some lymphocytes, but they also respond to antigen-antibody complexes, some parts of complement, soluble products of some bacteria and products of neutrophils. They respond to both immune and nonimmune stimuli. Macrophages and neutrophils carry out regular patrols of mucous membranes and cross the epithelium into the lumen or onto the surface of the mucosa. Macrophages have two major functions, phagocytosis and secretion. Some primarily act as phagocytes whereas others become epithelioid cells, are primarily secretory and can live from one to three weeks. ***Macrophages may divide in tissue to form other macrophages or may form epithelioid cells or giant cells.*** There may be different functional populations of macrophages in lesions, such as those with slow or rapid turnover. Inert particles cause lesions in which macrophages are replaced slowly, and they live a long time in the lesion. Many lesions caused by microorganisms have a high turnover rate, and macrophages are replaced by mitosis in the lesion and exudation from the blood. Lesions with a high turnover rate tend to have giant cells present.

The presence of macrophages in a lesion may have several interpretations. They tend to appear with, or somewhat later than, neutrophils and remain longer. They may indicate a chronic lesion or a stage of cleanup after an acute battle has ended. Their role in chronic inflammation and their direction by lymphocytes in immune-mediated lesions will be discussed later; this may be their most common function. The appearance of macrophages in different kinds of lesions may be quite variable, with great differences in size, amount and color of the cytoplasm and in size and density of the nucleus being commonly observed (Figs. 4–20 through 4–23). Some organs and tissues contain large numbers of resident macrophages for protection, and they form the phagocytic component of the ***reticuloendothelial system*** in the sinusoids of the spleen, lymph nodes, microglia of the nervous system, alveolar macrophages and Kupffer cells of the liver.

Macrophages have the ability to destroy tumor cells by means that apparently are independent of the immune system. This mechanism will probably place much research emphasis on the role of macrophages in nonspecific inflammatory reactions.

4. Epithelioid and Giant Cells. ***Epithelioid and giant cells*** are formed from macrophages and are often found together in lesions. Epithelioid cells have an appearance similar to that of macrophages (Fig. 4–24), but their surface properties seem to be changed so that they lie closer to each other and take on shapes and arrangements that are reminiscent of prickle cells in the squa-

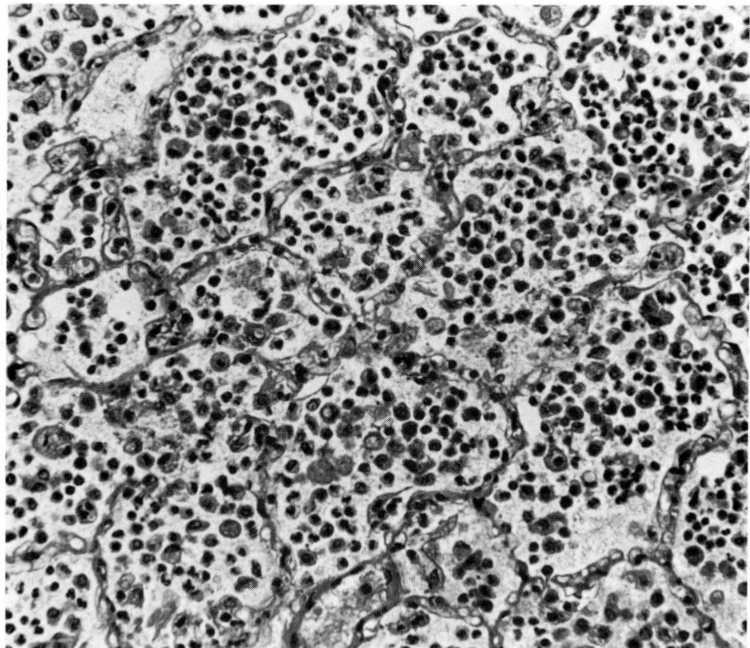

Figure 4–20. Alveoli of the lung containing neutrophils and many macrophages. The latter vary markedly in size, density of cytoplasm and location of nuclei.

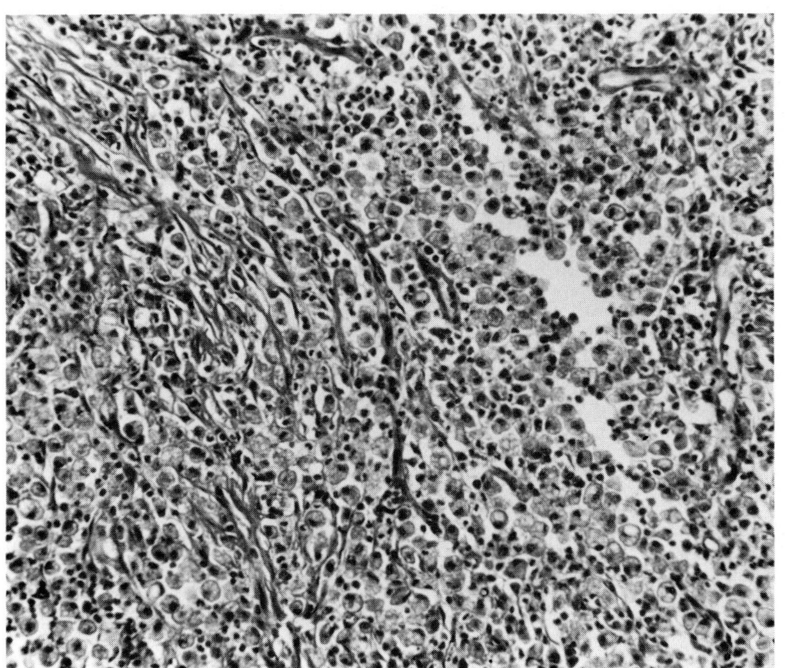

Figure 4–21. Foamy macrophages and a few neutrophils in a subcutaneous lesion in a dog.

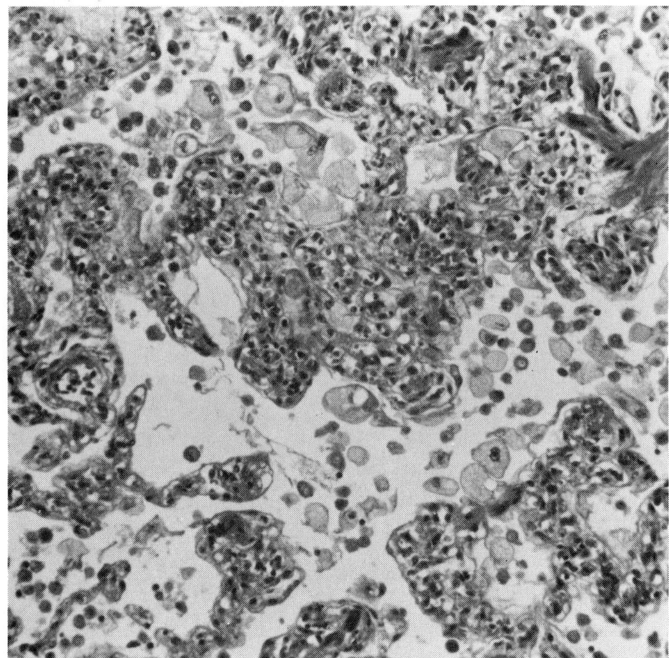

Figure 4–22

Figures 4–22 and 4–23. Very large foamy macrophages in a lipid pneumonia in a cat. Some are binucleate. View of the same lesion at a higher power is seen in Figure 4–23.

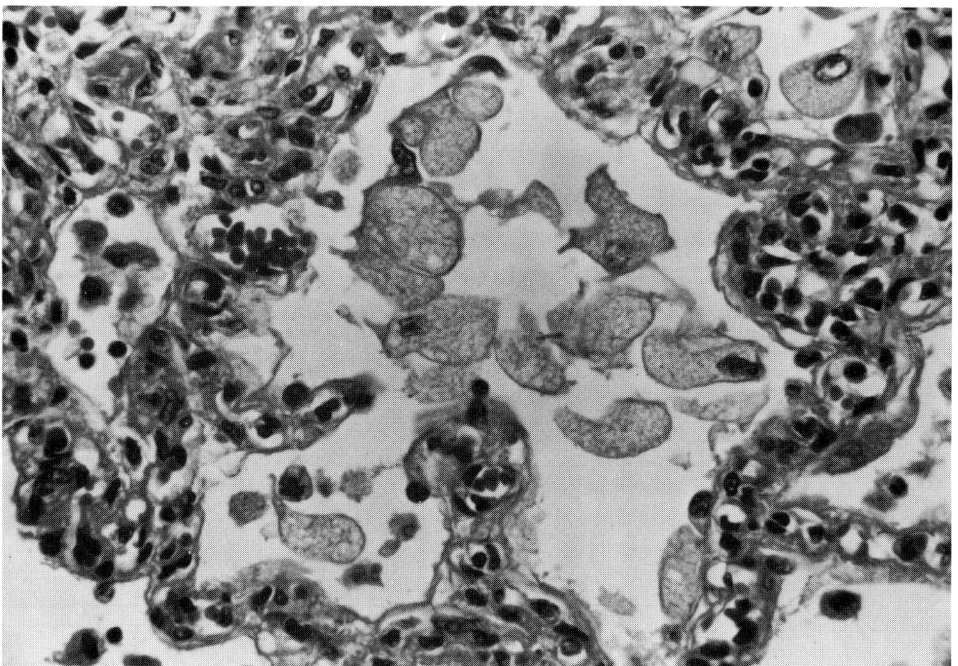

Figure 4–23

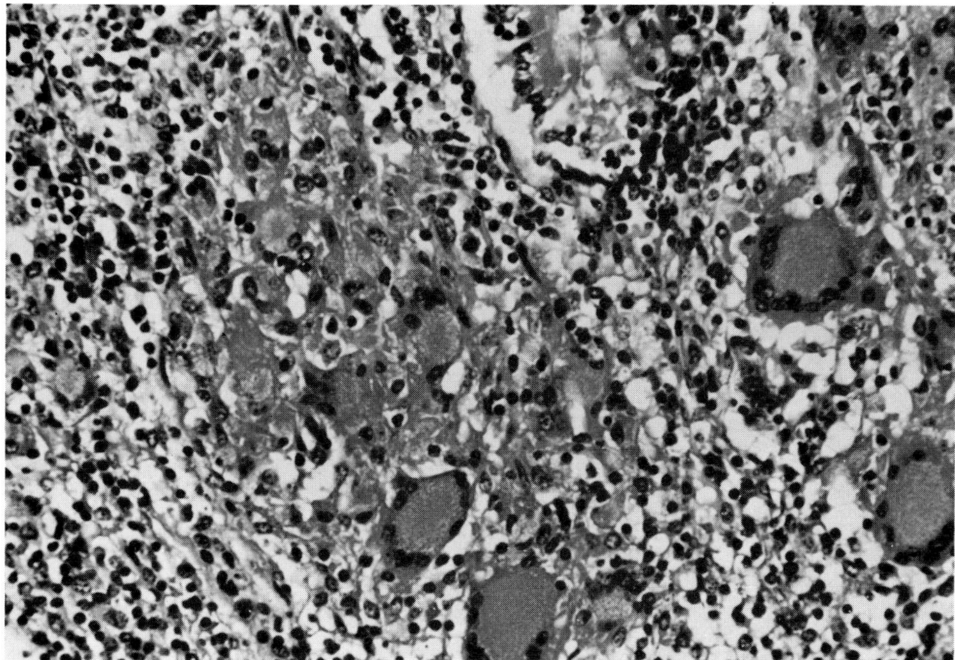

Figure 4–24. Giant cells and epithelioid cells in the intestinal mucosa of a cow with Johne's disease. The epithelioid cells have indistinct boundaries, but with some imagination, their transition to giant cells may be visualized.

mous epithelium—thus the name ***epithelioid.*** The cytoplasm is eosinophilic, but cell membranes are indistinct. These cells contain much endoplasmic reticulum, an active Golgi zone, many lysosomes but few phagocytic vacuoles, giving the appearance of a secretory cell. The cell membrane interdigitates extensively with neighboring cells of the same kind, which accounts for their indistinct cell outline under light microscopy. Some are binucleate. Apparently, differentiation to epithelioid cells occurs in macrophages that are in chronic lesions but are ***not required to phagocytize.*** Probably, they work at destruction of the irritant from the outside by ***secretions*** instead of from the inside as in phagocytosis. They divide to produce new immature macrophages. They are common in many granulomatous lesions, especially in tuberculosis and Johne's disease.

Giant cells form by the fusion of the cytoplasms of macrophages. There may be from two or three to two hundred nuclei in one cell. Their shape may be round, oblong or quite irregular (Figs. 4–25 through 4–28). Traditionally, there have been two types of giant cells: Langhans' cells with nuclei around the periphery and foreign-body giant cells with the nuclei arranged throughout. This distinction is not valid; both types are found in the same lesion and there seems to be no relationship between the type and an etiological agent (Fig. 4–29). Giant cell nuclei can undergo mitosis. The arrangement of nuclei in the cell is related to the actions of contractile proteins in the cytoplasm and has no particular functional significance. Giant cells are a removal system for macrophages, particularly those which have recently arrived at the scene and have not become either secretory or phagocytic. Giant cells secrete lysosomal enzymes directly by exocytosis or through or into the intracytoplasmic membranous labyrinth. Experimentally, some macrophages begin division but then they fuse to form giant cells. Chromosomal abnormalities and polyploidy have been found in these macrophages, suggesting that the abnormalities influence surface properties and are recognized as foreign by new macrophages. ***Fusion may be a means for disposal of these abnormal cells.*** Another recent mechanism suggested for the formation of giant cells is the attempt by two or more cells to take up particles simultaneously by endocytosis. The cell membranes contact each other in the process and parts of each are taken in by the other, resulting in fusion

Text continued on page 188

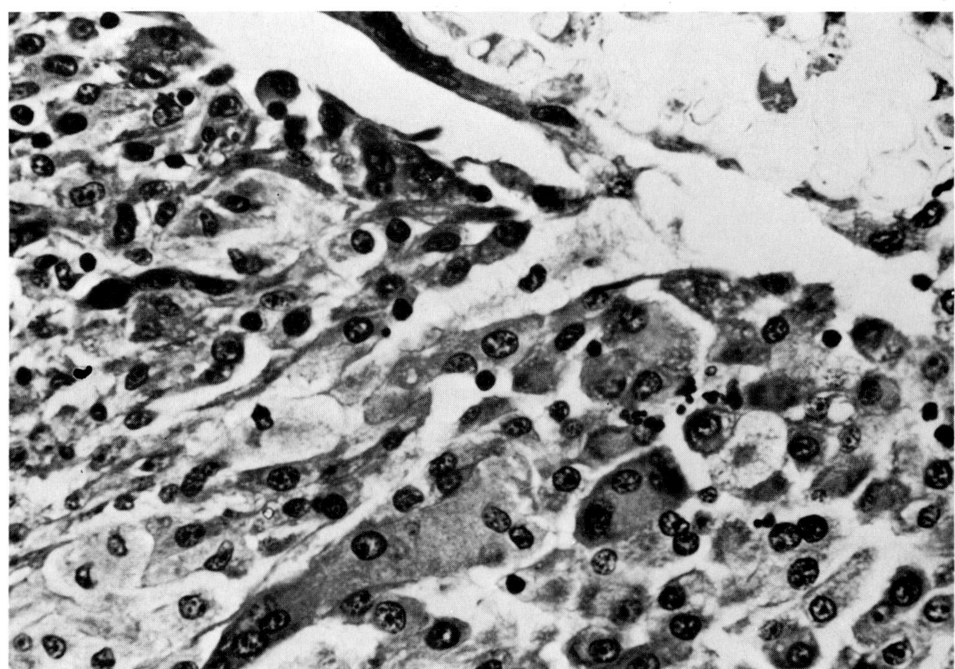

Figure 4–25

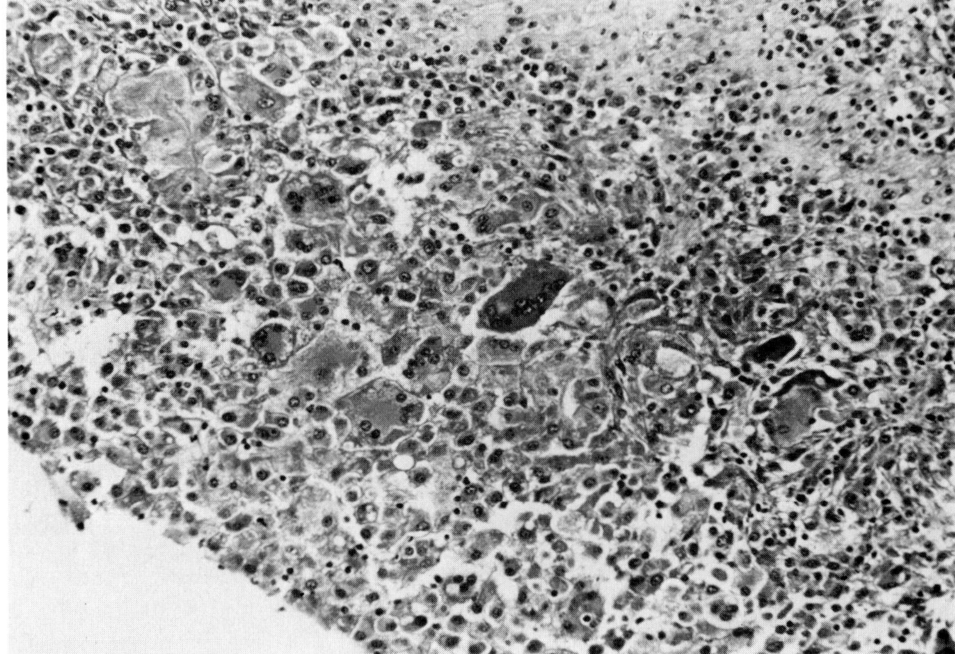

Figure 4–26

Figures 4–25 through 4–28. The transition from macrophages or epithelioid cells to giant cells may be visualized in this foreign body reaction in a dog's lung. Figures 4–26, 4–27 and 4–28 are from the same lesion and demonstrate variations in the morphological aspects of the cells involved. Plant fiber is present in the same lesion in Figure 4–28 toward the right (arrow).

Illustration continued on opposite page

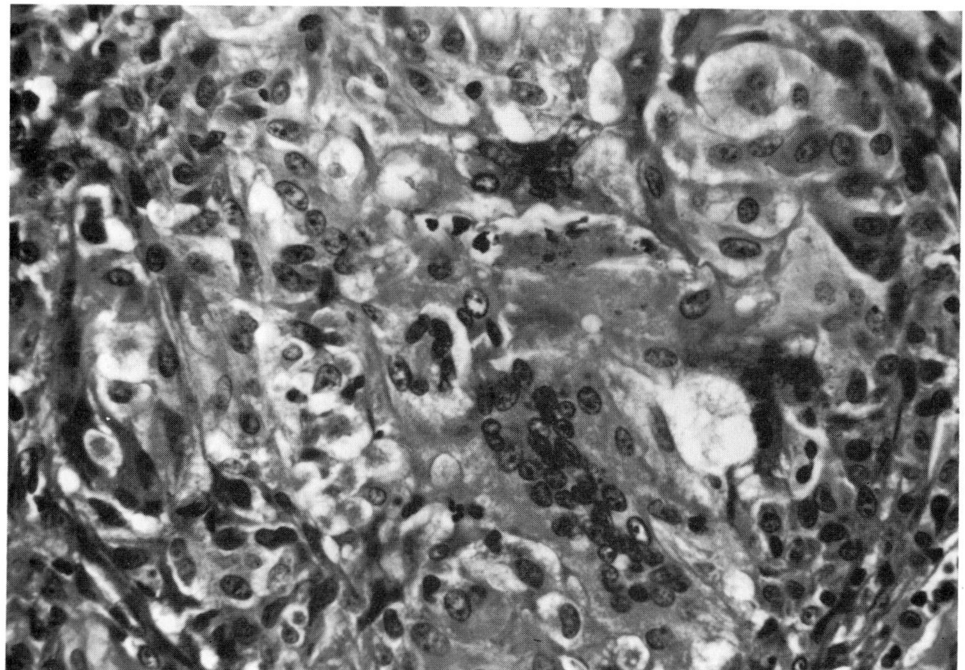

Figure 4–27

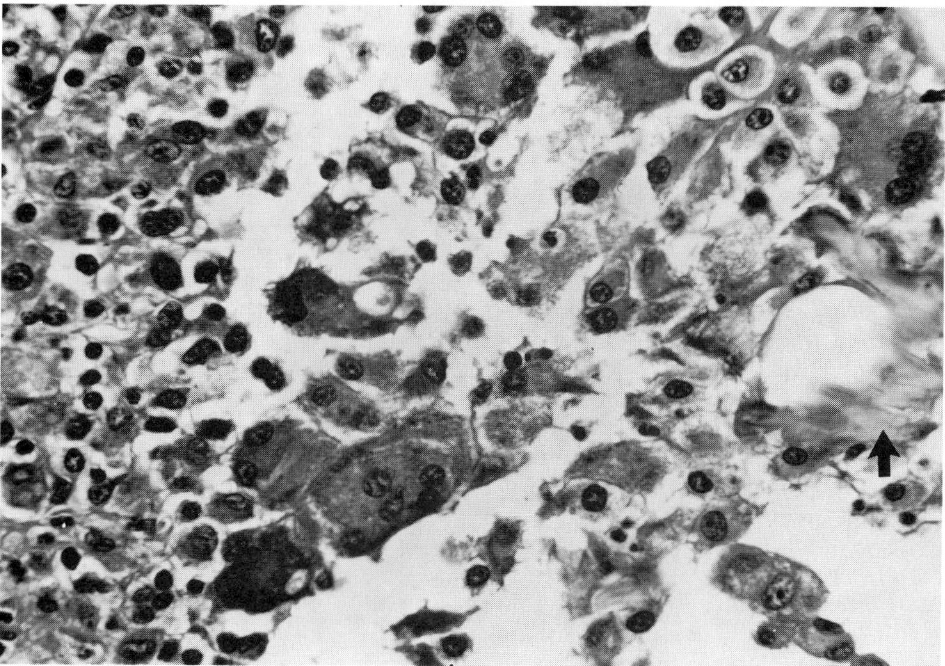

Figure 4–28

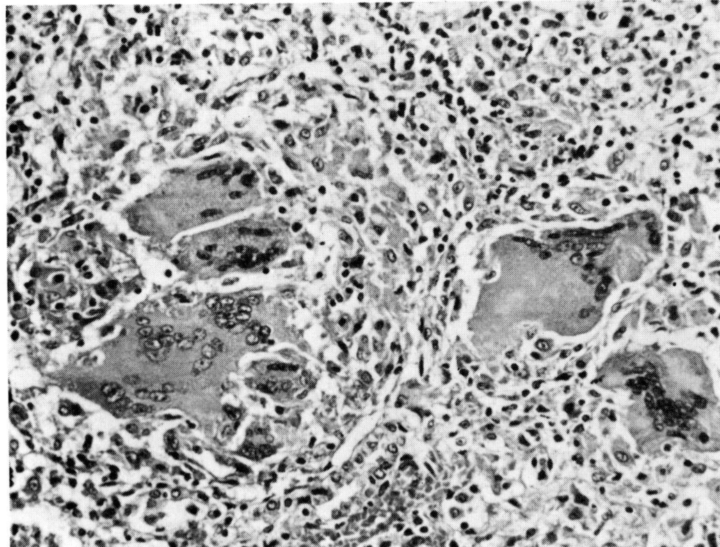

Figure 4–29. Variations in form, structure and number of nuclei in giant cells in a bovine lung infected with tuberculosis.

of the cell membranes, which is called simultaneous interiorization. The process may be stimulated by agents in the environment of the inflammatory reaction that promote endocytosis. Giant cells are poorly phagocytic and probably have a life span of only a few days. Some viral infections characteristically induce giant cells in tissue, presumably by altering surface properties.

CLASSIFICATION OF EXUDATES

The functions and appearances of the individual cellular and fluid components of the inflammatory exudate have been described. Rather than describing every inflammatory lesion separately, a ***system of classification of exudates*** based on certain circumstances and characteristic features can be formulated and used in various organs and tissues. Once this system is established and learned, the use of the term for a particular exudate conveys the predominant components present. The purpose now is to ***define these classifications*** so that they will have the same meanings for all who use them—thus one language.

Exudates are classified by time and appearance of the exudate.

Time

The terms used for classification by time are ***acute, subacute*** and ***chronic.*** These are arbitrary terms and may be parts of one spectrum, with the names conveying the lesion's ***main feature at a particular time.*** In general, acute refers to a period of time lasting from a few to several days, and chronic refers to a period of weeks, months or years. Subacute lies between the other two and usually pertains to between one and two or three weeks. An acute lesion usually has some or most of the features of the classic acute response, that is, hyperemia, edema and exudate. The components may vary considerably. There may be much edema and cellular exudation with little hyperemia, or there may be much hyperemia with little exudation.

It seems that all the components of acute inflammation are expected in every acute lesion—the textbook picture—but often this does not occur.

In general, the presence of fluid and neutrophils microscopically suggests an acute lesion, whereas mononuclear cells and fibrosis suggest chronic lesions. There may be small acute foci within a large chronic lesion, however. The presence of lymphocytes and plasma cells suggests an immunologically based pathogenesis, and macrophages may suggest a nonantigenic irritant. A preponderance of neutrophils does not, however, necessarily indicate an acute situation, and mononuclear cells do not necessarily indicate a chronic one. Lymphocytes and macrophages may be very prominent in a lesion two days after its initiation. A lesion may appear chronic microscopically but be relatively acute in a clinical context.

The lesion is named according to the predominant feature. Some lesions begin as acute and end quickly so that the whole process is acute. Some begin as acute lesions, but the offense persists and chronicity develops. There may be acute flare-ups during the chronic stage. Some lesions start as chronic lesions and remain so.

Whether a lesion is acute or chronic, it is controlled by the release of chemical mediators and is dependent upon the type of mediator and the time it is present. In chronic inflammation, it must be concluded that the offending agent or antigen is still present and causing the release of mediators to generate and often attract more inflammatory cells to the site. The mediators may be ***dependent*** upon and part of the immune system or may be ***independent.*** Figure 4–30 provides an ***overview of chronic inflammation.*** Key points are the modified proteins that may be antigenic and the mitogenic factors that stimulate the proliferation of connective tissue and inflammatory cells. This rather simple figure conveys the essence of chronic inflammation very well.

Exudate

The classification used here is one of convenience with somewhat ill-defined borders but nonetheless is very useful.

Certain predominant features of exudate appear when certain components of the exudate are present in large amounts or in particular combinations. Different factors cause different types of responses, and there may be lesions in which fluid and fibrin predominate and others in which neutrophils or mononuclear cells predominate. Since these differ in appearance, names can be used to describe the different appearances—thus, the classification. ***The terms apply best to the gross appearance***

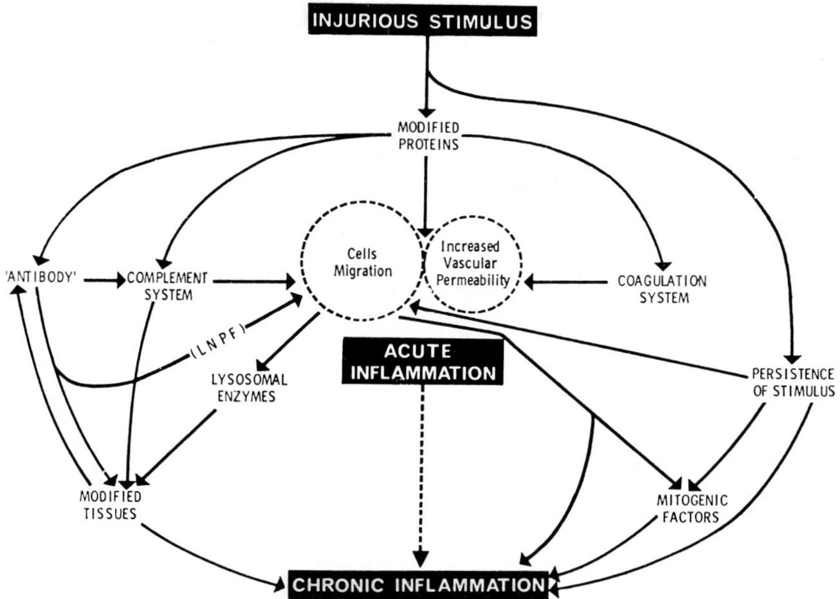

Figure 4–30. Development of chronic inflammation. (From Forscher, B. K., and Houck, J. C.: Immunopathology of Inflammation. Amsterdam, Excerpta Medica, 1971. Reprinted by permission.)

and have limitations when used microscopically. The reason for this is that the name applies to the ***predominant features.*** The microscopic features may vary considerably within a particularly large lesion depending on selection of tissues. ***It is important to develop the ability to visualize the probable microscopic composition and appearance of exudate from observation of the gross lesion, and the reverse.*** It is equally important to be able to ***visualize the pathogenesis of the formation of the exudate.***

There are characteristic locations for different types of exudate.

SEROUS EXUDATE

Serous exudate is composed primarily of clear fluid, and its presence indicates mild injury. Edema due to injury of vessels could be considered a form of serous exudation. Mild irritation of a serosal or mucosal surface would increase fluid exudation. Even mild injury, however, usually results in some exudation of neutrophils. ***If neutrophils occur in considerable numbers, the color will become whitish.*** The runny nose with excess clear or cloudy fluid is an example. The location of serous exudate may be within organs or on surfaces. It is usually acute and is a reflection of vascular injury. Hyperemia may or may not be present.

FIBRINOUS EXUDATE

Fibrinous exudate is so named because fibrin is a main feature in the exudate, which is an indication of ***severe acute vascular injury.*** The exudate will be a yellowish fluid, gel or solid rubbery mat. It usually occurs on serosal or mucosal surfaces and is prominent on intestinal mucosa, peritoneum, pleura, synovial membranes and meninges and in the lungs. Fibrinous ***polyserositis*** refers to this type of exudate on the pleura, peritoneum, pericardium, meninges and synovial membranes in the same animal. Since fibrin is chemotactic, neutrophils are soon found in large numbers in the fibrin, which changes the color toward white. When viewed microscopically, the neutrophils may appear to be predominant, but grossly, the appearance and texture of the fibrin may predominate. The neutrophils will eventually assist with lysis of the fibrin for removal. Cattle have higher levels of plasma fibrinogen than most other species, and fibrinous exudates are voluminous and common in that species.

Hyperemia and some hemorrhage may be apparent with fibrinous exudates, but surprisingly, these features may be absent even in a voluminous fibrinous exudate. An early lesion on a serosal surface gives a roughened ***ground-glass*** appearance that is easily overlooked (Figs. 4–31 through 4–35). When present in large quantities, it takes on a ***"bread and butter"*** appearance that is supposed to resemble the surface appearance of two pieces of heavily buttered bread after being placed together and then separated (Fig. 4–36). Microscopically, the fibrin is very eosinophilic on hematoxylin-eosin slides and may be in solid clumps or long delicate strands (Figs. 4–37 through 4–39). There is usually much edema as well, and both are voluminous in lymphatic vessels.

Considerable quantities of fibrin may occur on an intact epithelial surface, such as the intestine. Presumably, the fibrinogen crossed in fluid form and congealed later. Such a layer of fibrin may line an entire section of the lumen and literally form a cast of it; such a structure is called a ***fibrin cast*** (Fig. 4–40). These are characteristic of salmonella enteritis. At times, casts develop in cattle with what appears to be a mild disease clinically, but several meters of cast may be passed with the feces. Some observers would think that the whole mucosa of the gut has sloughed off, but not so.

In more severe intestinal damage, the epithelium may be lost and a fibrin layer may accumulate on the surface of the lesion. Connective tissue from the lamina propria will grow into the fibrin and organize the exudate to the mucosa. The layer cannot be easily removed at this stage and is named a ***diphtheritic membrane*** after the characteristic tracheal lesions of diphtheria in humans (Fig. 4–41 through 4–46). The term applies to organization of any fibrinous or necrotic exudate on a mucosal surface. Organization of the fibrinous exudate between any two serosal surfaces results in an ***adhesion.*** Both may markedly inhibit normal functions and end in fatality, such as by malabsorption in the intestinal lumen or by intestinal accident because of the immobility caused by peritoneal adhesions. Fibrinous exudates are typical of acute mycoplasmal polyserositis and also of Glasser's disease in swine, meningitis and arthritis in coliform septicemia in calves, fibrinous pneu-

Text continued on page 199

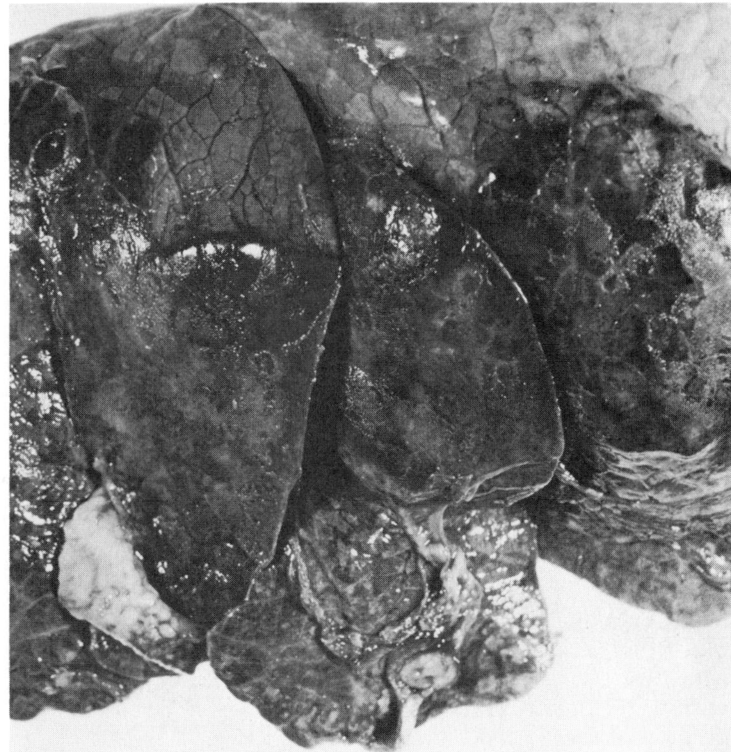

Figure 4–31. Acute fibrinous pleuritis and pneumonia in a bovine lung in a case of shipping fever. Note the ground-glass appearance of the pleura where fibrin is beginning to accumulate over the dark red areas of inflammation.

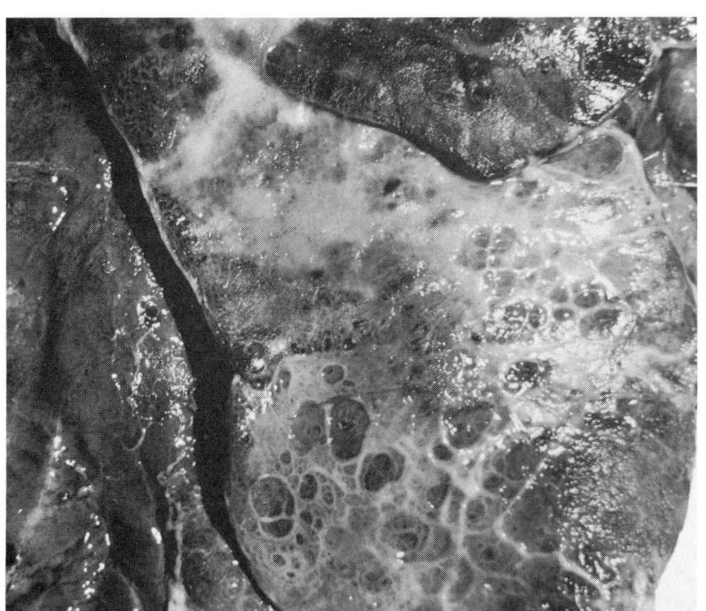

Figure 4–32. Close-up of a lesion similar to that seen in Figure 4–31.

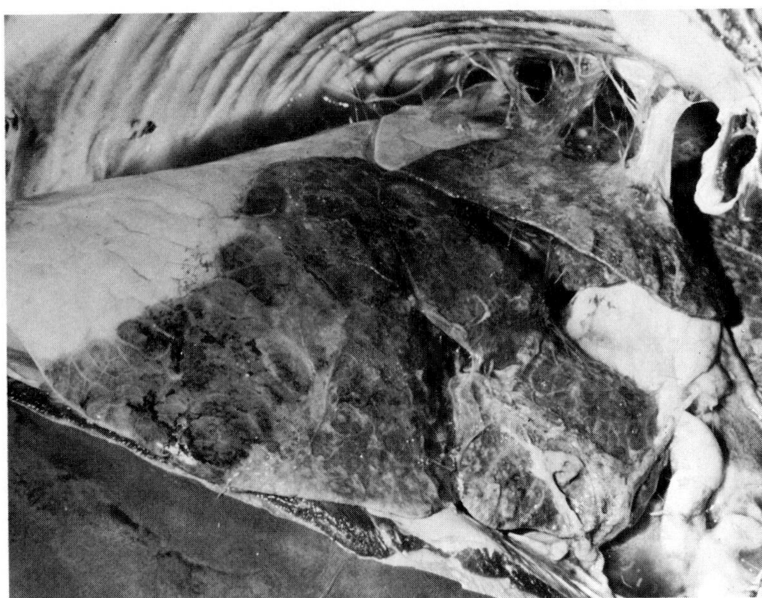

Figure 4–33. This lesion is similar to those seen in Figures 4–31 and 4–32, but there is more extensive exudation, with fibrin sticking to the parietal and visceral pleura.

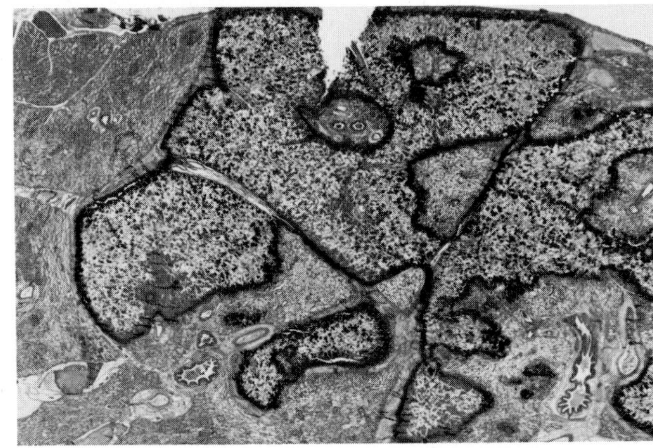

Figure 4–34. An acute fibrinous pneumonia which also has discrete areas of coagulation necrosis in the lung parenchyma. Note the dark line around the areas of necrotic parenchyma. These lines would appear pale in the gross lesion.

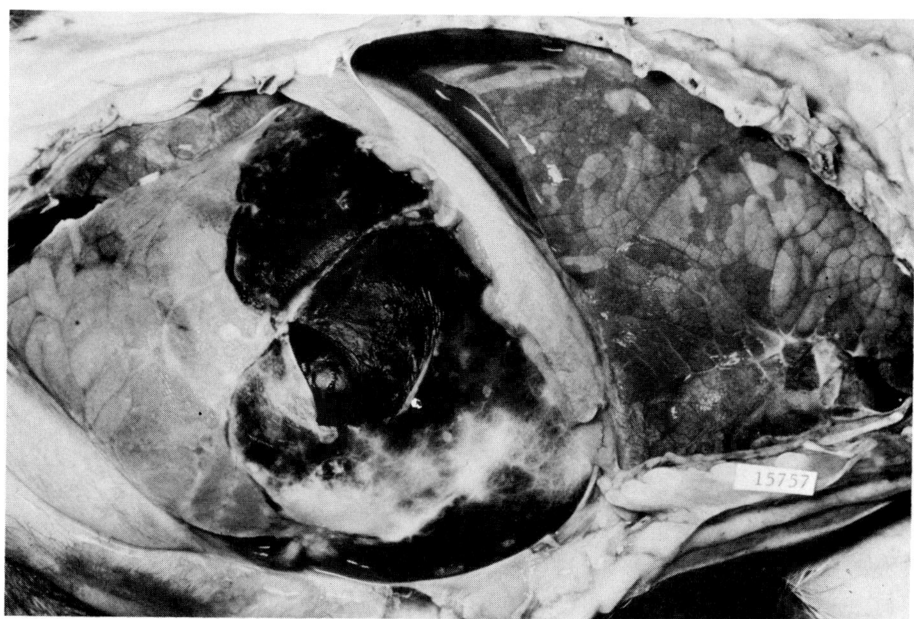

Figure 4–35. Acute fibrinous peritonitis and pleuritis in a pig. If several serous surfaces are affected in this manner, the term polyserositis is appropriate. This lesion may be caused by *Mycoplasma hyorrhinis*.

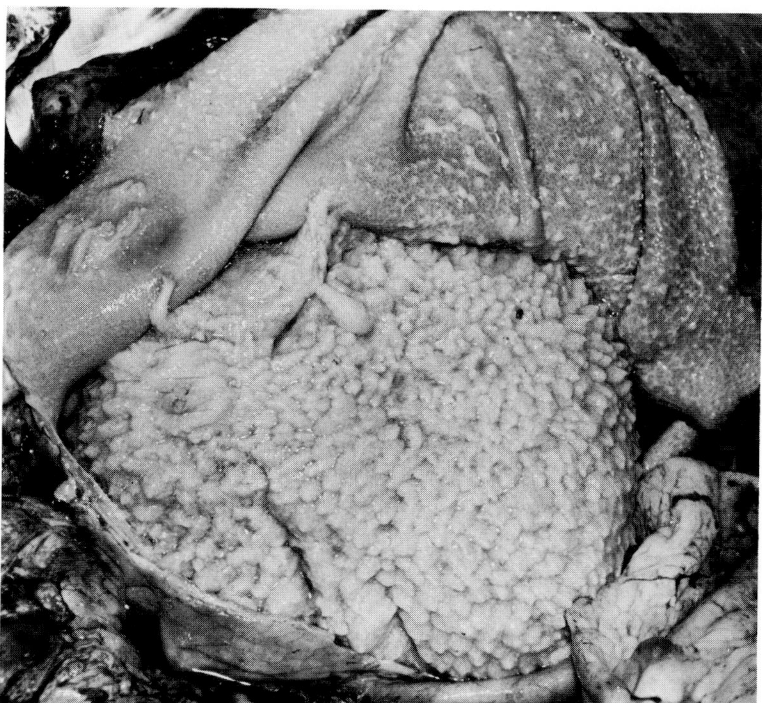

Figure 4–36. Subacute fibrinous pericarditis in which the fibrin is thick enough to resemble the so-called "bread and butter" appearance.

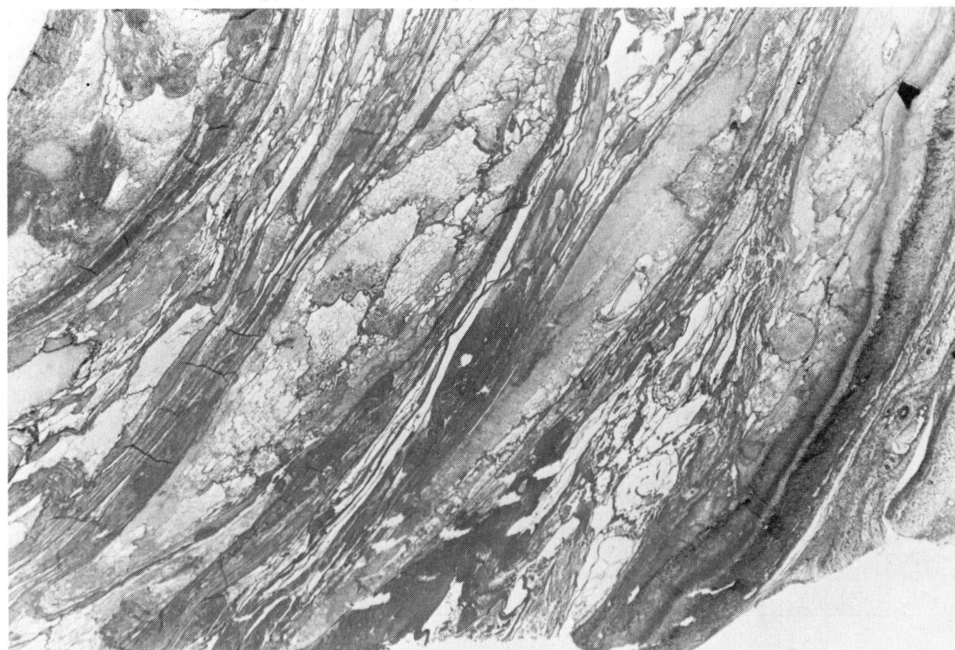

Figure 4–37

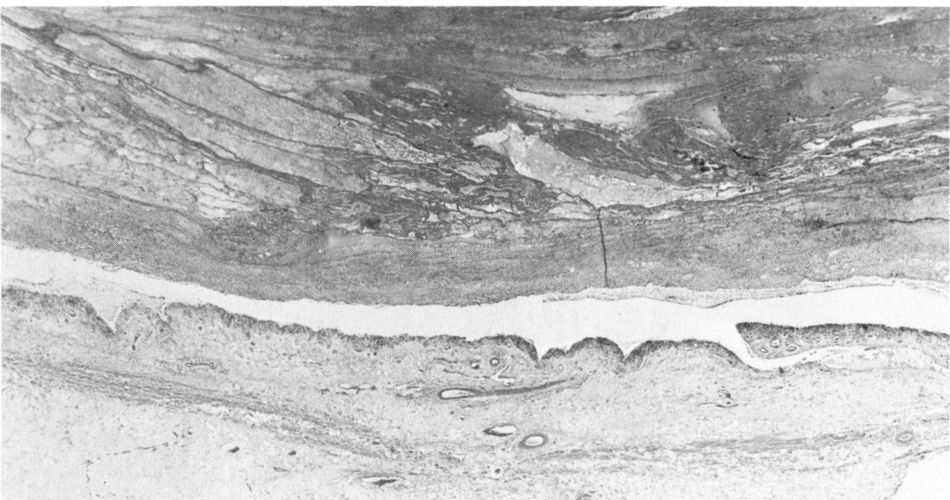

Figure 4–38

Figures 4–37 and 4–38. Acute fibrinous arthritis due to mycoplasma organisms in a calf. The fibrin is very loosely arranged and contains fluid and cells between strands of fibrin. The synovial membrane, from which all the exudate arose, is at the right. In Figure 4–38, a similar lesion, the fibrin is more compact. The synovial membrane is at the bottom and the separation from the exudate occurred in processing. Note the rather minimal reaction in the synovial membrane in comparison to the amount of exudate in the joint space.

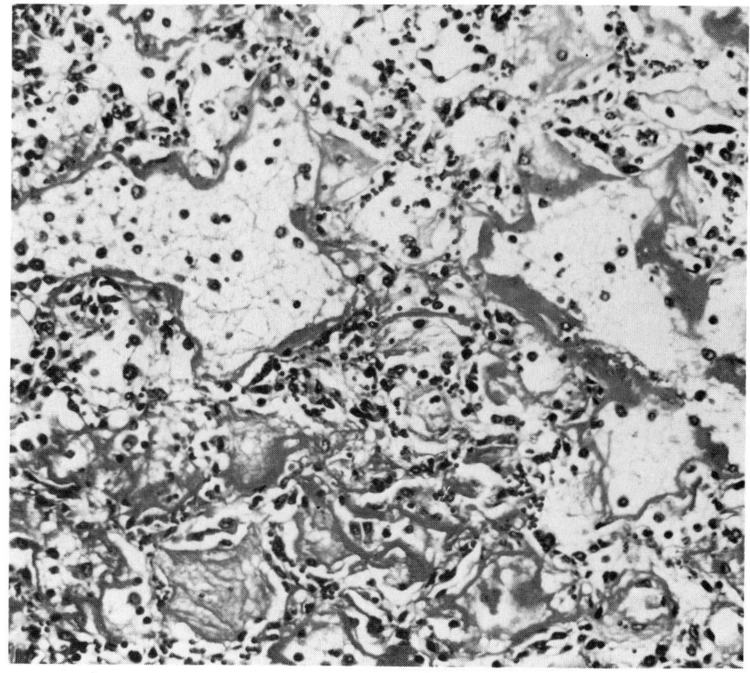

Figure 4–39. Acute inflammation in the lungs. Alveoli contain edema and strands of fibrin that tend to line alveolar ducts and walls as so-called hyaline membranes. Fibrin is present as hyaline membranes but also fills some alveoli.

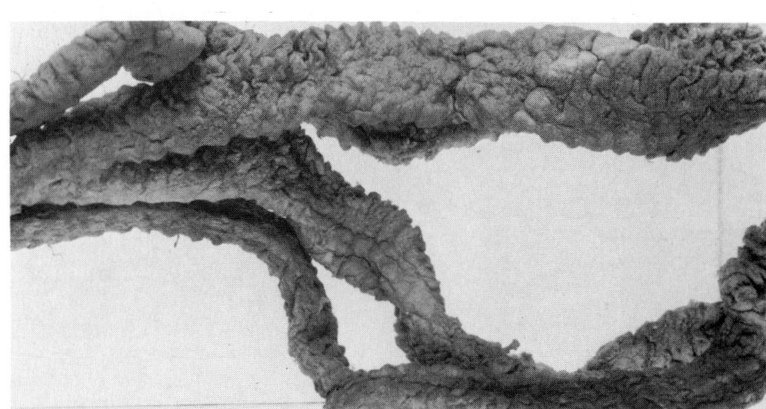

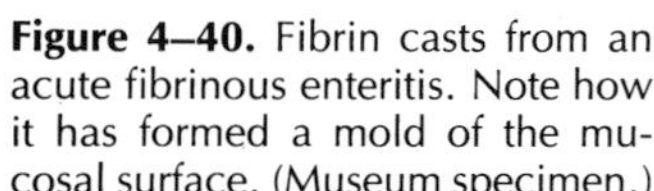

Figure 4–40. Fibrin casts from an acute fibrinous enteritis. Note how it has formed a mold of the mucosal surface. (Museum specimen.)

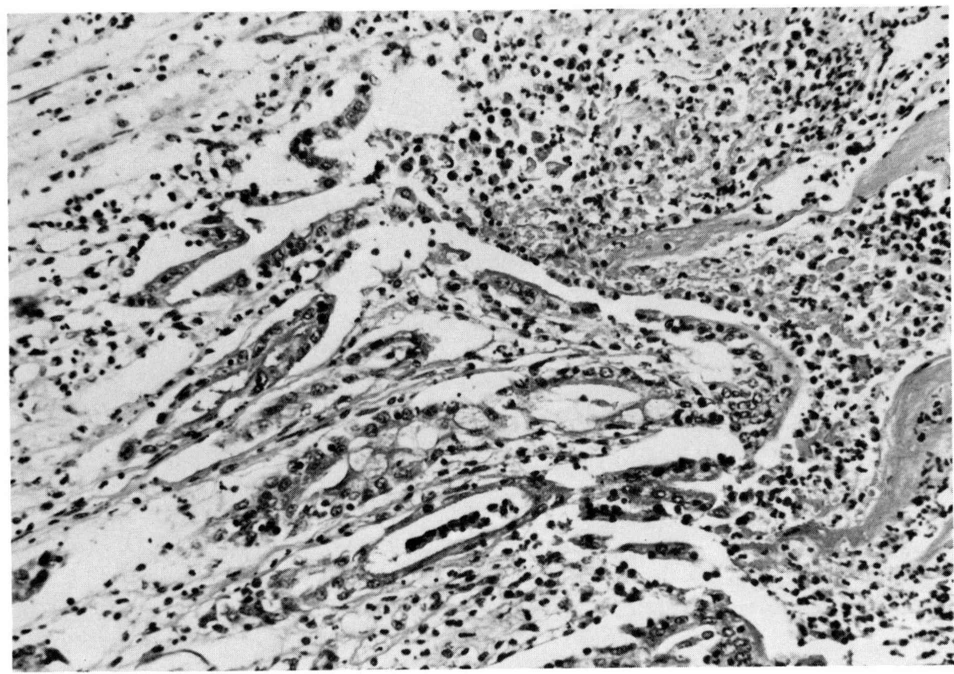

Figure 4–41. Acute necrotizing fibrinous enteritis. The lumen of the intestine is located toward the right and contains fibrin neutrophils and necrotic epithelial cells. There is marked destruction of glandular epithelium, but the epithelium on the villi is partially intact.

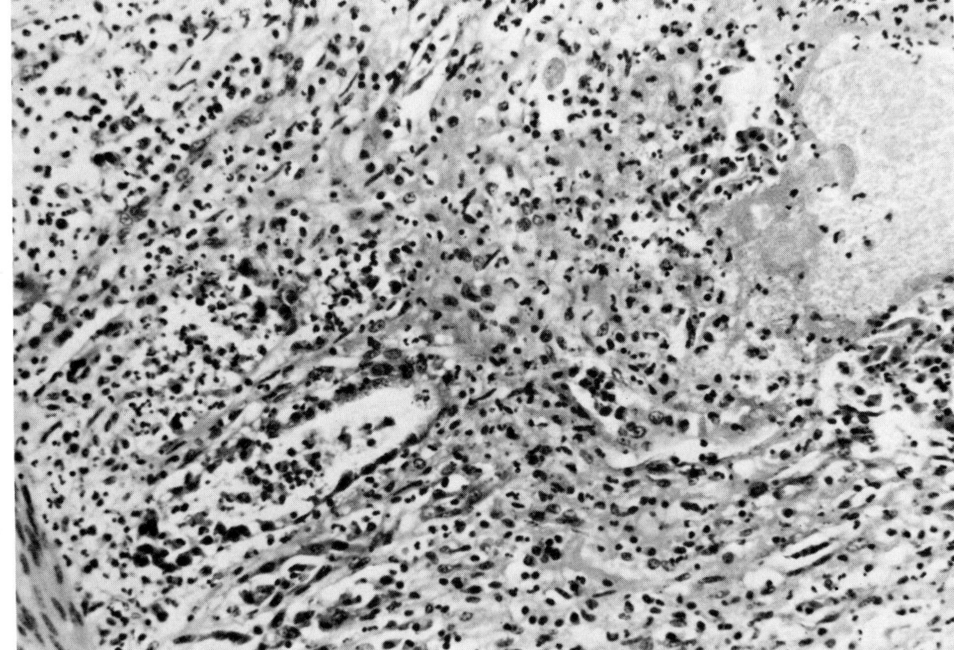

Figure 4–42. Same case as that seen in Figure 4–41. There are remnants of mucosal glands but there is much necrosis of the mucosa and fibrinous exudate in the intestinal lumen (toward the top, right). The lesion will become diphtheritic.

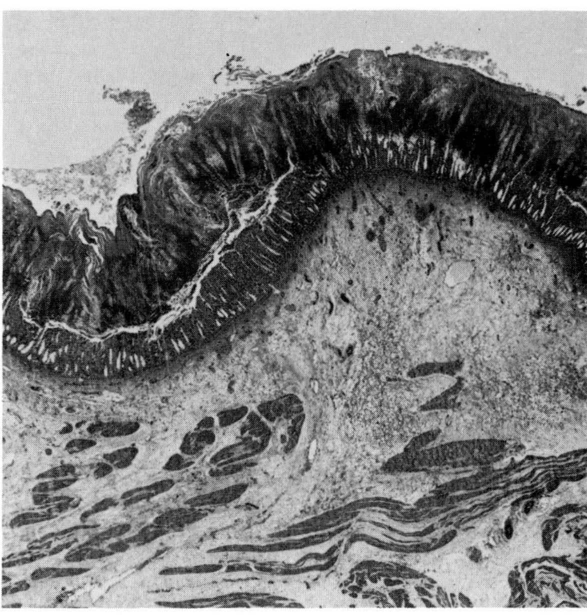

Figure 4–43. Acute fibrinohemorrhagic enteritis in a calf with salmonellosis. Note the thick layer of exudate on and partly attached to the mucosa. Dilated epithelial crypts are visible just above the edematous submucosa. The material above the mucosa is a mixture of fibrin, mucus and necrotic debris, which composes the exudate in the lumen. The exudate remains partially attached to the right and is forming a diphtheritic membrane.

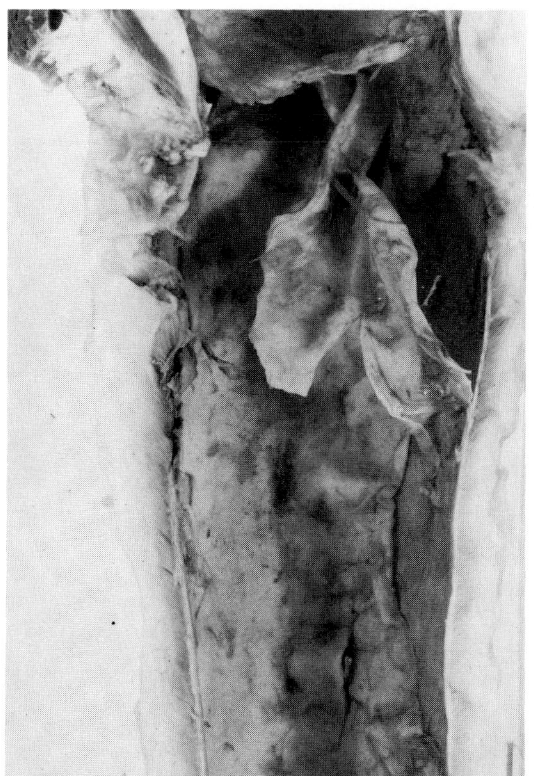

Figure 4–44. Diphtheritic membrane in the trachea of a cow with malignant catarrhal fever.

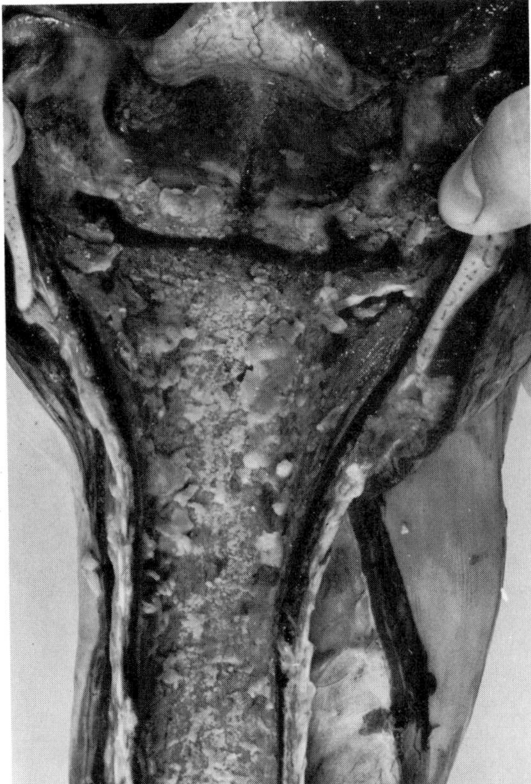

Figure 4–45

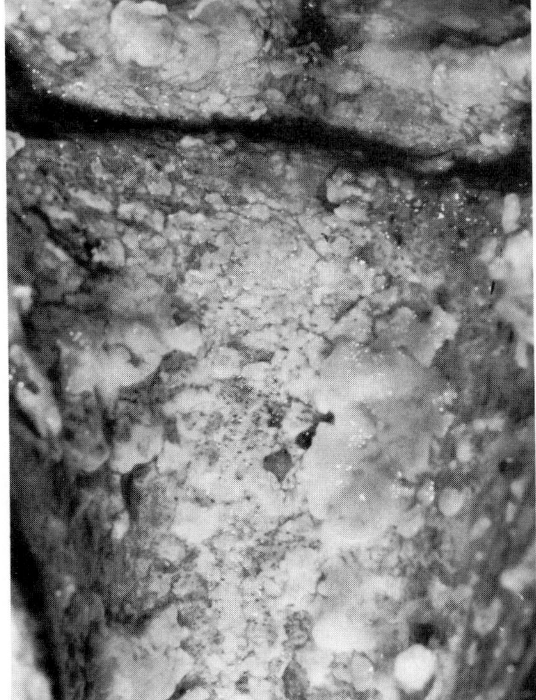

Figure 4–46

Figures 4–45 and 4–46. Acute necrotizing, almost diphtheritic, tracheitis in a steer with infectious bovine rhinotracheitis. Closer view is seen in Figure 4–46.

monia of shipping fever in cattle, peritonitis from perforated ulceration in the digestive tract of all species and pleuritis in horses.

HEMORRHAGIC EXUDATE

The term ***hemorrhagic*** is used to classify the exudate if hemorrhage is the predominant component. This usually occurs in organs with an abundant blood supply and much surface area, such as the lungs and the intestines (Figs. 4–47 through 4–49). The lesion implies a severe peracute reaction. ***Free as well as clotted blood, fibrin and tissue debris are often present.*** Microscopically, hemorrhage and necrosis of the acute caseous type are prominent features. This type of exudate occurs in aspiration pneumonia and in severe acute enteritis caused by agents such as diarrhea virus. Actually, this type of lesion is not as common as some others, but the classification is often erroneously used for the presence of red blood cells in noninflammatory lesions, such as visceral pooling in the intestine of cattle, hemorrhage of various types unassociated with inflammation or just congestion. It is one of the most ***commonly misused terms in pathology*** and compounds the problems associated with the use of the term hemorrhagic, which should be avoided as an adverb.

CATARRHAL EXUDATE

Catarrhal exudate occurs on ***mucous membranes,*** and the term is derived from words meaning to flow down. Mucus should be a prominent feature, but neutrophils, bits of tissue debris, flecks of fibrin and a few red blood cells may be present (Figs. 4–50, 4–51 and 4–52). The term covers a broad range of ***both acute and chronic lesions*** and will vary with the location and the etiologic factors. The exudate has a gross appearance of clear to cloudy to pink color, has a fluid to mucoid consistency and may contain tiny clumps of clotted blood, bits of white to grey viscid mucus and a few yellow to white strands or clumps of fibrin. This is ***one of the most common exudates*** and is associated particularly with the mucosal surfaces of all levels of the tubular respiratory, reproductive and digestive tracts where glands or goblet cells are numerous. Amazing amounts of mucus can be generated from some of these surfaces. Rhinitis, sinusitis, tracheitis, bronchitis, endometritis, gastritis and enteritis often are catarrhal in nature.

PURULENT EXUDATE

Purulent exudate means that ***pus*** is the predominant feature of the exudate. ***Suppuration*** is the process of pus formation and requires necrosis, neutrophils and proteolytic enzymes. The presence of neutrophils alone does not qualify, but if they are present in large numbers for very long, pus will form. Pus may vary greatly in color from green to yellow, brown or white or any combination of these and may also vary in consistency from fluid to semisolid to gelatinous. It occurs on mucosal, serosal, integumentary and other types of surfaces or within solid organs. On a mucosal surface, there will probably also be considerable mucus present and ***mucopurulent*** may be an appropriate term, or on a serosal surface, ***fibrinopurulent*** may be appropriate. An acute purulent exudate in subcutaneous tissues is called ***cellulitis*** (Fig. 4–53).

A ***pustule*** is a visible collection of pus within or beneath the epidermis. Within a solid tissue, purulent exudate may be confined in an ***abscess,*** usually in response to a bacterium said to be ***pyogenic,*** that is, causing pus to be produced. When such organisms locate in tissues, they cause neutrophils to appear in great numbers, presumably by chemotaxis. The neutrophils or the organism or a combination of the two cause necrosis of surrounding tissue. Soon, there is an island of neutrophils in the tissue that increases in size as more neutrophils come and surrounding tissue becomes necrotic. At this point, the lesion is a ***microabscess*** (Figs. 4–54 and 4–55). An effort is made to confine this process, and a wall of connective tissue is gradually formed around the lesion, which is then an ***abscess.*** This occurs gradually and begins with proliferation of connective tissue in the immediate area from stroma or from perivascular fibroblasts if there is little stroma available. The connective tissue layer may become very thick or remain thin. Capillaries and venules in the connective tissue supply neutrophils that cross into the cavity of the abscess. The wall is called a ***pyogenic membrane*** (Figs. 4–56 through 4–59).

The process will not stop until the agent is overcome by neutrophils, antibody or

Text continued on page 207

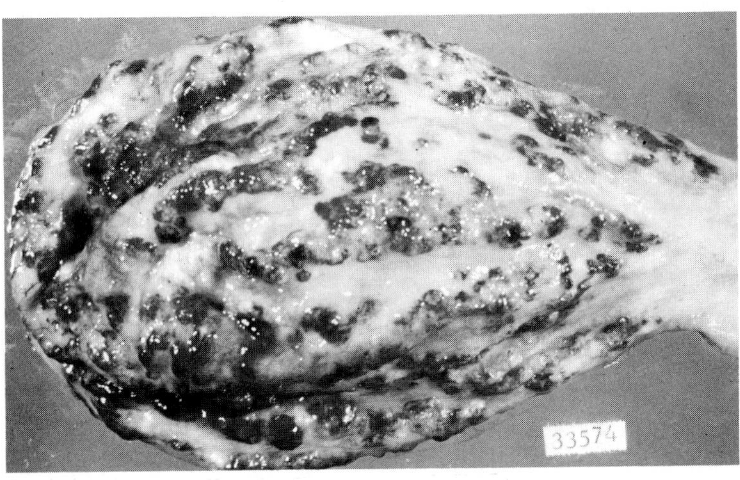

A

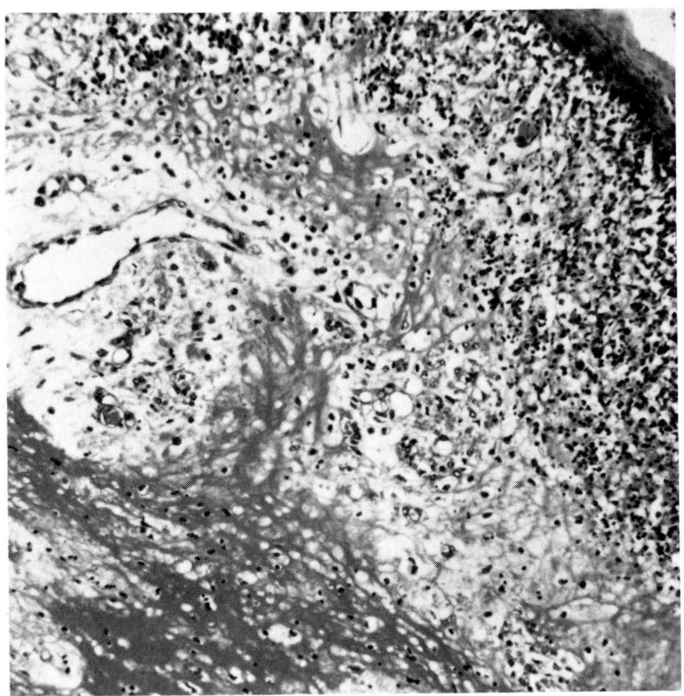

B

Figure 4–47. *A,* Acute hemorrhagic cystitis in a dog. The mucosa is raised and red in affected areas. *B,* Microscopic view of a case such as seen in *A.* There are numerous neutrophils, much fibrin and some hemorrhage in the mucosa below the epithelium (top right).

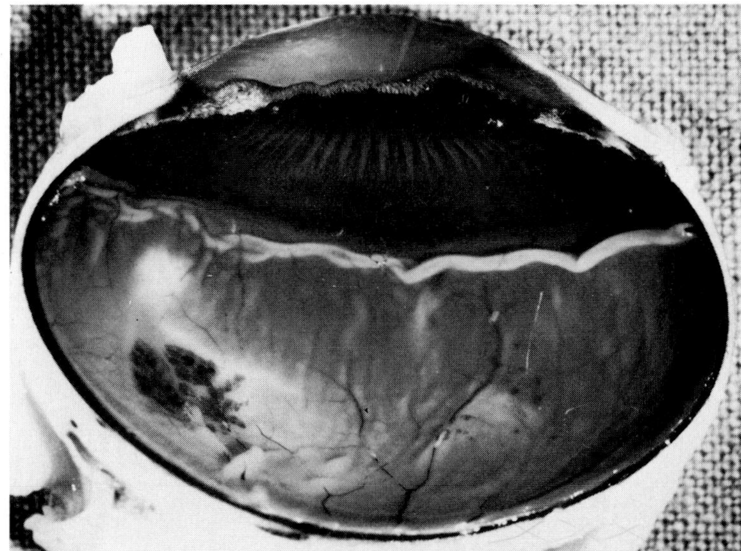

Figure 4–48. Acute hemorrhagic retinitis in a steer caused by *Hemophilus somnus.*

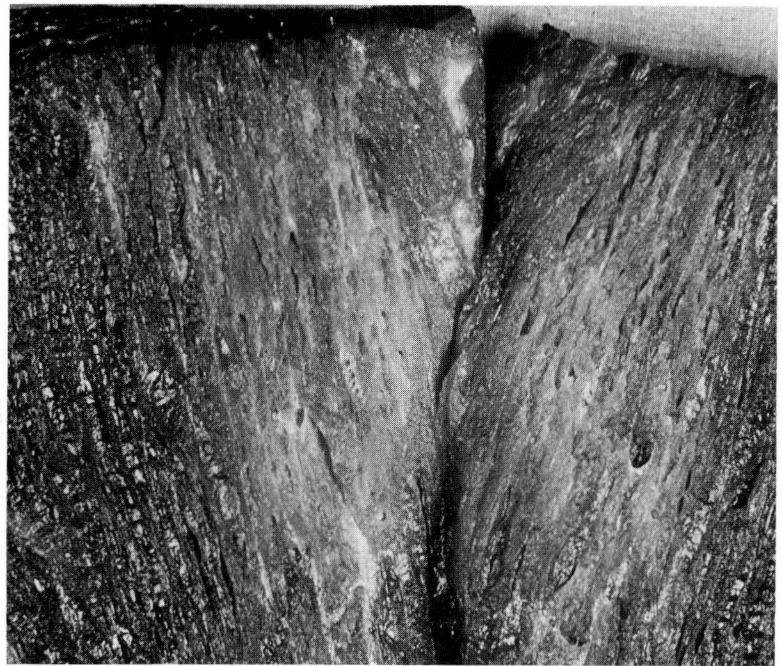

Figure 4–49. Acute hemorrhagic myositis in blackleg in cattle. The central area has a dry, cooked appearance, whereas the top area is very dark red. The dark color is from hemorrhage and lysis of red cells.

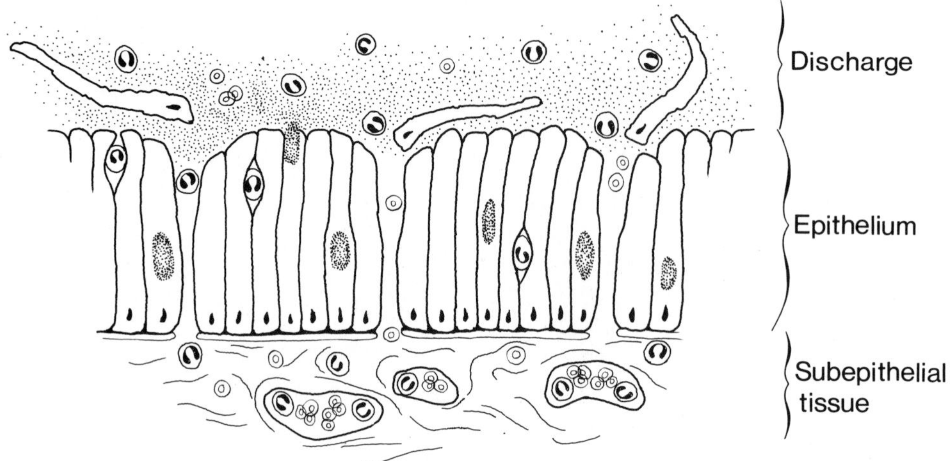

Figure 4–50. Diagrammatic representation of catarrhal exudate. The exudate contains mucus, necrotic epithelial cells, red cells and neutrophils. (Modified from Willis, R. A.: Principles of Pathology. 2nd ed. New York, Plenum Publishing Corp. [Butterworth], 1961. Reprinted by permission.)

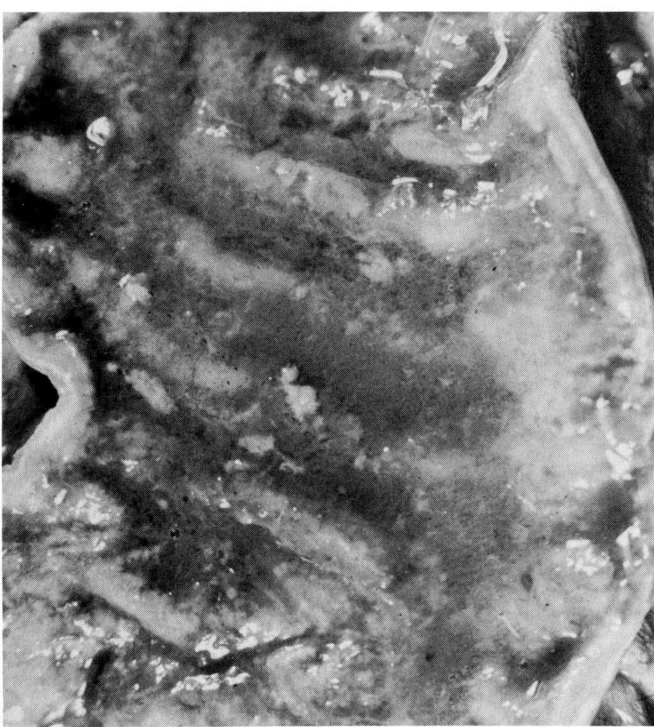

Figure 4–51. Catarrhal exudate in the colon of a pig with swine dysentery. Note the clumps of mucus and dark color of the fluid exudate.

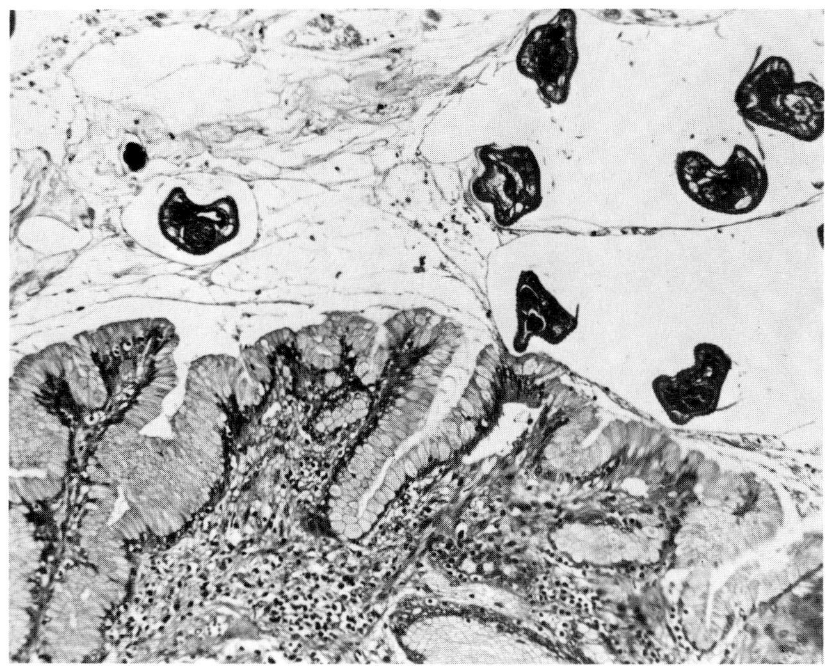

Figure 4–52. *Hyostrongylus rubidus* in the stomach of a pig. The parasites are partially surrounded by mucus in a catarrhal gastritis.

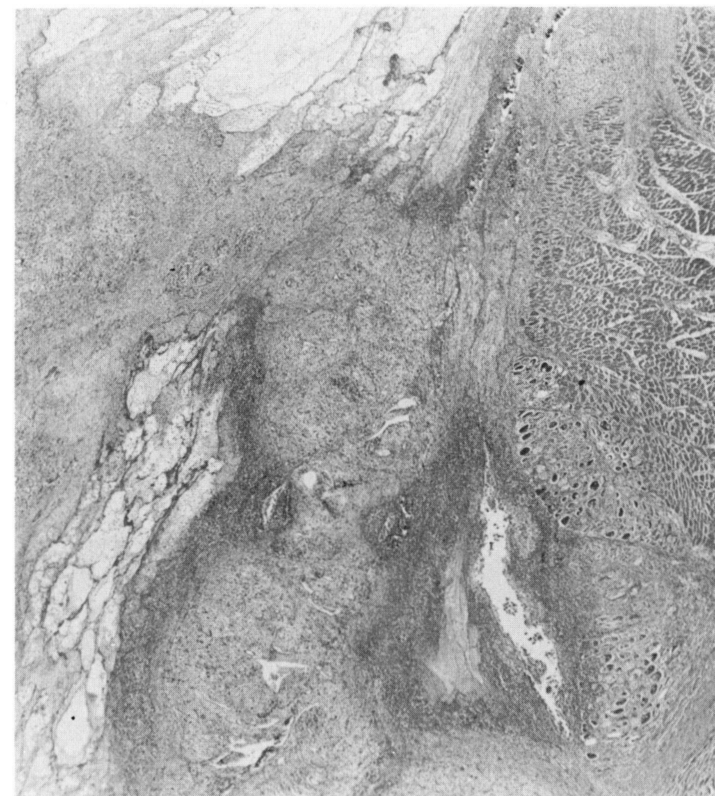

Figure 4–53. Diffuse inflammation with fibrin and pus in connective tissue (left) progressing into and causing necrosis of muscle (right). This lesion could qualify as cellulitis.

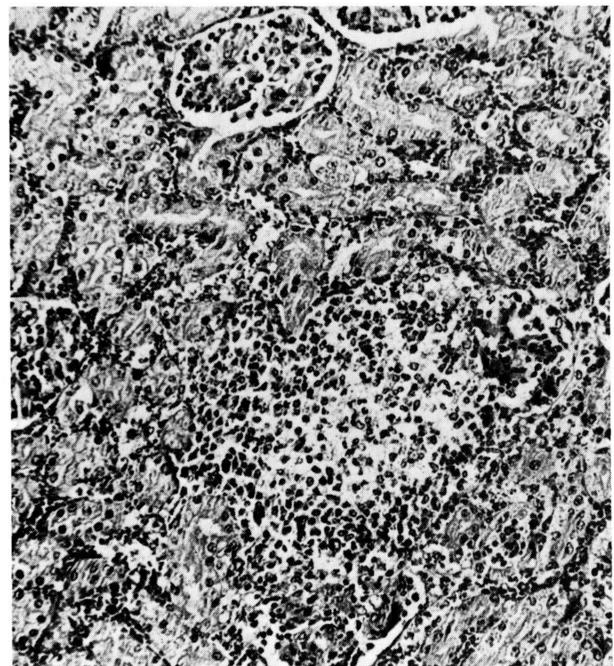

Figure 4–54. Microabscess in the kidney of a foal with neonatal septicemia. Note the necrosis of renal tissue in the area containing neutrophils.

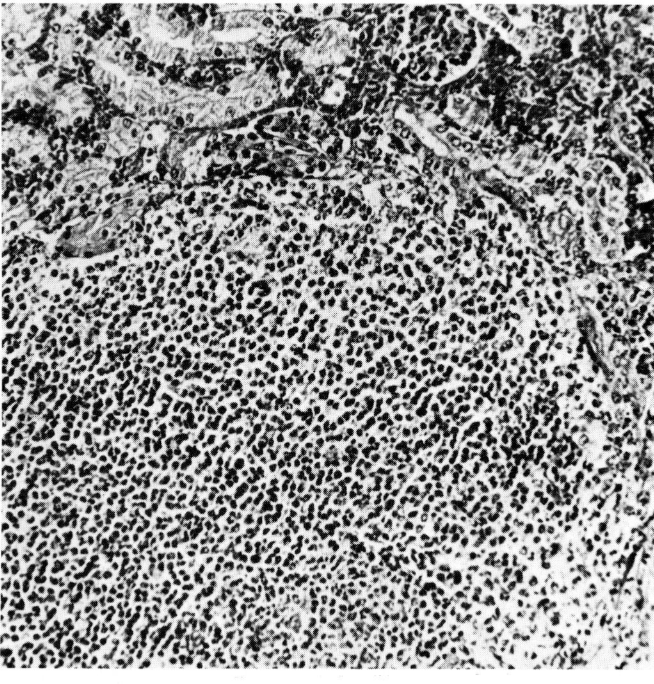

Figure 4–55. More advanced lesion than that seen in Figure 4–54. There is no connective tissue formation around the lesion at this stage, and the animal died from an overwhelming infection before a pyogenic membrane could form. Grossly, these two lesions would appear as focal necrosis.

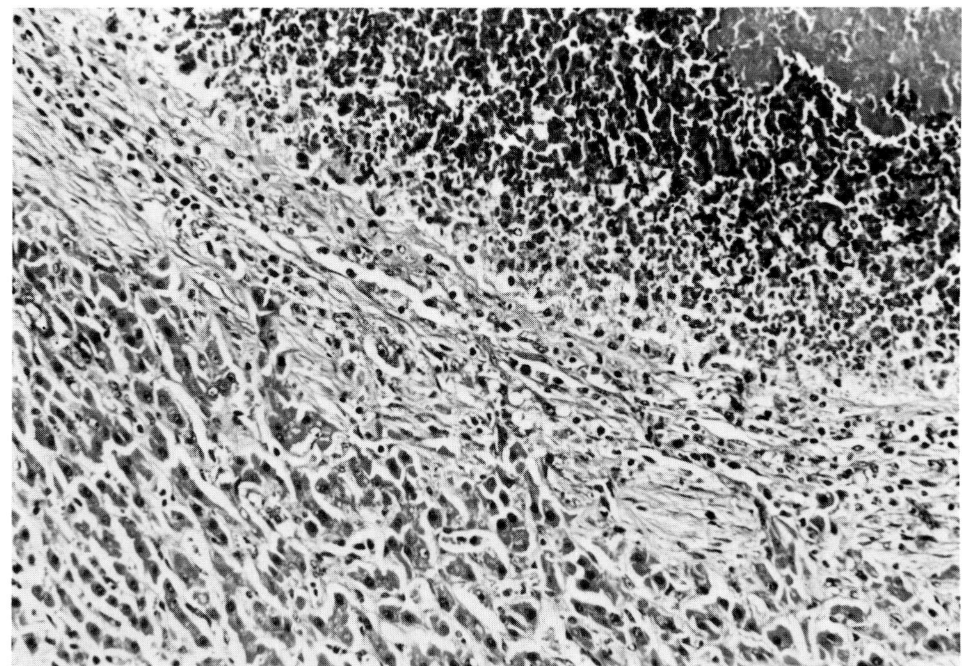

Figure 4–56. Liver abscess with a narrow pyogenic membrane (middle) around the purulent exudate (top right). The exudate is caseous and amorphous at the top right. Next are degenerate and necrotic neutrophils. The pyogenic membrane arises from proliferation of stromal fibroblasts.

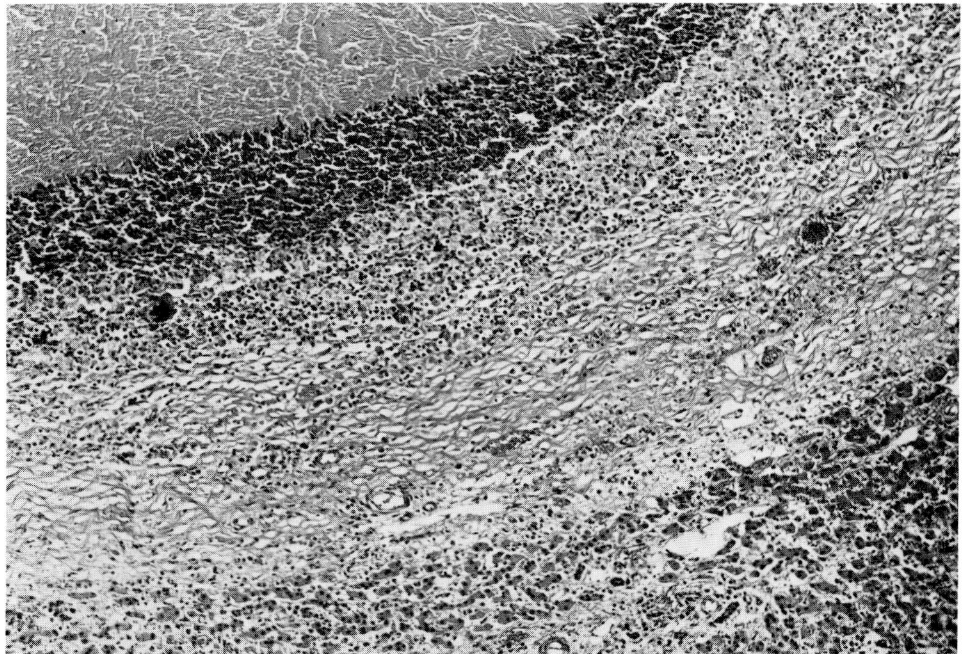

Figure 4–57. Liver abscess with a thicker pyogenic membrane. Note the mononuclear cells in the inner part of the membrane, the zone of neutrophils inside the pyogenic membrane and the liquefactive necrosis toward the center of the abscess (top left). The thickness of the pyogenic membrane varies with the rate of growth of the abscess and its age. Probably the causative agent is also influential in the thickness of the wall.

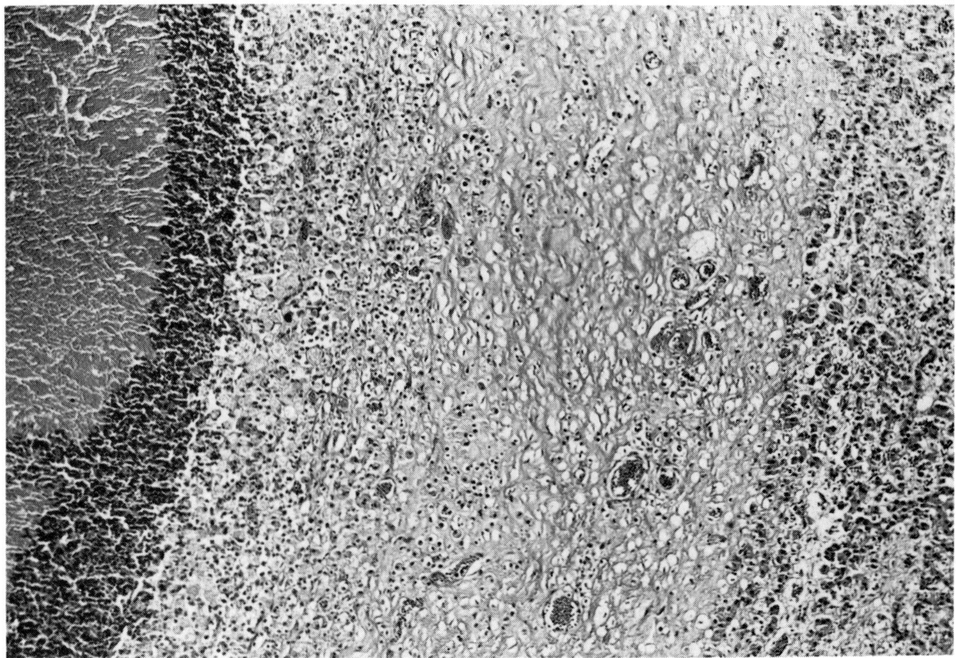

Figure 4–58. An abscess similar to that seen in Figure 4–57 but with more collagen (middle), which is quite mature, in the pyogenic membrane.

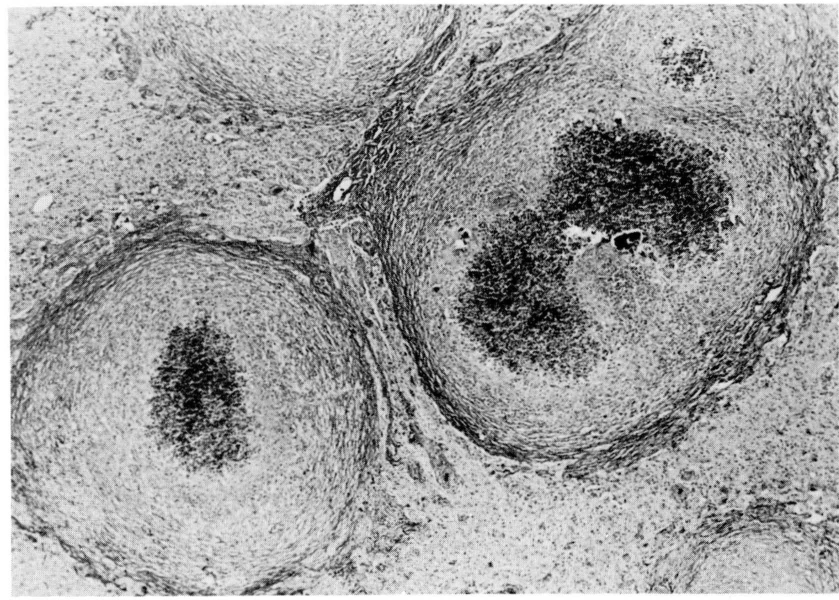

Figure 4–59. Abscesses in a bovine brain.

therapy. The abscess may grow to a huge size to accommodate the increase in pressure as more content accumulates inside. This process involves formation of ***more connective tissue*** in the middle and outer areas of the pyogenic membrane and lysis of the inner layer. If the agent is overcome, the abscess will heal by ***absorption of the fluid contents and removal and shrinkage of the membrane.*** The center is filled in by connective tissue, with only a scar eventually remaining.

An abscess may remain active for prolonged periods. If the pressure exceeds the ability to form connective tissue fast enough, the abscess may ***rupture*** along the lines of least resistance. If such an abscess is on the surface of an organ, it may rupture into a body cavity; if it is beside a major vein, it may rupture into the blood stream; if it is in a joint space, it may rupture through the skin. ***Pressure necrosis*** assists the process of rupture. Sometimes, an abscess will send out a branch or a tract from the main mass along a line of least resistance as pressure builds. The tract may travel some distance before finding a surface on which to empty in order to release the pressure. Such a tract is called a ***sinus tract.*** Thus, abscesses can grow and undergo atrophy to heal (Fig. 4–60).

Pus within a body cavity is called ***empyema*** and is best known in the thorax (Fig. 4–61). Chronic empyema is a common cause of death in mature cats and horses.

Purulent exudates may be acute but usually are chronic. Certain bacterial species characteristically cause abscesses; these species include ***Corynebacterium pyogenes*** in cattle, ***Corynebacterium ovis*** in sheep and ***Streptococcus*** spp. in horses and swine (Figs. 4–62 through 4–70). Many abscesses contain predominantly anaerobes, however, particularly with organisms from oral or intestinal flora. Some chronic purulent lesions on mucosal surfaces induce formation of lymph follicles in the mucosa (Fig. 4–71).

GRANULOMATOUS EXUDATE

Granulomatous inflammation is always chronic and may contain all types of inflammatory cells, but lymphocytes and macrophages usually predominate. Some definitions suggest that any exudate in which macrophages predominate is granulomatous, but most definitions include ***macrophages, epithelioid cells*** and ***giant cells,*** together with a rather diffuse healing component of ***connective tissue*** formation. ***The presence of numerous macrophages seems to be the main prerequisite.*** Granulomatous inflammatory lesions may have three types of macrophages: those that multiply in the lesion, those that have a long life and a slow turnover rate in lesions with a relatively inert target to attach, and those that have a high turnover rate with many new recruits arriving and many macrophages being killed in the battle. The latter is caused by agents which are particularly toxic to macrophages.

The proportion of the components varies markedly in different lesions, which provides a wide range of lesions that qualify as granulomatous. Some specific etiologic agents always induce a granulomatous response, and the lesion is an indication of a prolonged struggle between the host and some material that is disposed of with great difficulty. The reaction persists as long as the foreign material or antigen persists. Usually, three reactions occur together in the same lesion: ***inflammatory,*** as indicated by mononuclear cells; ***reparative,*** as indicated by slow persistent connective tissue production; and ***degenerative,*** as indicated by degeneration and necrosis in components of the reaction. The three may be rather clearly distinct from each other in a lesion or may be mixed together and visually inseparable.

The granulomatous reaction often causes a lump to form in the tissue and this is called a ***granuloma.*** Actually, this granuloma, which is often apparent grossly, may be made up of many smaller but somewhat confluent granulomas. The gross lesion may be a discrete or rather diffuse enlargement. It may be solid on cut surface or may contain small foci of pus or caseous necrosis throughout (Figs. 4–72 through 4–76).

When viewed microscopically, a ***classic granuloma contains the agent in the center surrounded by a somewhat layered but, to some extent, diffuse mixture of macrophages that is surrounded first by lymphocytes and then by connective tissue.*** The mental picture of concentric rings of macrophages, lymphocytes and connective tissue is too literal; the successive layers blend into each other. Neutrophils and pus may often be present around the agent. Epithelioid cells

Text continued on page 217

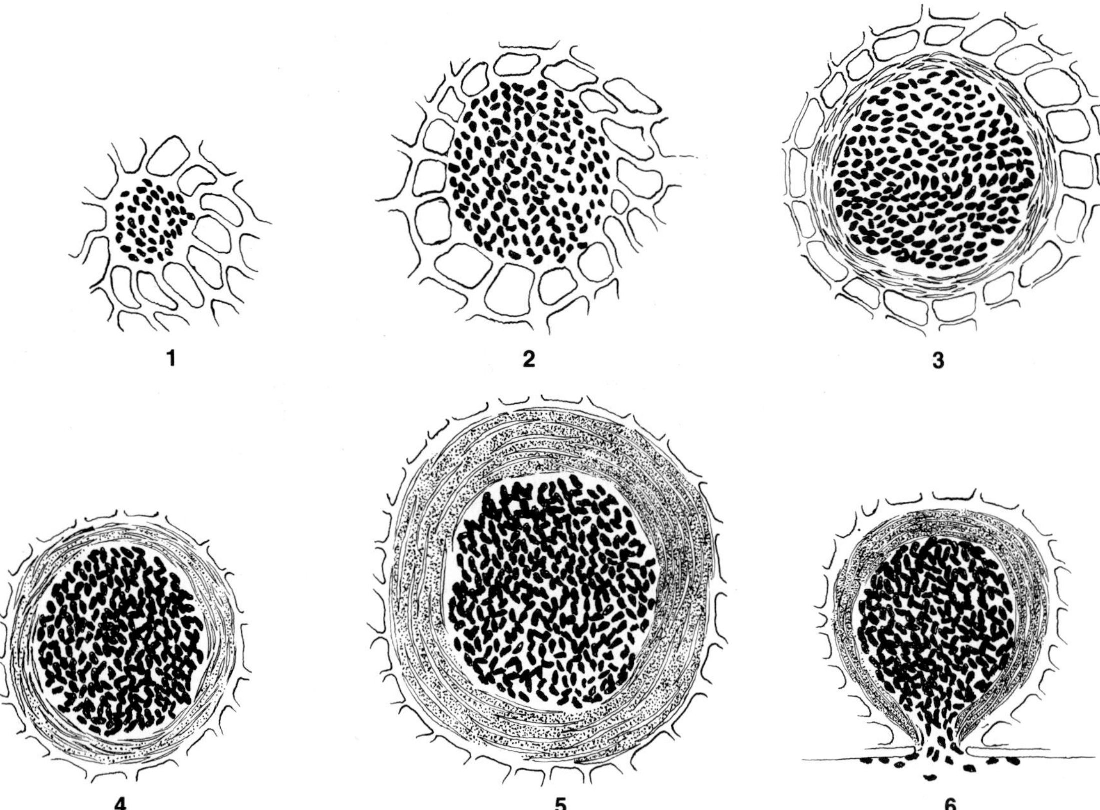

Figure 4–60. Diagrammatic representation of the growth of an abscess. *1,* Microabscess with focal necrosis. *2,* A more advanced state. *3,* Pyogenic membrane is present. The abscess may decrease in size *(4),* or enlarge *(5),* and may develop a very thick capsule. *6,* The build-up of exudate may create sufficient pressure to cause rupture through to a surface.

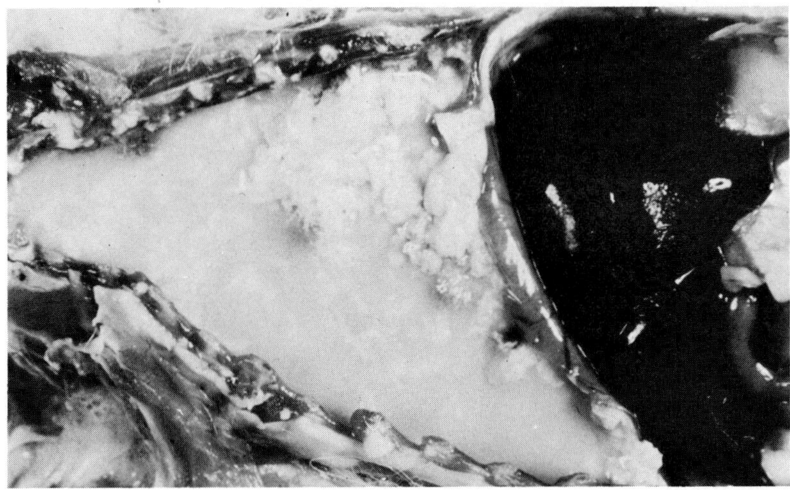

Figure 4–61. Empyema in a cat. The lungs are still in the thorax but are covered by fibrinopurulent exudate. This is a common lesion in cats.

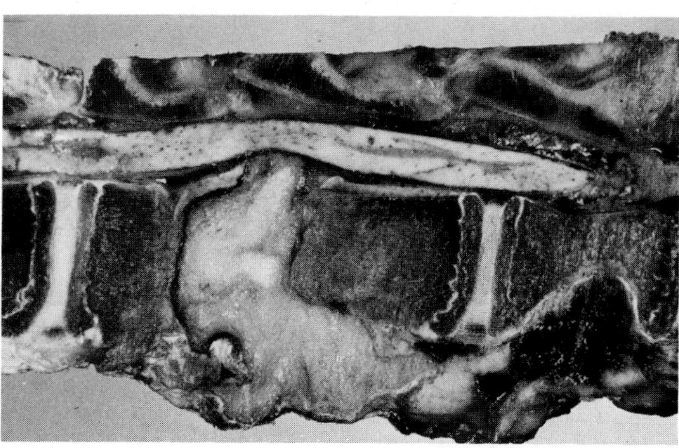

Figure 4–62. Chronic purulent osteomyelitis caused by *Corynebacterium pyogenes* in a cow. The exudate is causing pressure on the spinal cord, and the clinical signs would relate to this pressure.

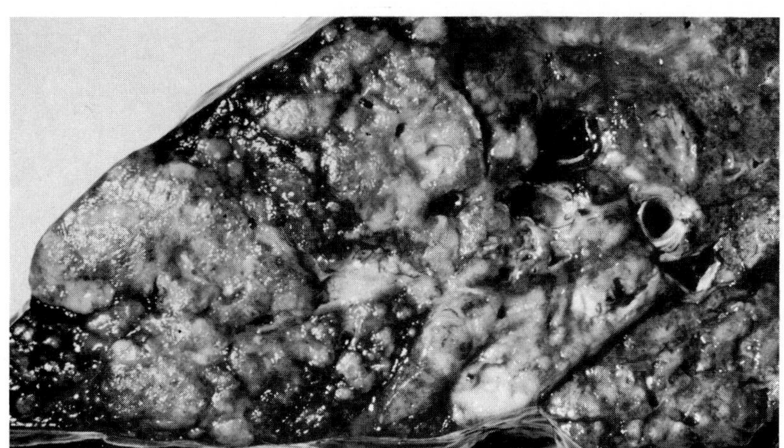

Figure 4–63. Chronic purulent pneumonia caused by *Corynebacterium equi* in a foal. Most of the lung contains purulent exudate. The cut surface reveals many individual lesions, but many tend to become confluent into an almost granulomatous lesion.

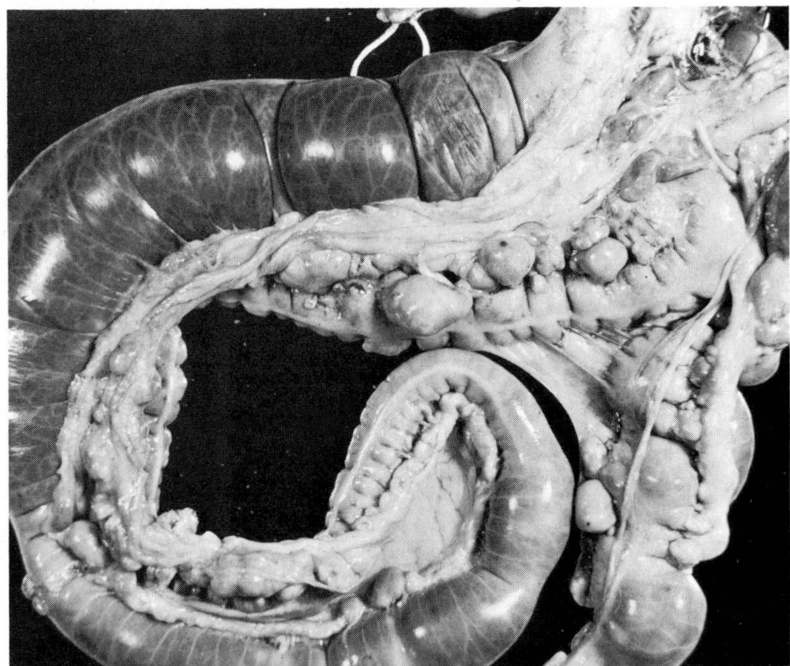

Figure 4–64. Multiple abscesses in mesenteric lymph nodes in a foal.

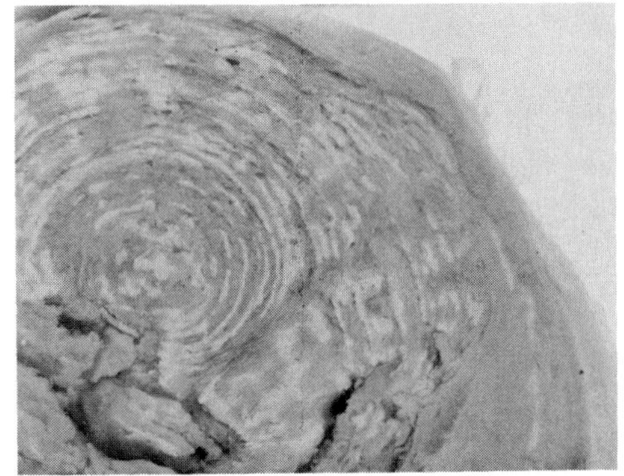

Figure 4–65. Laminated abscess caused by *Corynebacterium ovis* in a sheep. (Museum specimen.)

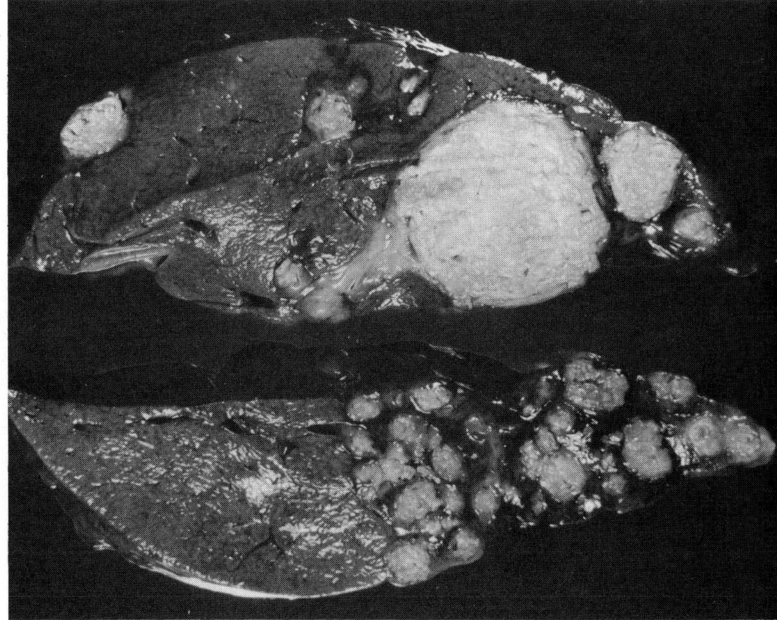

Figure 4–66. Multiple liver abscesses caused by *Corynebacterium ovis* in a sheep.

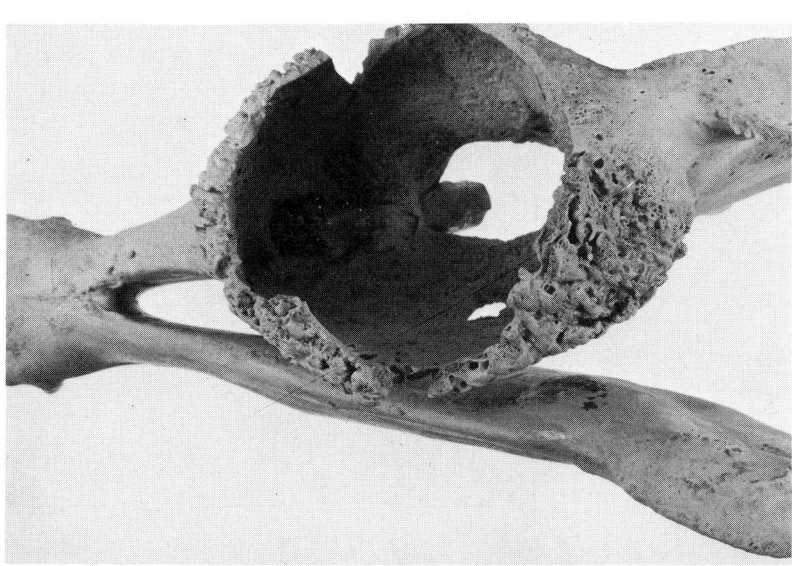

Figure 4–67. Chronic purulent osteomyelitis in a horse's mandible. The abscess expanded and caused the bone to be removed, with the result that more formed around the edge of the abscess in an effort to maintain strength. The new bone has taken the shape of the abscess.

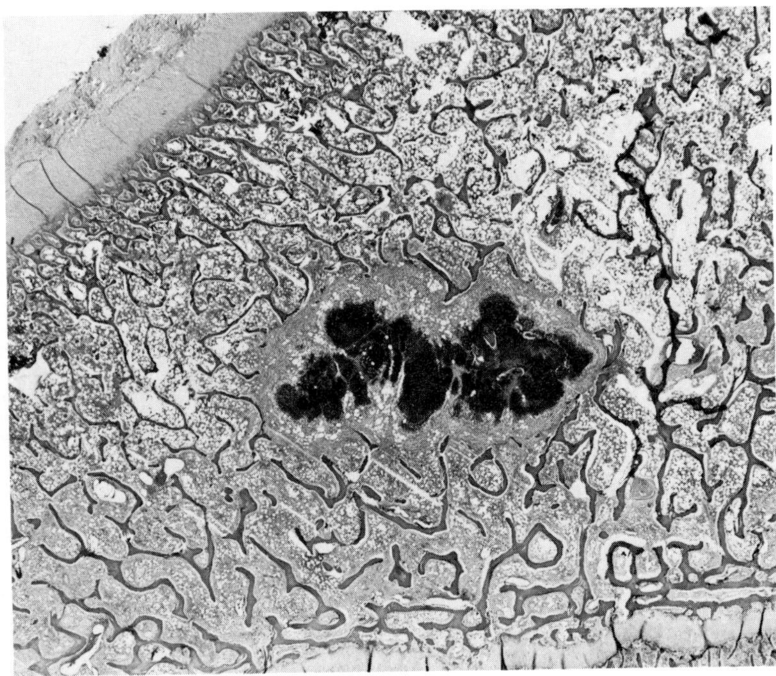

Figure 4–68. Subacute purulent osteomyelitis in a pig. Joint surface is at the top left, and epiphyseal cartilage is at the bottom. Purulent exudate is present in the epiphysis, which is causing resorption of bone spicules as the exudate expands. This lesion could lead to an abscess.

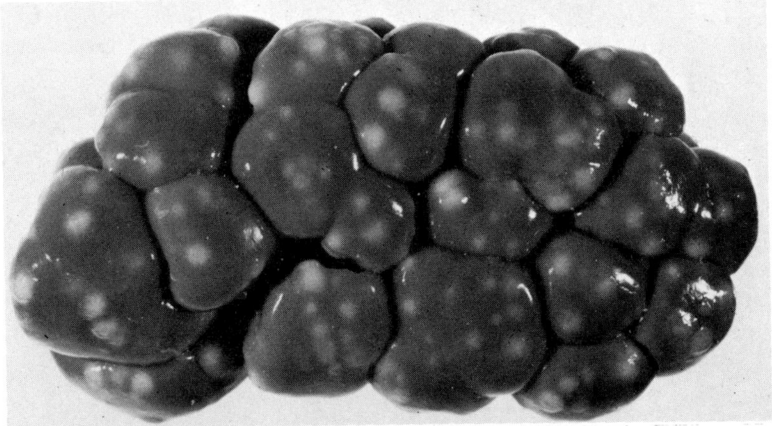

Figure 4–69. So-called white-spotted kidney in a calf. The white foci are areas of purulent inflammation, some of which occurs as microabscesses and some of which is diffuse in the tissue. The lesion is a result of localization of infection in young calves and is quite common. Healed lesions leave depressed scars.

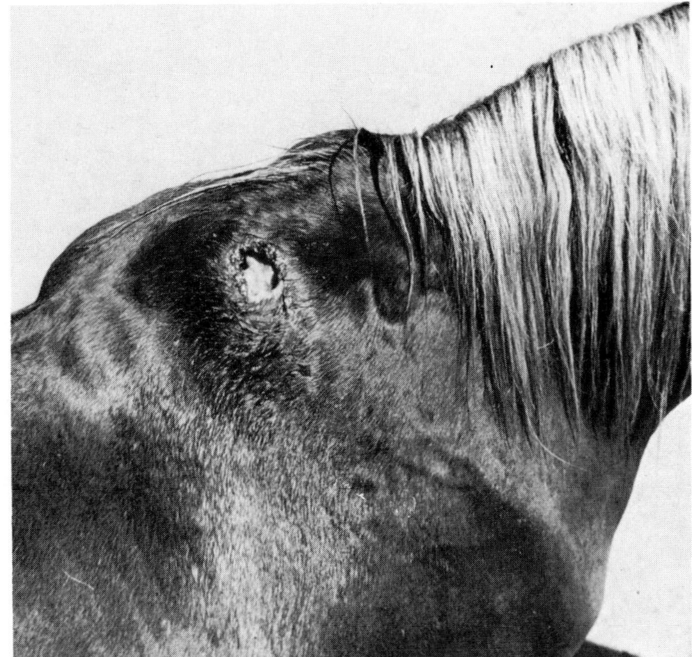

Figure 4–70. Chronic purulent exudate extending deep into the withers to the bursa between the nuchal ligament and the thoracic spine in so-called fistulous withers.

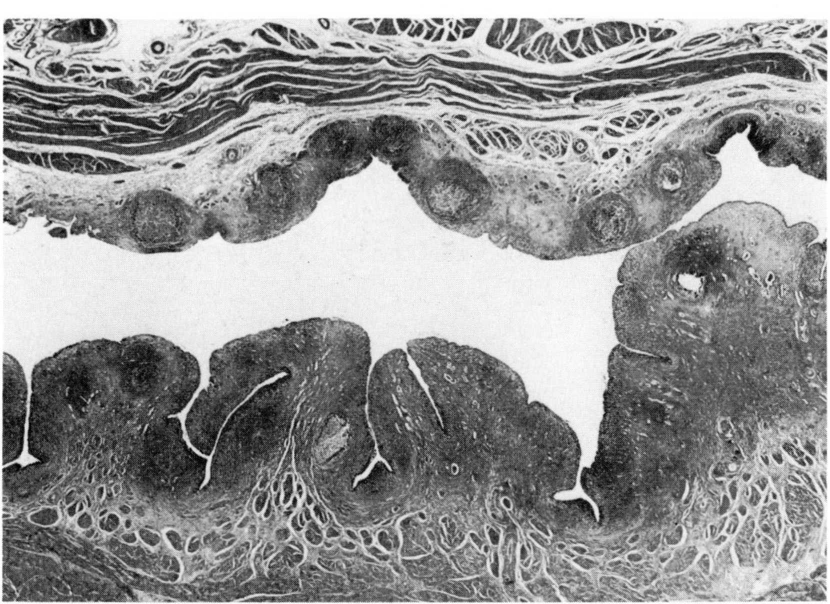

Figure 4–71. Chronic cystitis in a dog. Note the diffuse fibrosis in the submucosa and also the lymphoid follicles in the mucosa. These lesions indicate a long-standing chronic lesion.

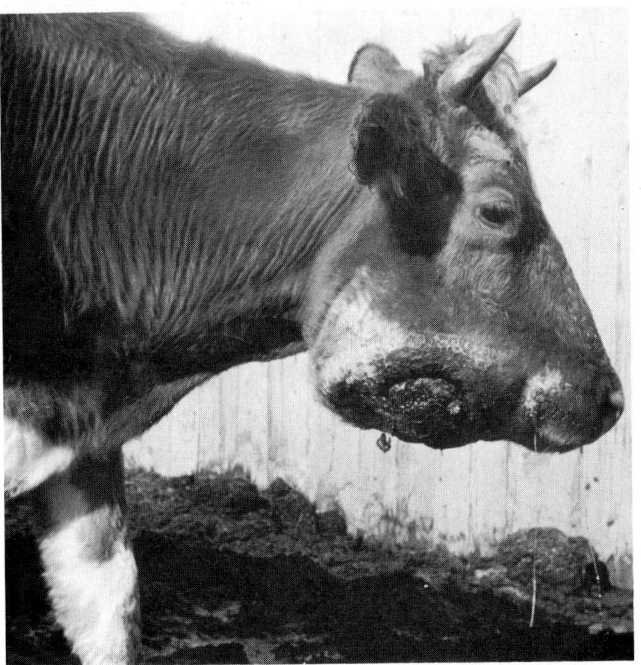

Figure 4–72

Figures 4–72, 4–73, and 4–74. Actinomycosis or lumpy jaw. The basic lesion is a chronic granulomatous osteomyelitis (Fig. 4–73). The bone is quite distorted from its normal shape. The spaces represent focal areas of chronic inflammation that so weaken the bone that more bone forms in an effort to maintain strength within the bone tissue. Figure 4–74 is a cross section of a mandible from another case of the same disease.

Illustration continued on following page.

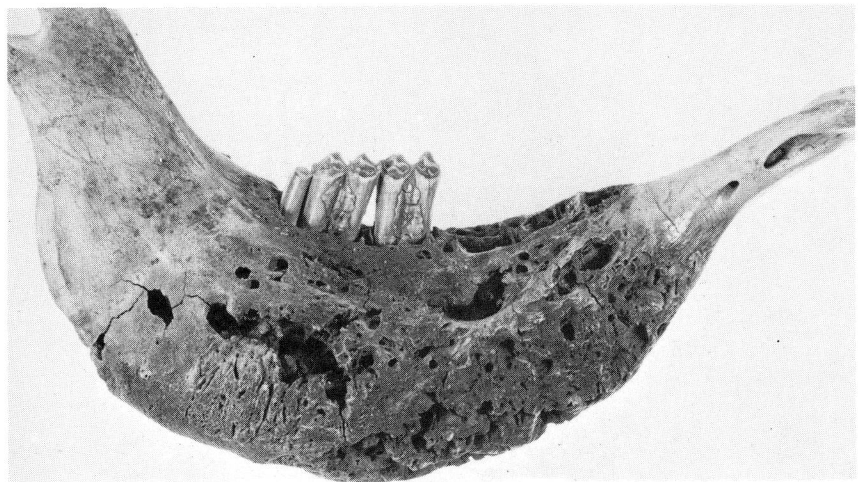

Figure 4–73

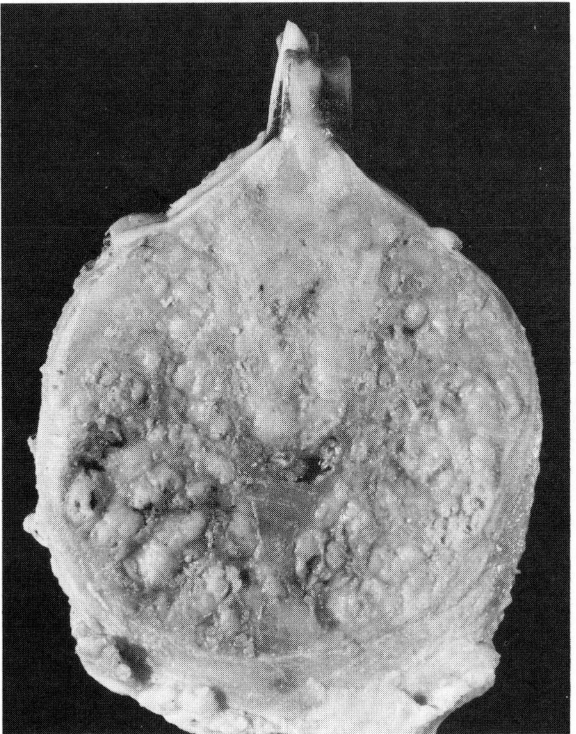

Figure 4–74

Figures 4–73 and 4–74. See legend on preceding page.

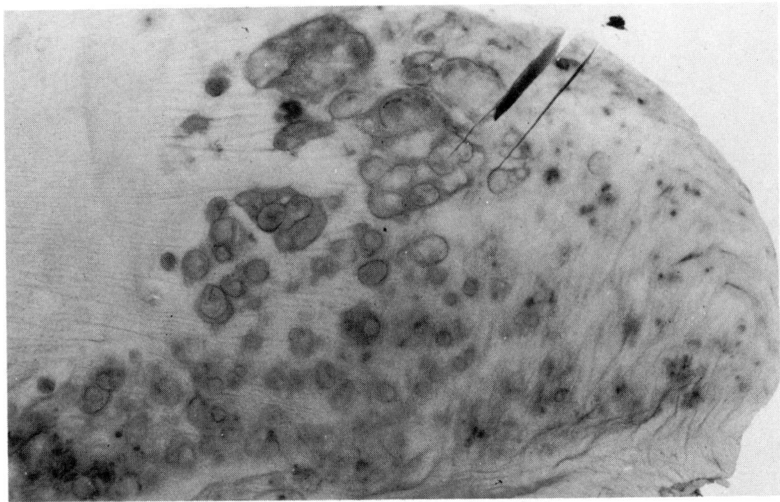

Figure 4–75. Actinobacillosis in the tongue of a cow. There are numerous foci of granulomatous inflammation contributing to the overall enlargement in the tongue. Many small granulomas are visible on the surface. (Museum specimen.)

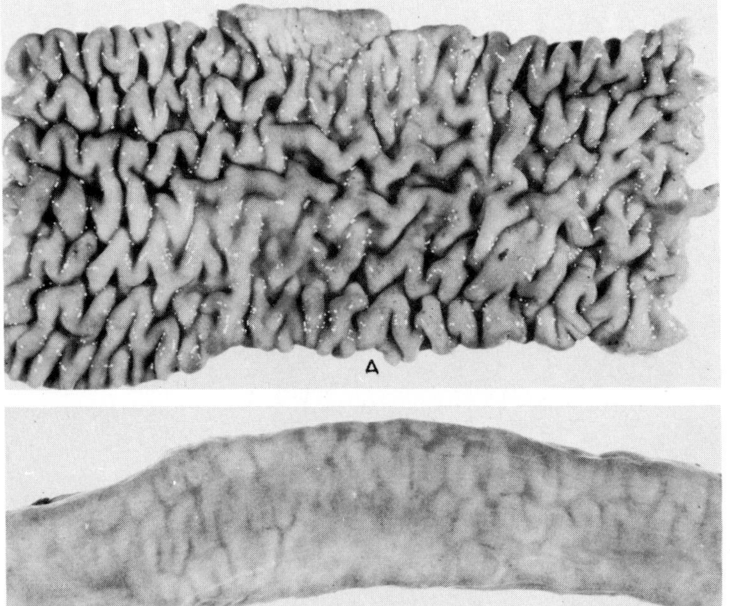

Figure 4–76. *A,* Small intestine from a cow with Johne's disease. The mucosa is thickened and corrugated by diffuse granulomatous inflammation, characterized mainly by epithelioid cells. *B,* Note the corrugated appearance reflected in the serosal surfaces.

and giant cells may be closest to the agent or spread throughout the lesion (Figs. 4–77 through 4–88).

Avian species produce giant cells rapidly and in large numbers and seem to form granulomas filled with caseous necrosis rather than liquid pus in response to many agents that would induce pus in mammals (Figs. 4–89 and 4–90).

Some infectious agents, particularly bacterial and fungal agents, develop a ring of dense eosinophilic material around them. This material is often arranged like a row of rectangles parallel to each other, and the width and height of the rectangle vary. This provides a ring of eosinophilic blocks around the agent, which has resulted in the name ***club colony*** or ***asteroid body*** for the eosinophilic material. Certain agents always have these in some species; the best known occur in actinobacillosis and actinomycosis in cattle. The eosinophilic material is composed of remnants of collagen and antigen-antibody complexes and is indicative of intense incompatibility between the agent and the host (Figs. 4–91 and 4–92).

The appearance of macrophages may vary markedly in the same granulomatous lesion or in different ones. Plasma cells may be numerous and mixed with the lymphocytes. The connective tissue component may be sparse or dominant, and its rather mature appearance is often deceptive. It is induced slowly over a long period and blends well with the normal resident connective tissue. The amount is often best appreciated on ***gross examination*** rather than on microscopic examination. The connective tissue is diffuse around the agent, however, and is not a discrete wall, which distinguishes the connective tissue of a granuloma from that of the pyogenic membrane of an abscess. It is important to recognize the ***circumscribed nature of the lesion*** near the agent; it is suggestive of a granulomatous response. Numerous such circumscribed areas give the overall view of confluent circumscribed areas composing the gross granuloma (Figs. 4–93 through 4–96). Granulomas may be tiny or huge, depending on the agent and the host. As in other types of chronic inflammation, the key to their persistence is the presence of antigen that generates the release of chemical mediators that bring the inflammatory cells to the site.

There should be three components in the name of an inflammatory lesion: *time, type of exudate* and *location.* For example, the following lesions might occur: acute fibrinous enteritis, subacute catarrhal rhinitis, chronic granulomatous hepatitis, acute mucopurulent tracheitis, acute hemorrhagic mastitis, acute necrotizing bronchitis. It is not always easy to name all three components in all inflammatory lesions in all tissues, but it is possible in most instances. In learning to name lesions accurately, it is necessary to *recognize the components of the exudate* and to actually *interpret what is happening in the pathogenesis* of the lesion. It is a goal well worth mastering.

MECHANISMS OF TISSUE INJURY

This seems an appropriate point to relate the inflammatory reaction in a general way to types of tissue injury, including some of the responses mentioned under exudates and cell types, as well as to necrosis and infectious disease.

Trauma and Necrosis

Trauma from the following types of injury may result in tissue damage: mechanical contact; compression-decompression, as in blast injury; sonic, thermal and electrical injuries; cold; sunburn; and irradiation. ***Irradiation*** concentrates an increase in energy to cells or parts of cells. Metabolic processes and specific components of the cell may be altered by the increase in energy. The primary action is ionization and excitation of molecules that results in rupture of bonds and production of chemical changes in the cell. Key steps in the metabolism or structural components of the cell may be altered by these chemical changes.

The ***main effect of trauma is direct tissue injury, resulting in hemorrhage and necrosis,*** and if severe injury occurs, shock becomes the major problem. Clinicians speak of reversible and irreversible types of shock that relate to the severity of injury and the amount of time between injury and ade-

Text continued on page 229

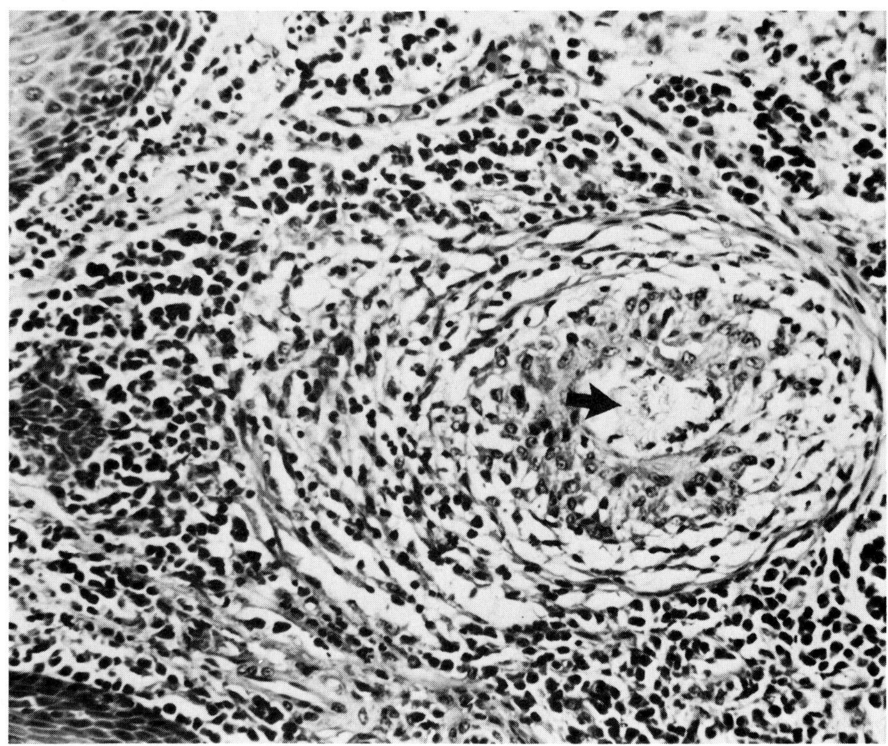

Figure 4–77. A typical foreign body type of granuloma (arrow) due to penetration of the tongue of a dog by plant fibers. Macrophages surround the plant material in the center of the circumscribed lesion. Note the rather loose connective tissue border around the lesion and the mononuclear cells nearby.

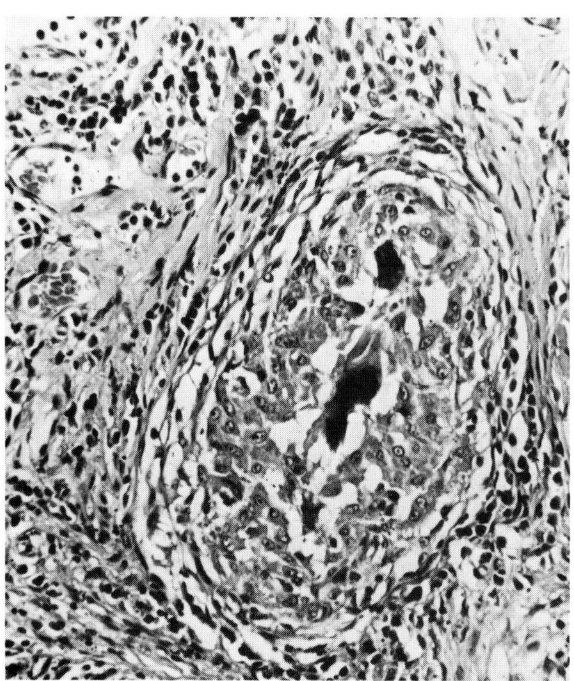

Figure 4–78. Same case as seen in Figure 4–77. The granuloma is more compact and epithelioid cells surround the agent.

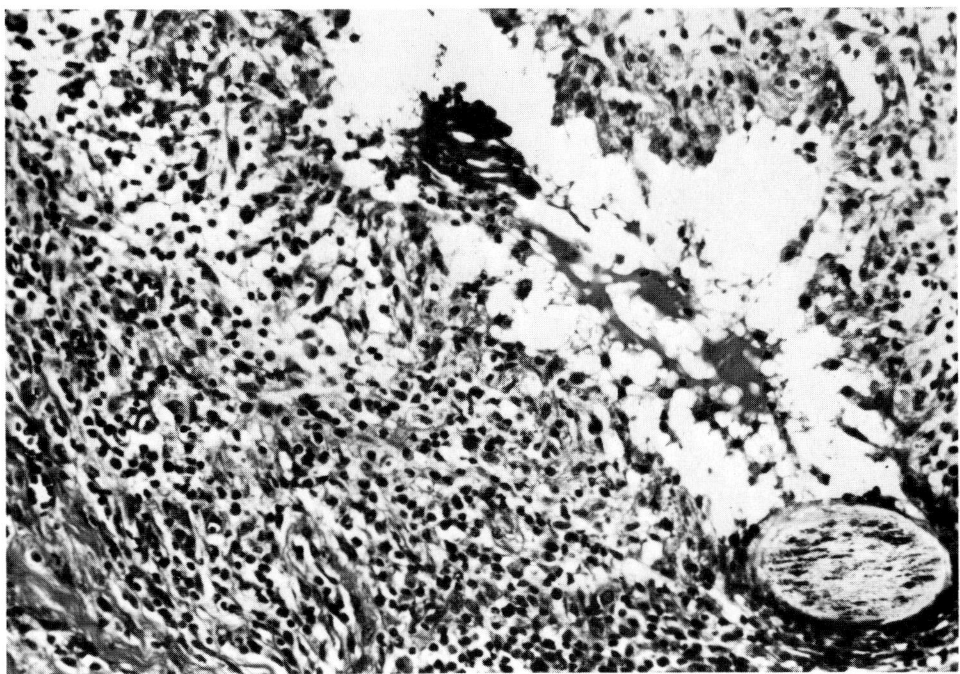

Figure 4–79. Granuloma in the skin of a dog in which a displaced piece of hair is acting as a foreign body (lower right). The cellular reaction is quite mixed.

Figure 4–80. A different perspective on a lesion similar to that in Figure 4–72. Note the chronic granulomatous or perhaps pyogranulomatous inflammation in the dermis. Pieces of hair are present in the central area of the lesions (arrows).

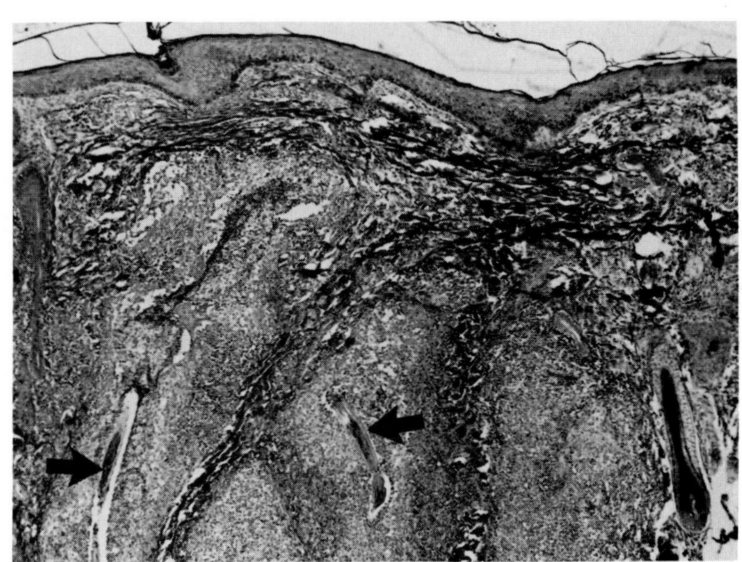

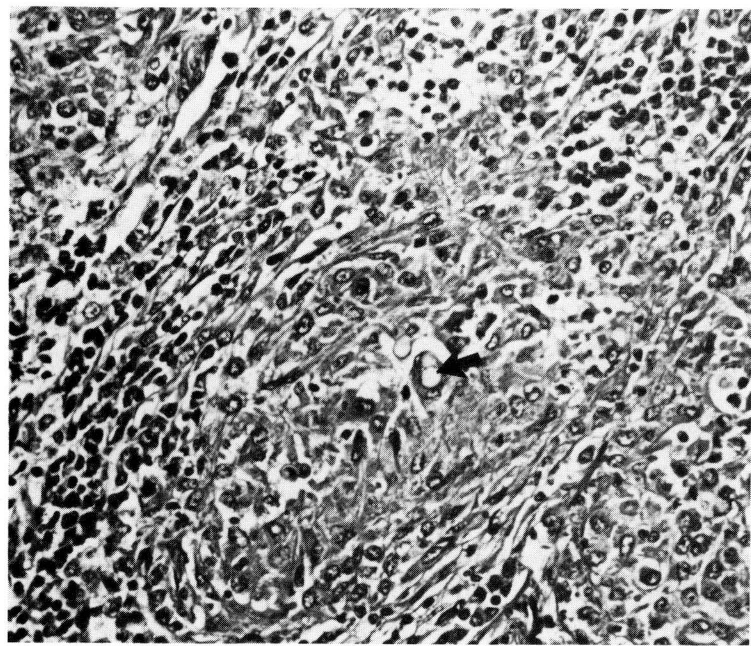

Figure 4–81. A granuloma in a dog's brain due to blastomycosis (arrow). The circumscribed nature of the lesion is less obvious but still apparent as a ring of macrophages and epithelioid cells. Connective tissue is sparse.

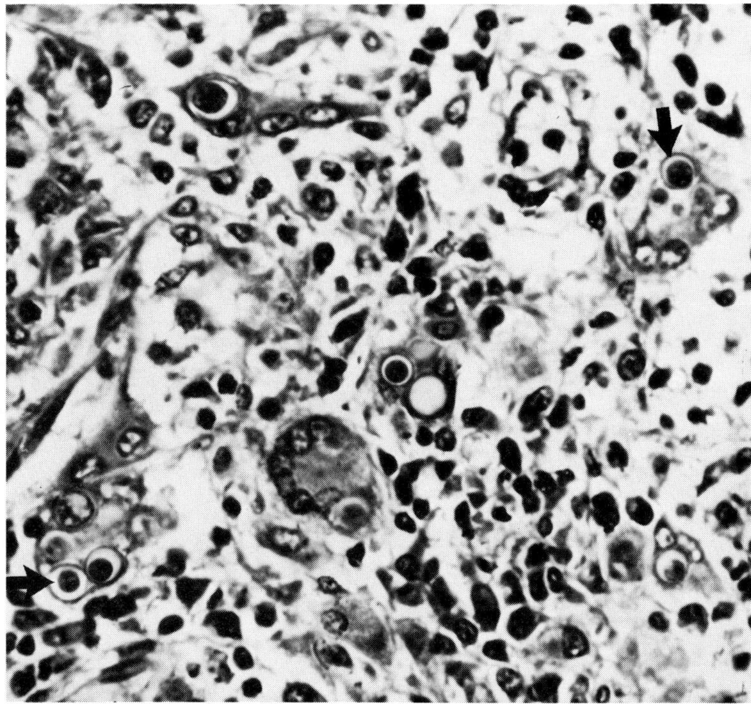

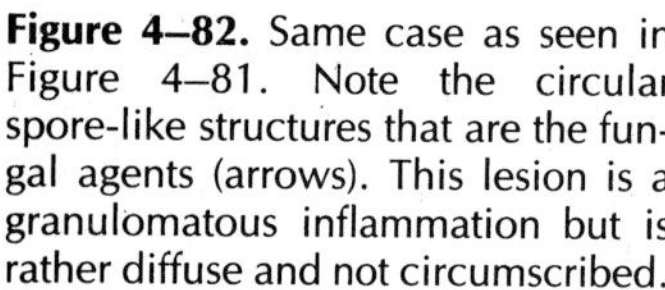

Figure 4–82. Same case as seen in Figure 4–81. Note the circular spore-like structures that are the fungal agents (arrows). This lesion is a granulomatous inflammation but is rather diffuse and not circumscribed.

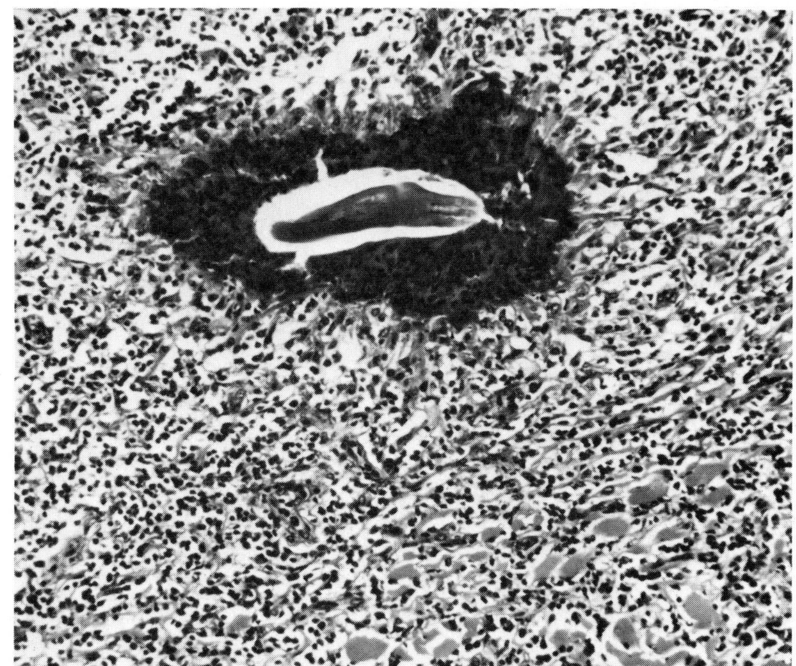

Figure 4–83. A *Habronema* larva in the skin of a horse. Pus is present around the larva, and a diffuse mononuclear response spreads into surrounding tissue. Other larvae in the same lesion are surrounded by giant cells (not shown), indicating considerable variation between focal areas, but the overall reaction is granulomatous.

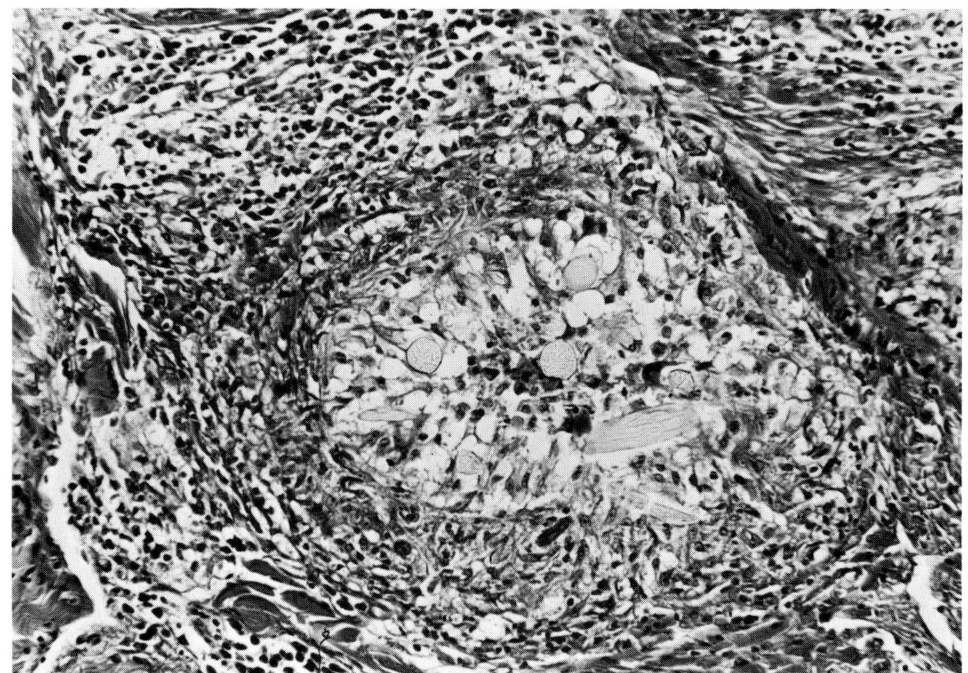

Figure 4–84

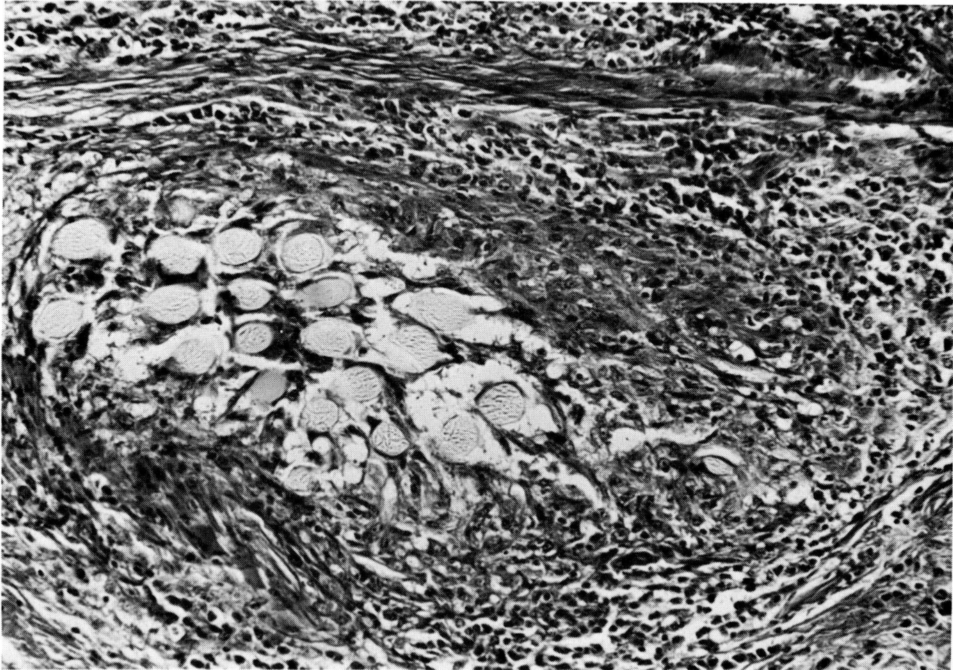

Figure 4–85

Figures 4–84 and 4–85. Subcutaneous granuloma found in a dog and caused by retained suture material—a so-called suture granuloma (Fig. 4–84). The degree of encapsulation varies between this lesion and the lesion in Figure 4–85.

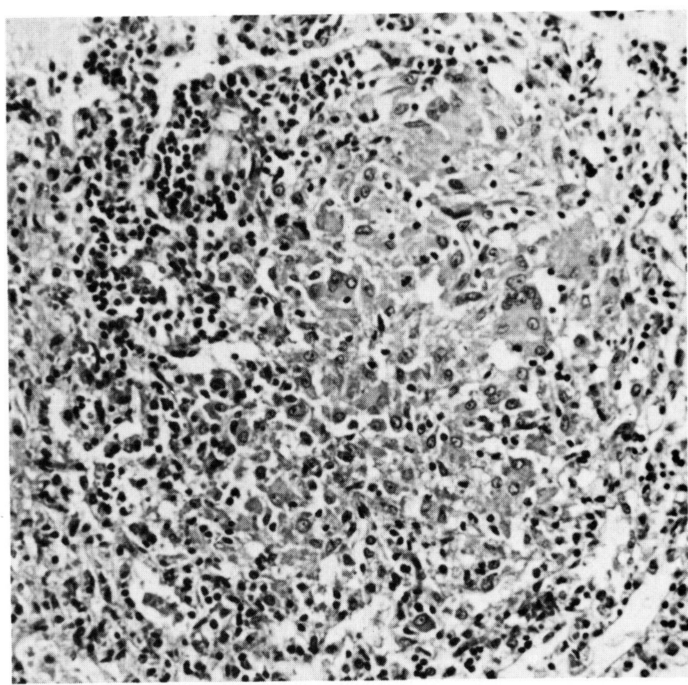

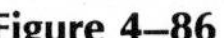

Figure 4–86

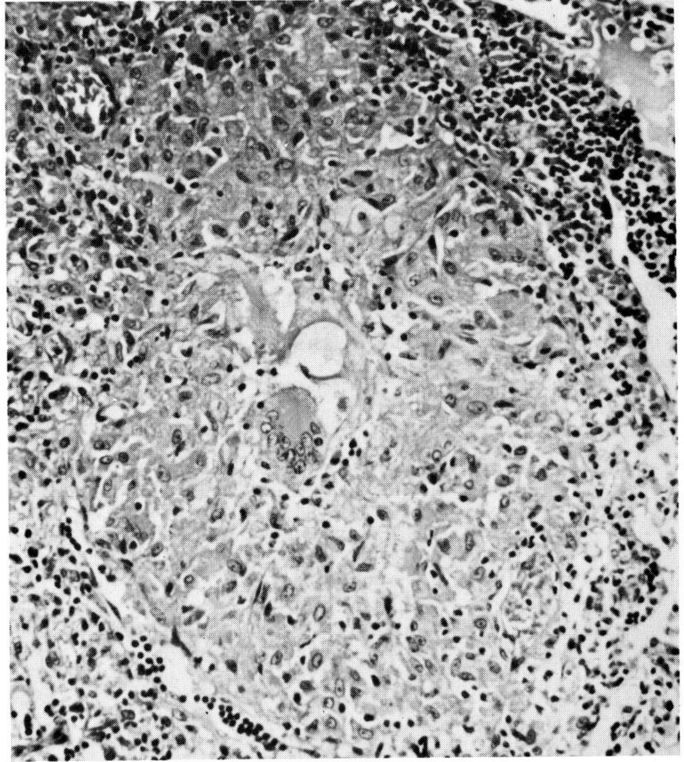

Figure 4–87

Figures 4–86 and 4–87. Two granulomas in a tuberculous bovine lung. The first granuloma has a rather loose arrangement and contains several types of mononuclear cells and a few small giant cells. The second granuloma is a more discrete lesion with epithelioid cells predominating (Fig. 4–87). Their cytoplasmic borders are indistinct.

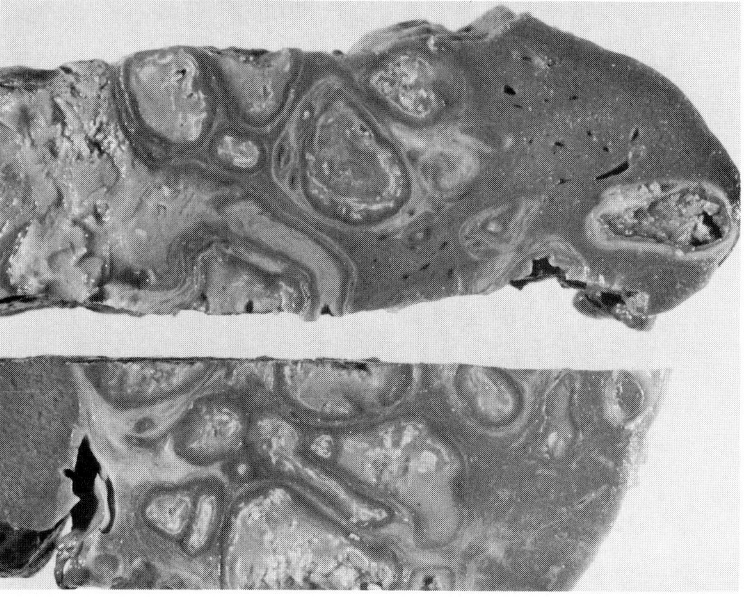

Figure 4–88. Some tuberculous granulomas develop extensive central areas of caseous necrosis, and many of these have large deposits of dystrophic calcification. Note the white areas of calcification within some of the lesions in this bovine liver.

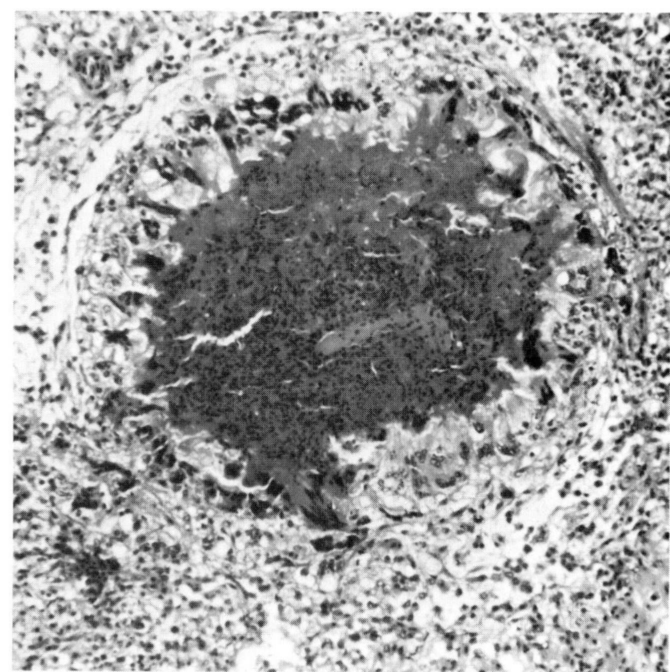

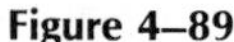

Figure 4–89

Figures 4–89 and 4–90. In avian species, giant cells are prominent around areas of caseous exudate and form a type of granuloma under circumstances in which mammals would form an abscess. These two lesions are in a bird's lung.

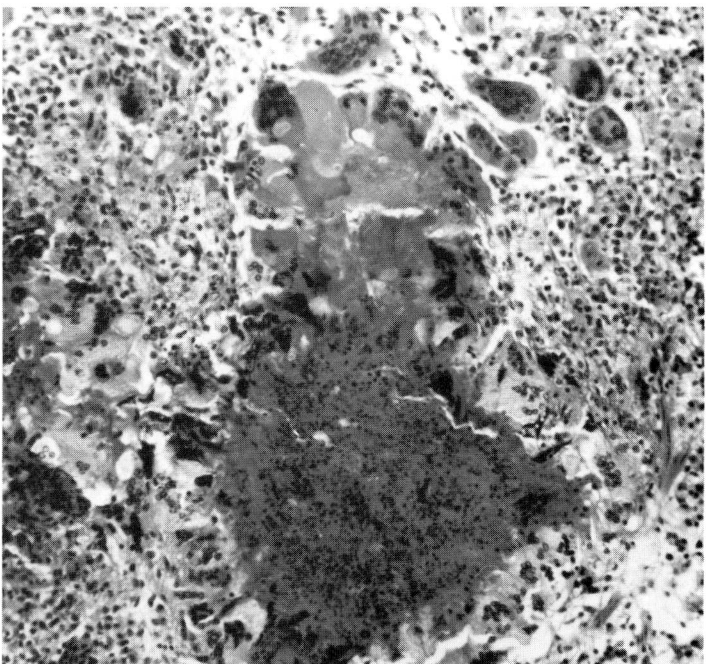

Figure 4–90

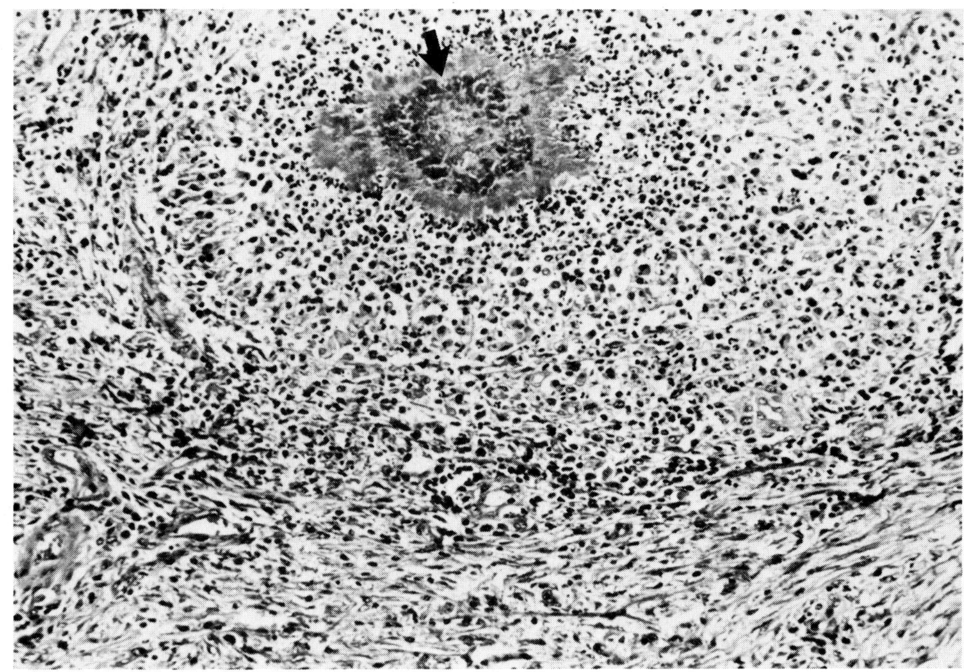

Figure 4–91. A colony of bacteria surrounded by dense eosinophilic material and then by neutrophils, mononuclear cells and connective tissue from a case of actinobacillosis.

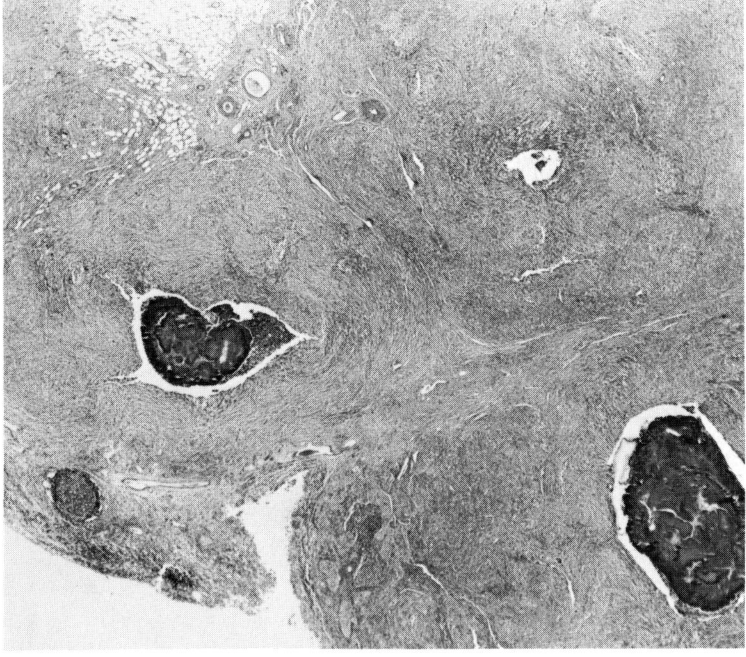

Figure 4–92. Large masses of bacteria and club colonies in a dog with thoracic nocardiosis. Connective tissue around the colonies is very prominent.

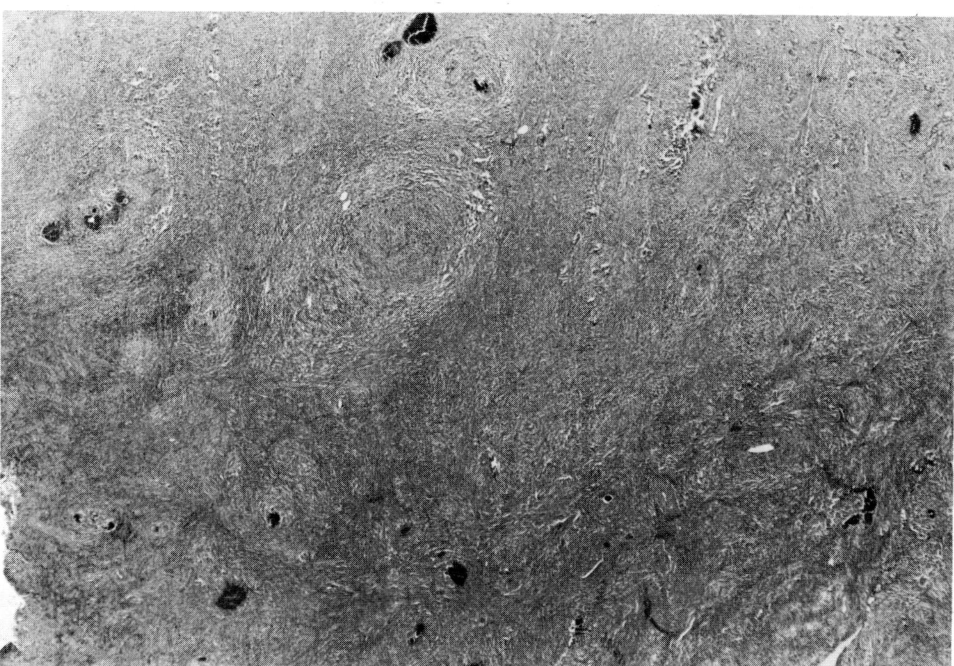

Figure 4–93. View at a lower power of a *Habronema* lesion. The dark foci are areas that contain larvae and pus or areas that had recently contained larvae. Note the circumscribed nature of the individual lesions and the great amount of connective tissue. The amount of connective tissue in granulomas, as demonstrated here, is typical of many granulomatous lesions and accounts for the gross appearance of a firm lump in the tissue.

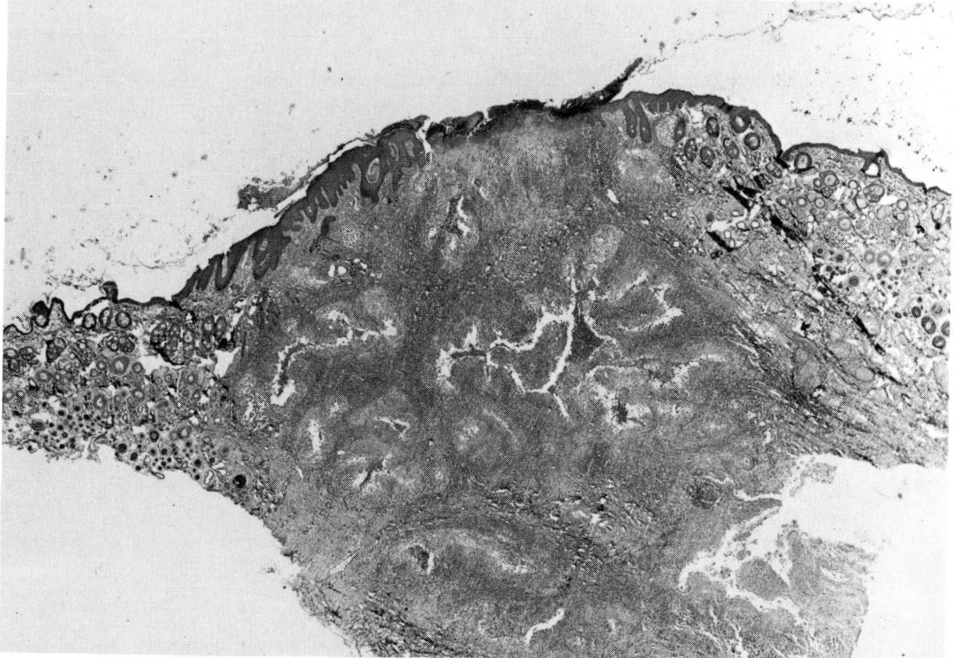

Figure 4–94. Blastomycosis in a dog's skin. This view demonstrates the lump in the skin that is composed of numerous foci and tracts, some of which contain purulent exudate and some of which are as shown in Figure 4–82. The surface epithelium over the lesion is thickened and is ulcerated in one area. This picture gives an overview of the extent of disruption of the normal architecture of the skin by the granulomatous inflammation.

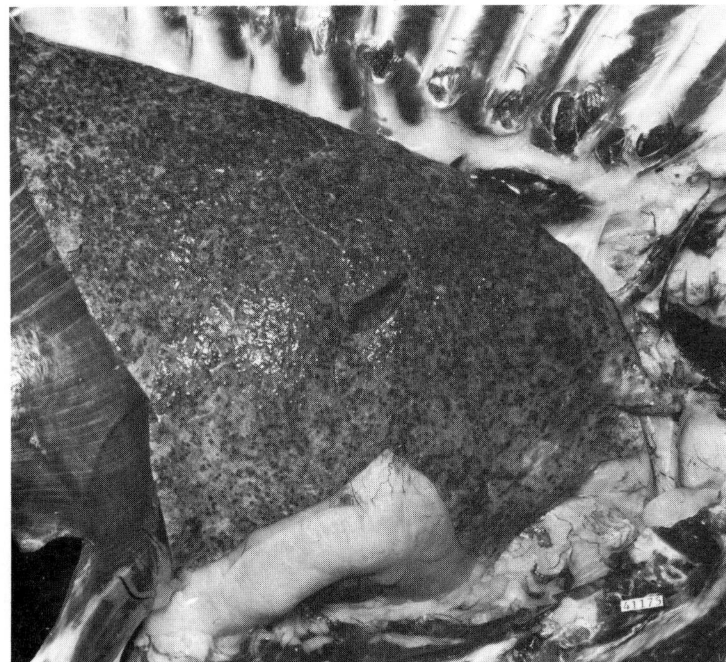

Figure 4–95. Numerous small granulomas in a case of blastomycosis in a dog's lung.

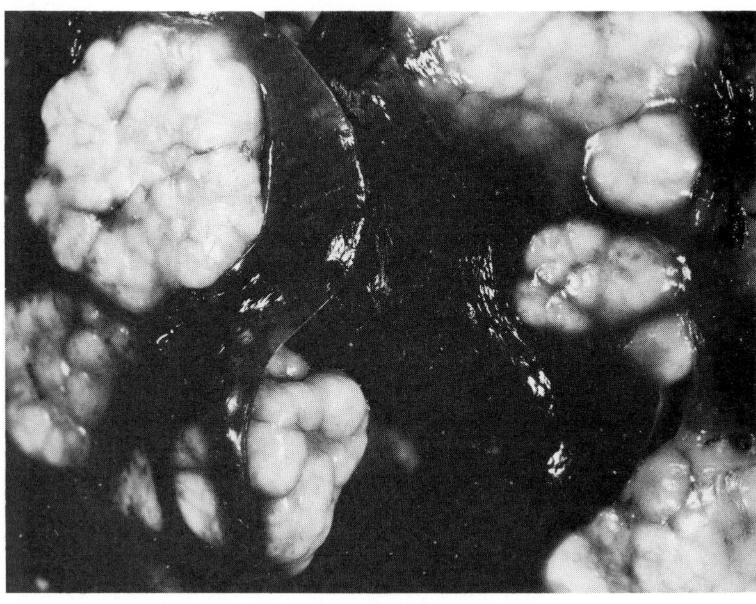

Figure 4–96. Close-up view of granulomatous inflammation caused by *Mycobacterium avium* in the liver of a partridge. Note the discrete lesions.

quate therapy. Irreversible shock occurs when anoxia, sludging and intravascular coagulation result in necrosis or irreparable damage in the kidneys, liver, heart or lungs. The endocrine system plays a major role in adaptation following trauma, mainly regulating normal circulation, conserving fluids and energy and activating alternate energy pathways.

Specific definition of traumatic lesions is required particularly in ***forensic or legal cases.*** Some of the following definitions relate especially to trauma, but some relate to other types of injuries as well. ***Trauma*** is defined as a wound or injury that is either physical or psychic. A ***wound*** is bodily injury caused by physical means with disruption of the normal continuity of structures. An ***abrasion*** is an area of the body denuded of skin or mucous membrane by abnormal or unusual mechanical processes. ***Contusion*** is a bruise or injury without a break in the skin or surface of the tissue. ***Laceration*** is a tearing of tissue that results in torn, ragged or mangled tissue. An ***incision*** is the act of cutting open or through. ***Concussion*** is a violent jar or shock or a condition that results from such injuries. A ***blast*** is a wave of high air pressure at high velocity usually followed by a negative wave resulting in suction.

Types of direct tissue injury leading to ***necrosis*** include trauma, heat, cold, irradiation, infection, pressure, abnormal metabolism, thrombosis, anoxia and toxic and immune reactions. Some of these may result in abnormalities in growth, but most involve ***necrosis of tissue*** and the presence of abnormal materials or antigens ***foreign*** to the host as well as to the immune system. ***In many instances, inflammation in a tissue causes considerable necrosis and loss of functional tissue. This is one of the most important effects of the inflammatory process in tissue. Figures 4–97 through 4–110 draw attention to the functional and morphological effects of primary inflammatory reactions on tissues.***

Necrosis results in the release of thromboplastins that not only initiate clotting and thrombosis because of local vascular injury but also attract neutrophils by chemotaxis. The chemotaxis may also occur via the complement system, which is activated by compounds released from dead and dying cells unassociated with direct immune involvement, by kinins or plasmin. These mechanisms are partially responsible for the neutrophils around an infarct, in focal necrosis or on the surface of an ulcer. The neutrophils release compounds that are also chemotactic. The main objective is to lyse and remove the necrotic tissue by means of the enzymes contained in the neutrophils. In some instances, the necrosis and thrombosis that occur together are self-perpetuating.

Immune Injury

The immune system is beneficial to the host and is designed to protect it from any foreign material by humoral and cellular responses. Ideally, an agent enters and stimulates antibody production or cellular immune response, which destroys the agent, and the memory cells guard against any further exposure. The response to re-exposure, called the ***anamnestic response,*** is intended to produce more protection faster than that produced at the first exposure (Fig. 4–111). Figure 4–112 depicts entry of organisms into the tissues, from which they are carried to a lymph node and become exposed to the immune system (Fig. 4–113). Re-entry of the same organism results in a much more effective response by the body's defenses (Fig. 4–114). The general responses to acute infection are indicated in Figure 4–115, and the responses to chronic infection are shown in Figure 4–116. The reactions to toxins or organisms are demonstrated in Figure 4–117.

Instances occur, however, in which the host's immune system responds to re-exposure with good intentions but the results may cause more harm than good by inducing tissue injury. ***The harmful effects of the immune response are called hypersensitivity***. The host might make more antibody than is needed or produce antibody that is not protective, antigen-antibody complexes may themselves initiate inflammation or the agent may persist for prolonged periods and maintain a harmful immune response. Also, the host may be unduly sensitive to a particular antigen of an agent and therefore react differently in different diseases. Hypersensitivity involves both the humoral and the cellular responses and is reflected as well-known clinical allergies. Allergies usually result from contact between exoge-

Text continued on page 240

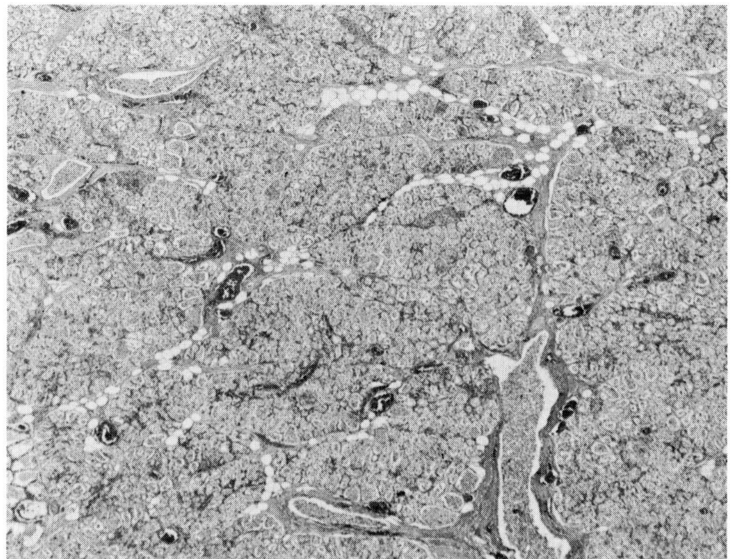

Figure 4–97

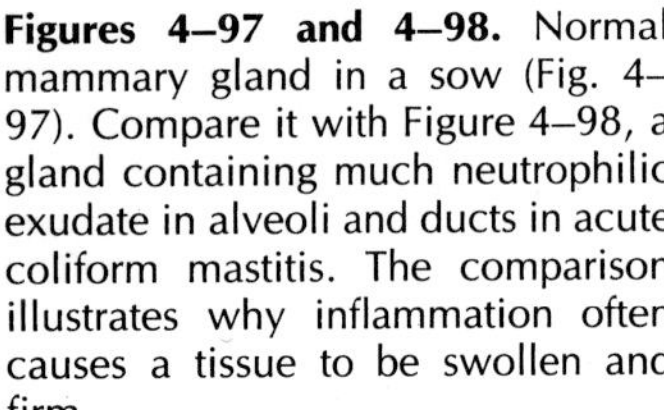

Figures 4–97 and 4–98. Normal mammary gland in a sow (Fig. 4–97). Compare it with Figure 4–98, a gland containing much neutrophilic exudate in alveoli and ducts in acute coliform mastitis. The comparison illustrates why inflammation often causes a tissue to be swollen and firm.

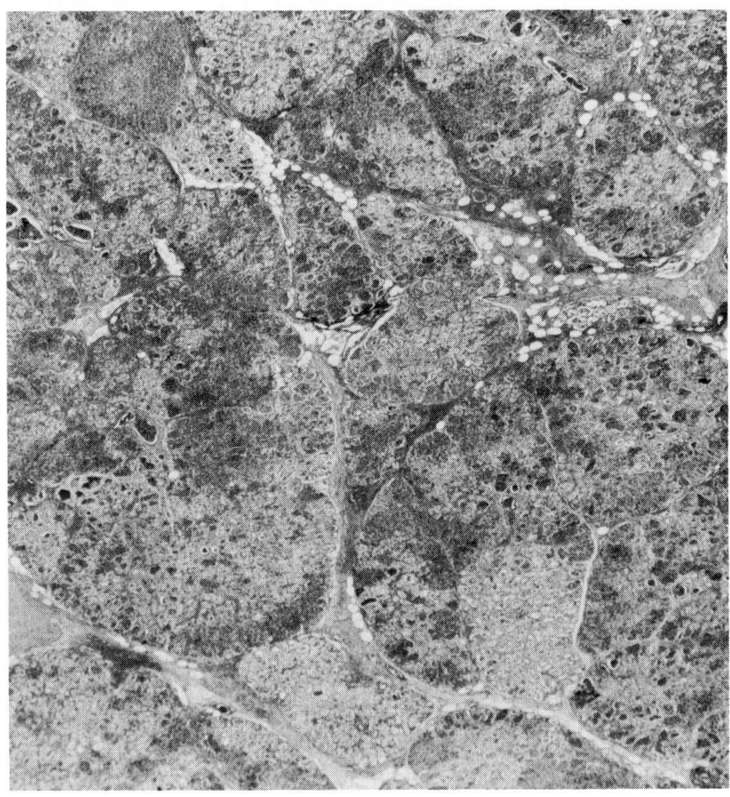

Figure 4–98

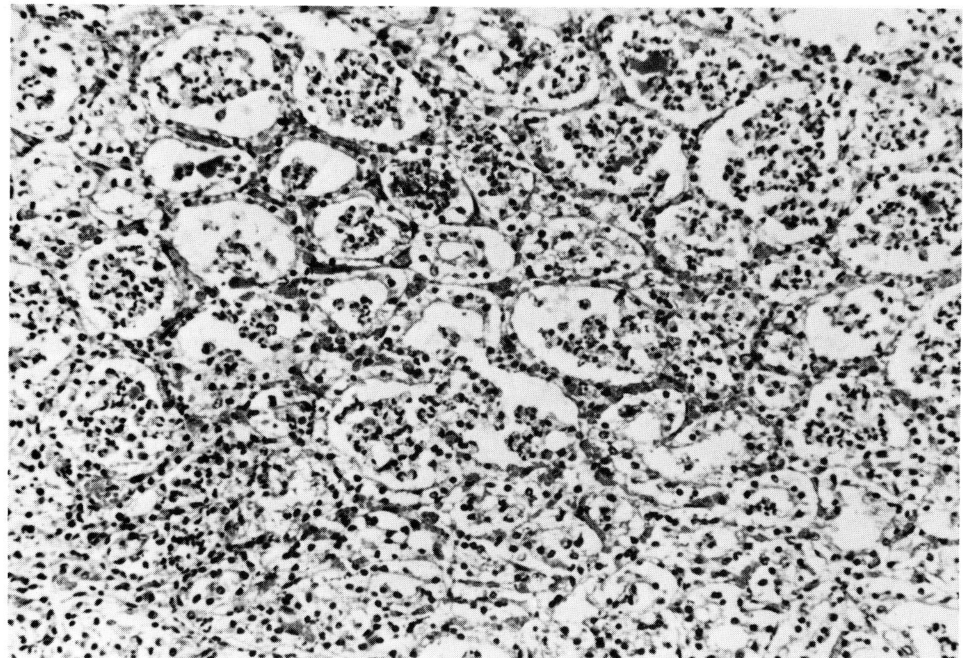

Figure 4–99

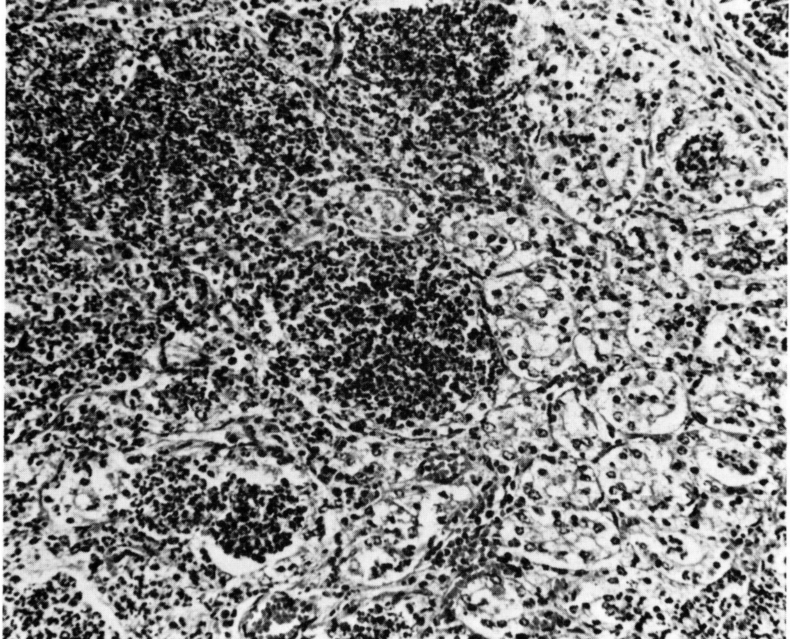

Figure 4–100

Figures 4–99 and 4–100. Same case as seen in Figure 4–98. Note the early exudation of neutrophils into acini and necrosis of acinar epithelium. The exudate is increased, and necrosis of acini is more extensive in Figure 4–100.

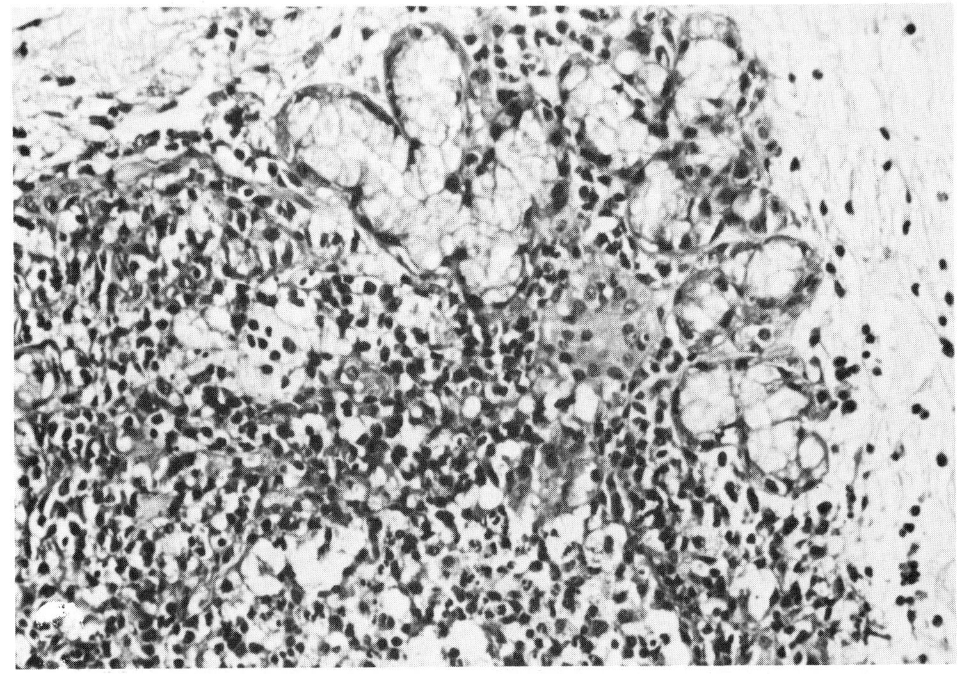

Figure 4–101 Subacute salivary gland adenitis in a dog. A large part of a lobule is necrotic and replaced by debris, neutrophils and mononuclear cells with only a few acini remaining.

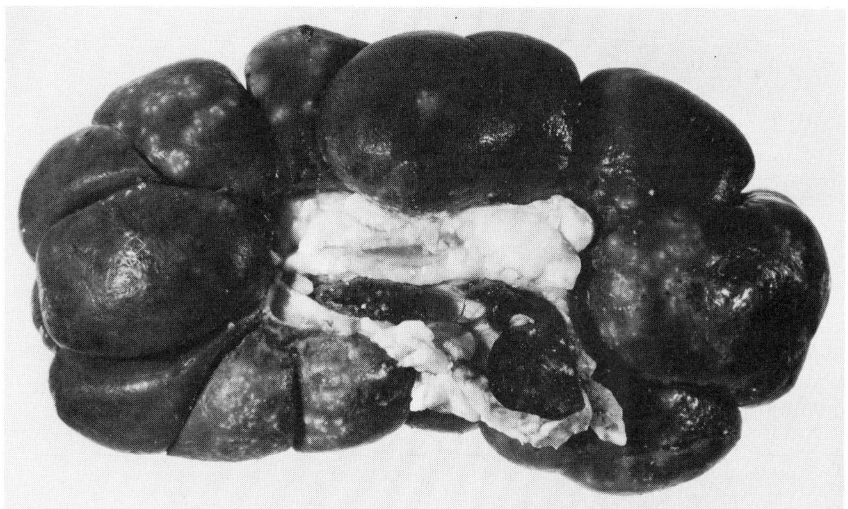

Figure 4–102

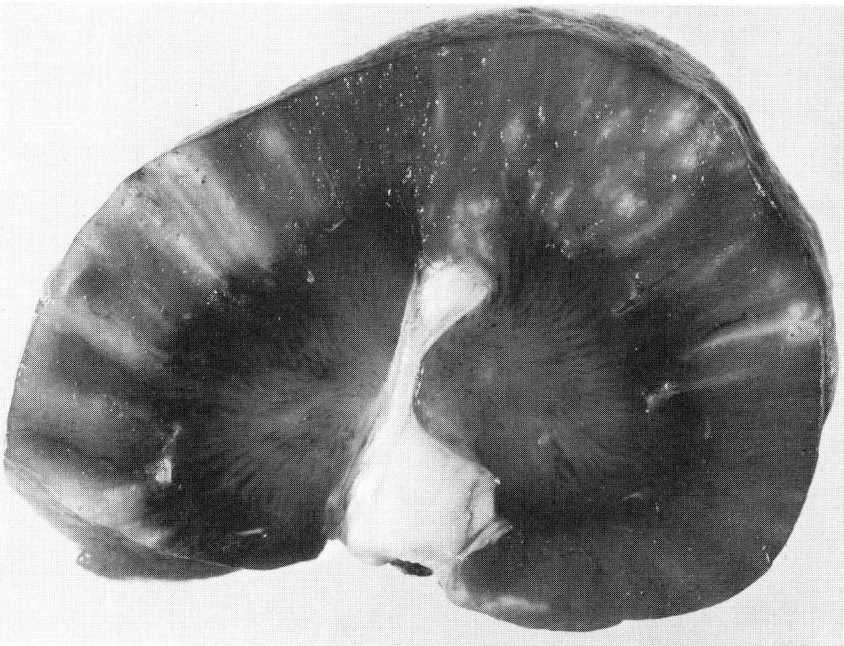

Figure 4–103

Figures 4–102 and 4–103. Focal necrosis and microabscesses on the surface of a calf's kidney as well as a thrombus in the renal vein. On the cut surface of the kidney (Fig. 4–103), the extent of the lesion is more apparent. The pale areas are inflammatory cells in the tissue. If the calf lived there would eventually be considerable scarring in the kidney.

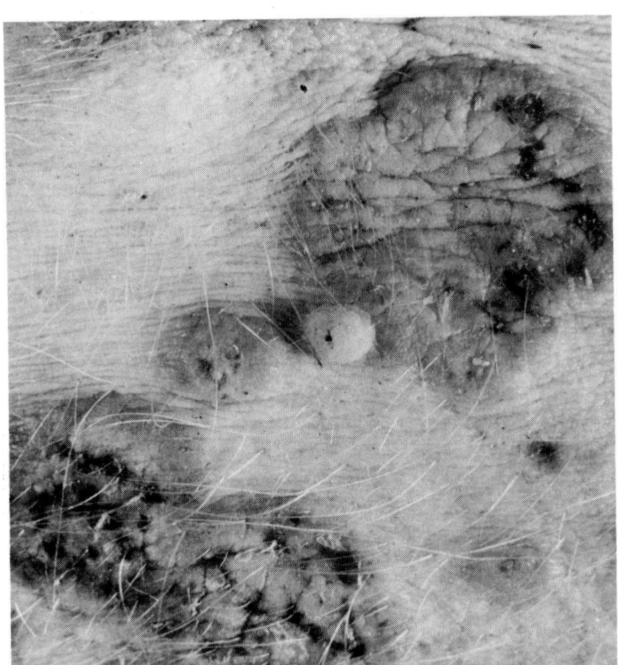

Figure 4–104

Figures 4–104 and 4–105. Raised thickened areas in the skin of a pig with swine pox. Microscopic view of a similar lesion in which a normal area is seen at the right (Fig. 4–105).

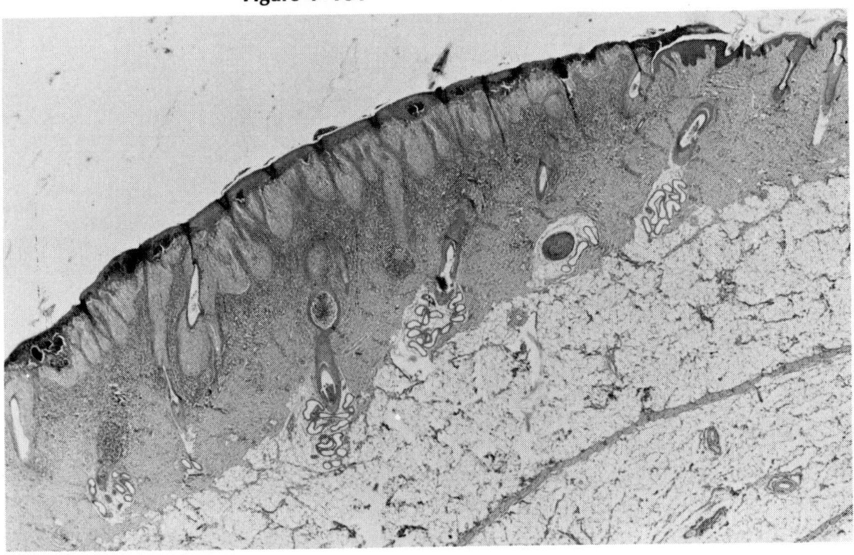

Figure 4–105

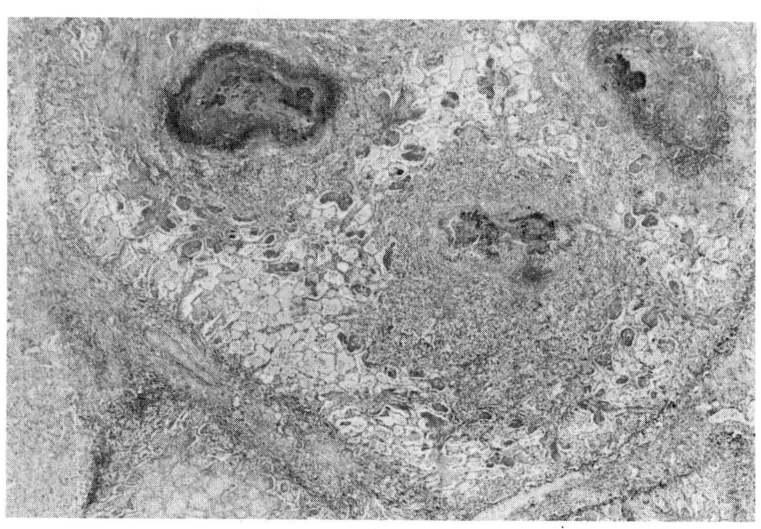

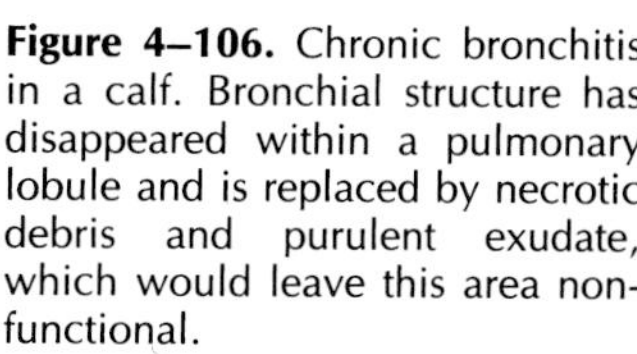
Figure 4–106. Chronic bronchitis in a calf. Bronchial structure has disappeared within a pulmonary lobule and is replaced by necrotic debris and purulent exudate, which would leave this area nonfunctional.

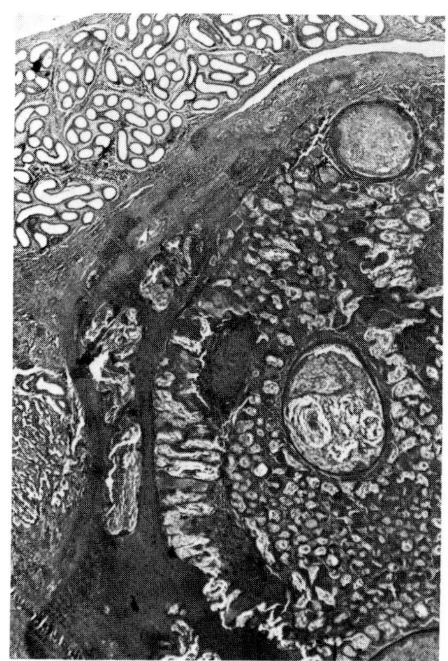

Figure 4–107. Extensive necrosis and inflammation of a calf's testicle. Epididymis is at the top.

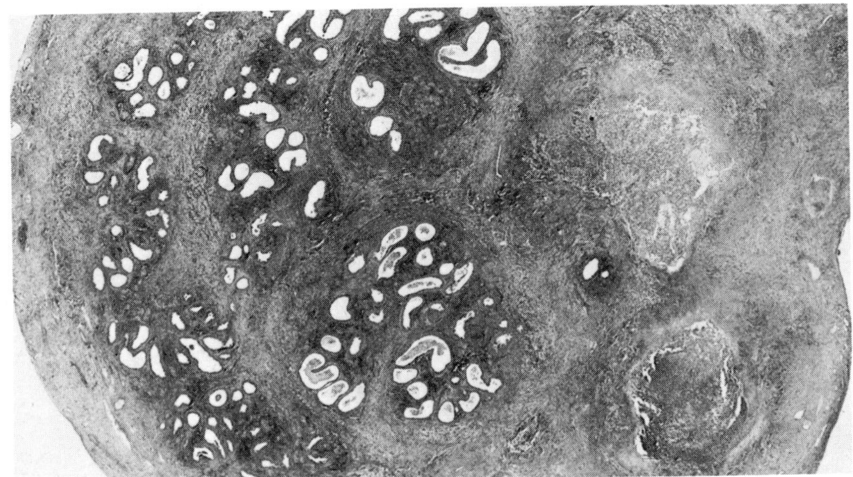

Figure 4–108. Diffuse inflammation necrosis and fibrosis in the epididymis of a dog.

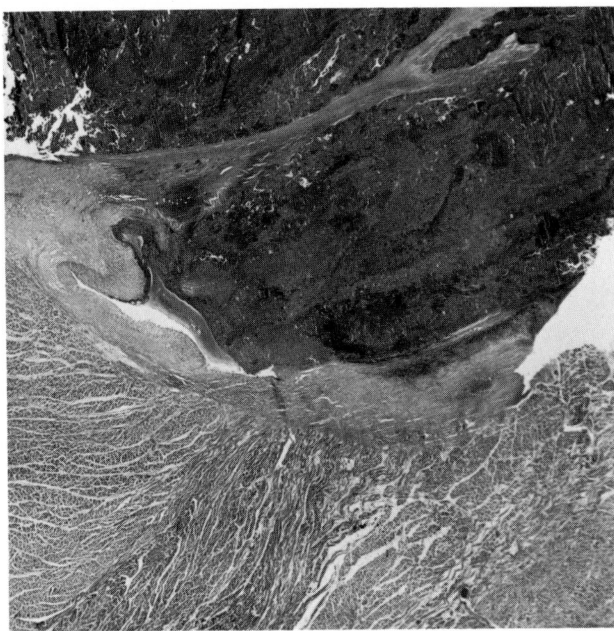

Figure 4–109. Extensive thrombosis and inflammation of the heart valves of a deer. Part of the valve is visible, toward the top, with thrombus and exudate above and below.

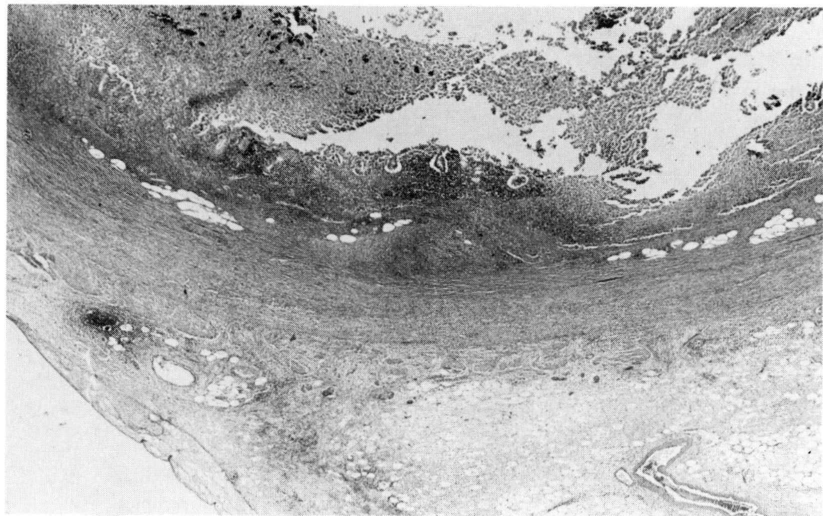

Figure 4–110. Acute appendicitis. Exudate is in the lumen to the top, and the mucosa is mostly necrotic with only remnants of glands remaining. Inflammation has spread into and through the muscle layers and into the mesenteric fat. Acute fibrinous peritonitis is present at the lower left. This lesion demonstrates how inflammation leads to necrosis in the intestinal wall and to possible perforation.

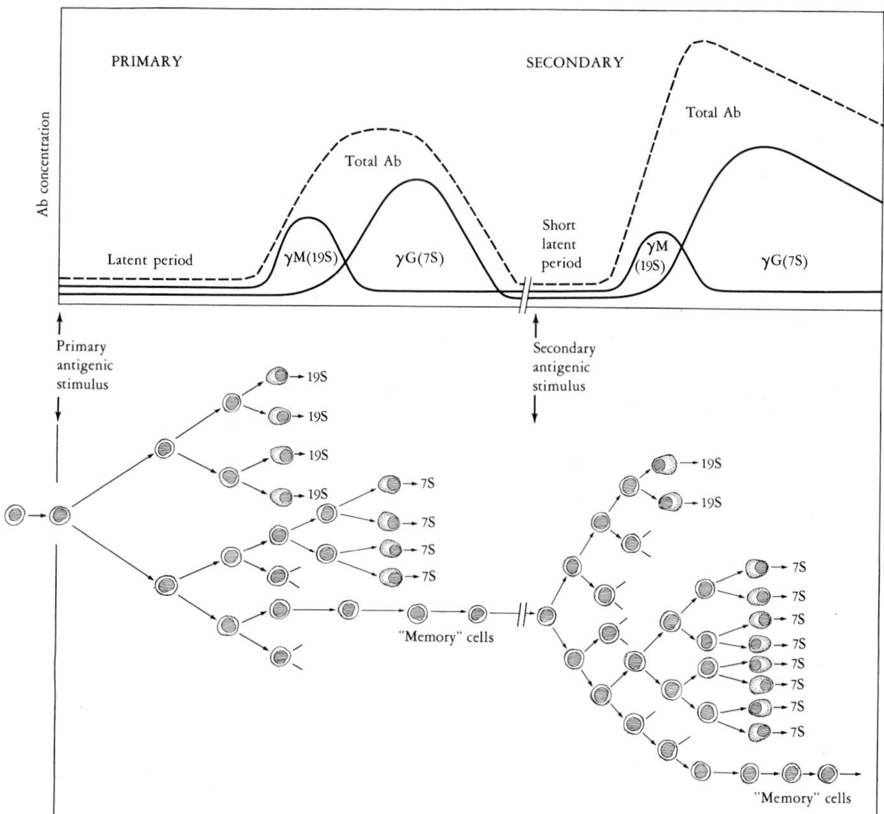

Figure 4–111. Schematic representation of primary and secondary (anamnestic) antibody responses. Note the shorter latent period, greater antibody production and enhanced cellular activity seen during anamnestic response. (From Bellanti, J. A.: Immunology II. Philadelphia, W. B. Saunders Company, 1978.)

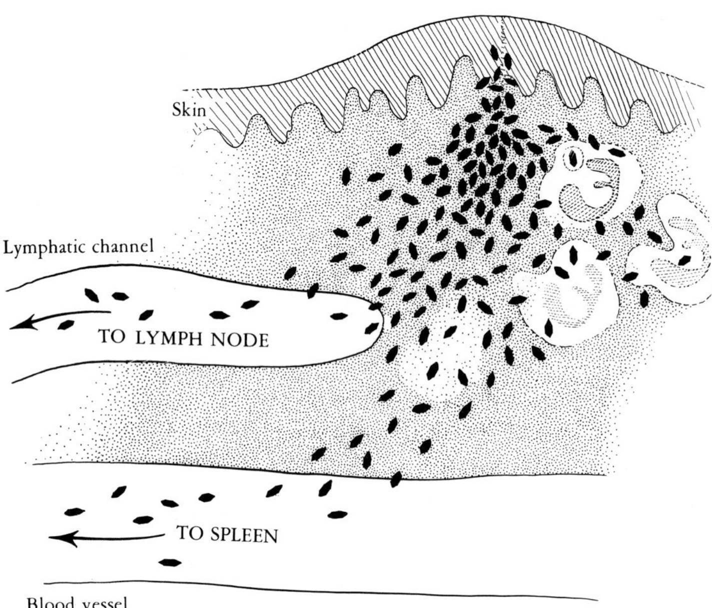

Figure 4–112. Schematic representation of the cellular events occurring if the polymorphonuclear leukocytes are unsuccessful in killing the bacteria. The organisms are shown replicating in the tissues and entering a lymphatic channel and a blood vessel. (From Bellanti, J. A.: Immunology II. Philadelphia, W. B. Saunders Company, 1978.)

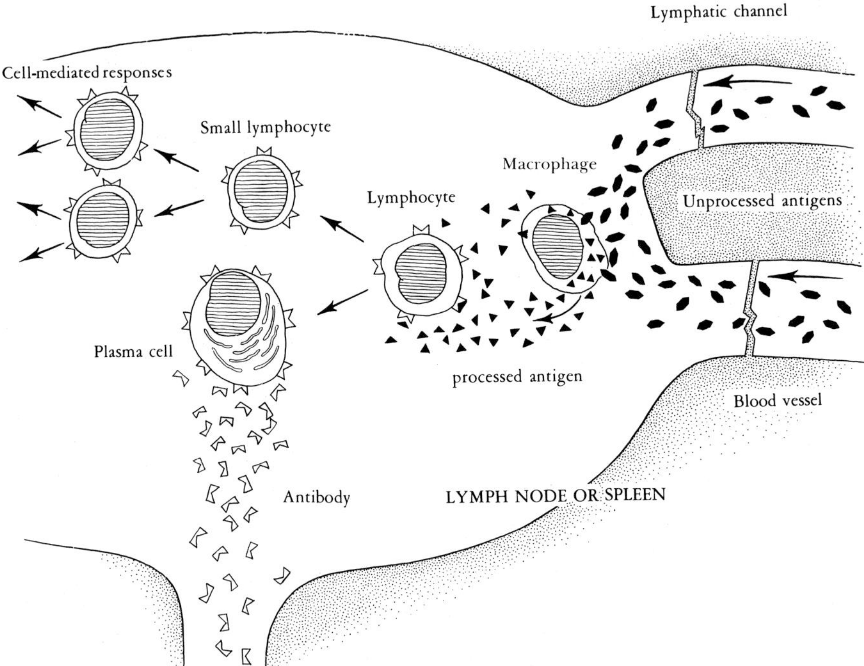

Figure 4–113. Schematic representation of the induction of a specific immune response in a lymph node or the spleen with elaboration of cell-mediated (delayed hypersensitivity) response and antibody. (From Bellanti, J. A.: Immunology II. Philadelphia, W. B. Saunders Company, 1978.)

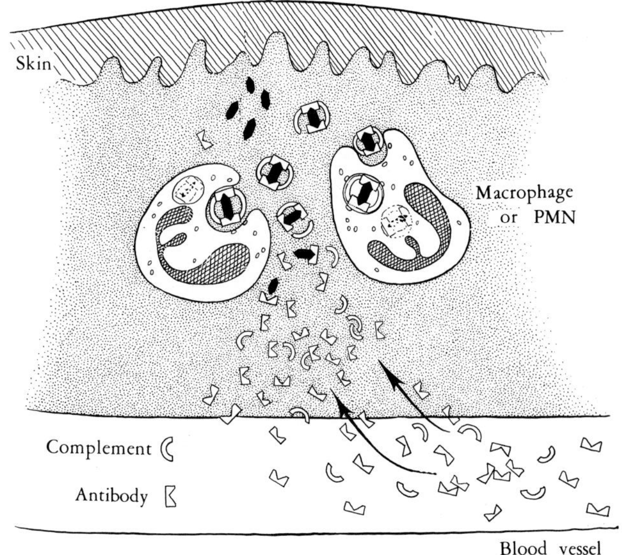

Figure 4–114. Schematic representation of the enhancement of phagocytosis, occurring with the development of specific antibody together with the participation of complement. (From Bellanti, J. A.: Immunology II. Philadelphia, W. B. Saunders Company, 1978.)

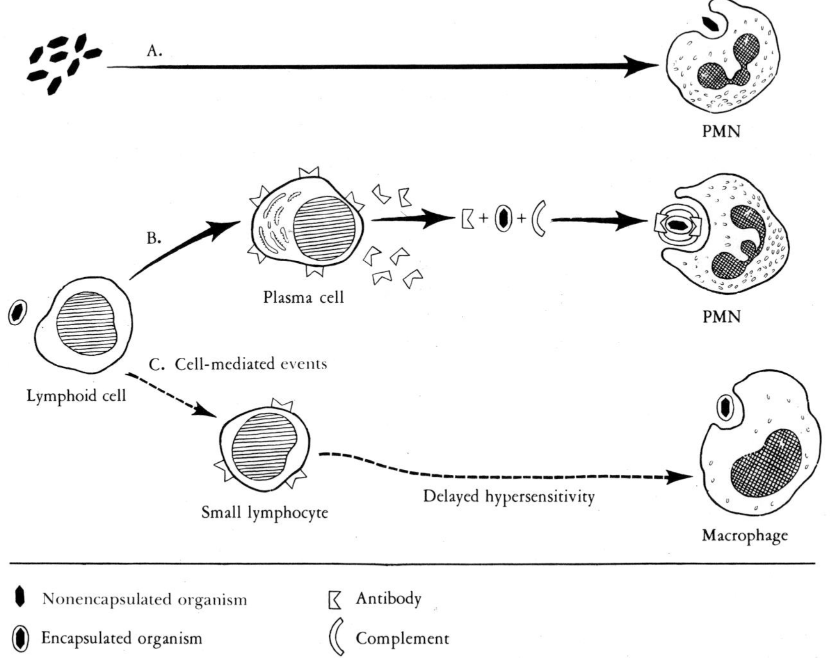

Figure 4–115. Schematic representation of relative roles of antibody and cell-mediated events in enhancement of phagocytosis in *acute bacterial infections. A,* Phagocytosis of an unencapsulated organism through an unenhanced process. *B,* The enhanced process of phagocytosis through antibody and complement. *C,* The relatively lesser importance of cell-mediated events during acute infection. Note the interrelationship of antibody and phagocytosis of polymorphonuclear leukocytes (PMN) and its relatively greater importance than cell-mediated events during acute infections. (From Bellanti, J. A.: Immunology II. Philadelphia, W. B. Saunders Company, 1978.)

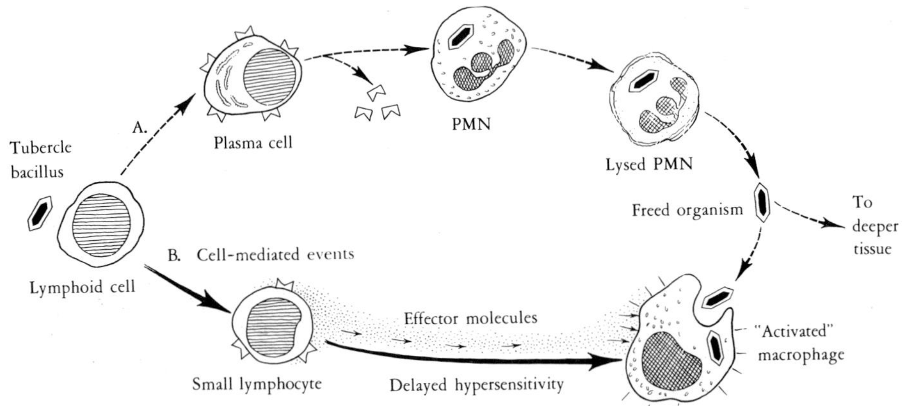

Figure 4–116. Schematic representation of the relative roles of antibody and cell-mediated events in enhancement of phagocytosis during *chronic bacterial infections. A,* Limited activity of the polymorphonuclear leukocytes. *B,* The major cellular response in chronic infection, carried out through macrophages with simultaneous stimulation of cell-mediated events, further enhancing immunity. Note the interrelationship between the cell-mediated immunity effector molecules with phagocytosis by macrophages and its relatively greater importance than antibody-enhanced phagocytosis by polymorphonuclear leukocytes (PMN) in chronic infection. (From Bellanti, J. A.: Immunology II. Philadelphia, W. B. Saunders Company, 1978.)

nous antigens and the respiratory, gastrointestinal or integumentary systems. The emphasis here will be on ***tissue damage***.

There are four groups of reactions that underlie the ***mechanisms of immunological tissue injury*** and are generally known as Types I, II, III and IV allergic or hypersensitivity reactions (Table 4–3). These have been defined through years of experimental immunopathology. It is only through knowledge of these experimental lesions that progress can be made in recognition of similar types of lesions in naturally occurring diseases. These observations are useful to further investigation of the pathogenetic mechanisms of naturally occurring diseases as a means of determining control, prevention or treatment.

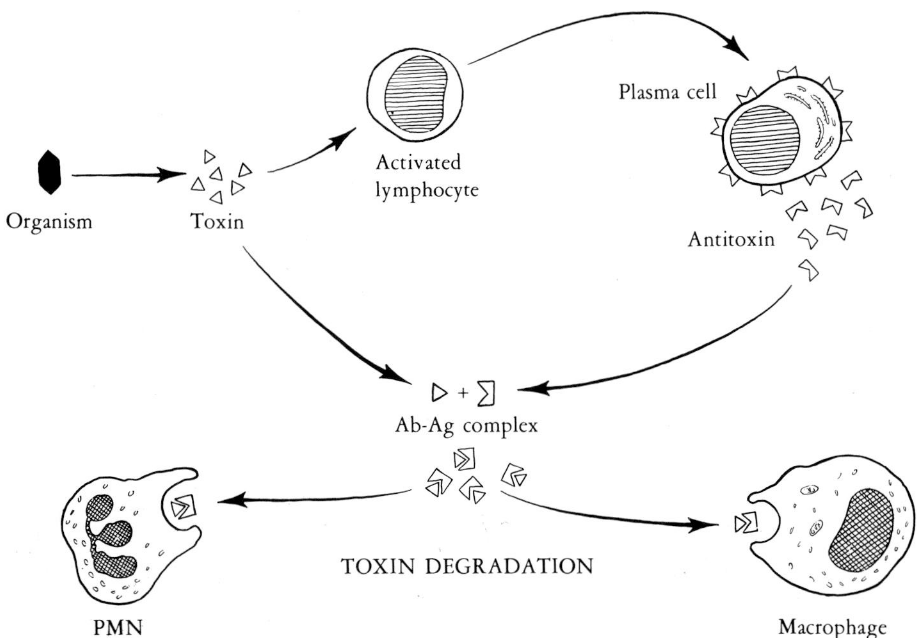

Figure 4–117. Schematic representation of the immunologic mechanism of toxin neutralization by antibody. The neutralized toxin-antitoxin complexes are shown being taken up and degraded within both types of phagocytic cells. (From Bellanti, J. A.: Immunology II. Philadelphia, W. B. Saunders Company, 1978.)

TABLE 4–3. CLASSIFICATION OF IMMUNOLOGICALLY MEDIATED DISEASES

Reaction Type	Reaction Time	Immunologic Mediator	Mechanism
Type I	Immediate (10–20 minutes)	IgE (Reagin)	Antigen: IgE-induced release of pharmacologic mediators from mast cells
Type II	Variable	IgM, IgG	"Autoantibodies" ± complement lyse host's tissues
Type III	Intermediate (6–18 hours)	IgM, IgG	Precipitating antigen-antibody complex and complement produce an Arthus reaction
Type IV	Delayed (48 hours)	T-lymphocytes (cell-mediated)	Sensitized thymus-dependent lymphocytes plus antigen lead to release of lymphokines or cellular cytotoxicity

IMMEDIATE HYPERSENSITIVITY (TYPE I)

This type of lesion results from exposure to a soluble antigen in a previously sensitized host and may be local or generalized. It is called anaphylaxis, allergy or immediate hypersensitivity, depending on the chemical expression, and involves primarily IgE antibody. The reaction may be systemic or localized and edema is a major manifestation in the tissue involved. Examples are allergies to food, inhaled antigens, internal parasites and ectoparasites. The main effect is to cause the release of vasoactive substances from mast cells, basophils and platelets in order to increase vascular permeability and to contract smooth muscle. Species vary in their expressions of anaphylaxis; for example, they may develop pulmonary edema, as in cattle, or bronchospasm, as in guinea pigs. The type of expression is dose-dependent to some extent.

ANTITISSUE ANTIBODY INJURY (TYPE II)

These injuries occur through direct damage to cells by antibody causing activation of complement and cytolysis. Injury may also occur by phagocytosis of the cells possessing the antigens when antibody is present on the surface of the cells. ***Autoimmune diseases result from production of antibody to cell antigens of the host.*** The host literally causes its own tissue cells to be destroyed by its own immune system. The designation of a disease as autoimmune is somewhat arbitrary and is based on evidence of an autoimmune reaction, on a judgment that the immunological findings are not secondary and on the lack of another identified cause for the disease. These conditions have been recognized in humans, and naturally occurring counterparts exist in animals. Some are single organ or single cell types of disorders, and some are multisystem disorders involving a multiplicity of autoantibodies or cell-mediated responses or a combination of the two. In canine ***autoimmune hemolytic anemia,*** the red cells are lysed when antibody attaches to the cell membrane. The antibody may be due to altered antigens on the cell membrane or antibody to a viral protein or drug attached to the membrane. Usually, the lysis occurs via phagocytosis in the reticuloendothelial system. Diagnosis is confirmed by demonstration of antiglobulin on the red cells and evidence of anemia. Thrombocytopenia often occurs in the disease and may result in purpura. A clear example of ***autoimmune thyroiditis*** occurs in chickens in which lymphocytic infiltration and atrophy are present; lymph follicles develop in the thyroid gland. Thyroiditis occurs in dogs and may be a clinical problem. The lesion is suggestive of an autoimmune pathogenesis (Fig. 4–118).

Canine systemic lupus erythematosus is a syndrome of hemolytic anemia, thrombocytopenic purpura, proteinuria and polyarthritis. The basic problem is due to antinuclear antibody, that is, antibody against the host's DNA. Phagocytes take in red blood cells, nuclei and nuclear debris, and these phagocytic cells are called LE cells. Circulating antigen-antibody complexes probably account for glomerular lesions and purpura. The lesions are partly Type II and partly Type III.

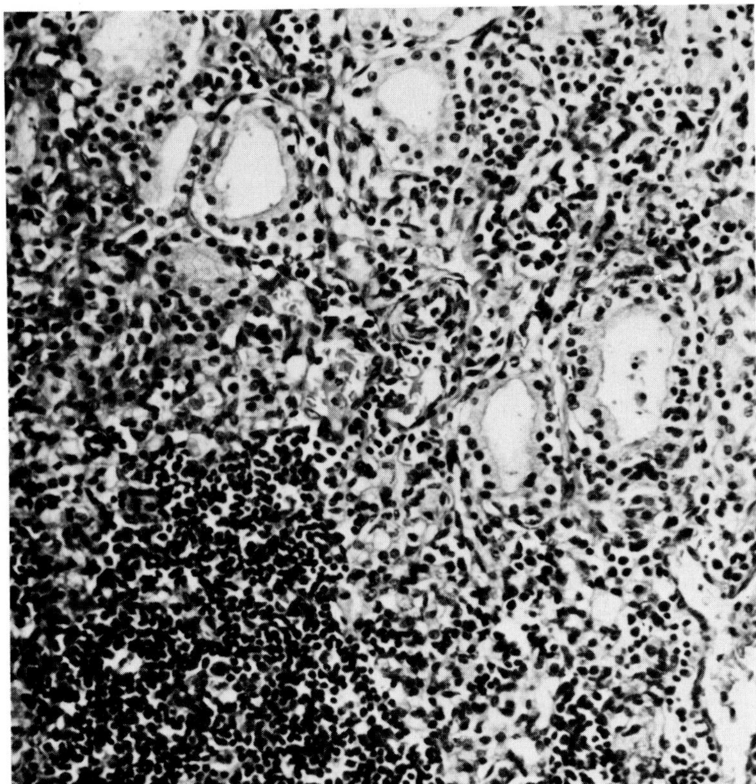

Figure 4–118. Chronic autoimmune thyroiditis in a dog with diffuse and focal accumulations of neutrophils.

Recently, authentic cases of ***rheumatoid arthritis*** have been diagnosed in dogs with chronic shifting lameness, particularly involving peripheral joints. The etiological factors are not clear, but the lesion involves bone, articular cartilage and synovial membranes. Proliferative synovitis with lymphocytic and plasma cell infiltration is prominent. Cells in the synovial membrane produce IgG that is abnormal in structure and therefore antigenic, leading to the production of so-called rheumatoid factors that are detectable antibodies to the altered IgG. Again Type II and Type III reactions are present. Several features of lupus erythematosus and rheumatoid arthritis overlap and they may be difficult to differentiate. They represent clinical syndromes that express themselves in a variety of ways.

At times, ***allergic encephalitis*** occurs in dogs after rabies vaccination if the virus has been grown in nervous tissue. ***Idiopathic*** polyneuritis, or so-called coonhound paralysis, is apparently an ***autoimmune demyelination*** in peripheral nerves and ganglia.

In addition, evidence is accumulating that suggests that some common lesions, such as diffuse interstitial nephritis, may have an antitubular–basement membrane component involving both immune complex deposition and cell-mediated aspects. No doubt the role of cell-mediated influences in many lesions will be further elucidated in the near future.

INJURY BY ANTIGEN-ANTIBODY COMPLEXES (TYPE III)

The pathogenesis of this type of injury involves four phases: combination of antibody with antigen to produce the complexes, localization of complexes at specific sites in tissue, accumulation at these sites of humoral and cellular mediators attracted by the complexes and the induction of tissue injury. The experimental ***Arthus reaction*** is characteristic of this type of injury. The striking feature is the accumulation of neutrophils by chemotaxis when complement is activated by the union of antigen and antibody. The neutrophils cause the damage (Fig. 4–119). The reaction will not occur if either complement or neutrophils are not available. Complement becomes

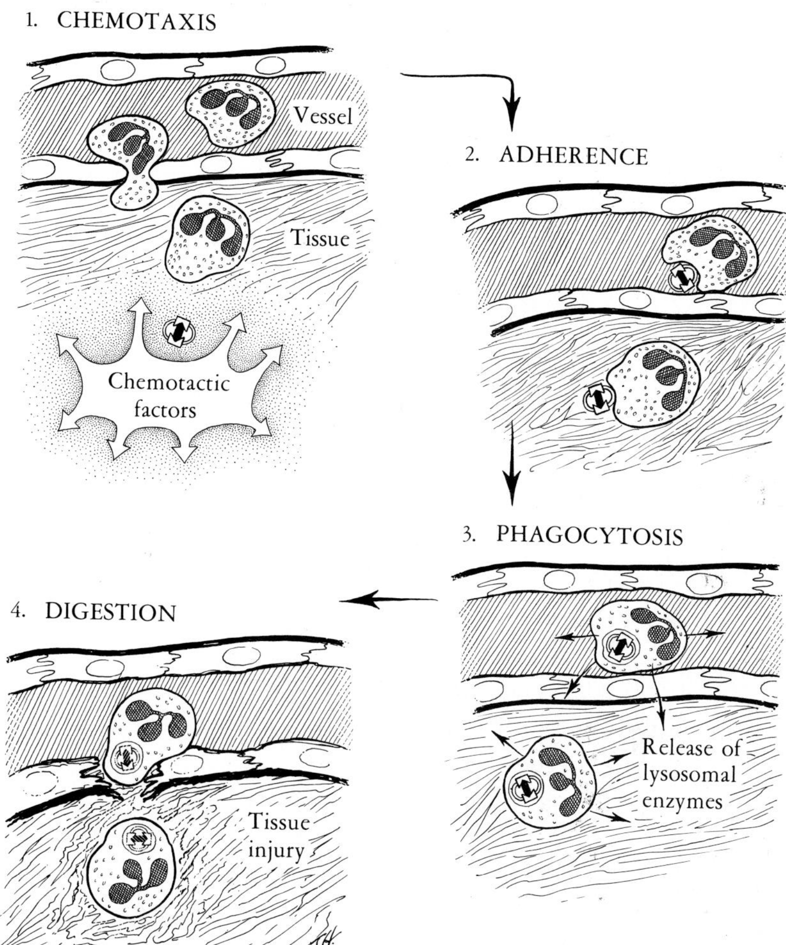

Figure 4–119. Sequence of reactions leading to tissue injury associated with polymorphonuclear leukocyte influx. Note that in addition to chemotaxis, adherence, phagocytosis and digestion processes that normally result in particle inactivation, there may also be the release of neutrophilic constituents (lysosomal enzymes), which results in tissue injury. (From Bellanti, J. A.: Immunology II. Philadelphia, W. B. Saunders Company, 1978.)

toxic to cells by altering the cell membrane and upsetting osmotic gradients and results in osmotic lysis. Hageman factor is also activated in this type of reaction, with accumulation of platelets and release of their contents. The lesion may occur in a vessel wall or be free in tissue. The presence of ***fibrinoid*** and neutrophils in vessel walls is usually indicative of this type of reaction (Fig. 4–120). All the features of acute inflammation are present in these lesions, and ideally the neutrophils will destroy the immune complexes so that the reaction will stop (Fig. 4–121).

Immune complexes formed in the blood stream may produce generalized effects when they become localized in particular tissues, and the problem may be acute or chronic, depending on the time period over which the complexes are formed. Disease from such complexes is called ***immune-complex disease***. An example of this lesion is the deposition of complexes in an ***uneven patchy distribution*** on glomerular capillary basement membranes. The endothelial cells proliferate and the capillaries leak proteins (Fig. 4–122). Glomerulonephritis is a common but nonspecific lesion and may be caused by bacterial antigens, viral antigens or autoantigens, which induce the complexes to form (Fig. 4–123). Another form of immune-complex disease occurs when antibodies against basement membranes occur. The complexes deposit in a ***uniform smooth pattern*** on capillaries, such as in the glomeruli.

The relative amounts of antigen and antibody influence the formation of immune

Text continued on page 246

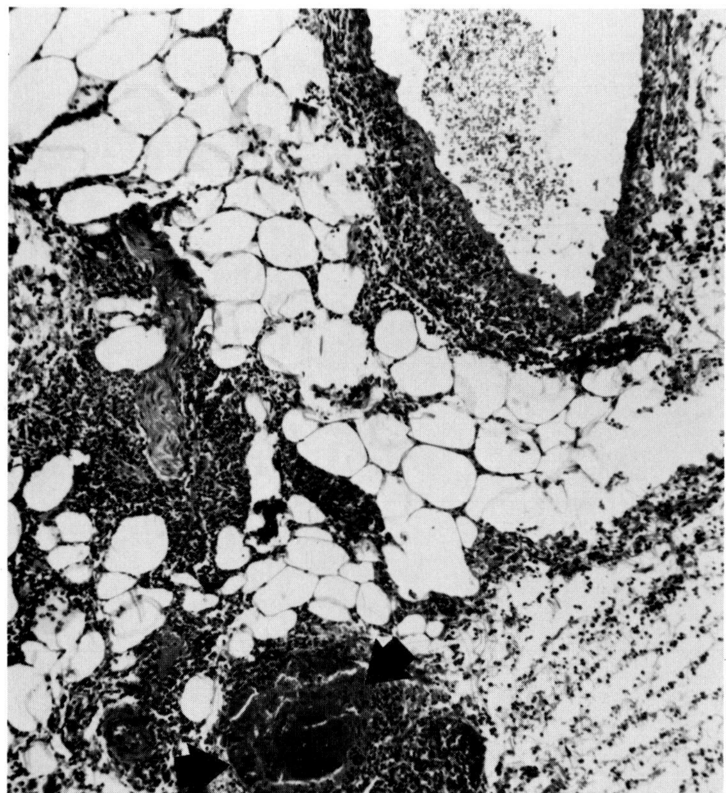

Figure 4–120. Experimental Arthus reaction in a rabbit's skin. The vessel is thrombosed, and fibrinoid material is in the wall as well as outside. Neutrophils are numerous in the vessel walls and in the stroma around the vessels.

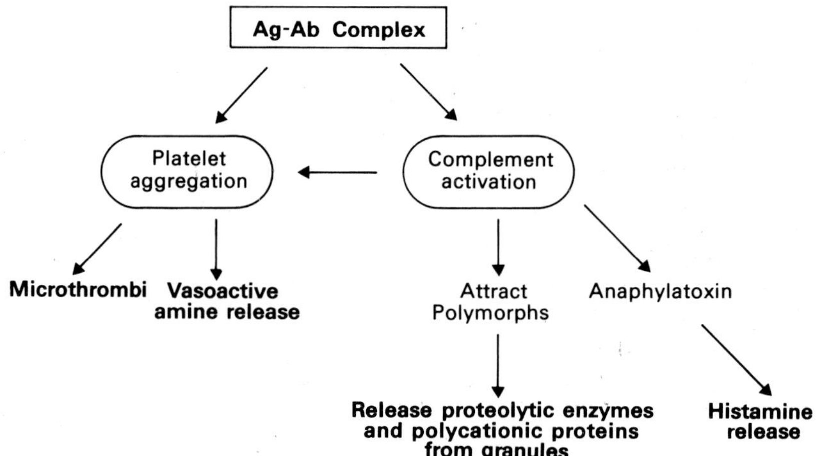

Figure 4–121. Complex-mediated hypersensitivity. (From Roitt, I.: Essential Immunology. Philadelphia, F. A. Davis Company [Blackwell Scientific Publications], 1971. Reprinted by permission.)

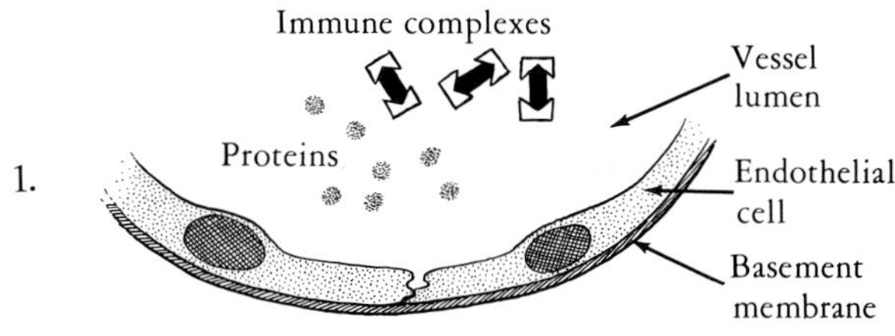

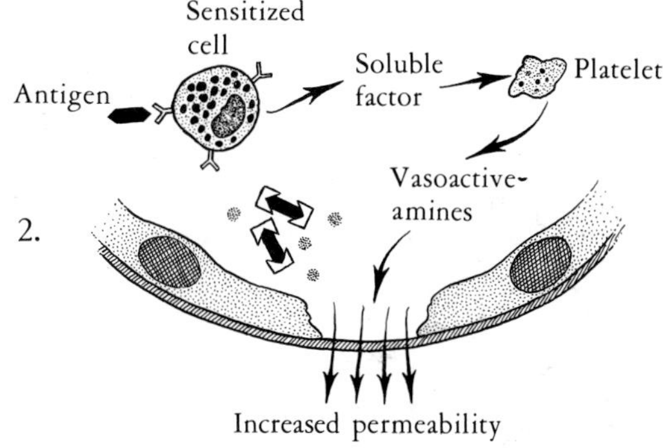

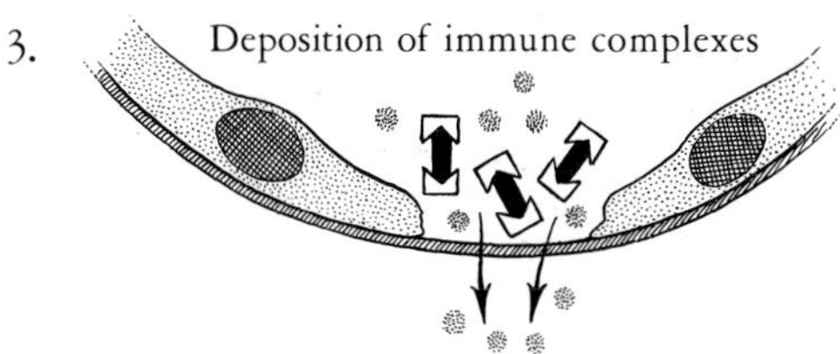

Figure 4–122. Hypothetical scheme for deposition of immune complexes in acute immune-complex disease. *1*, Constituents of the deposition process. *2*, Release of vasoactive amines from platelets induces increased vascular permeability. The sensitized cell appears to be a basophil sensitized with IgE antibody. *3*, With the outflow of fluid, the larger immune complexes become trapped by the filtering basement membrane. (From Bellanti, J. A.: Immunology II. Philadelphia, W. B. Saunders Company, 1978.)

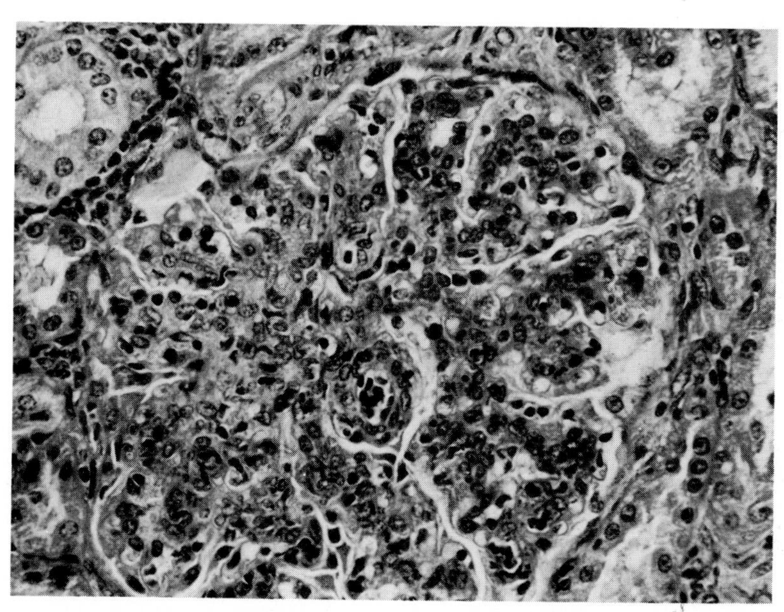

Figure 4–123. Glomerulitis induced experimentally in a sheep by repeated injections of Freund's adjuvant. Note the increased cellularity, thickened basement membranes and adhesions of glomerular loops to the glomerular capsule. (Courtesy of B. Schiefer.)

complexes *in vivo* and the type of lesions that might develop. If antibody is present in excess of antigen, the precipitates form at the site of antigen introduction, as in the Arthus reaction. If antigen is in excess, soluble complexes are formed in the blood stream and they may cause systemic reactions and be widely deposited throughout the body. The latter is termed ***serum sickness***. The effects depend upon the extent of tissue injury caused by the immune complexes.

DELAYED HYPERSENSITIVITY (TYPE IV)

This type of reaction is more difficult to define or quantitate than humoral responses. It is best known as the basis of the tuberculin reaction (Figs. 4–124, 4–125 and 4–126). In contrast to the humoral responses, these reactions contain predominantly mononuclear cells. Sensitized lymphocytes recognize the antigen, and when they meet, the lymphocytes become metabolically active and secrete various factors called ***lymphokines*** that have a variety of functions (Table 4–4). Macrophages are attracted and remain at the site. Lymphocytes replicate at the site, as do macrophages, and both may be cytotoxic to cells in the area. Macrophages may release harmful enzymes into the tissue. Many granulomas are generated and maintained by delayed-type hypersensitivity when antigen persists.

TABLE 4–4. Factors Released from Lymphocytes

Macrophage migration inhibition factor (MIF)
Macrophage aggregation factor (MAF)
Macrophage-spreading inhibitory factor
Factors chemotactic for macrophages and PMN's
Mitogenic factor
Lymphotoxin
Inhibitors of proliferation, DNA synthesis, and so forth
Skin reactive factor
Interferon
(Lymph node permeability factor)

From Bellanti, J. A.: Immunology II. Philadelphia, W. B. Saunders Company, 1978.)

Dermatitis in dogs and other species is often thought to be caused by allergies, but substantiation of the diagnosis is often difficult. Figure 4–127 illustrates the sites of lymphocytic accumulation in the two types of lesion. Note that some aspects are quite similar. In the contact type of lesions, mast cells degenerate and also proliferate and have a marked effect on endothelial injury and edema formation along with the lymphokines.

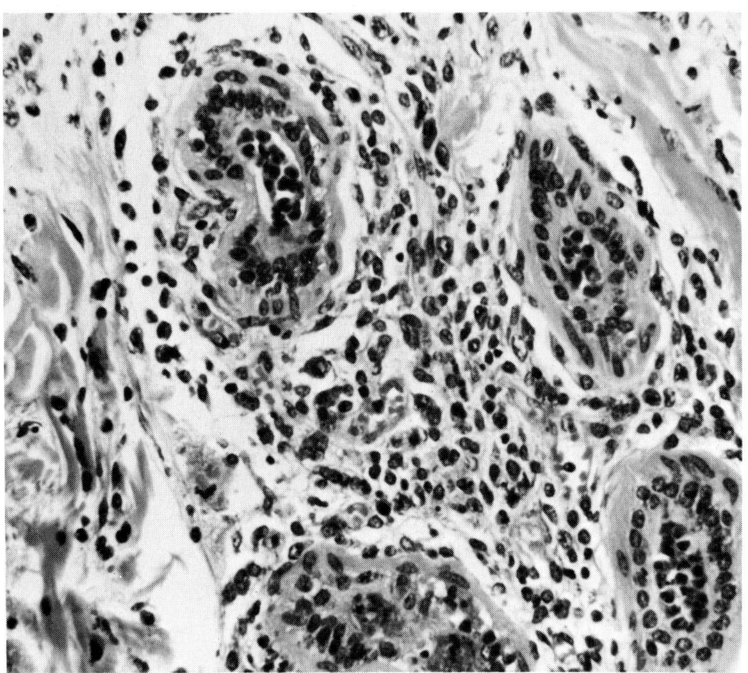

Figure 4–124

Figures 4–124, 4–125 and 4–126. Positive tuberculin reaction in bovine skin. Note the perivascular accumulation of mononuclear cells. The mononuclear cells are quite variable in appearance (Fig. 4–125). The perivascular distribution is quite evident in a low power view (Fig. 4–126), and why the area is grossly swollen is apparent. *(Illustration continued on opposite page)*

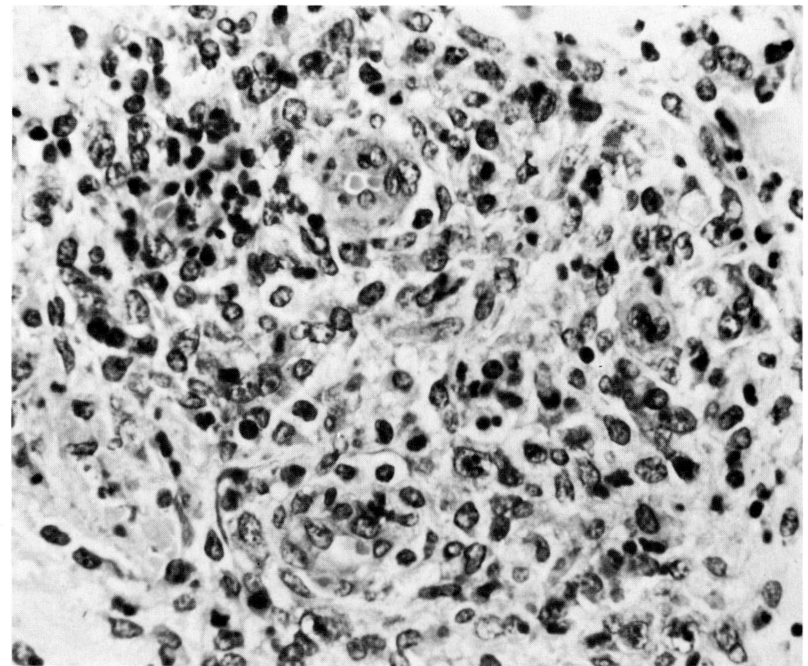

Figure 4–125

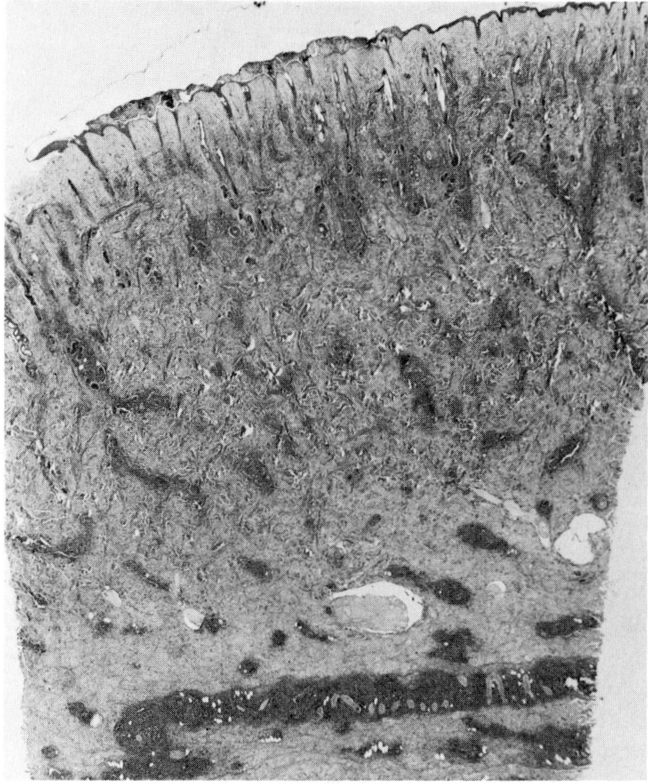

Figure 4–126

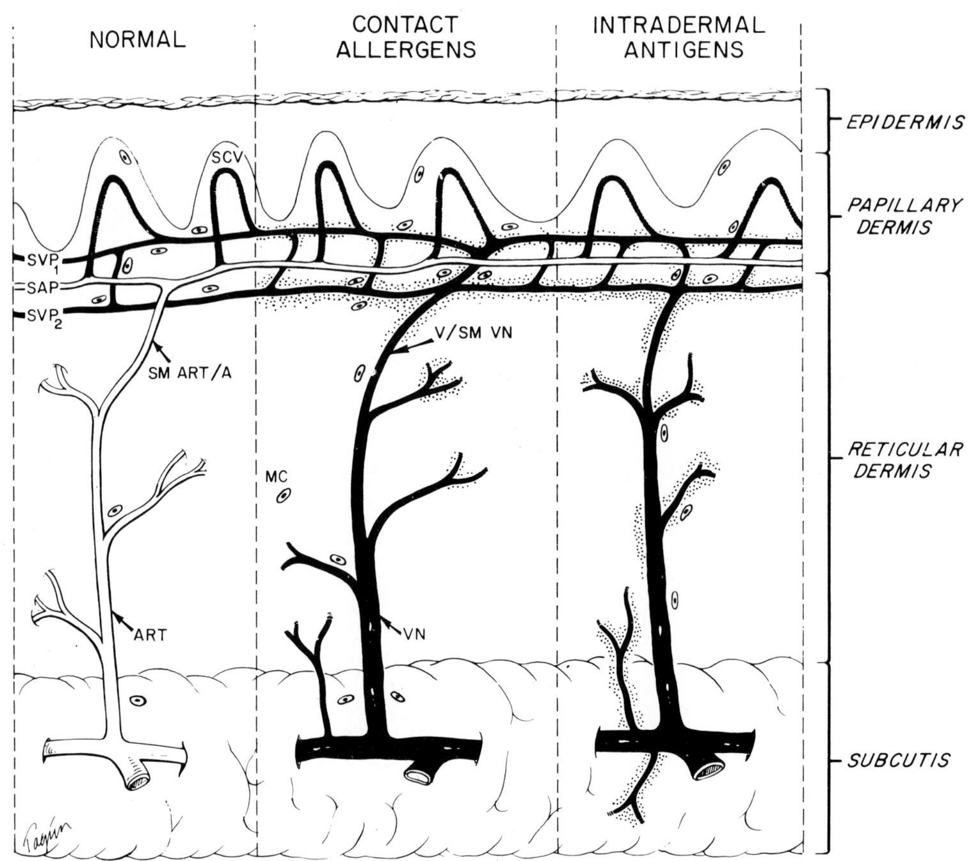

Figure 4–127. Schematic diagram of the microvasculature and distribution of the cellular infiltrate in skin from the arm of a normal human and in the lesions of allergic contact dermatitis. For comparison, lesions of delayed-type hypersensitivity reactions to intradermally injected microbial antigens are also included. SCV, Superficial capillary venule; SAP, superficial arteriolar plexus, SVP_1 and SVP_2, superficial and deep layers of superficial venular plexus; SM ART/A, small artery/arteriole; ART, artery; V/SM VN, venule/small vein; VN, vein; MC, mast cell. The cellular infiltrate in contact dermatitis largely spares the SCV and only mildly envelops the SVP_1, whereas the SVP_2 is principally affected. In delayed-hypersensitivity reactions to microbial antigens, deeper venules and small veins are also enveloped by cuffs of inflammatory cells. (From Dvorak, A. M., Martin, C., and Dvorak, H. F.: Morphology of delayed-type hypersensitivity reactions in man. II. Ultrastructural alterations affecting the microvasculature and the tissue mast cells. Lab. Invest., *34*:179–191, 1976. Reprinted by permission.)

The various types of immune mechanisms of injury do not always occur independently or separately, and in some instances, ***all four types may occur in the same lesion by response to different antigens or by multiple response to the same antigens.*** These complexities make specific interpretations of pathogenesis difficult or impossible in many naturally occurring or experimental lesions (Figs. 4–128, 4–129, and 4–130). The point is, however, to be aware of the mechanisms that may be involved in a lesion as a means of understanding how and why certain cells are present. ***Too often, the presence of cells is recorded very accurately in descriptions but with little thought as to why they came, where they came from, how they got there or how the lesion is likely to progress.****

The immune mechanisms initiate or contribute to inflammation by triggering reactions, which have already been described under inflammation, such as release of mediators, permeability changes, chemotaxis, phagocytosis, cytotoxicity, fixation of complement, release of lymphokines, release of lysosomal enzymes and tissue necrosis. Most of the reactions relate to antigen-antibody interactions and to lymphokines.

The inflammatory reaction in a fetus varies with the age of the fetus and in part relates to the ***development of immune competence.*** The earliest response in a fetus is by mononuclear cells, and there is an absence of or only very few neutrophils in young fetuses. In older fetuses, neutrophils respond slowly. Edema and fibrin are absent in inflammatory lesions in early fetal life but develop gradually with age. These factors seem to relate to a minimal vascular response in the inflammatory process in young fetuses.

*Many lesions caused by infectious agents are immune mediated. Specific immune mediated lesions are illustrated in the following illustrations—Chapter 2: Figures 2–38, 2–40, 2–41, 2–118, 2–120, 2–121, 2–122, 2–123; Chapter 4, Figures 4–124, 4–125, 4–126, 4–127, 4–128.

FEVER

Elevation of body temperature, or fever, is associated with many disease states. Since the hypothalamus is the control center for thermal regulation, alterations that influence that center must occur. It is generally considered that chemicals called pyrogens can influence and alter the control center. ***Pyrogen*** refers to any substance that will alter body temperature. Pyrogens are divided into ***exogenous*** or ***endogenous,*** although the exogenous may actually carry out their actions via the endogenous route. Certain bacteria contain, secrete or excrete pyrogens with the result that infection with such agents will cause fever. The endogenous factors are ***released from body tissues and fluids when either or both are injured.*** Necrosis causes release of pyrogens. There is a tendency to think that fever means infection, but this is not always so. Large amounts of necrosis in a tumor will cause release of pyrogens and cause persistent fever. Neutrophils release pyrogens and are one of their main sources. There is some argument as to whether pyrogens are released from damaged tissue or from the neutrophils that arrive in response to the damaged tissue. The neutrophils can release pyrogens from their location in exudate or while still in the blood stream. Immune mechanisms may induce release of pyrogens but, again, probably by damaging tissue or drawing neutrophils to a site of injury or just with antigen-antibody complexes. The process of phagocytosis by neutrophils, macrophages, monocytes or eosinophils causes release of pyrogens. Gram-negative bacteria contain pyrogens in their cell walls, whereas, in general, gram-positive bacteria do not. Thus, endotoxin is strongly associated with pyrogenic activity. There is a possibility that neoplastic cells may secrete pyrogens.

The detailed explanation of mechanisms that cause fever awaits elucidation. Cases occur in which fever persists for unknown reasons or perhaps as an unusual expression of a common disease. Considerable debate regarding the beneficial or deleterious effect of fever to the patient continues in the literature.

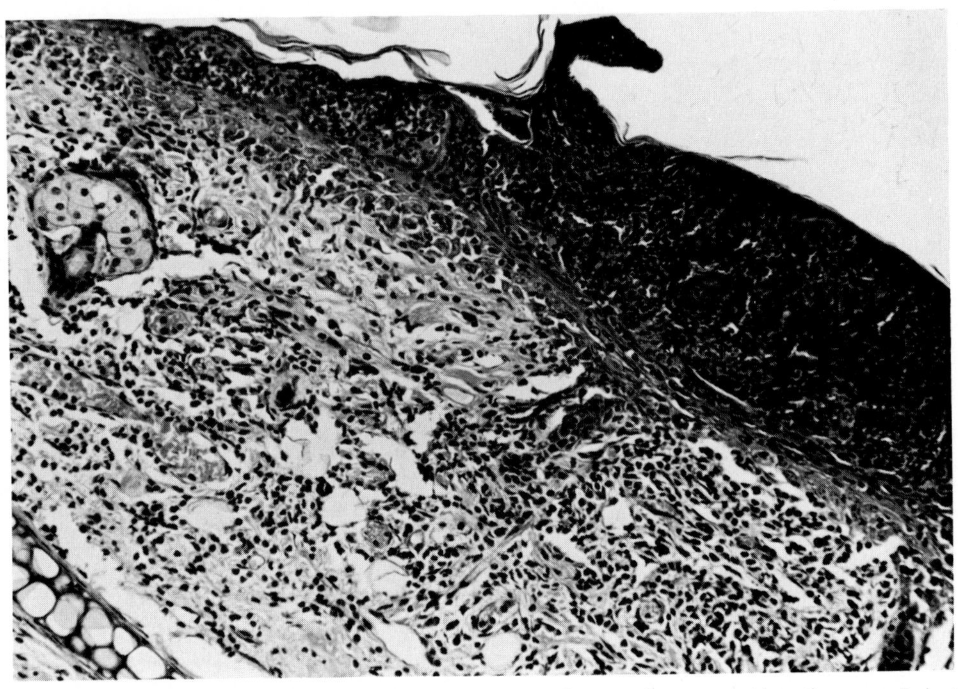

Figure 4–128. Experimentally induced contact hypersensitivity in the ear of a mouse. Note the necrosis in the skin. Cartilage of the ear is at lower left.

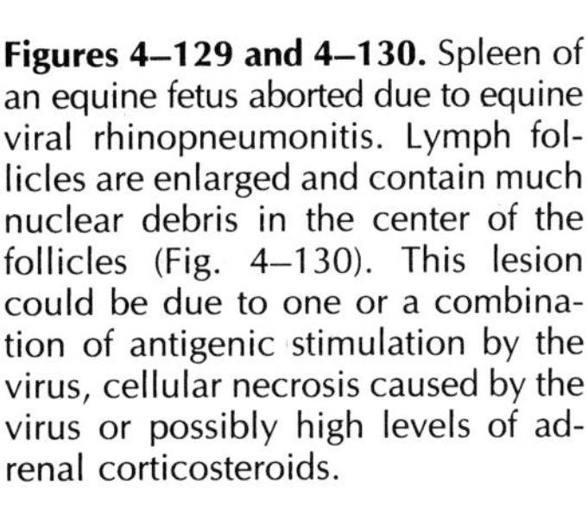

Figures 4–129 and 4–130. Spleen of an equine fetus aborted due to equine viral rhinopneumonitis. Lymph follicles are enlarged and contain much nuclear debris in the center of the follicles (Fig. 4–130). This lesion could be due to one or a combination of antigenic stimulation by the virus, cellular necrosis caused by the virus or possibly high levels of adrenal corticosteroids.

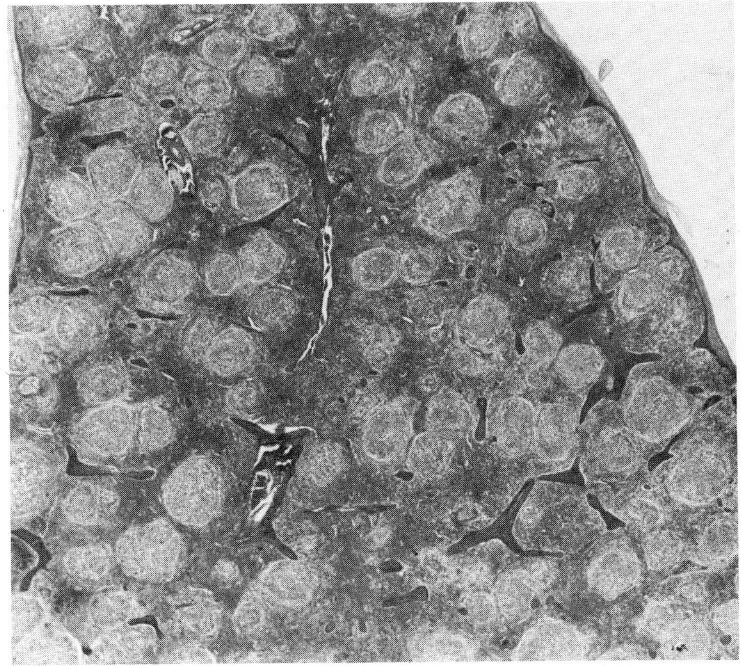

Figure 4–129

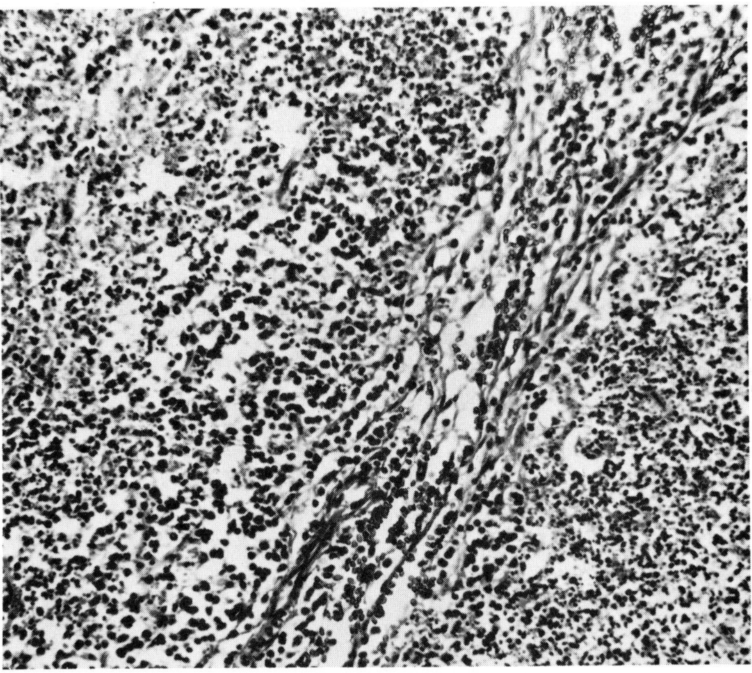

Figure 4–130

REPAIR

Repair begins soon after injury occurs, but, as mentioned earlier, it was not discussed in any detail in the previous chapters and was arbitrarily kept separate. Since repair occurs in all forms of tissue injury and inflammation, it is necessary to first ***describe its general aspects*** and then ***integrate that information back into the major topics of injury discussed in earlier chapters***.

Repair occurs throughout the plant and animal kingdoms, often in the form of ***regeneration*** in lower orders of species. Regeneration is significant at the tissue level in mammals and birds, but regeneration of organs tends not to occur. The regenerative ability of tissues will be discussed later, and the emphasis here will be on healing by the proliferation of fibroblasts and endothelial cells.

Almost any injury will involve fibrocytes and fibroblasts. Even when very few seem to be present in a normal tissue, the few that are present in stroma or around capillaries have tremendous capabilities to proliferate. In minor injuries, there will probably be some contribution by fibroblasts to repair, whereas in major injuries, they form the greatest contribution. The objective in repair is to return ***normal anatomical and functional integrity*** to the tissue. In major injuries, full functional integrity is not likely to be restored, but through connective tissue healing and a degree of tissue regeneration, an attempt to maintain anatomical integrity is made.

Repair begins with the proliferation of fibroblasts and endothelial cells in injured tissue, usually within two or three days of injury caused by necrosis or inflammation or a combination of the two. ***Repair, necrosis and inflammation occur concurrently***, and this is often difficult to recognize in some lesions but is usually quite clear in wound healing at a clean surgical site. The discussion here will emphasize healing in surgical sites since the events and time associations can be followed rather easily. Surgeons refer to healing of wounds by first intention or second intention. In first intention healing, there is proper ***apposition*** of the edges of the incision with no loss of tissue. In second intention, there is considerable ***tissue loss***, so that a degree of filling in of space must occur. The main events that occur in healing are proliferation of fibroblasts and endothelial cells and production of matrix and filaments by these cells. Each will be discussed separately.

GRANULATION TISSUE AND WOUND HEALING

Following an incision, there is sudden but intensive ***hyperplasia of fibroblasts*** from resident fibrocytes. These proliferating cells are numerous and have very large nuclei with little cytoplasm. The nuclei and cytoplasm are irregular in shape and have features suggestive of malignant cells. They begin to form matrix, which is mainly mucopolysaccaride and collagen. The collagen initially is scanty and stains lightly. Over a period of several days, the nuclei gradually elongate, reduce in size and take on the appearance of normal but active fibroblasts. They fill in any space in the tissue and bind the two edges of the incision together.

At the same time that the fibroblasts go through these processes, the endothelial cells from around capillaries and cut ends of vessels undergo ***similar hypertrophy and hyperplasia*** and become intermixed with the fibroblasts. It is difficult to distinguish the fibroblasts from endothelial cells by light microscopy at the most active period of proliferation. Many large and active macrophages in the lesion further complicate attempts to identify individual cells (Figs. 4–131 through 4–134). Gradually, capillary loops become apparent from the buds of endothelial proliferation on each side of the wound, and they grow across or meet in the middle of the line of the incision and form anastomoses that become functional blood vessels. Over two to three weeks, the number and size of nuclei gradually decrease and the new vessels and fibroblasts begin to resemble normal tissue nearby. Their architectural arrangement and staining properties in the site of incision distinguish them from the original resident tissue for some time, however. The whole process might be thought of as sewing two pieces of cloth together or closing a zipper.

In ***second intention healing***, the process is similar but more extensive. It is easiest to think of this process as filling in a broad

Inflammation

X-- inflammation is the vascular + cellular responses of living tissue to injury

Injury results in chemical changes in the injured cells or tissue that call forth the inflammatory reaction

Inflammation is generally manifested as redness, heat, swelling + pain.

Any inflammatory lesion carries the suffix "-itis"

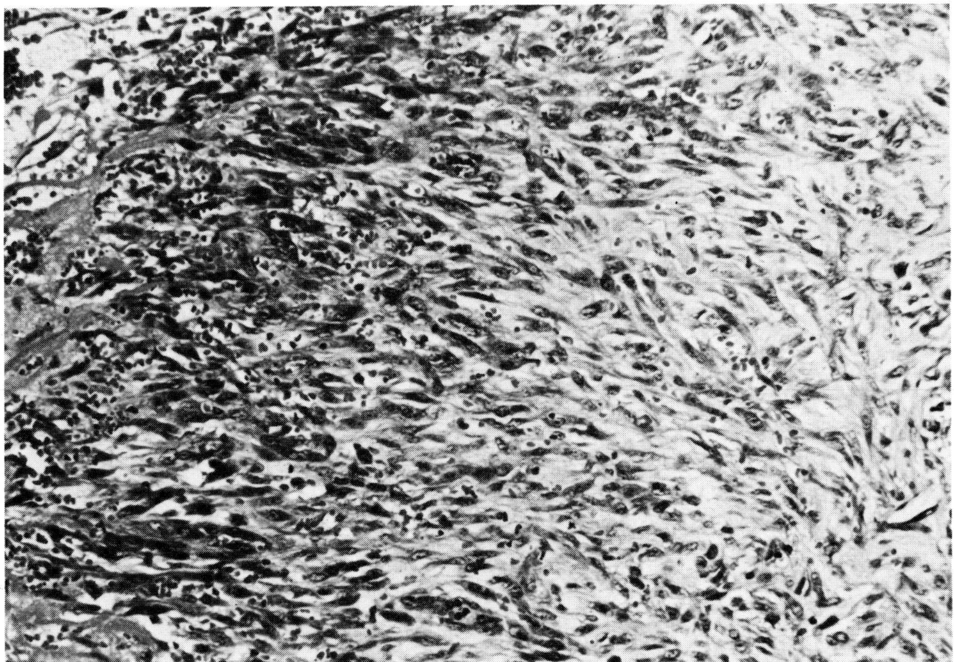

Figure 4–131

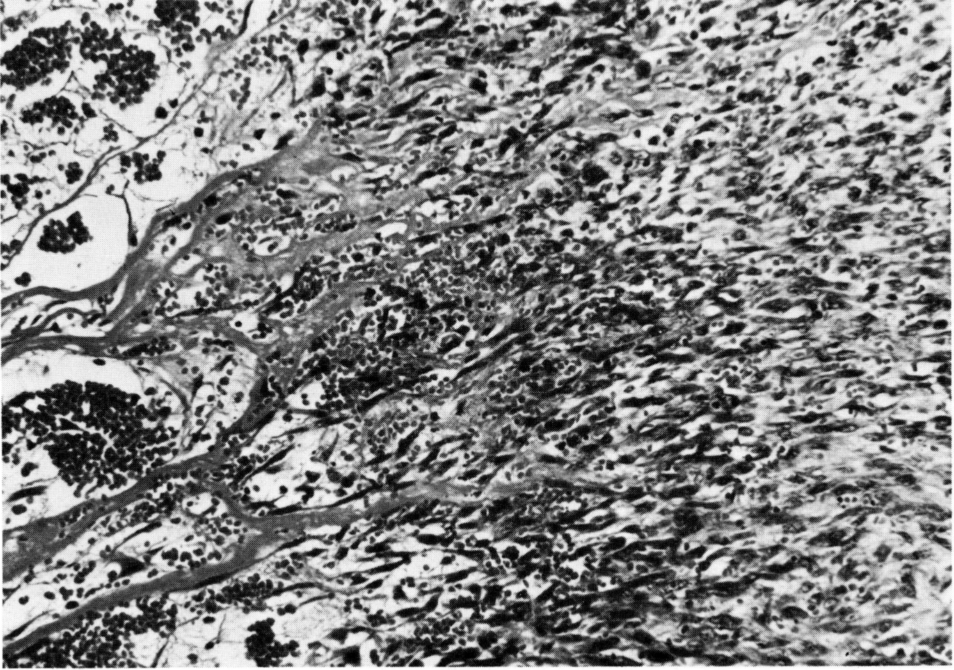

Figure 4–132

Figures 4–131, 4–132 and 4–133. Granulation tissue. More mature collagen is to the right and active growth is to the left. The identity of specific cells is not clear, since fibroblasts, endothelial cells and macrophages appear to be similar when examined with light microscopy at this stage in the lesion. In Figure 4–132, fibroblasts and endothelial cells grow into the fibrin, which is resorbed in the process. Figure 4–133 demonstrates individual fibroblasts and endothelial cells far from the tissue surface and growing into the fibrin.

Illustration continued on following page

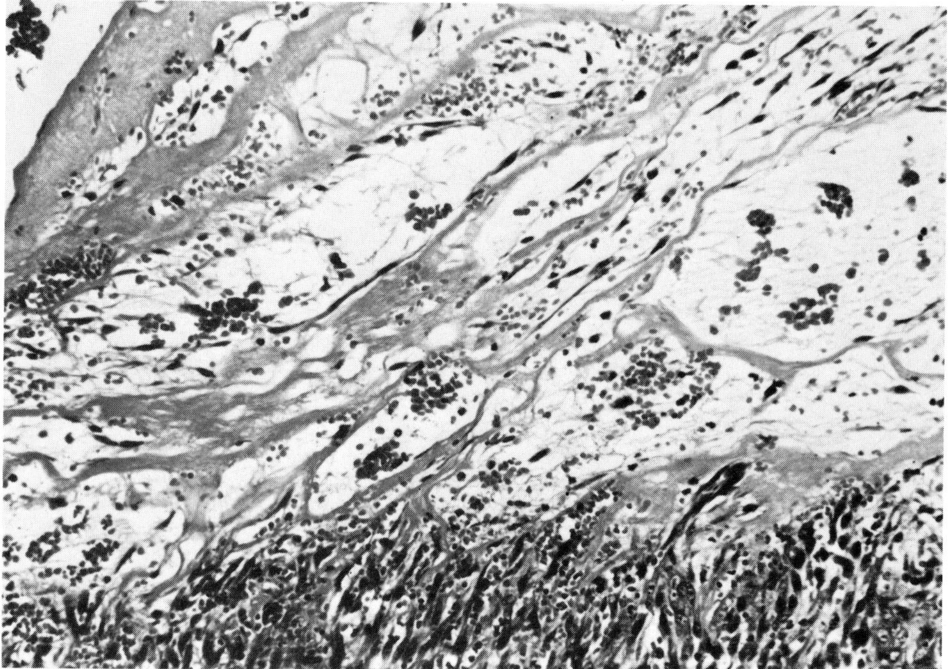

Figure 4–133 *See legend on* *page253*

hole. The fibroblasts and endothelial cells reach out into the hole as elongated projections in apparent haphazard fashion. They grow out by mitosis. Soon they take on a different arrangement, with the fibroblasts aligning themselves parallel with the surface and the endothelial cells perpendicular to the surface. The endothelial cells reach up alone first, then form tubes that reach up and later anastomose with other tubes

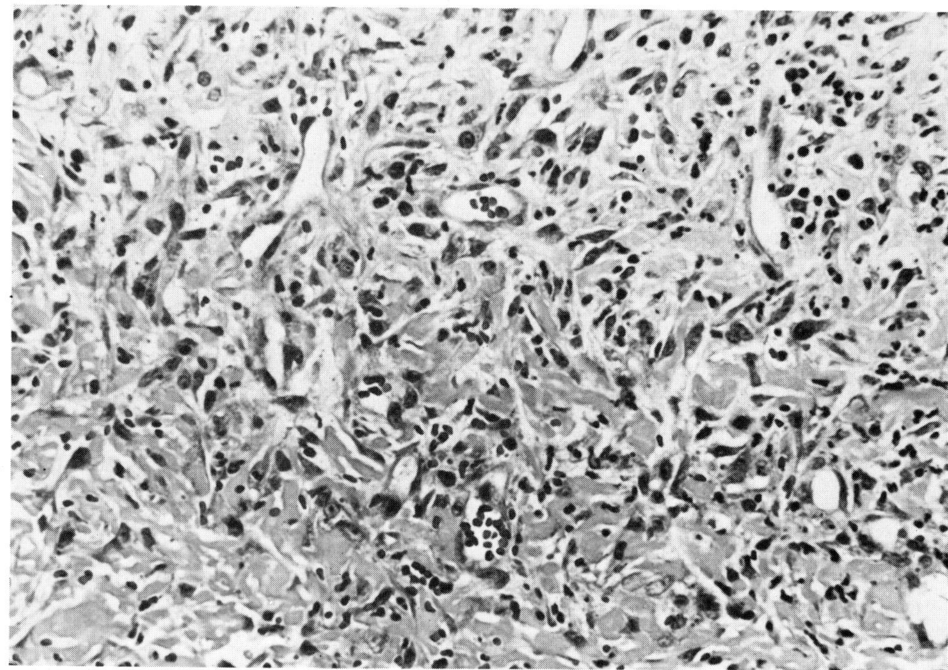

Figure 4–134. Somewhat older granulation tissue than that seen in Figure 4–133. Vessels are evident and many cells are mixed with the fibrin, which is being removed.

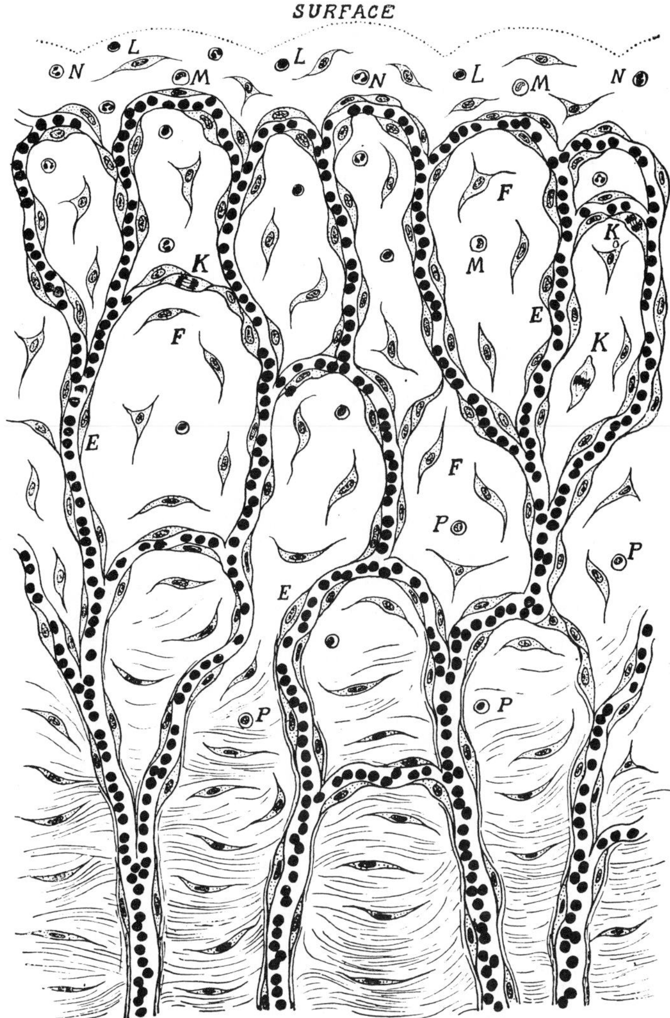

Figure 4–135. Diagram of structure of granulation tissue. *E,* Capillary endothelial cells; *F,* fibroblasts; *K,* cells in mitosis; *L,* lymphocytes; *M,* macrophages; *N,* granulocytes; *P,* plasma cells. Note horizontal orientation of fibroblasts and fibers in the deeper part. (From Willis, R.: Principles of Pathology. 2nd ed. New York, Plenum Publishing Corp. [Butterworth], 1961. Reprinted by permission.)

near the surface to become functional vessels (Fig. 4–135). Maturation reduces the size and number of nuclei and increases cytoplasmic content. Again, the architectural arrangement in the tissue distinguishes the new tissue from the original. The loops of capillaries, when viewed from the surface, have a ***granular*** appearance (Fig. 4–136). It is this appearance that probably accounts for the name ***granulation tissue,*** which refers to the new growth of fibroblasts and endothelial cells just described. New granulation tissue has ***collagenolytic properties*** that participate in cleanup of debris and in renewal or remodeling of collagen.

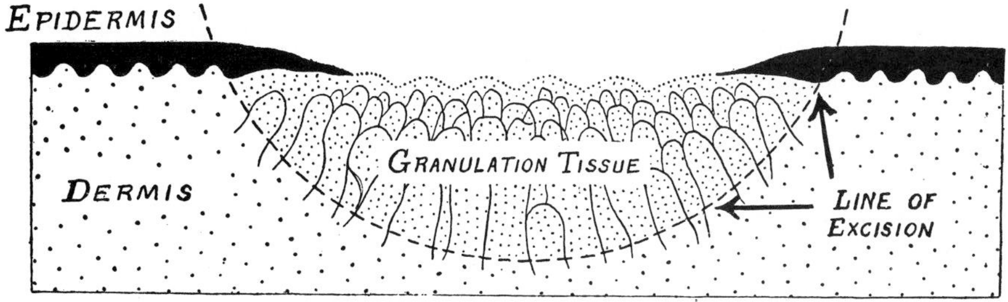

Figure 4–136. Diagram of a granulating excised wound of the skin. (From Willis, R.: Principles of Pathology. 2nd ed. New York, Plenum Publishing Corp. [Butterworth], 1961. Reprinted by permission.)

There are two other components of these lesions: the ***epithelial covering*** and the ***scab***. Very early after the incision in first intention healing, the ***epithelial cells*** begin to proliferate and grow down the sides of the wound and meet inside within about 48 hours (Fig. 4–137). The epithelial cells slide or migrate over the surface of a wound like a sheet. The cells take on phagocytic capabilities as well as collagenolytic functions to aid their progress in closing the surface. The migrating cells undergo mitosis and differentiation as the surface is covered for protection. The epithelium then recedes as

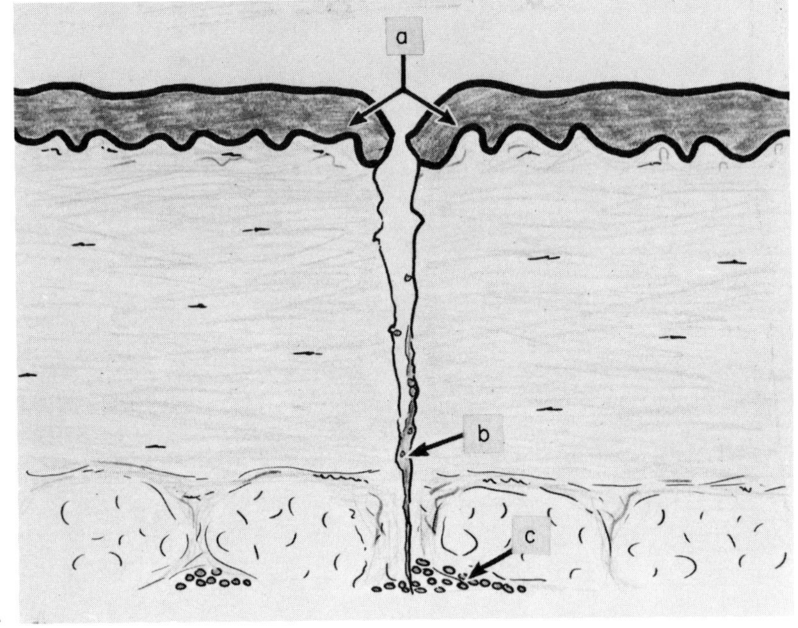

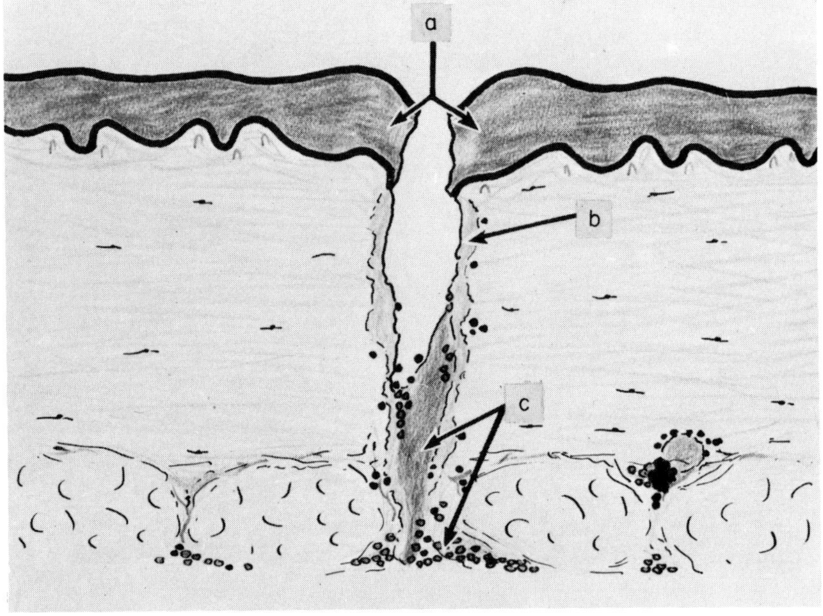

Figure 4–137. Diagrammatic representation of the healing of human skin incisions. *A*, At six hours: (a) epidermal margins inverted; (b) early clot; (c) subcutaneous hemorrhage. *B*, From six hours to two days; (a) epidermal thickening; (b) homogeneous coagulum lining wound walls; (c) further inflammatory reaction.

Illustration continued on opposite page

the fibroblasts and endothelial cells close the wound. The epithelium grows under the blood clot and tissue debris on the surface. This material dries as a scab and eventually falls off when the epithelium is intact. The proliferation and hyperplasia of the epithelium, which later returns to normal, are controlled by chalones. The new white tissue in a healed lesion is called a ***scar*** and is the new connective tissue visible below the epithelium. It is white because of the concentration of fibroblasts. The large disfiguring scars of severe injuries are also connective tissue. It is apparent that proper

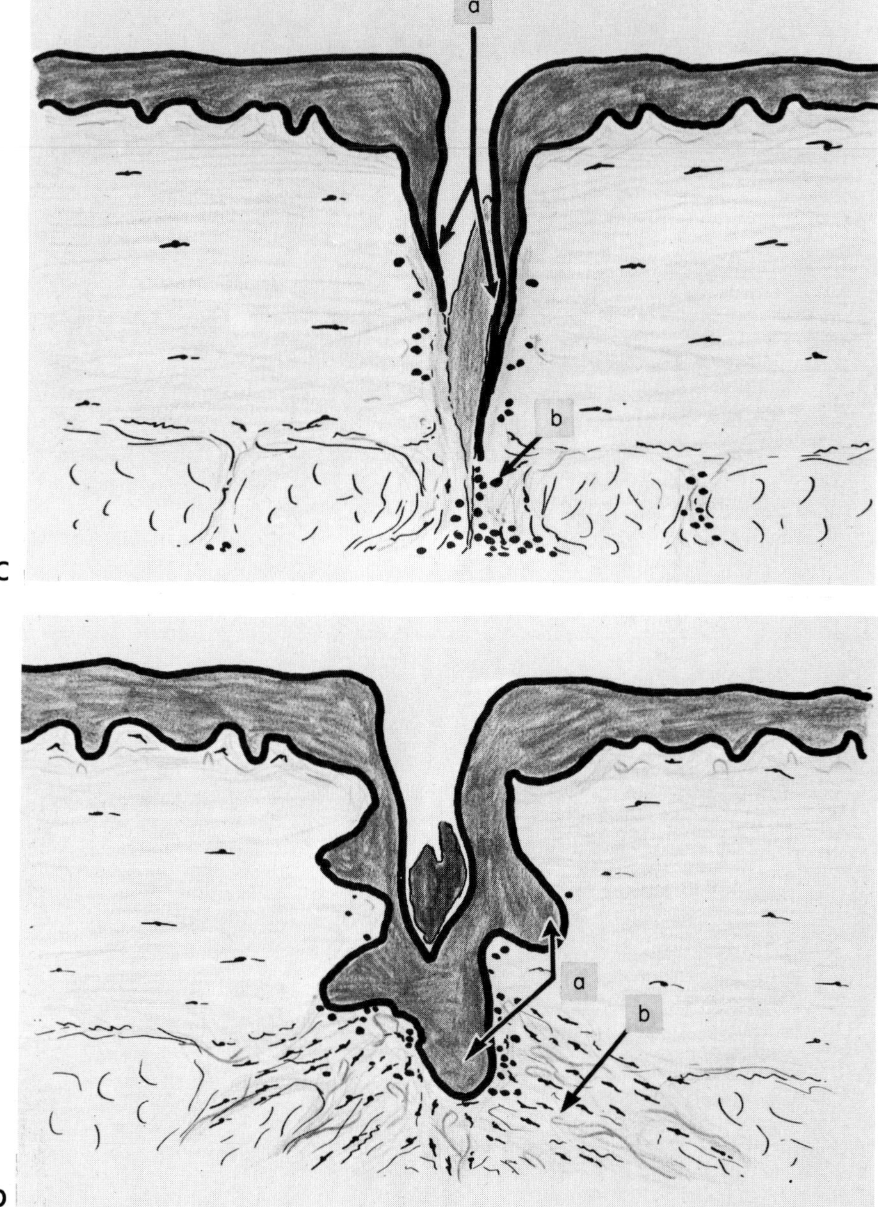

Figure 4–137 *Continued C,* From 2 to 14 days: (a) epidermis migrating down wound walls; (b) phagocytes removing debris. *D,* From 14 to 30 days: (a) epidermal proliferation into dermal and connective tissue defects; (b) granulation tissue ridge.

Illustration continued on following page

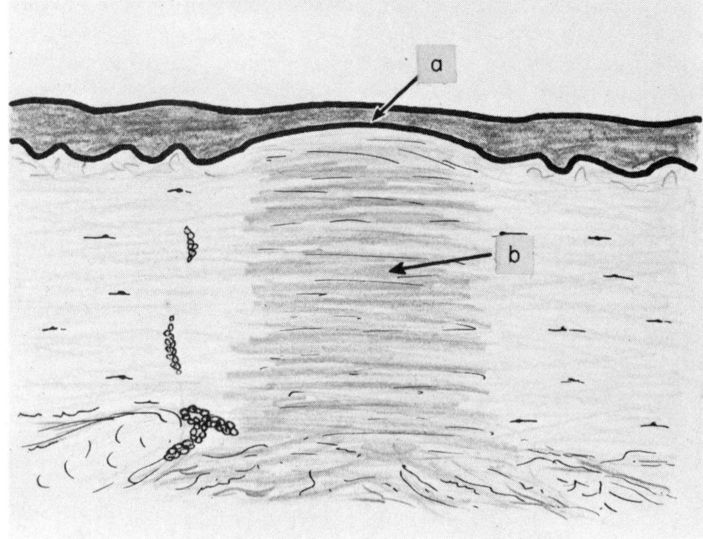

Figure 4–137 *Continued E*, After 30 days: (a) raised thin epidermis; (b) dense maturing scar. (From McMinn, R. H. M.: Tissue repair. New York, Academic Press, 1969. Reprinted by permission.)

apposition of incisions is essential, and grafts may be needed in large injuries (Figs. 4–138, 4–139 and 4–140).

It has been demonstrated that neutrophils and complement are not required for wound healing and that if they are removed experimentally, the wounds will heal normally. Research efforts are now directed at experimentally removing, one at a time, each of the cellular and humoral components that influence wound healing in order to determine which factors are significant and by what means. ***The macrophage is essential for wound débridement and promotes fibroblast proliferation.*** In fact, macrophages control débridement and collagen synthesis regulators. There are reports that macrophages can be transformed into fibroblasts. Platelets contain a factor that stimulates proliferation of fibroblasts and smooth

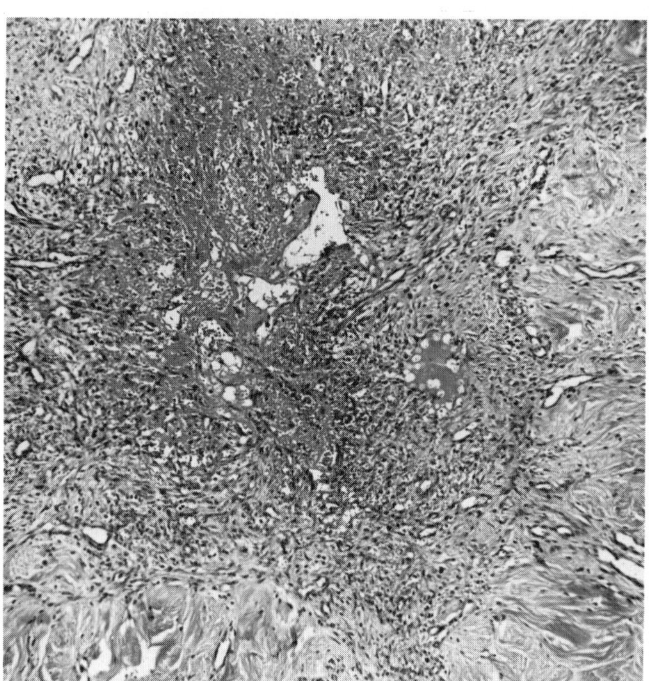

Figure 4–138. Six-day-old skin incision in a horse. Blood clot is in the center and mature collagen is at the edge. Note the relatively narrow area from which the granulation tissue originates and grows into the blood clot.

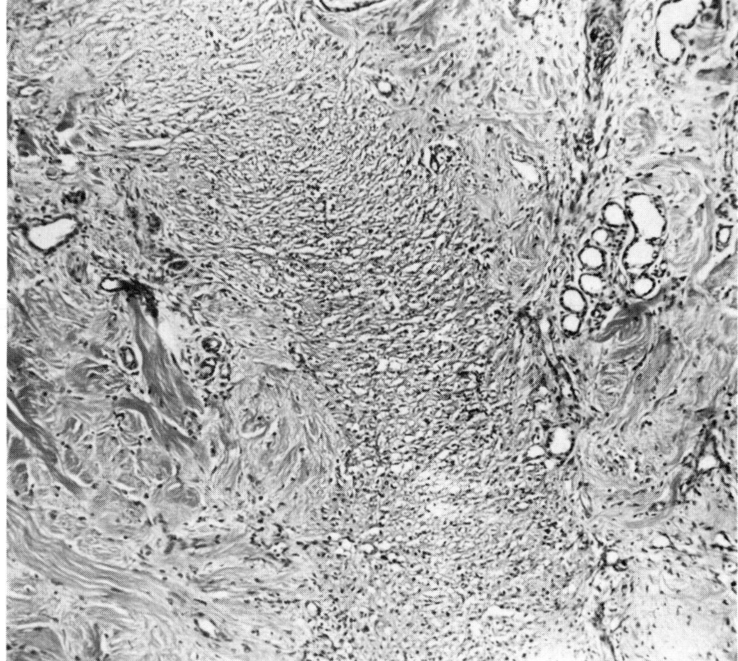

Figure 4–139. Ten-day-old skin incision in a horse. Note the sharp demarcation between mature collagen at the sides and the granulation tissue in the middle, which has now bridged the two sides of the incision.

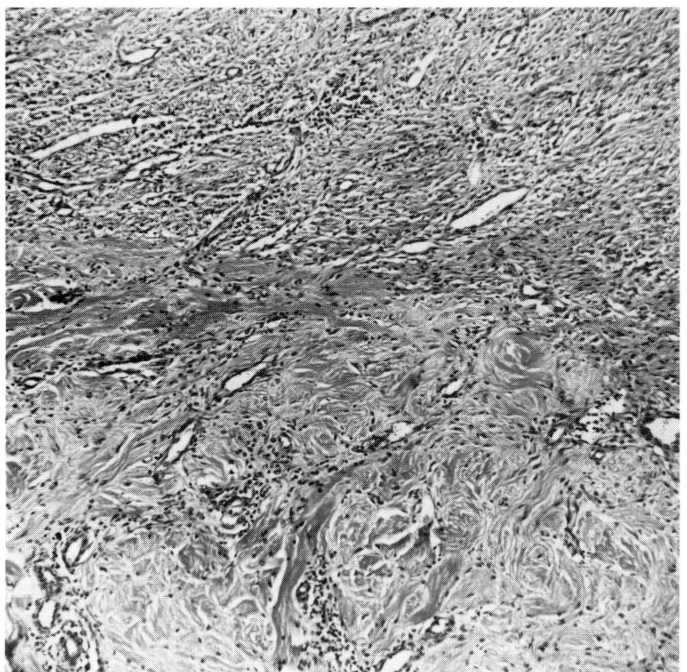

Figure 4–140. A closer view of the junction seen in Figure 4–139 with new collagen toward the top and old toward the bottom.

muscle cells. Plasma contains a ***mitogenic factor*** that stimulates proliferation of fibroblasts and that is present in any wound in which hemorrhage or extensive edema has occurred. A normal chalone feedback mechanism exists to control fibroblasts and is probably interfered with by the plasma.

Endothelial cells secrete ***plasmin,*** which lyses the fibrin in blood clots or fibrinous exudates and gives the impression that the fibrin is organized by connective tissue (Table 4–5). The contraction of wounds occurs by way of cells in the granulation tissue that are really part fibroblast and part smooth muscle cell. These cells make collagen but contain muscle fibrils. They are ***myofibroblasts.***

The collagen in a healing wound matures by ***internal restructuring,*** and a long time is required before the structure approaches that of normal mature collagen. It is possible to experimentally assess the strength of wounds by removing pieces of a surgically induced wound and measuring the force required to pull the two pieces apart at the incision line. In the early stages of healing, only the gluing effect of fibrin and serum proteins and the adhesion of migrating epithelium hold the wound together. Collagen secretion starting at three to four days markedly increases the strength of the wound, and a maximum of actual collagen content is reached at about 14 days. Thereafter, the strength increases primarily by ***remodeling*** through dissolution and reformation of collagen fibers that gives a stronger, more efficient bonding of collagen fibrils and fibers. Even though cells may have filled the space between the edges of an incision, it ***takes months for the strength to return to near normal.*** The healing rate is different in different species. It is also different in different tissues and at different sites in the same tissue.

There is a ***lack*** of correlation between ***collagen content and breaking strength of***

TABLE 4–5. ROLE OF BLOOD COAGULATION AND FIBRINOLYSIS IN TISSUE REPAIR

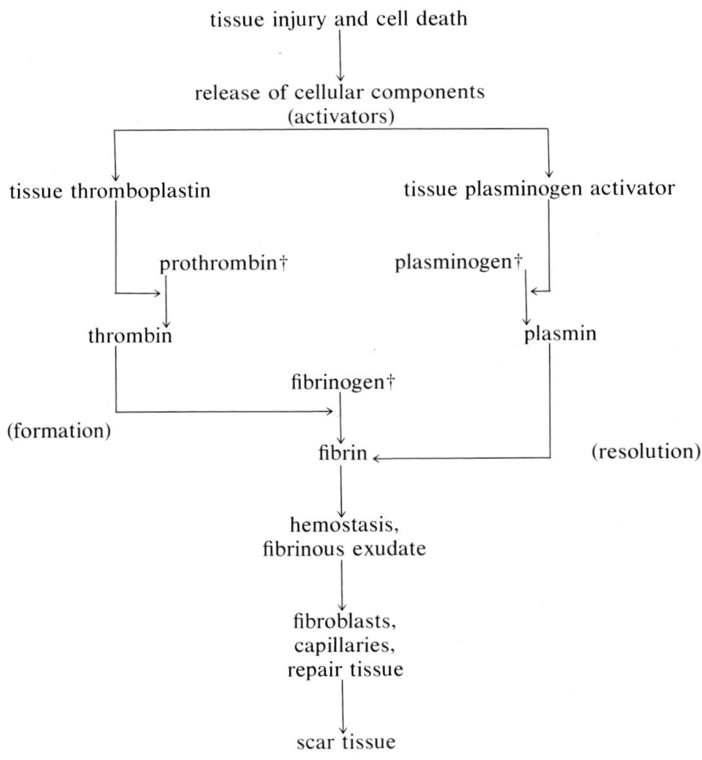

†Components of the humoral system.

(From Forscher, B. K. (ed.): Chemical Biology of Inflammation. New York, Pergamon Press, 1967. Modified from Astrup.)

wounds after the initial phases of collagen production. There ***is*** a correlation between ***breaking strength and the rate of collagen turnover and deposition*** for extended periods after the total collagen accumulation in the wound has leveled out. Tensile strength in most normal tissues is directly related to collagen content.

Collagen is not a static tissue but is gradually removed and replaced by synthesis of more collagen. The process of synthesis is well known, but the means of degradation is not entirely agreed upon and is therefore somewhat controversial. Recent evidence suggests that the fibroblast may be the means of degradation through phagocytosis of collagen into a phagosome and fusion of the phagosome with primary lysosomes to form a phagolysosome. Macrophages are known to contain remnants of collagen, and extracellular breakdown occurs in inflammatory lesions. The actual breakdown involves initial cleavage of the macromolecule by a specific ***collagenase***. There is considerable turnover of collagen in scars and remodeling at the junction of the old and new collagen in a wound. Collagenases have been identified in several tissues.

The most common problems associated with wound healing are (1) the presence of dead or dying tissue; (2) infection, often resulting from presence of dead tissue; (3) mechanical factors such as constant tearing of newly formed elements in wounds at the flexor and extensor aspects of joints or excessive licking or biting of the wound by the animal, or incorrectly applied dressings or bandages; (4) the anatomical site itself, such as one with a poor blood supply (for example, over superficial bone or where there is likely to be repeated injury); (5) the presence of an alien tissue such as serous membrane or omentum in a penetrating skin wound; (6) the existence of foreign bodies, either animate, such as parasites, inanimate, such as grit or wood splinters, or endogenous, such as detached bone chips; (7) tumor cells invading the wound; (8) imbalance between connective tissue and epidermal healing rates, which is a notable feature of horses; (9) persistent irritation; and (10) major trauma elsewhere.

HEALING IN VARIOUS TYPES OF LESIONS

In previous sections, reference was made to ***fibrosis*** and ***organization*** without specifying that they are in fact ***growth of granulation tissue***. Organization of a ***thrombus*** occurs by fibroblasts and sometimes by endothelial cells growing through the vessel wall and into the thrombus. The thrombus is replaced and removed by the granulation tissue, leaving a scar, and is then an organized thrombus. The fibrosis occurring around an ***infarct***, which results in the depressed pale scar, is granulation tissue that matures to form a scar. Organization of a ***diphtheritic membrane*** is by granulation tissue, as is the formation of an ***adhesion*** from a fibrinous exudate (Figs. 4–141 and 4–142). A ***pyogenic membrane*** is granulation tissue in which new connective tissue and

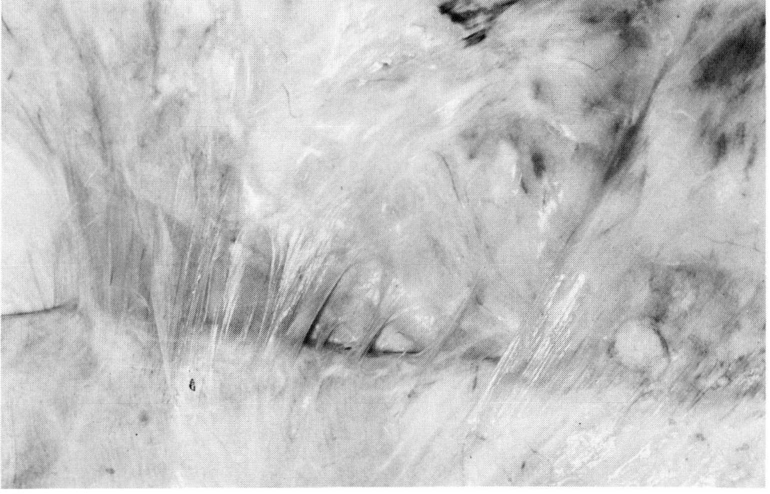

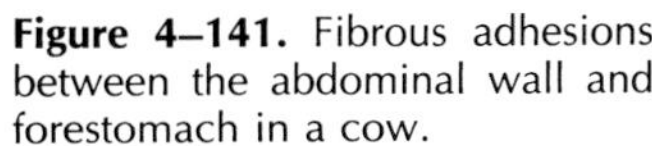

Figure 4–141. Fibrous adhesions between the abdominal wall and forestomach in a cow.

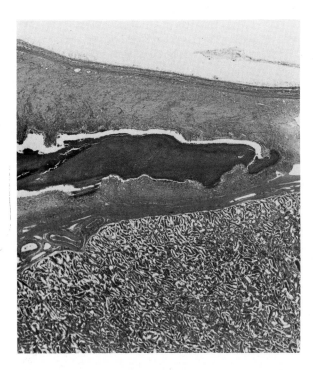

Figure 4–142. Organizing fibrinous exudate between the testicle and the tunica vaginalis. Note the thickness of the granulation tissue on each side, which would form an adhesion when the two sides met.

capillaries are very prominent (Figs. 4–56, 4–57 and 4–58). An ***abscess*** heals by absorption of its contents, by collapse and by being filled in with granulation tissue to leave a scar. The connective tissue in a ***granuloma and granulomatous inflammation*** is granulation tissue (Figs. 4–77 and 4–92). The diffuse fibrosis that occurs in lesions such as ***diffuse interstitial nephritis*** or ***diffuse hepatitis*** is also granulation tissue. The difference between some of these chronic lesions and a healing wound is only in time, location and stimulus to form the new connective tissue. If it happens slowly, the process is so gradual and subtle that the large nuclei of fibroblasts and endothelial cells do not develop and the recognition of acute granulation tissue is not possible.

The term ***fibrosis*** is very common and relates to the gradual, insidious hardening of a tissue by diffuse or focal proliferation of new connective tissue (Figs. 4–143 through 4–159). A small, pale, hard kidney becomes fibrotic through a process of degeneration and necrosis of renal tissue in an inflammatory or degenerative process, with healing by the stimulation of fibrous tissue. Fibrosis may be recognized grossly on the surface of organs as being ***pale and depressed*** (Fig. 4–151). Exudate in the tissue will usually result in ***pale raised*** areas (see Fig. 4–102). Combinations of fibrosis and exudate are visible as pale streaking on the serosal or cut surface of an organ. A large amount of scar tissue is called a ***scirrhous*** reaction, and another name for a scar is a ***cicatrix.***

There is a tendency to think that fibrosis is permanent and it may be, but scars often become smaller in time and fade away. There are enzymes that lyse and remove collagen, and in some instances, this collagenolytic mechanism can remove large quantities of connective tissue.

An overall, simplified concept of inflammation and healing is included in Figure 4–160.

THERAPEUTIC INFLUENCES ON INFLAMMATION AND REPAIR

There is considerable interest in the therapeutic agents that will speed up wound healing or increase the strength of wounds, but very few have had documented evidence of efficiency. Efforts to clinically control the formation of scar tissue by drugs make use of compounds that act by limiting collagen secretion, by increasing degradation of collagen, by inhibiting maturation by influencing polymerization of collagen

Text continued on page 272

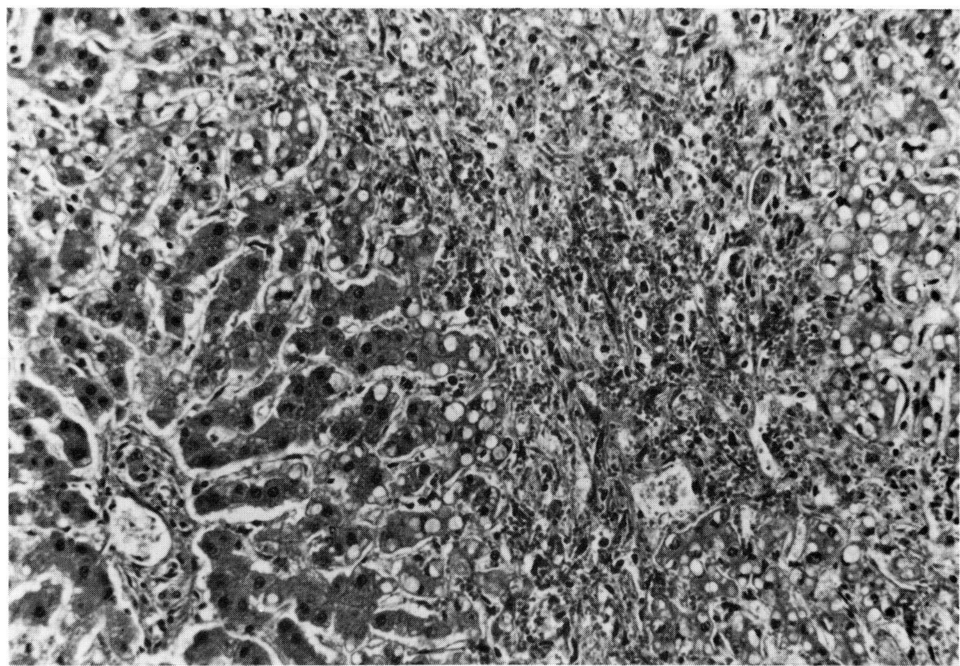

Figure 4–143. Early fibroplasia in the central vein area of a liver in chronic passive congestion. The central vein runs from top to bottom on the right. A portal area is to the left.

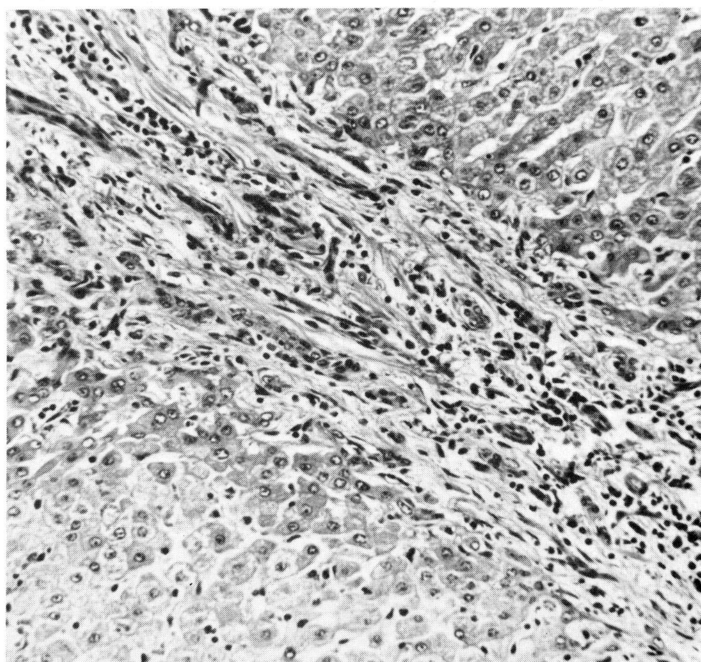

Figure 4–144. Diffuse interlobular hepatic fibrosis. The mononuclear cells suggest chronic inflammation as the cause.

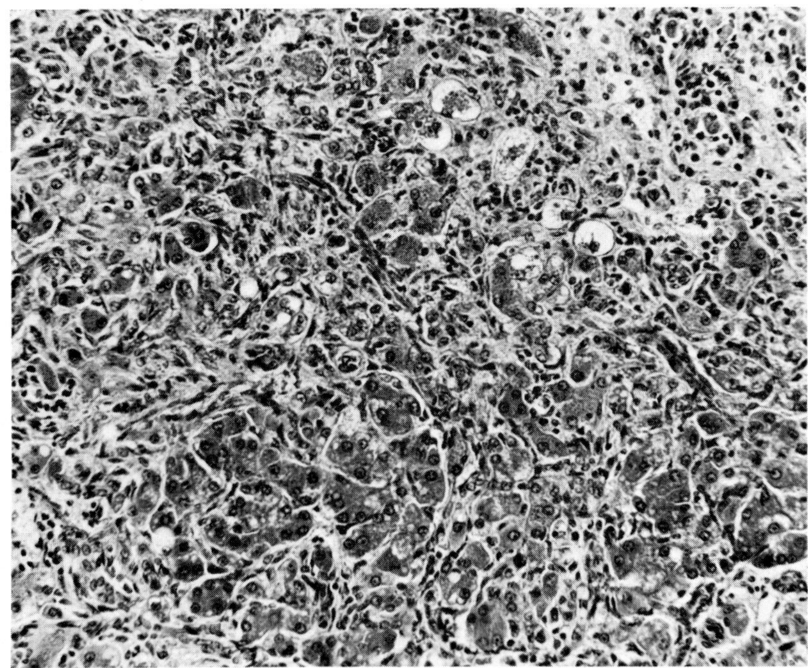

Figure 4–145. Diffuse hepatic fibrosis extending between individual hepatocytes and cords. Note the disruption of normal architecture. The three cases shown in Figures 4–143, 4–144 and 4–145 each have a different pathogenesis.

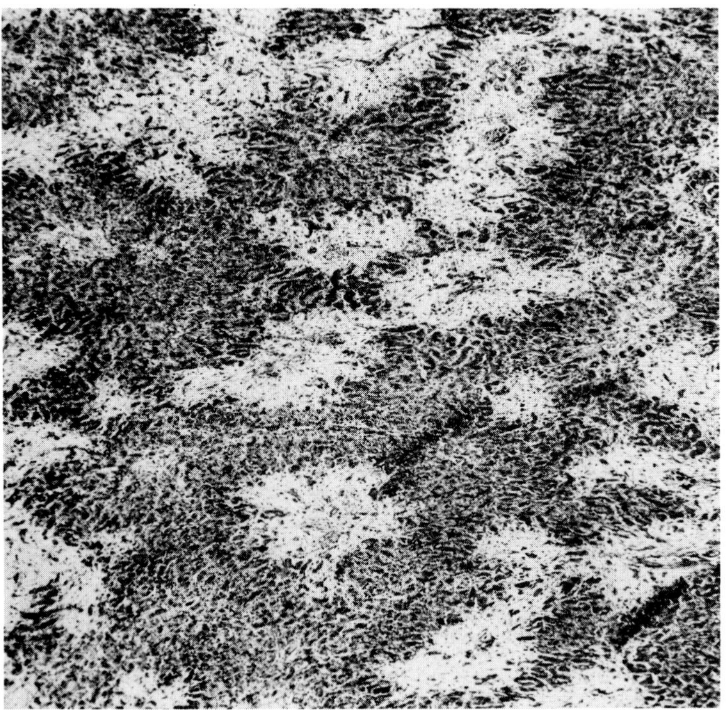

Figure 4–146. Hepatic fibrosis of the portal areas (pale areas). The cause would be a chronic inflammation in and around the bile duct system, probably induced by bacteria or parasites coming up from the intestine.

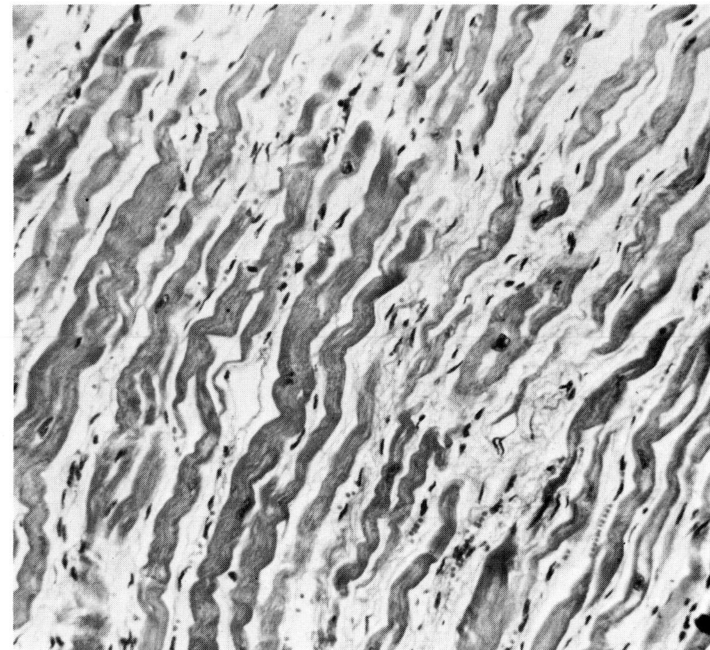

Figure 4–147. Diffuse myocardial fibrosis in a cow. Note the separation of muscle fibers by connective tissue.

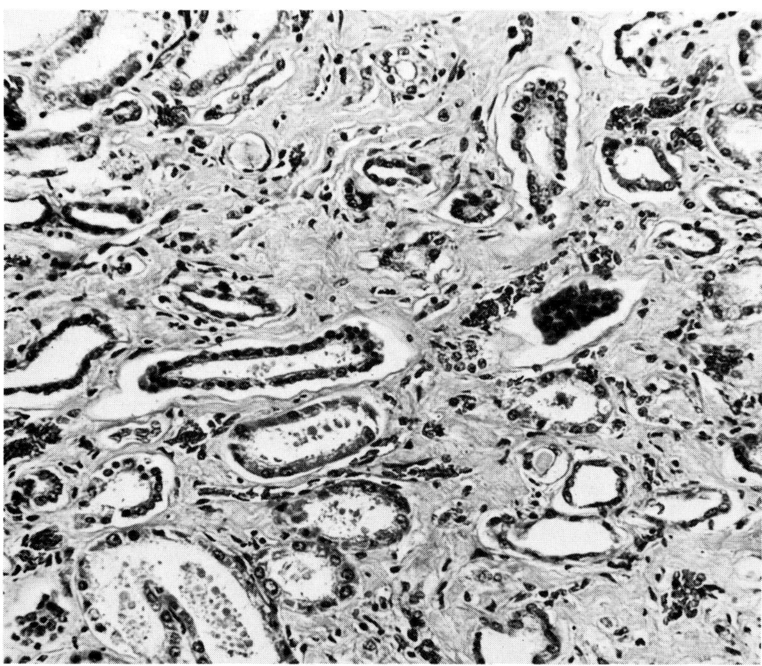

Figure 4–148. Diffuse renal fibrosis in a dog. Such a kidney would be smaller than normal, pale and hard.

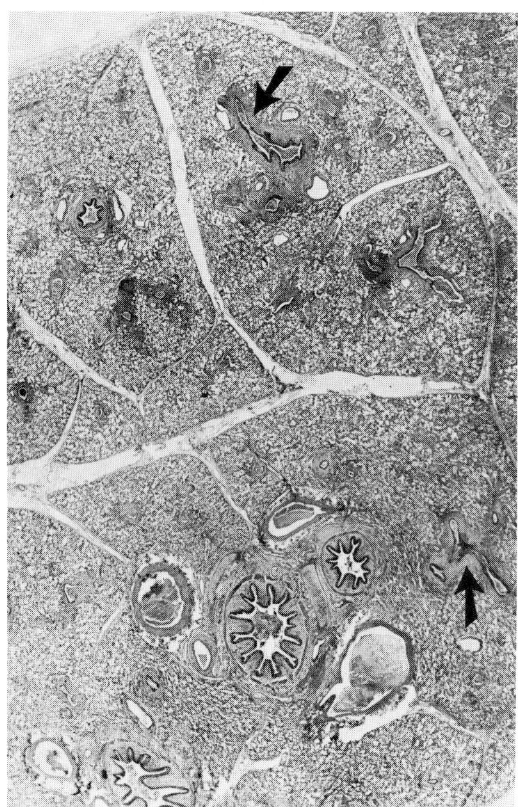

Figure 4–149. Chronic bronchiolitis in a calf. Note the fibrosis around bronchioles in several lobules (arrows). These bronchioles would be functionally impaired.

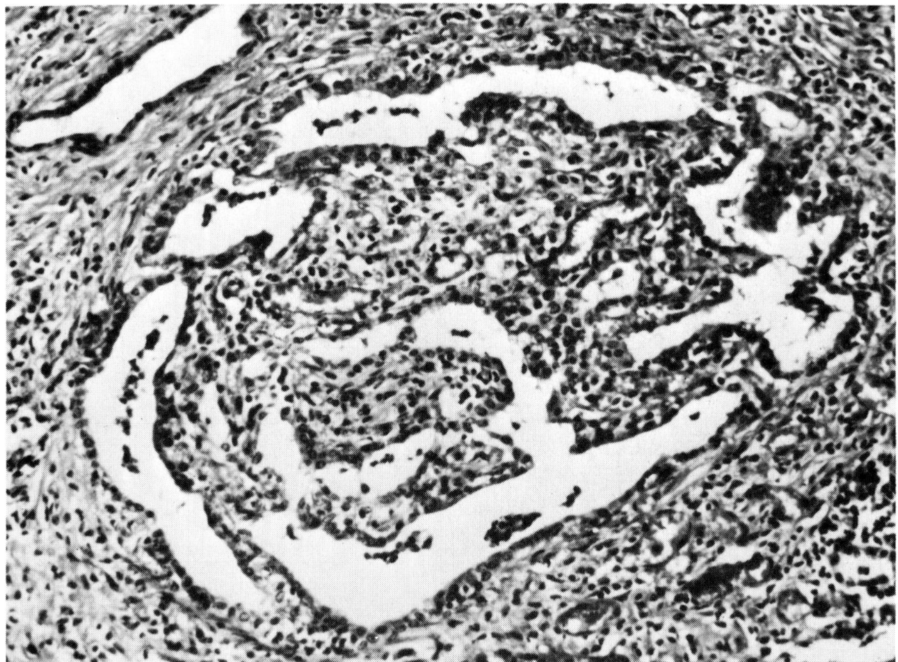

Figure 4–150. Another expression of chronic bronchitis in a calf in which erosion of epithelium has occurred along with accumulation of exudate in the lumen and subsequent organization of the exudate in the lumen. Surface epithelium covers part of the plug. This lesion has similarities to organization and recanalization of thrombi. Such a permanent plug causes marked functional impairment.

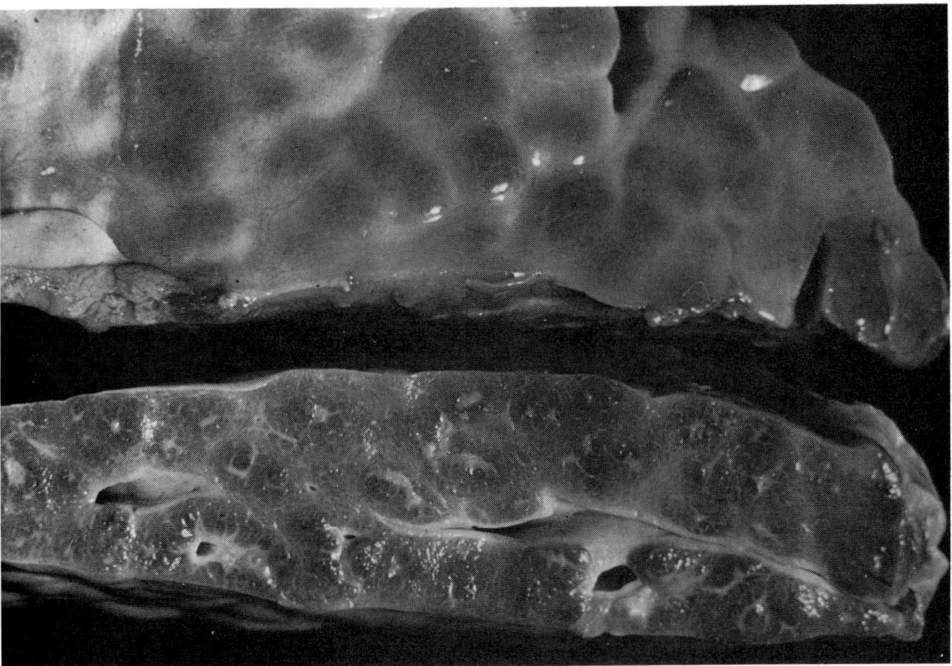

Figure 4–151

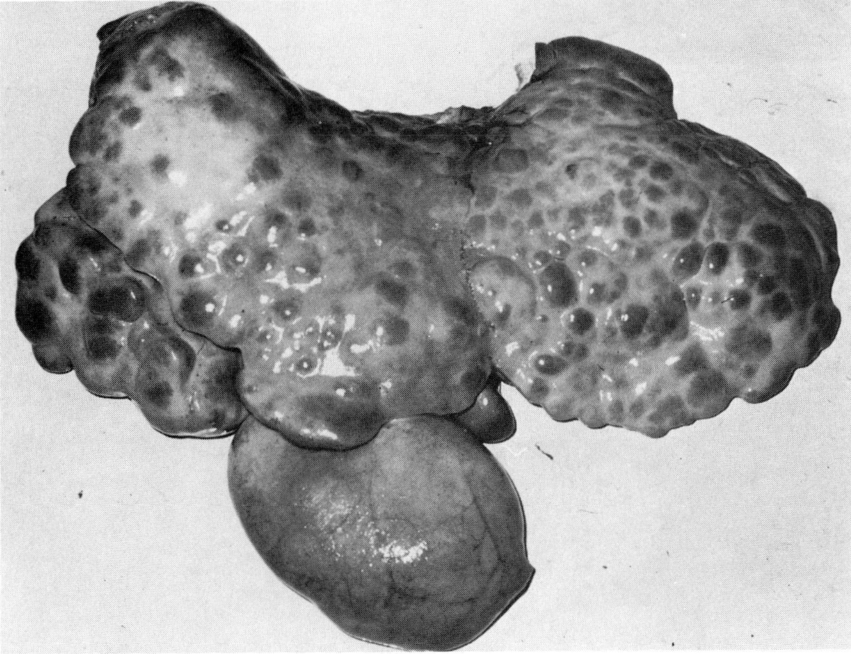

Figure 4–152

Figures 4–151 and 4–152. Serosal and cut surface of diffuse hepatic fibrosis in a cow with ragwort poisoning. The paleness is due to fibrosis. An extreme case of hepatic fibrosis is demonstrated in Figure 4–152. The liver is small, nodular, pale and hard.

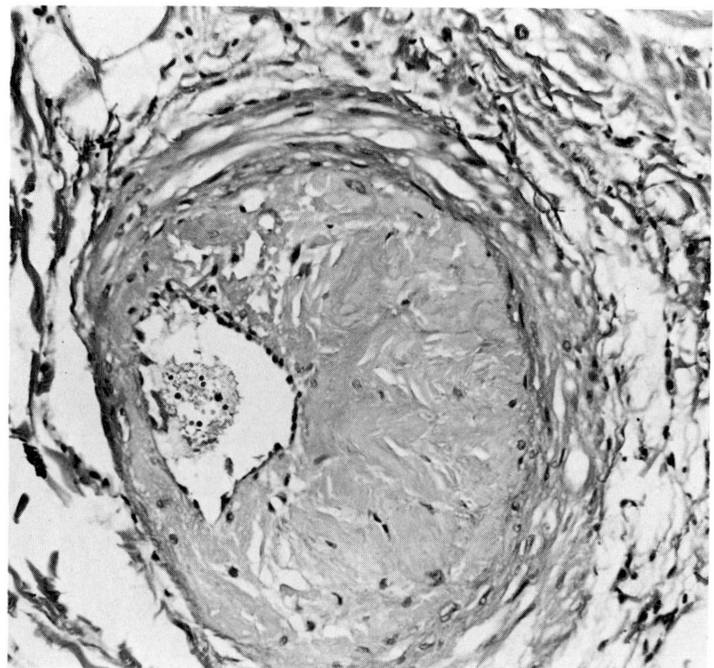

Figure 4–153. Fibrosis in the wall of a branch of the coronary artery in a dog. The original lumen is markedly reduced. This lesion may be called arteriosclerosis.

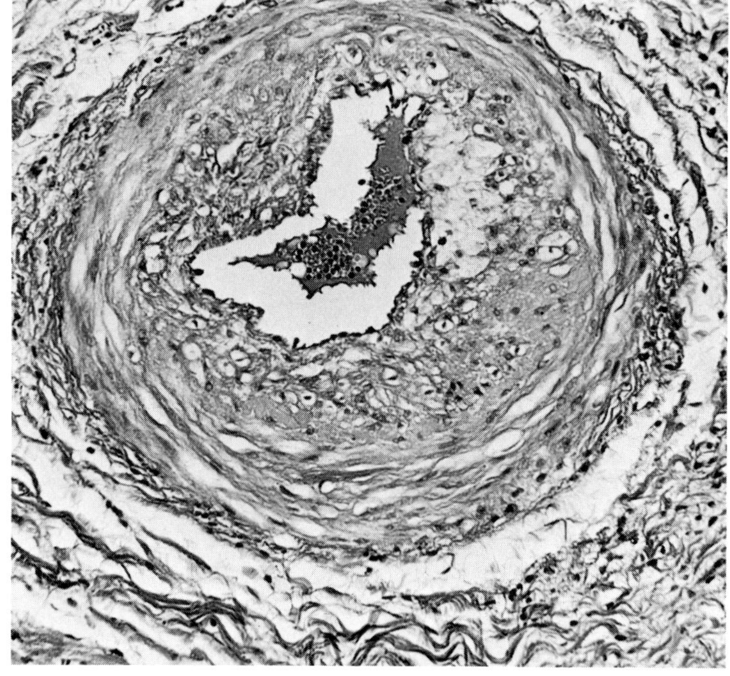

Figure 4–154. Another artery in the heart of the same dog as described in Figure 4–153. Note the foamy lipid in the fibrotic area. When lipid is present, the lesion is often called atherosclerosis.

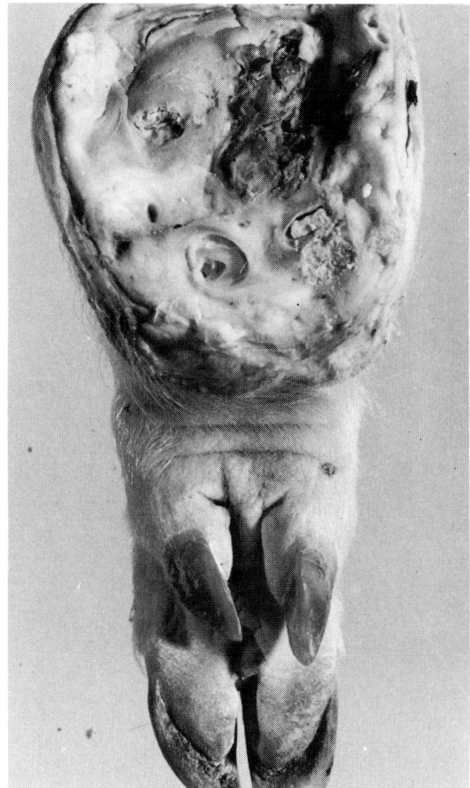

Figure 4–155. Pig's knee joint that was enlarged and hard. Note the extensive fibrosis around the subcutaneous tissue and pockets of purulent exudate in this case of chronic arthritis.

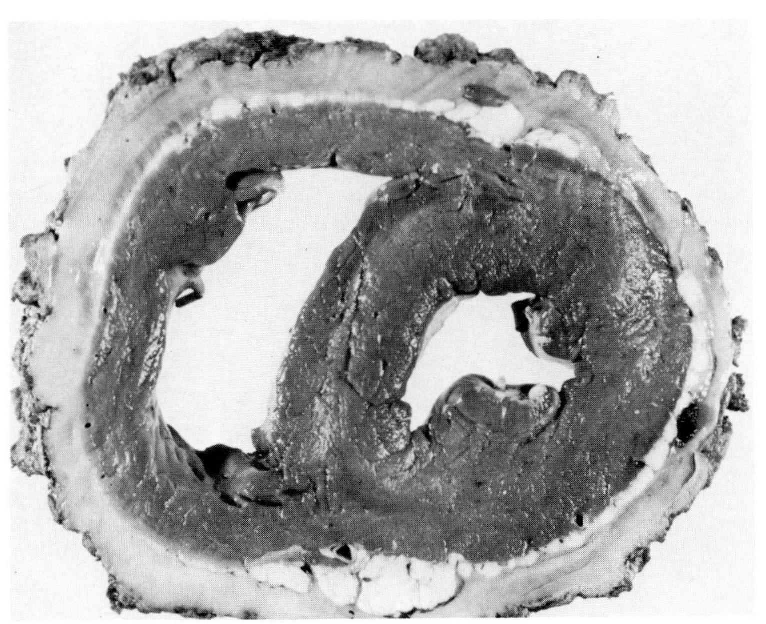

Figure 4–156. Chronic organizing pericarditis in a cow with traumatic pericarditis. Note the dense white layer of connective tissue around the myocardium. The white material between the connective tissue and the myocardium is fat.

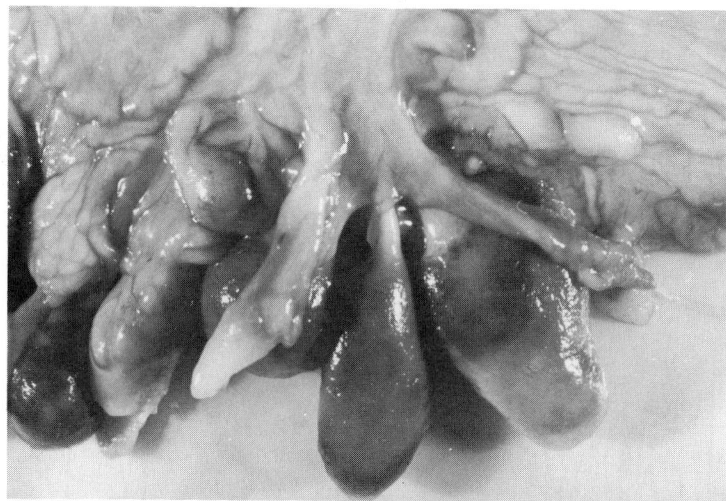

Figure 4–157. Chronic arthritis with proliferation and fibrosis of synovial membrane resulting in a villous appearance to the synovial membrane.

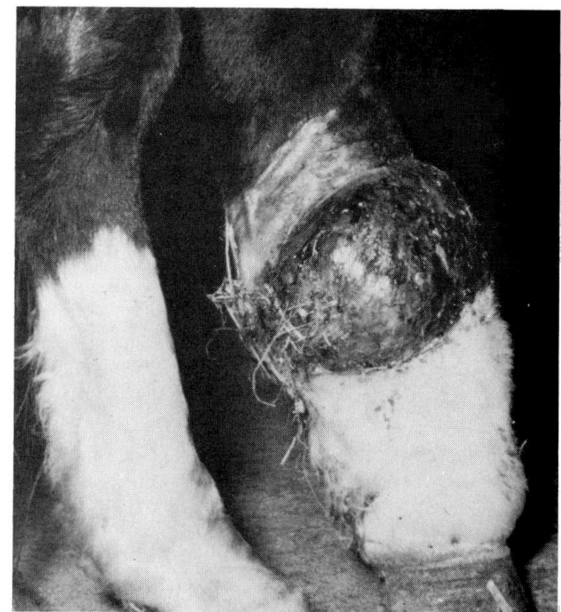

Figure 4–158. Extensive inflammation, fibrosis and granulation tissue production due to chronic inflammation in a horse's leg.

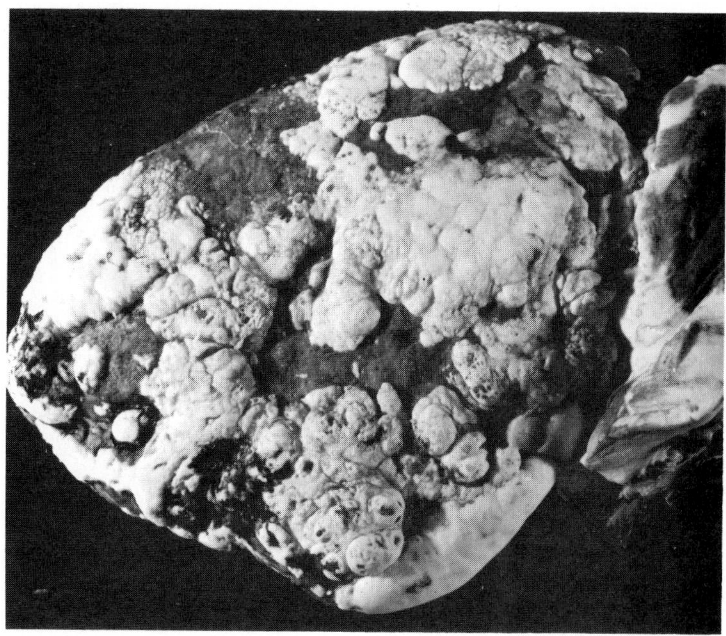

Figure 4–159. Pectoral flipper of a bottle-nosed dolphin. The distal two-thirds sloughed three months after extensive pressure necrosis due to prolonged improper restraint eleven years previously. The remaining stump is now rounded in shape, has white raised areas of fibrosis and active granulomatous inflammation between ulcerated dark areas. The animal died after prolonged (approximately five years) infection with *Mycobacterium marinum*. (Courtesy of J. R. Ceraci.)

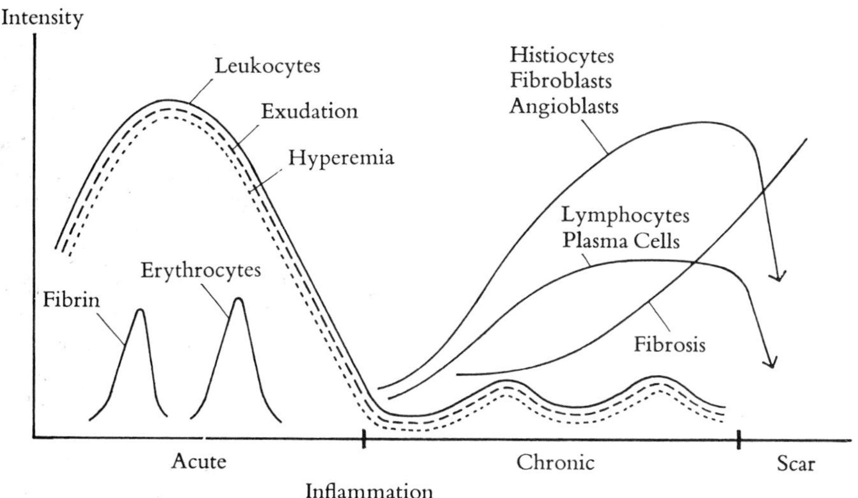

Figure 4–160. Schematic representation of the tissue reactions to inflammatory stimuli. (From Sandritter, W., and Wartman, W. B.: Color Atlas and Textbook of Pathology. Chicago, Year Book Medical Publications, 1969. Reprinted by permission.)

or by reducing the initial inflammatory response and thus the stimulus for connective tissue formation.

There are individuals that form excessive amounts of granulation tissue, which results in large amounts of scar tissue. This lesion is named a ***keloid*** (Fig. 4–158) and results from abnormal formation of whorls and nodules of collagen matrix rather than normal parallel arrangements. The problem seems to be caused by collagenase inhibitors. Such lesions retain characteristics of embryonic collagen. See the review by Shoshan (1981) regarding details of control factors for wound healing.

A wound or incision is protected by macrophages, neutrophils and plasma, which are present in the lesion secondarily, but infection is of great concern, since the inflammatory process in an infection would impair and break down any healing that had occurred. Considerable caution is required to prevent such infections in wounds. If a wound is not well cleaned and closed, pockets of fluid and tissue debris provide excellent media for bacterial growth and complications. The surgeon's principles are ***gentleness, hemostasis, adequate blood supply, asepsis and no tension***. At one hospital for humans, in a survey concerning 100 major complications of surgical treatment, the incidence of these complications was 12 per cent of total surgical procedures; half were wound complications, and half of these were ***wound infections***.

Anti-inflammatory agents such as corticosteroids act in general by decreasing vasodilation, adhesion of leukocytes, phagocytosis, mucopolysaccharide matrix production and immunological reactivity. Eosinophils and lymphocytes are depressed in the hemogram, whereas neutrophils are increased. In addition, there is less pain from lesions that would otherwise be more painful.

Corticosteroids seem to act primarily by stabilizing lysosomes, and nonsteroidal anti-inflammatory drugs such as aspirin inhibit the biosynthesis of prostaglandins. The specific mechanisms of action for the latter are not well understood, but they bind to plasma proteins and may compete with other exogenous compounds or with endogenous ones on cell membranes. More specifically, the actions of corticosteroids influence inflammation by suppressing vasodilation, edema formation and migration of cells out of vessels, as well as by decreasing collagen deposition and fibroblast and endothelial proliferation. These effects of corticosteroids occur in lesions induced by any etiological factor. Very minor chemical differences between some drugs may result in profound differences in their effects on inflammation. When these drugs are used in infectious diseases, concurrent antimicrobial therapy is advised to prevent possible spread or flare-up. Overall, the inflammatory response and healing processes are reduced by these agents.

The book by Peacock and Van Winkle (1976) provides detailed information on wounds and regeneration. The book has a well-illustrated chapter on burns and one on repair of skin wounds.

REGENERATION OF TISSUE

The regenerative capacities of tissues are quite variable; some tissues have almost unlimited capabilities, providing there is some normal tissue surviving. Regeneration may occur in the normal architectural pattern of the tissue or in nodules of new tissues with only partial normal architecture. Tissues with great potential for regeneration are as follows: connective tissue, blood vessel, lymph vessel, bone marrow, fat, ovary, some endocrine glands and liver. Bone tissue will remodel or form new periosteal bone but not a new bone as an organ (Fig. 4–161). Cartilage, ligament and tendon have limited capabilities. Synovial membranes will form over organized exudate, and endothelium will do the same over thrombi. The kidneys and pancreas have considerable compensatory activity but only moderate regenerative functions. Many organs, such as the lungs, have such a large functional reserve that regeneration is not often required and is limited when it is required. Surface epithelium has great capabilities but requires a surface over which to expand. All the adnexa in skin can regenerate. Intestinal and gastric epithelia regenerate well, and even villi and glands may form after severe injury and collapse of the lamina propria (Figs. 4–162 and 4–163). The testis does not make new tubules. Neural tissues can regenerate parts of axons but not neurons. Skeletal muscle will regen-

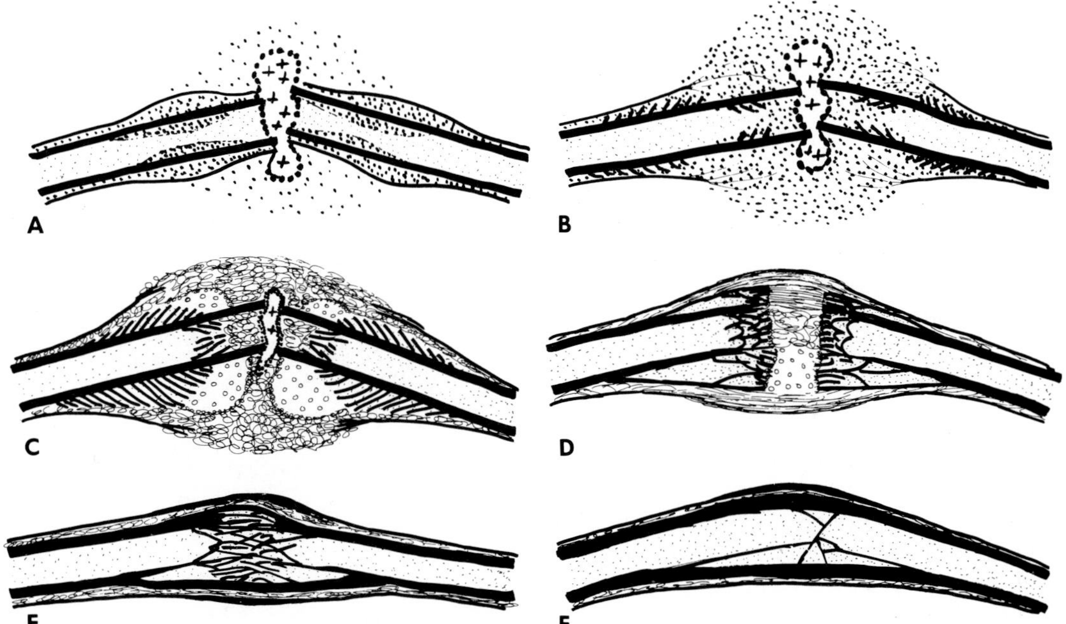

Figure 4–161. *A*, Sites of cellular proliferation in relation to the fracture site. Large dots, macrophages; Crosses, debris.

B, Blastema developing around the fracture site. Note bone formation (slanting lines) beginning under the fibrous periosteum and on the walls of the marrow cavity.

C, Sites of early bone and cartilage formation in the blastema. Oblique lines, new bone; circles, cartilage.

D, New bone at a later stage in repair. Ossification "fronts" face each other across a "no-man's-land" of fibrous and fibrillar tissue and cartilage. A fibrous capsule has formed externally.

E, Bony union. Note new cortical bone and partial atrophy of old cortex.

F, Advanced stage of repair with remodeled cortex and new marrow cavity.

(From McMinn, R. M. H.: Tissue Repair. New York, Academic Press, 1969. Reprinted by permission.)

erate fibers if the sarcolemmal sheath is intact, but cardiac muscle will not. Tubules in the kidney and acini in glands will repair if the basement membrane is intact and some epithelial cells remain to begin the process. The status of the basement membrane is of great significance in such organs. The eye and ear do not regenerate. ***The more specialized the tissue, the more limited the capability to regenerate***. The book by McMinn (1969) describes regenerative capacity of each tissue in detail, as does the book by Peacock and Van Winkle (1976), but the latter emphasizes the surgical aspects of repair as well.

The fact that tissues heal invites investigation of the control mechanisms that initiate and then stop the hyperplasia in healing. How does the epithelium in the skin know when to stop multiplying? The answer involves ***chalones***, the chemical messengers that control tissue mass. Chalones are chemical compounds present in cells that send messages from cell to cell and control mitosis. They have been found in many tissues and are tissue-specific. They are polypeptides and glycoproteins. ***Chalones act by inhibiting mitosis through a negative feedback system***. They are produced constantly, pass from cell to cell and are degraded constantly.

A component of plasma enhances or permits mitosis of fibroblasts in culture, perhaps by displacing the chalone from its binding site on the cell. This may account for the necessity of having serum in the media for successful tissue culture of cells.

The epidermal-dermal relationship will be discussed as an example of tissue interactions. The basal cells of the epithelium readily undergo mitosis; the cells above usually do not. Mitosis is inhibited by the epidermal chalone and promoted by a mesenchymal factor produced in the dermis. The basal cells are released from the control of their own chalone because of their location close to the dermis, and they undergo mitosis. When cells leave the basal layer and move toward the surface, the epidermal chalone maintains control. The speed of cell aging

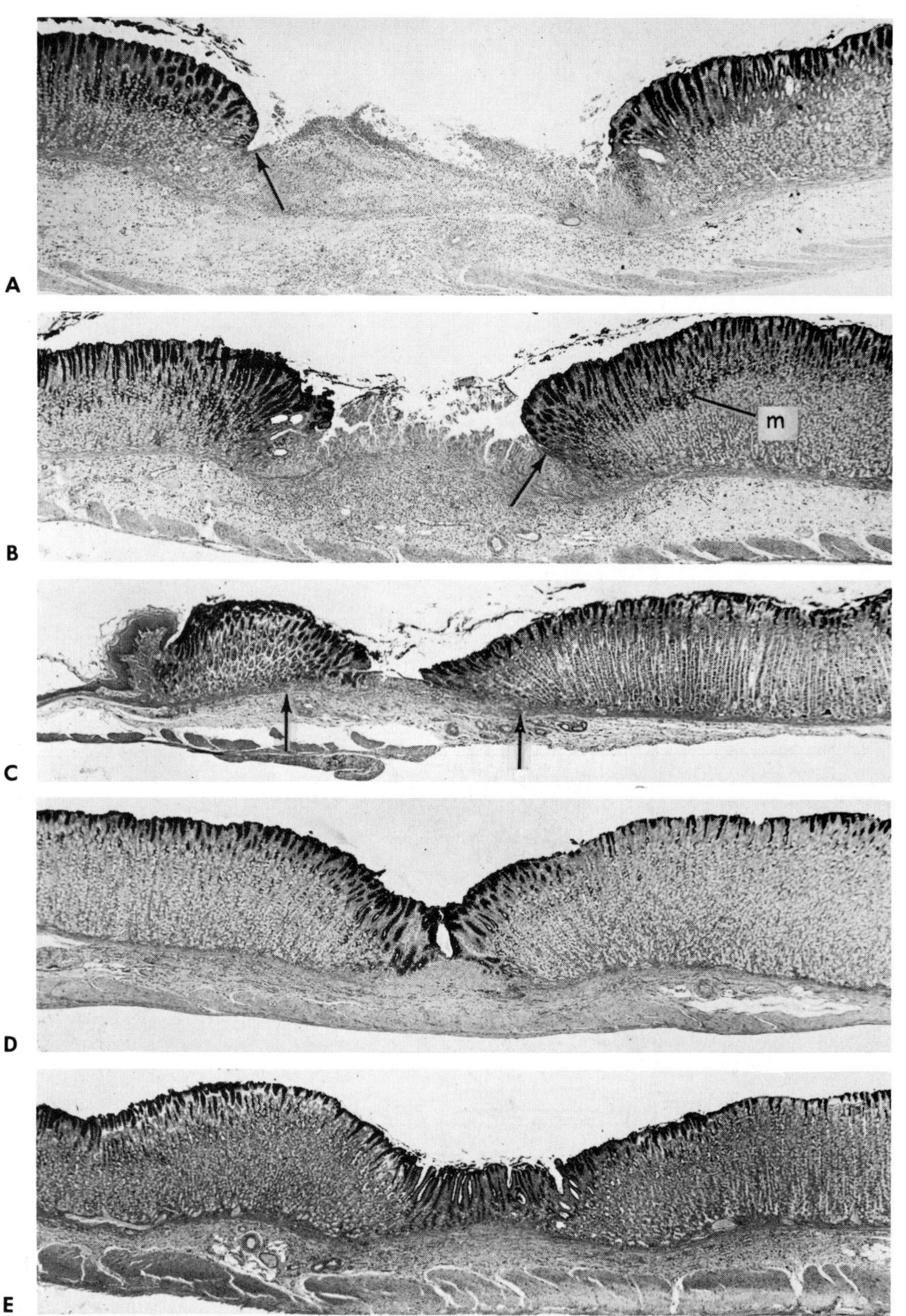

Figure 4–162. *A,* Section showing a defect in the mucosa of a rat stomach two days after injury. Note the deep foveolae and tongue of epithelial cells (arrow). Periodic acid–Schiff stain.

B, Mucosa on fifth day of regeneration. The foveolae are deep and mucous neck cells (m) are numerous. Note tongue of cells (arrow). Periodic acid–Schiff stain.

C, Mucosa on 10th day of regeneration. The foveolae are not so deep, and the mucous neck cells are not so numerous as in *B*. Arrows indicate the approximate extent of the original defect. Periodic acid–Schiff stain.

D, Mucosa on 18th day of regeneration. The most recently regenerated glands are composed of mucous neck cells. Periodic acid–Schiff stain.

E, Mucosa on 36th day of regeneration. Central regeneration zone is about one-third normal thickness with deep foveolae and contains glands with mucous neck and parietal cells. Periodic acid–Schiff stain.

(From Hunt, T. E.: Regeneration of the gastric mucosa in the rat. Anat. Rec., *131*:193–211, 1958. Reprinted by permission.)

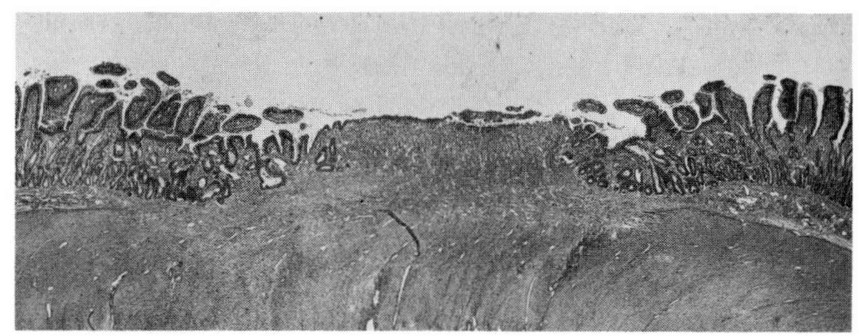
A

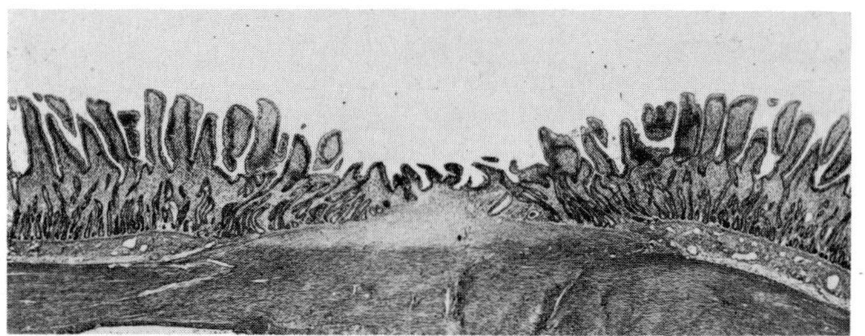
B

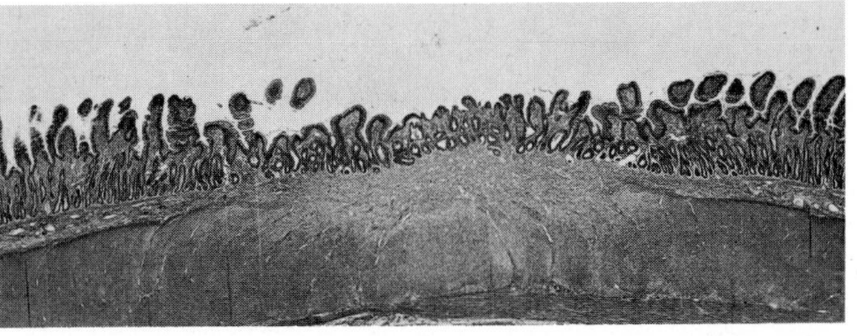
C

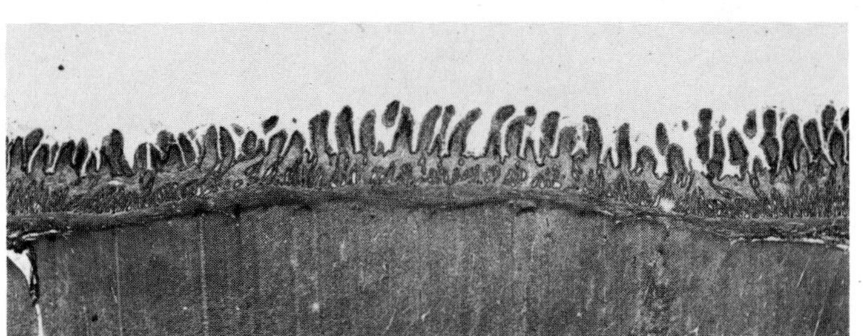
D

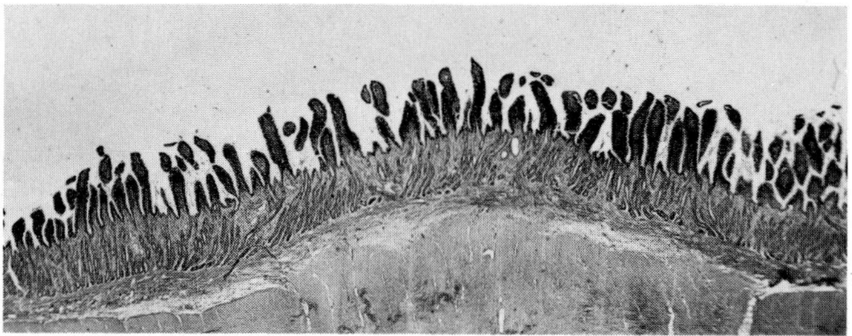
E

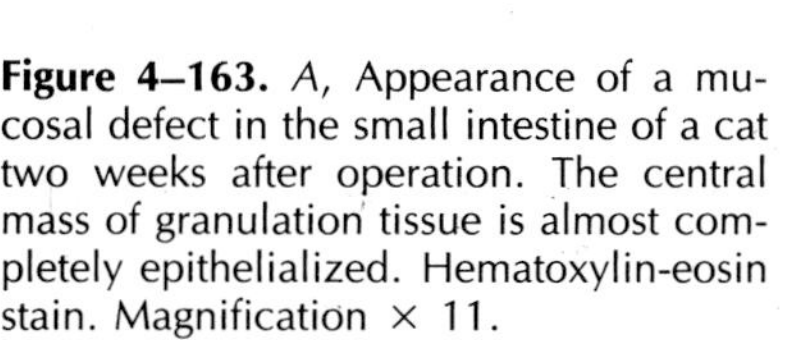
Figure 4–163. *A,* Appearance of a mucosal defect in the small intestine of a cat two weeks after operation. The central mass of granulation tissue is almost completely epithelialized. Hematoxylin-eosin stain. Magnification × 11.

B, Center of the healing site six weeks after operation. Hematoxylin-eosin stain. Magnification × 11.

C, Periphery of the healing site six weeks after operation. Note the irregular villi and glands. Hematoxylin-eosin stain. Magnification × 11.

D, Appearance of the lesion at the end of three months. Hematoxylin-eosin stain. Magnification × 11.

E, Site of the lesion one year after operation. The villi and glands have a normal appearance, but the muscularis mucosae has failed to regenerate. Compare with parts A through D. Hematoxylin-eosin stain. Magnification × 11.

(From McMinn, R. M., and Mitchell, J. E.: Formation of villi following artificial lesions of mucosa in small intestine of cat. J. Anat., *88*:99–107, 1954. Reprinted by permission.)

is controlled by the chalone, which inhibits aging by the strength of its influence. The balance between the inhibition of chalone by the dermis and the strength of the influence from within the epithelium maintains normal thickness. Therefore, the position of the cell within the epithelium seems to be the most significant factor. The influence of chalones would account for hyperplasia and atrophy. Epithelium requires connective tissue in apposition in order to undergo hyperplasia.

In some cancerous tissues, there is an excessive loss of chalone through abnormal cell membranes but production within the cell is normal. Abnormal levels of chalone are present in the blood in such situations, and there is evidence that chalones may be useful as mitotic inhibitors for therapeutic purposes in cases of cancer. The study of chalones is in its infancy. Probably, the pronounced influence on growth in hormone-dependent tissues is controlled in part by ***hormone-dependent chalone neutralization***. Hormones exert their influence through secretion of new proteins by the cell, and these influence growth (Fig. 4–164), perhaps by influencing chalones. The hormone is delivered to the target tissue, which has a specific hormone receptor. These receptors account for the tissue specificity of the action of hormones. The hormone-receptor complex is transported to the nucleus where it is bound to the target cell genome; this results in increased protein synthesis, some of which may influence chalones. Hormones have other mechanisms of action, such as by influence on cyclic AMP, water imbibition and changes in lysosomal distribution and permeability.

This chapter has outlined a host of normal biological and biochemical mechanisms, including many that have intricate interrelationships and can be initiated by several mechanisms for the protection of the host. It should be kept in mind that there are individuals that have ***congenital*** or ***acquired defects*** in these processes and are not able to respond to injury in a normal manner. Defects in the action of chemical mediators, phagocytosis or healing have been recognized in many individuals. The problem usually occurs in the form of the absence of a key enzyme in a sequential process. These

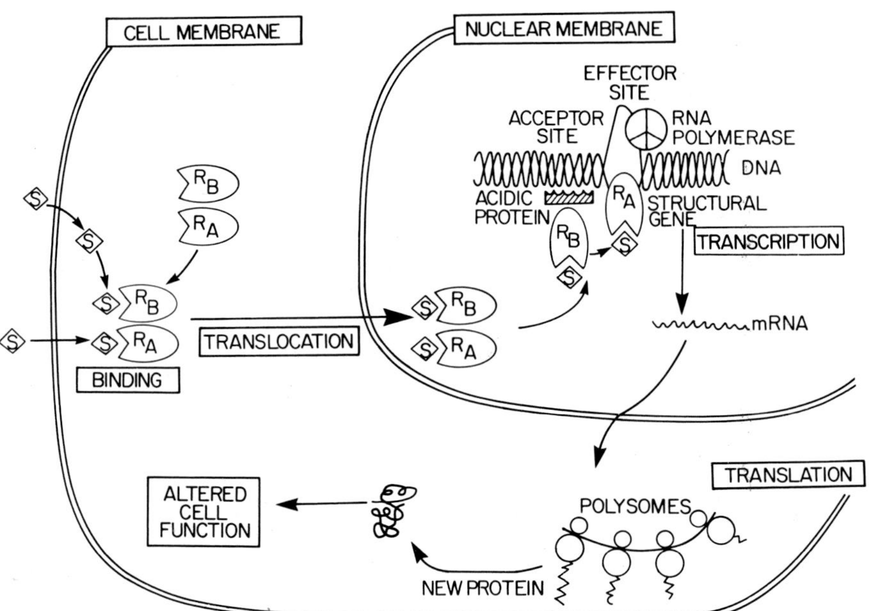

Figure 4–164. Molecular mechanism of sex steroid hormone action. The schematic representation of the subunit structure of steroid hormone receptor is based primarily on information from the progesterone receptor in the chick oviduct. It is likely, however, that the general concept applies to other steroid hormones as well. S represents steroid hormone, and R_A and R_B are steroid hormone receptor subunits. (From Chan, L., and O'Malley, B. W.: Mechanism of action of the sex steroid hormones. Reprinted by permission from New England Journal of Medicine, *294*:1322–1328, 1372–1381, 1430–1437, 1976.)

defects are often used to study the detail of interrelating processes.

SUGGESTIONS FOR FURTHER READING

General

Bach, M. K.: Mediators of anaphylaxis and inflammation. Ann. Rev. Microbiol., *36*:371–414, 1982.

Bélisle, C., and Sainte-Marie, G.: Topography of the deep cortex of the lymph nodes of various mammalian species. Anat. Rec., *201*:553–561, 1981.

Bourne, H. R., et al.: Modulation of inflammation and immunity by cyclic AMP. Science, *184*:19–28, 1974.

Braunstein, P. W., et al.: Platelets, fibroblasts, and inflammation-tissue reactions to platelets injected subcutaneously. Am. J. Pathol., *99*:53–62, 1980.

Carlson, H. C., and Allen, J. R.: The acute inflammatory reaction in chicken skin: blood cellular response. Avian Dis., *13*:817–833, 1969.

Cooper, K. E., et al.: Ontogeny of fever. Fed. Proc., *38*:35–38, 1979.

Feldman, B. F.: Fever of undetermined origin. Comp. Cont. Educ., *11*:970–977, 1980.

Finn, J. P., and Nielsen, N. O.: The inflammatory response of rainbow trout. J. Fish Biol., *3*:463–478, 1971.

Forscher, B. K., and Houck, J. C.: Immunopathology of Inflammation. Amsterdam, Excerpta Medica, 1971.

Gaffney, R. M., and Caseley-Smith, J. R.: Excess plasma proteins as a cause of chronic inflammation and lymphoedema: biochemical estimations. J. Pathol., *133*:229–242, 1981.

Haahr, S., and Mogensen, S.: Function of fever in infectious disease. Biomedicine, *28*:305–307, 1978.

Hirsch, R. L.: The complement system: its importance in the host response to viral infection. Microbiol. Rev., *46*:71–85, 1982.

Joiner, K. A., et al.: A quantitative model for subcutaneous abscess formation in mice. Br. J. Exp. Pathol., *61*:97–107, 1980.

Joiner, K. A., et al.: Host factors in the formation of abscesses. J. Infect. Dis., *142*:40–49, 1980.

Karnovsky, M. L., and Bolis, L. (eds.): Phagocytosis—Past and Future. New York, Academic Press, 1982.

Kluger, M. J.: Phylogeny of fever. Fed. Proc., *38*:30–34, 1979.

Leak, L. V., and Kato, F.: Electron microscopic studies of lymphatic capillaries during early inflammation. I. Mild and severe thermal injuries. Lab. Invest., *26*:572–588, 1972.

Lewis, G. P.: Prostaglandins in inflammation—a review. J. Reticuloendothel. Soc., *22*:389–402, 1977.

McQueen, E. G.: Acute-inflammatory drug mechanisms. Drugs, *6*:104–117, 1973.

Movat, H. Z.: Inflammation, Immunity and Hypersensitivity. New York, Harper & Row, 1971.

O'Flaherty, J. T.: Lipid mediators of inflammation and allergy. Lab. Invest., *46*:314–329, 1982.

Perryman, L. E., and Magnuson, N. S.: Immunodeficiency disease in animals. *In* Desnick, R. J., et al. (eds.): Animal Models of Inherited Metabolic Diseases. Progress in Clinical Biological Research. New York, Alan R. Liss, Inc., 1982, pp. 271–308.

Ratnoff, O. D.: Some relationships among hemostasis, fibrinolytic phenomena, immunity and the inflammatory response. Adv. Immunol., *10*:145–227, 1969.

Robbins, S. L., and Cotran, R. S.: Pathologic Basis of Disease. 2nd Ed. Philadelphia, W. B. Saunders Company, 1979.

Rocklin, R. E.: Modulation of inflammatory and immune responses by histamine. *In* Sirois, P. (ed.): Immunopharmacology. Amsterdam, Elsevier Biomedical Press, 1982, pp. 49–74.

Ryan, G. B.: Inflammation and localization of infection. Surg. Clin. North Am., *56*:831–846, 1976.

Ryan, G. B., and Majno, G.: Acute inflammation. Am. J. Pathol., *86*:183–276, 1977.

Samuelsson, B.: Leukotrienes: Mediators of immediate hypersensitivity reactions and inflammation. Science, *222*:568–575, 1983.

Schachter, M.: Kallikreins (kininogenases)—a group of serine proteases with bioregulatory actions. Pharmacol. Rev., *31*:1–17, 1980.

Schalm, O. W., et al.: Veterinary Hematology. 3rd ed. Philadelphia, Lea & Febiger, 1975.

Schwartz, L. W., and Osburn, B. I.: An ontogenic study of the acute inflammatory reaction in the fetal rhesus monkey. I. Cellular response to bacterial and nonbacterial irritants. Lab. Invest., *31*:441–453, 1974.

Silva, M., and Rocha, E.: A brief survey of the history of inflammation. Agents Actions, *8*:45–49, 1978.

Spragg, J.: Complement, coagulation and kinin generation. *In* Sirois, P. (ed.): Immunopharmacology. Amsterdam, Elsevier Biomedical Press, 1982, pp. 113–144.

Ward, P. A.: Leukotaxis and leukotactic disorders: a review. Am. J. Pathol., *77*:520–538, 1974.

Weissmann, G.: Cell Biology of Inflammation: Handbook of Inflammation. Vol. 2, Amsterdam, Elsevier North-Holland Biomedical Press, 1980.

Weissmann, G., et al. (eds.): Advances in Inflammation Research. Vol. 1. New York, Raven Press, 1978.

Wood, S. L., and Hurley, J. V.: The role of blood capillaries in the formation of inflammatory exudate. J. Pathol., *127*:73–87, 1979.

Zweifach, B. W., et al.: The Inflammatory Process. Vol. III. 2nd ed. New York, Academic Press, 1974.

Granulocytes

Bachner, R. L.: Disorders of leukocytes leading to recurrent infection. Pediatr. Clin. North Am., *19*:935–956, 1972.

Becker, E. L.: Some interrelations of neutrophil chemotaxis, lysosomal enzyme secretion, and phagocytosis as revealed by synthetic peptides. Am. J. Pathol., *85*:386–394, 1976.

Bellanti, J. A., and Dayton, D. H.: The Phagocytic Cell in Host Resistance. New York, Raven Press, 1975.

Fantone, J. C., and Ward, P. A.: Role of oxygen-derived free radicals and metabolites in leukocyte-dependent inflammatory reactions. Am. J. Pathol., *107*:397–414, 1982.

Gallin, J. T., and Quie, P. G.: Leukocyte Chemotaxis. Methods, Physiology and Clinical Implications. New York, Raven Press, 1978.

Goetzl, E. J.: Modulation of human eosinophil polymorphonuclear leukocyte migration and function. Am. J. Pathol., *85*:419–436, 1976.

Henson, P. M.: Pathologic mechanisms in neutrophil-mediated injury. Am. J. Pathol., *68*:593–605, 1972.

Lazarus, G. S., et al.: Role of granulocyte collagenase in collagen degradation. Am. J. Pathol., *68*:565–576, 1972.

Malech, H. L., et al.: Structural analysis of human

neutrophil migration. J. Cell Biol., *75*:666–693, 1977.

Martin, M. W.: The globule leukocyte and parasitic infection—brief review. Vet. Bull., *49*:821–827, 1979.

O'Flaherty, J. T., and Ward, P. A.: Chemotactic factors and the neutrophil. Semin. Hematol., *16*:163–174, 1979.

Oliver, J. M.: Cell biology of leukocyte abnormalities. Membrane and cytoskeletal function in normal and defective cells. A review. Am. J. Pathol., *93*:221–260, 1978.

Quie, P. G., and Cates, K. L.: Clinical conditions associated with defective polymorphonuclear leukocyte chemotaxis. Am. J. Pathol., *88*:711–725, 1977.

Rebuck, J. W., and Crowley, J. H.: A method of studying leukocytic functions *in vivo*. Ann. N.Y. Acad. Sci., *59*:757–805, 1955.

Snyderman, R., and Goetzl, E. J.: Molecular and cellular mechanisms of leukocyte chemotaxis. Science, *213*:830–837, 1981.

Stossel, T. P.: Phagocytosis: clinical disorders of recognition and ingestion. Am. J. Pathol., *88*:741–751, 1977.

Wade, B. H., and Mandell, G. L.: Polymorphonuclear leukocytes: dedicated professional phagocytes. Am. J. Med., *74*:686–693, 1983.

Ward, P. A., et al.: Leukotactic factors elaborated by virus-infected tissues. J. Exp. Med., *135*:1095–1103, 1972.

Ward, P. A., et al.: Regulatory dysfunction in leukotaxis. Am. J. Pathol., *88*:701–708, 1977.

Zuzel, L. F., et al.: Changes in the concentration of leukocytes and platelets in the peripheral blood during sterile inflammation in rabbits. Br. J. Exp. Pathol., *58*:200–208, 1977.

Mononuclear Leukocytes

Allison, A. C.: Macrophage activation and nonspecific immunity. Int. Rev. Exp. Pathol., *18*:303–346, 1978.

Allison, A. C., et al.: The role of macrophage activation in chronic inflammation. Agents Actions, *8*:27–35, 1978.

Asherson, G. L., and Allwood, G. G.: Inflammatory lymphoid cells. Cells in immunized lymph nodes that move to sites of inflammation. Immunology, *22*:493–502, 1972.

Bersani, Amado C. A., and Garcia, L. J.: Some characteristics of the participation of lymphocytes in nonimmune inflammation. Br. J. Exp. Pathol. *63*:463–471, 1982.

Boros, D. L.: Granulomatous inflammation. Prog. Allergy, *24*:183–267, 1978.

Carr, I.: The Macrophage. A Review of Ultrastructure and Function. New York, Academic Press, 1973.

Chambers, T. J.: Studies on the phagocytic capacity of macrophage polykaryons. J. Pathol., *123*:65–77, 1977.

Issekutz, T. B., et al.: The *in vivo* quantitation and kinetics of monocyte migration into acute inflammatory tissue. Am. J. Pathol., *103*:47–55, 1981.

Jones, T. C.: Macrophages and intracellular parasitism. J. Reticuloendothel. Soc., *15*:439–450, 1974.

Kambara, T., et al.: The chemical mediation of delayed hypersensitivity skin reactions. Am. J. Pathol., *87*:359–370, 1977.

Lasser, A.: The mononuclear phagocytic system—a review. Hum. Pathol., *14*:108–126, 1983.

Mariano, M., and Spector, W. G.: The formation and properties of macrophage polykaryons (inflammatory giant cells). J. Pathol., *113*:1–19, 1974.

Nathan, C. F., et al.: The macrophage as an effector cell. New Engl. J. Med., *303*:622–626, 1980.

Nelson, D. S. (ed.): Immunobiology of the Macrophage. New York, Academic Press, 1976.

Papadimitriou, J. M.: Endocytosis and formation of macrophage polykarya: an ultrastructural study. J. Pathol., *126*:215–219, 1979.

Papadimitriou, J. M.: The role of resident and exudate macrophages in multinucleate giant cell formation. J. Pathol., *128*:93–97, 1979.

Papadimitriou, J. M., and Robertson, T. A.: Exocytosis by macrophage polykarya: an ultrastructural study. J. Pathol., *130*:75–81, 1980.

Papadimitriou, J. M., et al.: Kinetics of multinucleate giant cell formation and their modification by various agents in foreign reactions. Am. J. Pathol., *73*:349–361, 1973.

Rydgren, L., et al.: Lymphocyte locomotion. I. The initiation, velocity, pattern and path of locomotion *in vitro*. Lymphology, *9*:89–96, 1976.

Rydgren, L., et al.: Lymphocyte locomotion. II. The lymphocyte traffic over the post-capillary venules analysed by phase contrast microscopy of thin sections of rat lymph nodes. Lymphology, *9*:96–100, 1976.

Sainte-Marie, G.: Study on plasmocytopoiesis. I. Description of plasmocytes and of their mitoses in the mediastinal lymph nodes of ten-week-old rats. Am. J. Anat., *114*:207–223, 1964.

Sainte-Marie, G.: A critical analysis of the validity of the experimental basis of current concept of the mode of lymphocyte recirculation. Bull. Inst. Pasteur, *73*:255–279, 1975.

Spector, W. G.: The macrophage: its origins and role in pathology. Pathobiol. Annu., *4*:33–64, 1974.

Stossel, T. P.: Phagocytosis. N. Engl. J. Med., *290*:717–723, 774–780, 833–839, 1974.

Tanaka, A., et al.: Epithelioid granuloma formation requiring no T-cell function. Am. J. Pathol., *106*:165–170, 1982.

Unanue, E. R.: Secretory function of mononuclear phagocytes: a review. Am. J. Pathol., *83*:396–417, 1976.

Unanue, E. R.: Cooperation between mononuclear phagocytes and lymphocytes in immunity. N. Engl. J. Med., *303*:977–985, 1980.

Yoffey, J. M., and Courtice, F. C.: Lymphatics, Lymph and the Lymphomyeloid Complex. New York, Academic Press, 1970.

Tissue Injury

Bellanti, J. A.: Immunology II. 2nd ed. Philadelphia, W. B. Saunders Company, 1978.

Bernstein, T.: Effects of electricity and lightning on man and animals. J. Forensic Sci., *18*:3–11, 1973.

Cheville, N. F.: Environmental factors affecting the immune response of birds—a review. Avian Dis., *23*:308–314, 1979.

Cochrane, C. G.: Immunologic tissue injury mediated by neutrophilic leukocytes. Adv. Immunol., *9*:97–162, 1968.

Cohen, S.: The role of cell-mediated immunity in the induction of inflammatory responses. (Park-Davis Lecture.) Am. J. Pathol., *88*:502–528, 1977.

Crane, S. W.: Trauma. Vet. Clin. North Am. [Small Anim. Pract.], *10*:513–751, 1980.

Day, S. B.: Trauma: Clinical and Biological Aspects. New York, Plenum Publishers, 1975.

Dvorak, A. M., et al.: Morphology of delayed-type

hypersensitivity reactions in man. II. Ultrastructural alterations affecting the microvasculature and the tissue mast cells. Lab. Invest., *34*:179–191, 1976.

Eisenbrandt, D. L., and Phemister, R. D.: Radiation injury in the neonatal canine kidney. I. Pathogenesis. Lab. Invest., *37*:437–446, 1977.

Eyre, P.: Pharmacological aspects of hypersensitivity in domestic animals: a review. Vet. Res. Commun., *4*:83–98, 1980.

Garfield, E.: The hazards of sunbathing. Curr. Cont., *22*:8:5–12, 1979.

Howard-Flanders, P.: Physical and chemical mechanisms in the injury of cells by ionizing radiations. Adv. Biol. Med. Phys., *6*:553–603, 1958.

Kaltreider, H. B.: Expression of immune mechanisms in the lung. Am. Rev. Resp. Dis., *113*:347–379, 1976.

Kolata, R. J., et al.: Patterns of trauma in urban dogs and cats: a study of 1,000 cases. J. Am. Vet. Med. Assoc., *164*:499–502, 1974.

Krohn, K., et al.: Immunologic observations in canine interstitial nephritis. Am. J. Pathol., *65*:157–168, 1971.

Krum, S. H., and Osborne, C. A.: Heatstroke in the dog: a polysystemic disorder. J. Am. Vet. Med. Assoc., *170*:531–535, 1977.

LaJoie, R. J.: Post-electroshock syndrome. Industr. Med. Surg., *31*:354–359, 1962.

Leithead, C. S., and Lind, A. R. (eds.): Heatstroke and heat pyrexia. *In* Heat Stress and Heat Disorders. Philadelphia, F. A. Davis (Cassell), 1964.

Lewis, R. M., and Schwartz, R. S.: Canine systemic lupus erythematosus. J. Exp. Med., *134*:417–438, 1971.

McCluskey, R. T., and Klassen, J.: Immunologically mediated glomerular, tubular and interstitial renal disease. N. Engl. J. Med., *288*:564–570, 1973.

Movat, H. S.: Pathways to allergic inflammation: the sequelae of antigen-antibody complex formation. Fed. Proc., *35*:2435–2441, 1976.

Muller, H. K.: Mechanisms of clearing injured tissue. *In* Glynn, L. E. (ed.): Tissue Repair and Regeneration. Amsterdam, Elsevier North-Holland Biomedical Press, 1981, pp. 145–175.

Newton, C. D., et al.: Rheumatoid arthritis in dogs. J. Am. Vet. Med. Assoc., *168*:113–122, 1976.

Pedersen, N. C., et al.: Noninfectious canine arthritis: the inflammatory nonerosive arthritides. J. Am. Vet. Med. Assoc., *169*:304–310, 1976.

Perryman, L. E.: Primary and secondary immune deficiencies of domestic animals. Adv. Vet. Sci. Comp. Med., *23*:23–52, 1979.

Pryor, W. A. (ed.): Free Radicals in Biology. New York, Academic Press, 1982.

Samuelsson, B.: Leukotrienes: Mediators of immediate hypersensitivity reactions and inflammation. Science, *220*:568–575, 1983.

Scott, D. W., et al.: The comparative pathology of nonviral bullous skin diseases in domestic animals. Vet. Pathol., *17*:257–281, 1980.

Scott, D. W.: Observations on canine atopy. J. Am. Anim. Hosp. Assoc., *17*:91–100, 1981.

Slauson, D. O., and Lewis, R. M.: Comparative pathology of glomerulonephritis in animals. Vet. Pathol., *16*:135–164, 1979.

Slauson, D. O., et al.: The pulmonary vascular pathology of experimental radiation pneumonitis. Am. J. Pathol., *88*:635–654, 1977.

Solem, R., et al.: The natural history of electrical injury. J. Trauma, *17*:487–492, 1977.

Talal, N. (ed.): Autoimmunity: Genetic, Immunologic, Virologic and Clinical Aspects. New York, Academic Press, 1977.

Theofilopoulos, A. N., and Dixon, F. J.: Immune complexes in human diseases. A review. Am. J. Pathol., *100*:531–591, 1980.

Theofilopoulos, A. N., and Dixon, F. J.: Autoimmune diseases, immunology, and etiopathogenesis. Am. J. Pathol., *108*:321–365, 1982.

Tizard, I. R.: An Introduction to Veterinary Immunology. 2nd ed. Philadelphia, W. B. Saunders Company, 1982.

Vaes, G.: 1. Cellular secretion and tissue breakdown. Cell-to-cell interactions in the secretion of enzymes of connective tissue breakdown, collagenase and proteoglycan-degrading neutral proteases. A review. Agents Actions, *10*:474–485, 1980.

Watson, G. M.: The nature of radiation injury. Pathology, *12*:155–160, 1980.

Weissmann, G., et al.: Leukocytic proteases and the immunologic release of lysosomal enzymes. Am. J. Pathol., *68*:539–559, 1972.

Wilkie, B. N.: Bovine allergic pneumonitis: an acute outbreak associated with mouldy hay. Can. J. Comp. Med., *42*:10–15, 1978.

Witebsky, E., et al.: Spontaneous thyroiditis in the obese strain of chickens. I. Demonstration of circulating autoantibodies. J. Immunol., *103*:708–715, 1969.

Zaleznik, D. F., and Kasper, D. L.: The role of anaerobic bacteria in abscess formation. Ann. Rev. Med., *33*:217–229, 1982.

Repair

Auerbach, R. : Angiogenesis-inducing factors: a review. Lymphokines, *4*:69–86, 1981.

Brandes, D., and Anton, E.: Lysosomes in uterine involution: intracytoplasmic degradation of myofilaments and collagen. J. Gerontol., *24*:55–69, 1969.

Bullough, W. S., et al.: The vertebrate epidermal chalone. Nature, *214*:578–580, 1967.

Chvapil, M.: Pharmacology of fibrosis: definitions, limits and perspectives. Life Sci., *16*:1345–1362, 1976.

Chvapil, M., et al.: Dynamics of the healing of skin wounds in the horse as compared with the rat. Exp. Mol. Pathol., *30*:349–359, 1979.

Gabbiani, G., and Montandon, D.: Reparative processes in mammalian wound healing: the role of contractile phenomena. Int. Rev. Cytol., *48*:187–219, 1977.

Gabbiani, G., et al.: Granulation tissue as a contractile organ: a study of structure and function. J. Exp. Med., *135*:719–734, 1972.

Gibbins, J. R.: Migration of stratified squamous epithelium *in vivo*. The development of phagocytic ability. Am. J. Pathol., *53*:929–941, 1968.

Gillman, T.: On some aspects of collagen formation in localized repair and in diffuse fibrotic reactions to injury. *In* Gould, B. S. (ed.): Treatise on Collagen. Vol. 2, Part B. Biology of Collagen. New York, Academic Press, 1968, pp. 331–409.

Glynn, L. F. (ed.): Tissue Repair and Regeneration: Handbook of Inflammation. Vol. 3. New York, Elsevier North-Holland Biomedical Press, 1981.

Hell, E., and Lawrence, J. C.: The initiation of epidermal wound healing in cuts and burns. Br. J. Exp. Pathol., *60*:171–179, 1979.

Knapp, T. R., et al.: Pathologic scar formation (morphologic and biochemical correlates). Am. J. Pathol., *86*:47–63, 1977.

Majno, G.: The Healing Hand. Man and Wound in the Ancient World. Cambridge, Harvard University Press, 1977.

McMinn, R. M. H.: Tissue Repair. New York, Academic Press, 1969.

Ordman, L. J., and Gillman, T.: Studies in the healing of cutaneous wounds. Arch. Surg., *93*:857–928, 1966.

Peacock, E. E., and Van Winkle, W.: Wound Repair. 2nd ed. Philadelphia, W. B. Saunders Company, 1976.

Popper, H., and Udenfriend, S.: Hepatic fibrosis. Correlation of biochemical and morphologic investigations. Am. J. Med., *49*:707–721, 1970.

Ross, R., and Benditt, E. P.: Wound healing and collagen formation. J. Biophys. Biochem. Cytol., *11*:677–700, 1961.

Sholley, M. M., et al.: Endothelial proliferation in inflammation. Am. J. Pathol., *89*:277–290, 1977.

Shoshan, S.: Wound healing. Int. Rev. Conn. Tiss. Res., *9*:1–26, 1981.

Silver, I. A.: The mechanics of wound healing. Equine Vet. J., *11*:93–96, 1979.

Smith, Q. T.: Collagen metabolism in wound healing. *In* Day, S. B. (ed.): Trauma: Clinical and Biological Aspects. New York, Plenum Publishers, 1975, pp. 31–45.

TenCate, A. R., and Deporter, D. A.: The degradative role of the fibroblast in remodelling and turnover of collagen in soft connective tissue. Anat. Rec., *182*:1–14, 1974.

Van Winkle, W.: The tensile strength of wounds and factors that influence it. Surg. Gynecol. Obstet., *129*:819–842, 1969.

Walton, G. S., and Neal, P. A.: Observations on wound healing in the horse (the role of wound contraction). Equine Vet. J., *4*:i–v, 1971.

5

DISTURBANCES OF GROWTH

AGENESIS, APLASIA, ATRESIA
HYPOPLASIA
ATROPHY
HYPERTROPHY
HYPERPLASIA
DYSPLASIA
METAPLASIA
ANOMALIES OR MALFORMATIONS
CYTOGENETICS
AGING

Disturbances of growth include a broad category of lesions that in general refer to ***excess growth, deficient growth*** or ***abnormal patterns of growth*** in a tissue or an organ. Although it is a disturbance of growth, neoplasia has been excluded here and will be discussed in a later chapter. In general terms, disturbances of growth usually involve the following factors: the ***number*** of cells in a tissue or an organ, the ***size*** of the cells, a ***combination of the number and size*** of the cells and a change from the normal in the ***relationship*** of cells or tissues to each other. ***Lesions associated with these changes are very common and require accurate interpretation.*** The terms used to name some of the lesions are derived from the Greek words ***troph,*** meaning nutrition, and ***plasia,*** meaning to form.

This area of study is so large that only definitions and principles will be discussed; examples will be cited. All anomalies and nutritional disorders fall within this general area. Without mentioning each specifically, the effects of most will be covered by the topics included in this chapter.

AGENESIS, APLASIA, ATRESIA

Agenesis, aplasia, hypoplasia and atresia refer to reduced growth and imply anomalous development. They can occur in any organ, and the references at the end of this chapter cite many examples. ***Agenesis*** means that the tissue or organ did not develop and is absent; for example, one kidney might be absent at birth. ***Aplasia*** means that the organ is present but is markedly reduced in size from normal. An example is the absence of the gonads or of one horn of the uterus; when it occurs in a localized region of a tubular structure it is referred to as ***segmental aplasia. Aplastic*** is sometimes used to mean that there is no tendency to form new tissue, as in failure to regenerate bone marrow in aplastic anemia. When the term is used in this context, the lesion is not a congenital anomaly. ***Atresia*** means absence, or closure, of a normal opening; for example, absence of a continuous lumen of the intestine is called intestinal atresia. If the anus is absent, which occurs in pigs, the lesion is called atresia ani.

HYPOPLASIA

Hypoplasia means incomplete growth and is an anomaly. A range of incomplete growth occurs, and the term refers to anything from just short of normal development to agenesis. If often is used in place of agenesis and aplasia, since their meanings do overlap. As mentioned earlier, segmental aplasia and atresia tend to indicate a localized anomaly in an organ rather than an anomaly of a whole organ. By definition, hypoplasia means that the tissue or organ did ***not reach its normal size or structure*** and differs from a situation in which the organ achieved normal growth but later decreased in size. ***Hypoplastic*** lesions are common, and the best known perhaps are hypoplastic cerebellum, hypoplastic kidney and hypoplastic testes (Fig. 5–1). The reasons why the lesion occurs are usually not known but a possible explanation is failure of organizers to coordinate functions and structures in embryonic development, either by accident or by absence of the normal genetic coding. Cerebellar hypoplasia, however, may be caused by viral infection of the fetus ***in utero*** through agents that particularly affect rapidly dividing cells at key points in development. The neural cells are killed, resulting in the absence of groups of cells at birth, and this in turn may result in either marked reduction in the size of the cerebellum or variations in its size up to normal. The viruses responsible for panleukopenia in cats and bovine virus diarrhea in cattle cause such lesions, and no doubt other examples await elucidation (Fig. 5–2). These are examples of disease conditions that were once thought to be genetically controlled; infection was not considered to be an etiological factor.

The results of all of these lesions referring to reduced growth are ***decreased function and lack of normal functional reserve*** (Figs. 5–3 and 5–4). Terminal renal disease in a young dog usually is an indication of renal hypoplasia and the lack of functional reserve. Hypoplastic testes may be obviously small but may also have normal gross appearance and defects in the final stages of sperm development that result in deficient functional reserve or abnormal sperm, depending upon the type of lesion present.

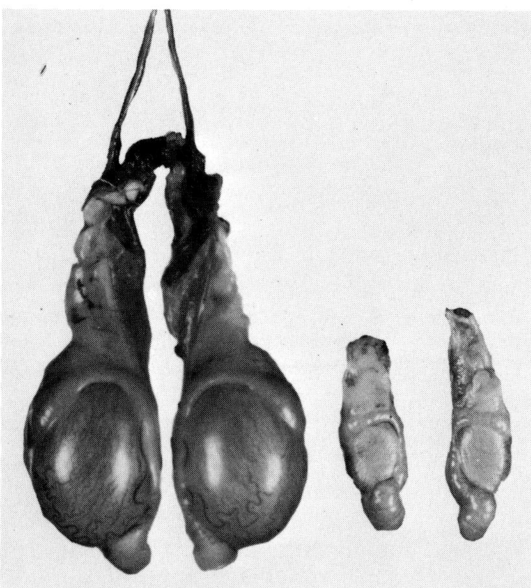

Figure 5–1. Hypoplasia of testes in goats. Normal on the left and hypoplastic on the right, from goats of similar ages. (Courtesy of C. A. V. Barker.)

ATROPHY

Atrophy means a decrease in the amount of tissue ***after*** normal growth has been achieved and as such is ***distinct from hypoplasia.*** Any tissue may atrophy and the cause is usually reduced number or size of cells or a combination of the two. These situations usually involve deficient nutritive supply to an area, lack of innervation, necrosis of cells, pressure, disuse or, in the case of endocrine glands, defective feedback mechanisms. A withered limb is the result of ***denervation atrophy,*** which is a classic response of muscle to denervation. Individual fibers become smaller and eventually disappear (Fig. 5–5). If necrosis of cells occurs slowly and diffusely in an organ, an imbalance between loss and replacement may occur and the organ will become

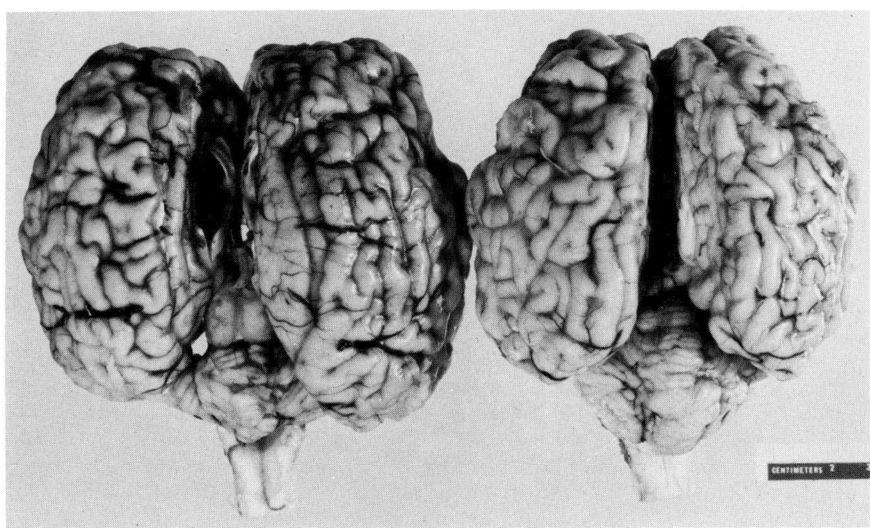

Figure 5–2. Cerebellar hypoplasia in the brain of a calf on the left, with a normal brain on the right for comparison.

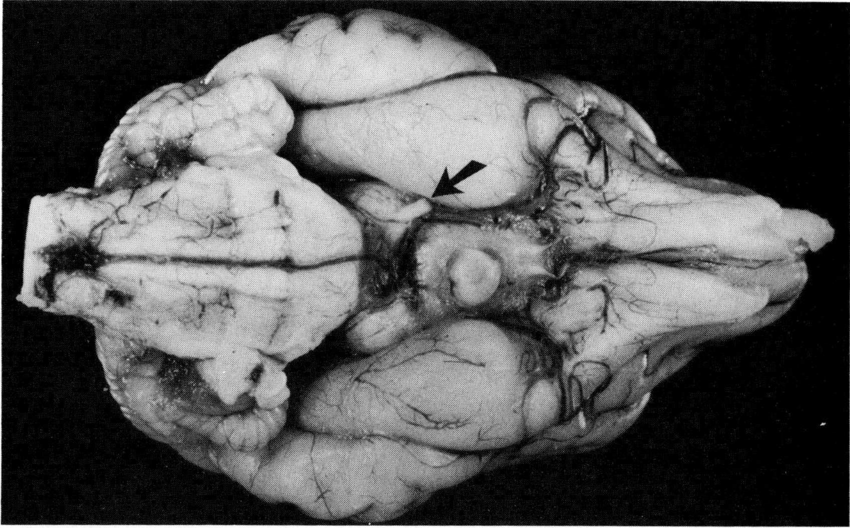

Figure 5–3. Congenital hypoplasia of the optic nerve in a dog. Note that only one optic nerve is present (arrow). (Courtesy of B. Schiefer.)

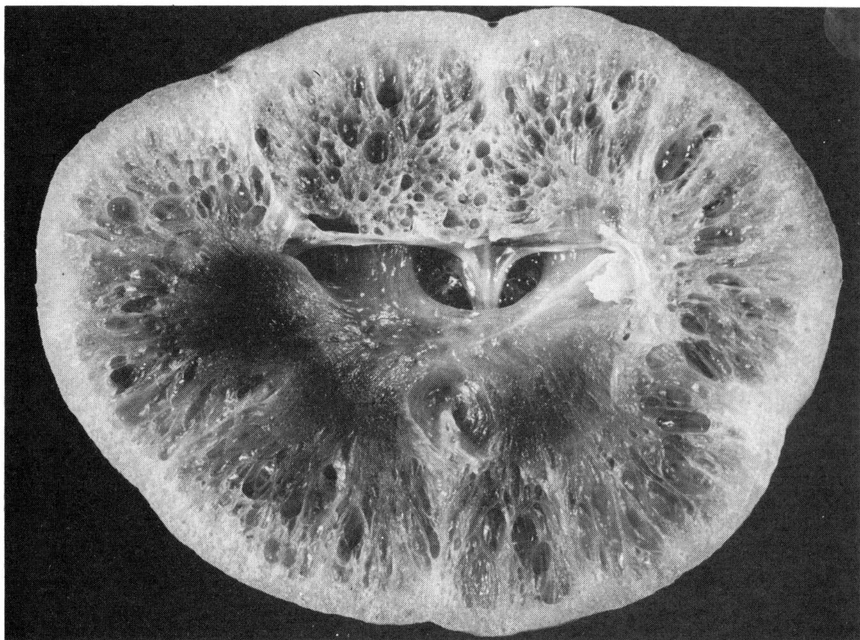

Figure 5–4. Congenital polycystic kidney in a cat. Uremia develops at a young age. (Courtesy of N. O. Nielsen.)

smaller. If normal loss of cells occurs and replacement is impaired by ***nutritive inadequacy,*** the organ may also become smaller. The involution of the normal corpus luteum may be considered atrophy. Pressure may also result in a slow localized loss of cells through degeneration and necrosis, as when an expanding testicular tumor presses on surrounding seminiferous tubules, causing ***pressure atrophy*** (Fig. 5–6). Keeping a limb in a cast will result in ***disuse atrophy*** because the muscle fibers become uniformly reduced in size as a result of inactivity. If thyrotropin is not available from the pituitary gland, the thyroid will atrophy (Fig. 5–7); if adrenocorticotropic hormone (ACTH) is reduced or absent, the adrenal cortex will atrophy (Fig.5–8). These two conditions are significant clinical problems in dogs. Adrenal cortical atrophy also occurs following

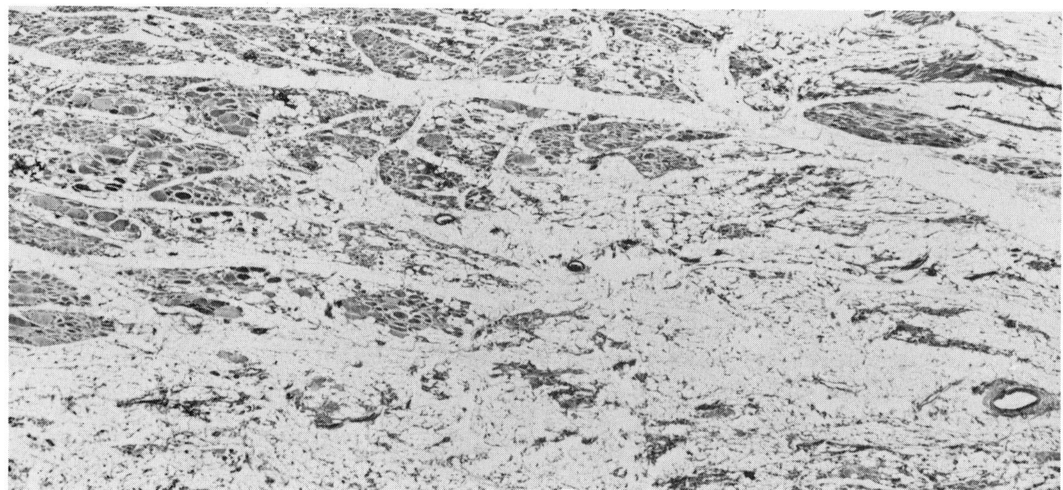

Figure 5–5. Neurogenic atrophy in skeletal muscle. Note the variation in size of muscle fibers and complete loss of fibers from some areas of the tissue.

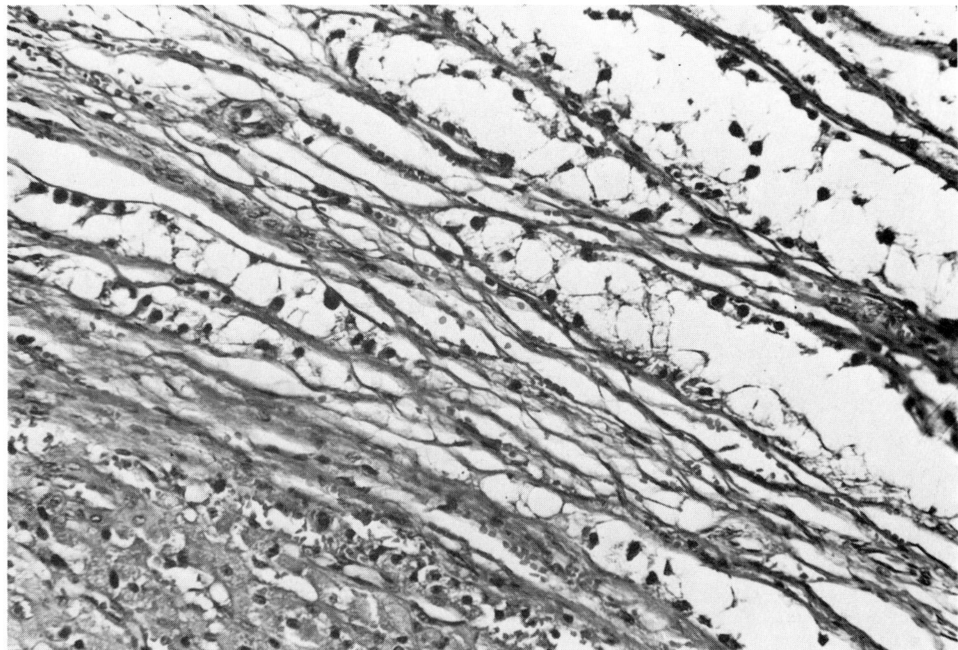

Figure 5–6. Pressure atrophy in the testicle of a dog with an interstitial cell tumor. The tumor is at the lower left. Pressure from the tumor is slowly causing degeneration and necrosis of seminiferous epithelium with subsequent collapse of the tubules. The collapsed stroma gives the impression of a capsule.

prolonged steroid therapy, during which the products of the adrenal gland are not needed and it atrophies. Also, a functional tumor in the cortex of one adrenal gland may produce so much hormone that atrophy occurs in the other gland. The discoverers of insulin tied off the pancreatic duct in dogs, and all acinar tissue underwent complete atrophy or ***involution,*** allowing a clean harvest of insulin from the islets. This type of atrophy tends to occur in glands drained by ducts. Metabolic disorders in bone may lead to atrophy of bone spicules and osteoporosis (Fig. 5–9). Malabsorption syndromes usually result from short atrophic intestinal villi, a lesion that may be caused by many different etiological factors (Fig. 5–10).

Serous atrophy of fat is a very important lesion to recognize during postmortem examination because it is an indication of ***emaciation*** and may therefore be the most significant lesion in an animal in terms of the immediate cause of death. The fat depots of the body are used up and all that remains is a clear or yellowish edematous or gelatinous material. ***The loss of fat from fat depots*** is the most significant finding. The lesion, therefore, is most evident on the heart and around the kidneys, as well as in mesenteries, which are all prominent normal fat depots. Serous atrophy of fat is an indication of what has happened but not why it happened and therefore is a nonspecific lesion. The etiology could be malnutrition, chronic infection, neoplasia, parasit-

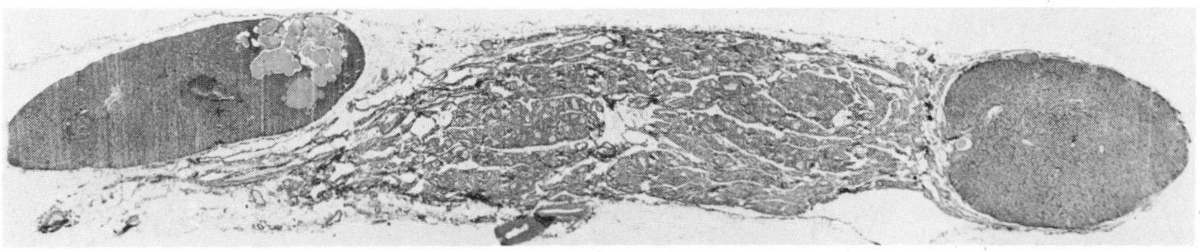

Figure 5–7. Thyroid gland of a dog in the middle, with parathyroids at each end. The thyroid is atrophic and the parathyroids may be hypertrophic.

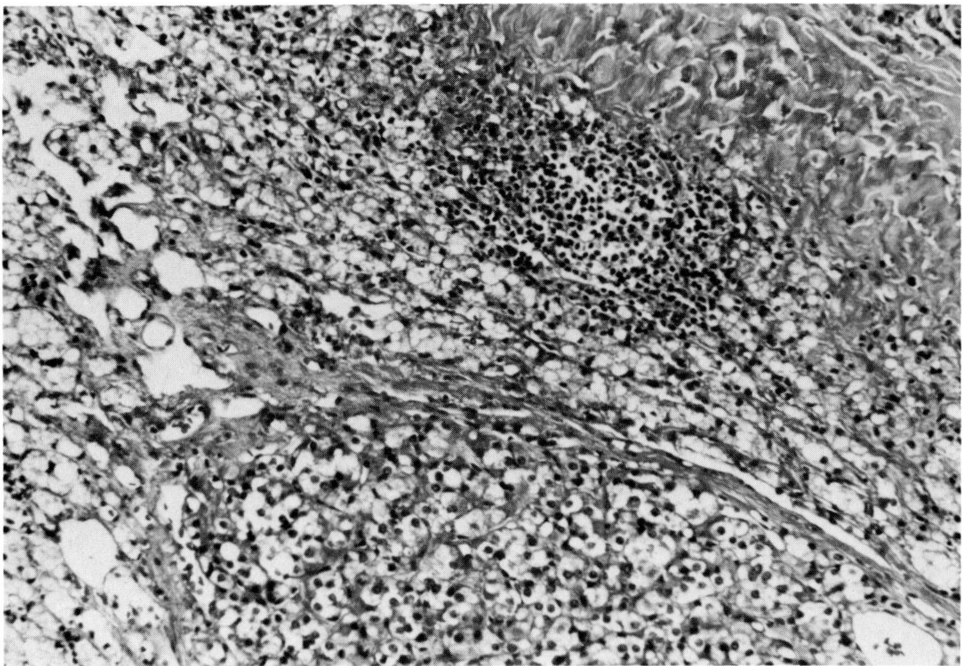

Figure 5–8. Adrenal gland in a dog. The capsule of connective tissue is at the top right and the medulla is at the bottom. Between the two is the markedly reduced atrophic cortex, which contains islands of lymphocytes. The normal medulla is at the lower middle.

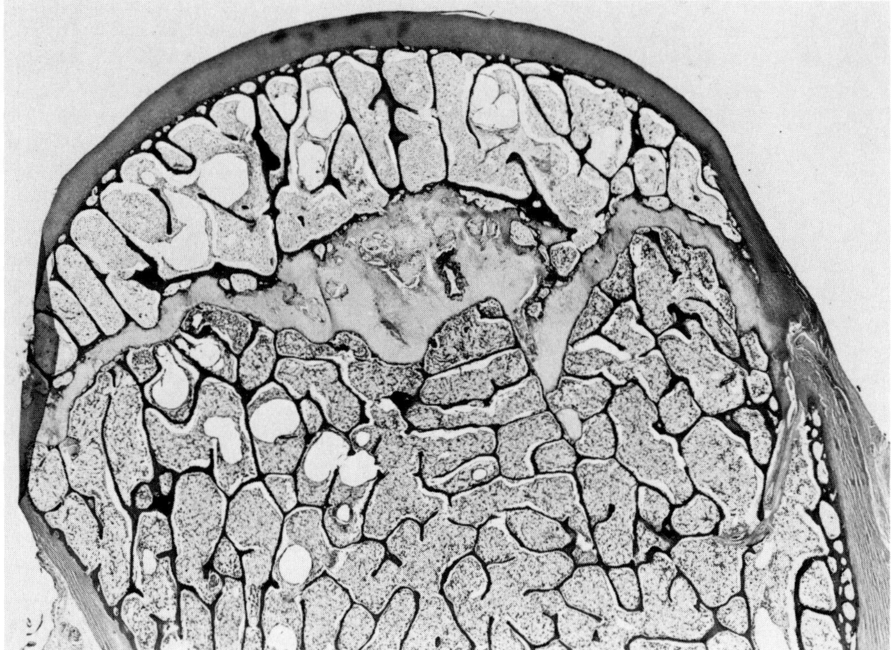

Figure 5–9. Bone of a pig. Note the irregularly shaped epiphyseal plate and reduction in size and number of bone spicules. Such atrophy of bone is called osteoporosis.

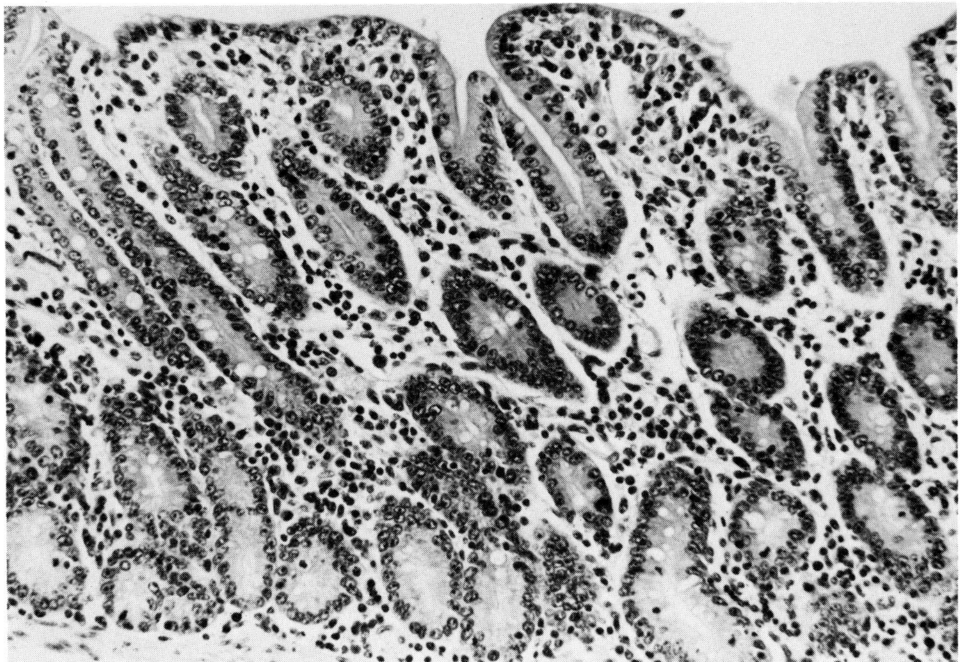

Figure 5–10. Small intestine having very short atrophic villi with flattened epithelium at the surface. Such lesions would lead to a malabsorption syndrome.

ism or many other conditions. ***Very often, the lesion is overlooked,*** especially in young animals.

HYPERTROPHY

Hypertrophy is an increase in tissue resulting from an increase in the ***size of individual cells.*** There is a range of normal physiological responses to be considered before the enlargement is noticeable as a lesion. The response of endocrine glands to excess stimulation involves, in part, hypertrophy of cells, which in turn may enlarge the organ. If part of an organ or one of a pair of organs (such as the kidneys) is lost, ***compensatory hypertrophy*** may occur in the remaining part or organ. The thickness of one of the ventricles in the heart may increase markedly in response to increased function, and this is called ventricular hypertrophy, a common lesion. The myocytes of the heart may double in size in a few days, as has been demonstrated by partial aortic occlusion close to the heart; the organelles retain normal proportions within these myocytes. Increase in muscle mass through exercise is hypertrophy of individual fibers. Physiological hypertrophy occurs in the uterus during pregnancy. The word hypertrophy is used for lesions in which there is more of a change than just an increase in the size of cells and tends to be used for any ***gross enlargement of an organ*** (Figs. 5–11 and 5–12).

HYPERPLASIA

Hyperplasia means an increase in the number of cells in a tissue or an organ and is a common lesion. Hyperplasia increases the size of a tissue or part of a tissue that, when observed grossly, might be considered hypertrophic. Thus, there is a degree of variability when using hypertrophy and hyperplasia for gross lesions, but there should be less when using them for microscopic lesions (Figs. 5–13 and 5–14). Other examples of hyperplasia are present in Figures 5–15 through 5–25. There may be a relatively uniform increase in the number of cells in an organ, perhaps combined with cellular hypertrophy, that will markedly increase the size of an organ, as in the case of a thyroid gland with a ***diffuse*** goiter. On the other hand, increase in the number of

Text continued on page 295

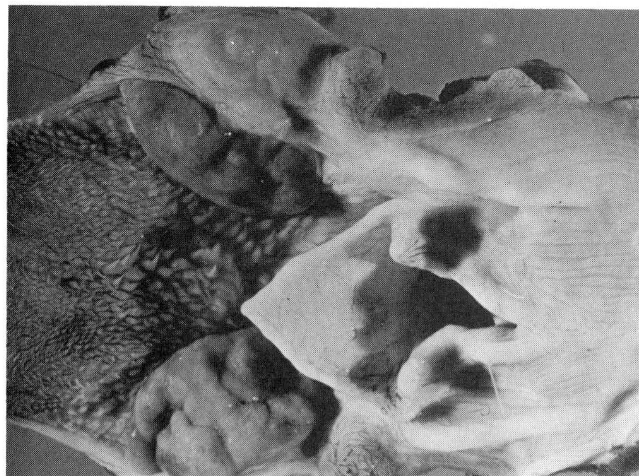

Figure 5–11. Hypertrophy of the tonsils in a dog. The enlargement is probably due to hyperplasia of lymphocytes.

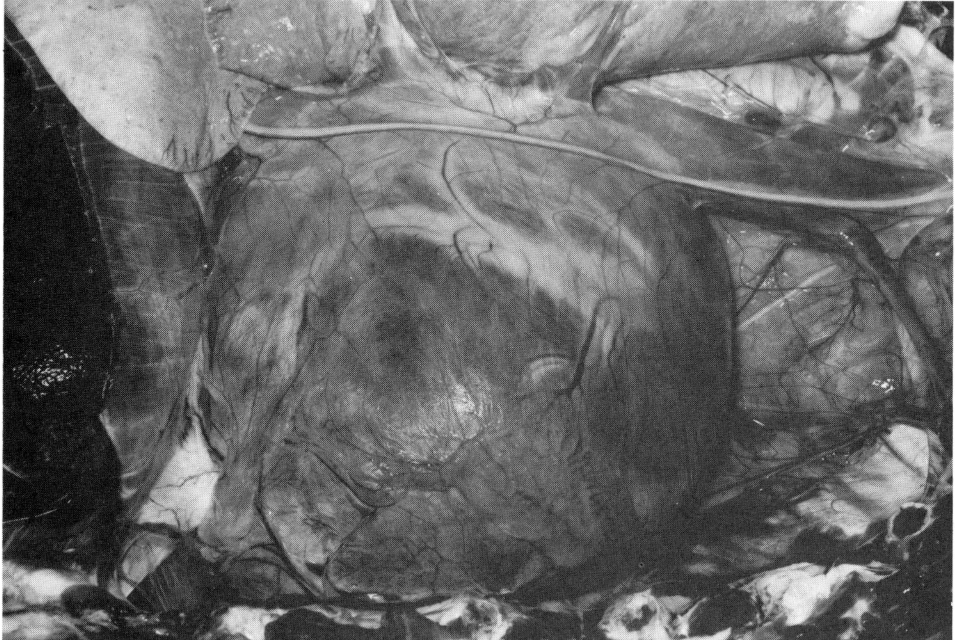

Figure 5–12. An enlarged globose-shaped heart in a dog. The heart may have hypertrophied ventricular walls or thin ventricular walls, but the entire heart is enlarged and this is called hypertrophy of the heart as a whole.

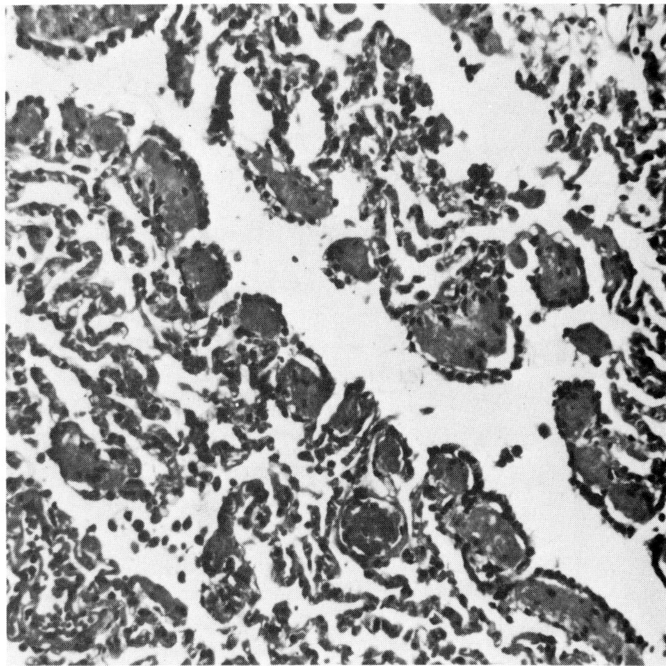

Figure 5–13. Fibromuscular hypertrophy and hyperplasia in alveolar ducts in a dog's lung. A closer view is shown in Figure 5–14. The structures are visibly enlarged and are probably a combination of hypertrophy and hyperplasia at the cellular level.

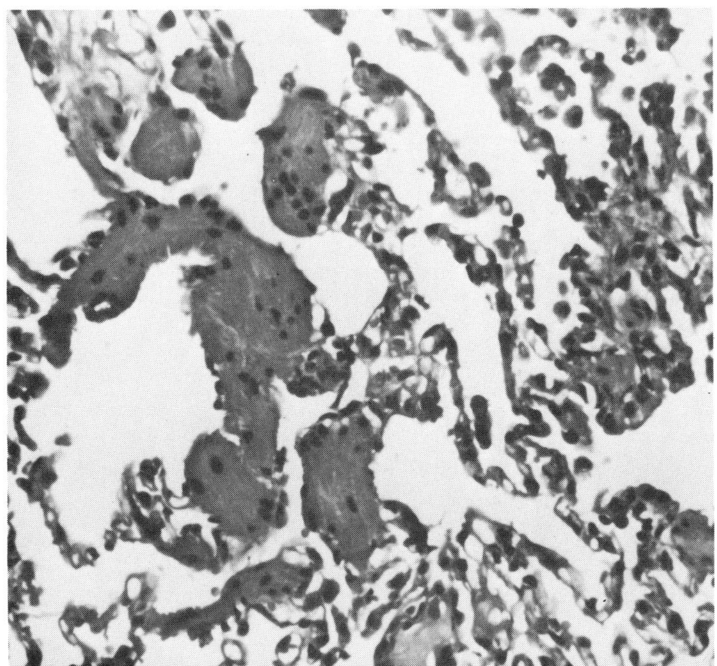

Figure 5–14. See the legend for Figure 5–13.

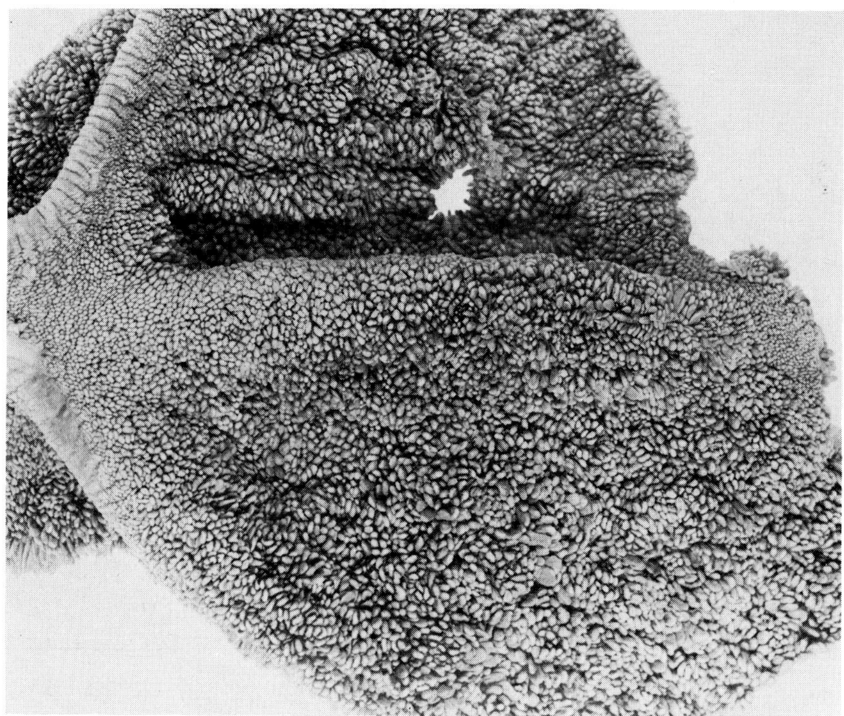

Figure 5–15. Enlargement of the rumen villi in a calf (hypertrophy) caused by excess accumulation of keratinized epithelium (Fig. 5–16), which is called hyperkeratosis. The basic lesion is hyperplasia of epithelium with retention of the upper layers and is caused by inadequate roughage in the diet.

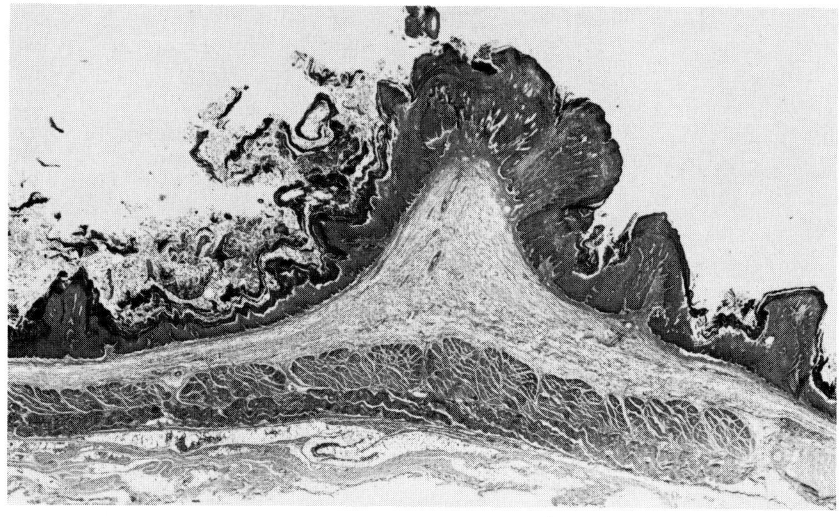

Figure 5–16. See the legend for Figure 5–15.

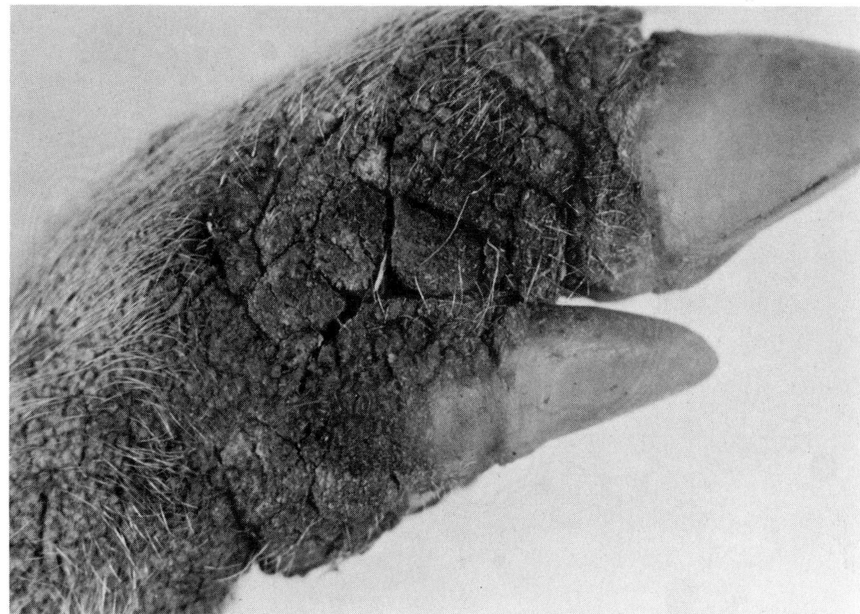

Figure 5–17

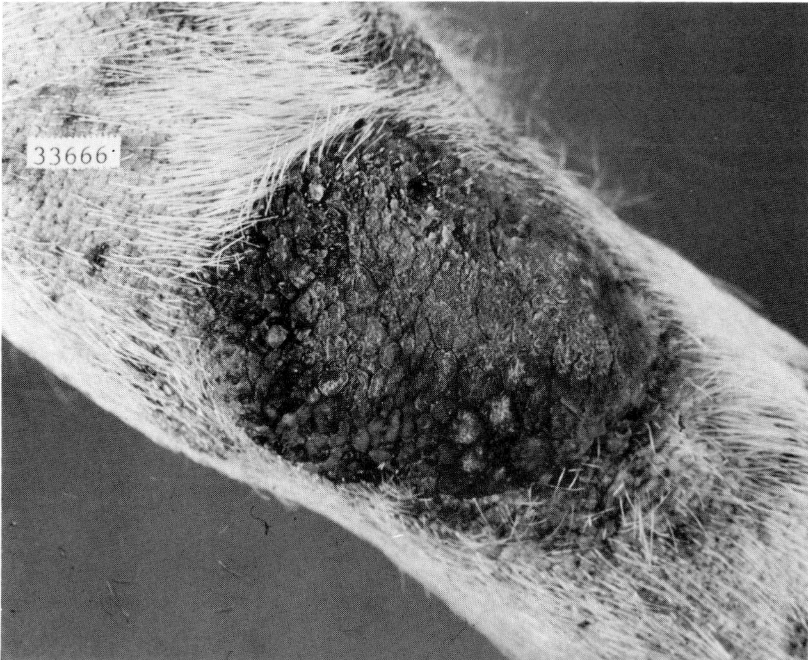

Figure 5–18

Figures 5–17 and 5–18. Hyperkeratosis or hyperplasia of the keratinized layer of epithelium in a pig caused by irritation from sarcoptic mange (Fig. 5–17) and, in another case in which a callus has developed from contact with a rough hard floor (Fig. 5–18).

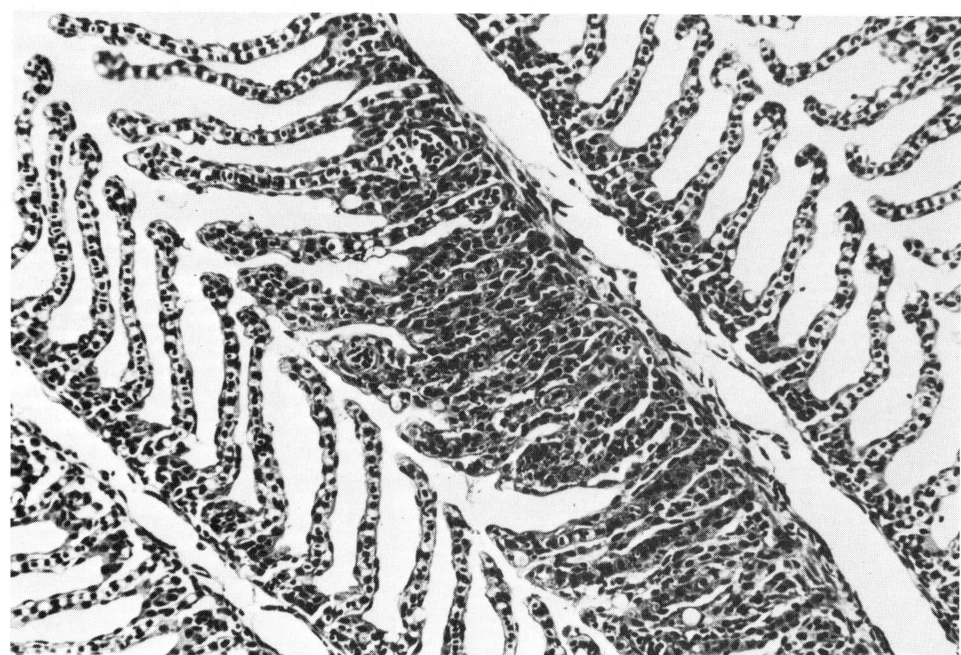

Figure 5–19. Hyperplasia of surface epithelium in the gills of a fish that causes the gills to thicken and fuse (Fig. 5–20). Oxygen exchange is markedly impaired in such a lesion.

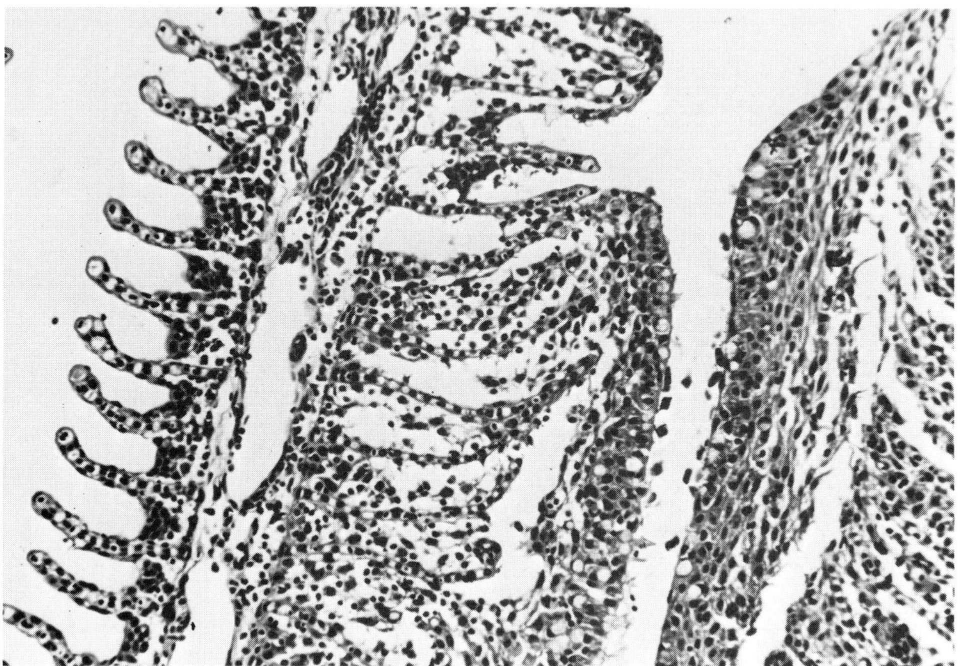

Figure 5–20. See the legend for Figure 5–19.

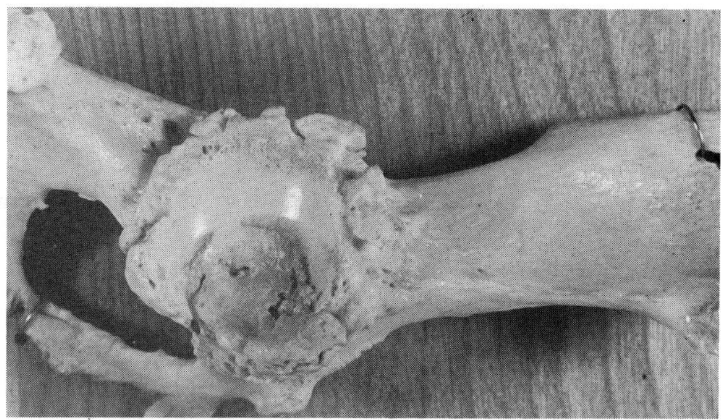

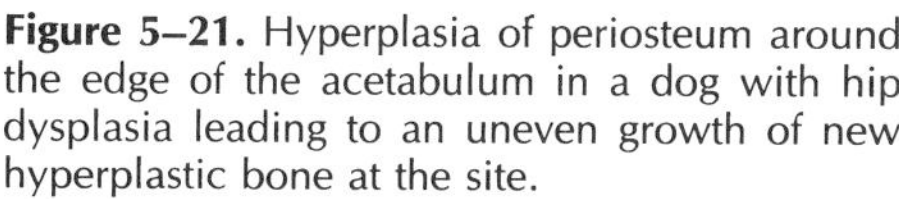

Figure 5–21. Hyperplasia of periosteum around the edge of the acetabulum in a dog with hip dysplasia leading to an uneven growth of new hyperplastic bone at the site.

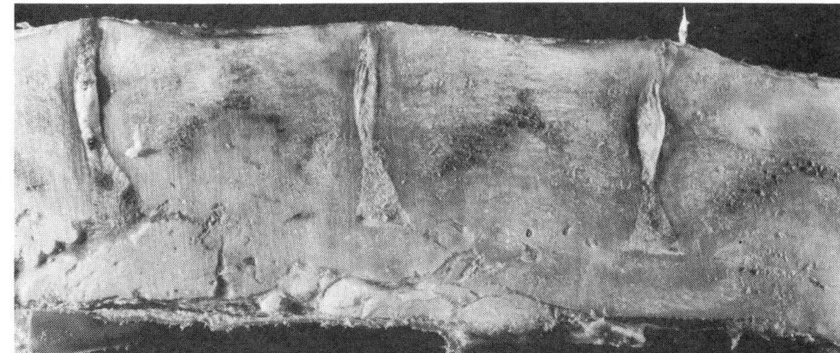

Figure 5–22. More extensive new growth of bone due to periosteal hyperplasia below the intervertebral space and along the ventral surface of the lumbar vertebral bodies in a midsaggital section of the spine of a bull with spondylosis.

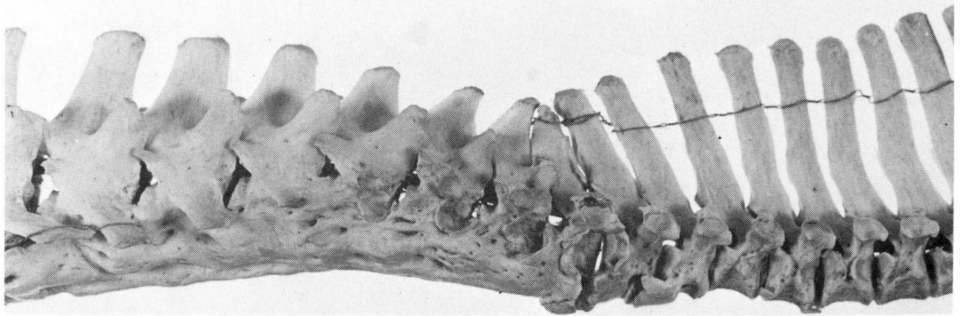

Figure 5–23. Varying degrees of periosteal new bone and bridging of intervertebral spaces in a dog. This lesion is similar to that shown in Figure 5–22 but demonstrates the lesion from the outside of the spine.

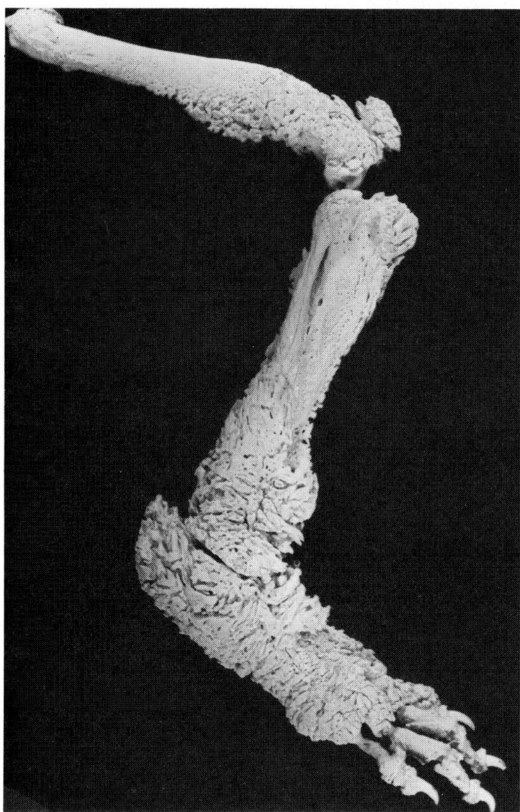

Figure 5–24. Extensive periosteal hyperplasia and production of new bone in the distal extremity of a dog's limb. This unusual lesion is caused by a space-occupying lesion in the thoracic cavity. (Courtesy of B. Schiefer.)

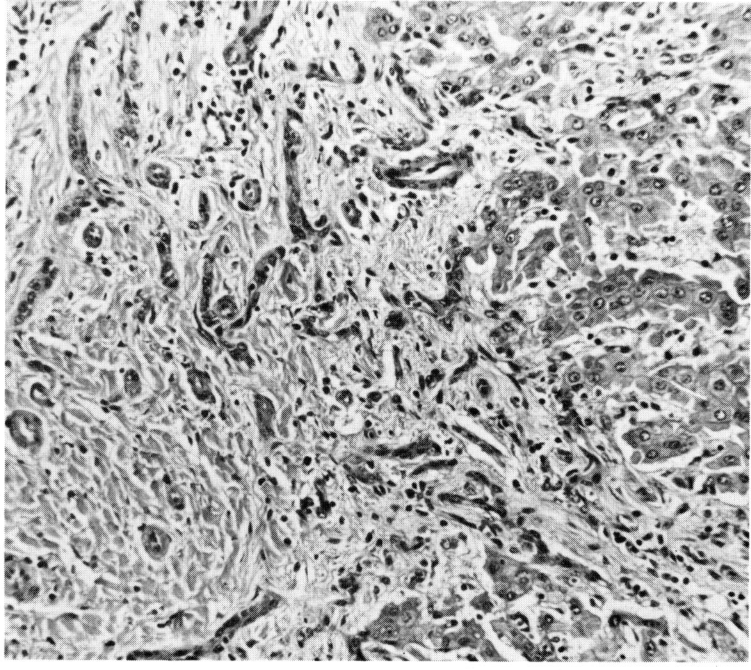

Figure 5–25. Hyperplasia of small bile ducts and of fibrous tissue in the interlobular area in a liver. Both are due to chronic inflammation.

cells may occur in a localized area within an organ and result in a localized nodule of new cells called ***nodular hyperplasia.*** Nodular hyperplasia may occur without known explanation and is common in the spleen and pancreas of old dogs. It is also common in the adrenal cortex, prostate gland and mammary glands of dogs. There is evidence that high fat–low protein diets result in a combination of nodular hyperplasia and atrophy of fatty areas to produce a small nodular liver, which is a common lesion in old dogs (Figs. 5–26 through 5–30).

In a secretory mucous membrane such as that lining the uterus, hyperplasia may result in focal folding of the epithelial lining because the increased number of cells causes the line of cells to bend. These foldings may expand to make space for more cells and may cause great thickening of the mucosa. In such situations, secretions are also increased but the folding of glands within the mucosa impairs the flow of secretions to the surface. These secretions accumulate and cause distention of some of the glands within the mucosa. These enlarging areas of retained secretion resemble ***retention cysts*** and the whole process is called ***cystic hyperplasia*** (Figs. 5–31 through 5–35). The usual cause of such lesions is excess or abnormal endocrine stimulation or markedly increased functional demands but is ***reversible*** if the etiological factors are withdrawn. In extreme cases, the tissue may not return to its normal morphological state. In addition, both hypertrophy and hyperplasia are present in neoplasms.

The extent of hyperplasia in an entire tissue is often not appreciated when examining selected pieces at random. The paper by Cameron and Faulkin (1971) describes ***all*** lesions in the mammary glands of eight beagles that were eight years old. These investigators found a total of 742 atypical nodules. Of these, 51 were inflammatory and 94 were neoplastic. There were 100 hyperplastic lobules with normal cellular proportions and 396 with disproportionate proliferative changes that could be considered as dysplasia, although they did not use this term. Of the 396, 31 were focal and 365 were diffuse epithelial lesions. Many of the hyperplastic lesions were probably preneoplastic. These findings also suggest that a tumor may not arise from just one lobule but perhaps develops from several.

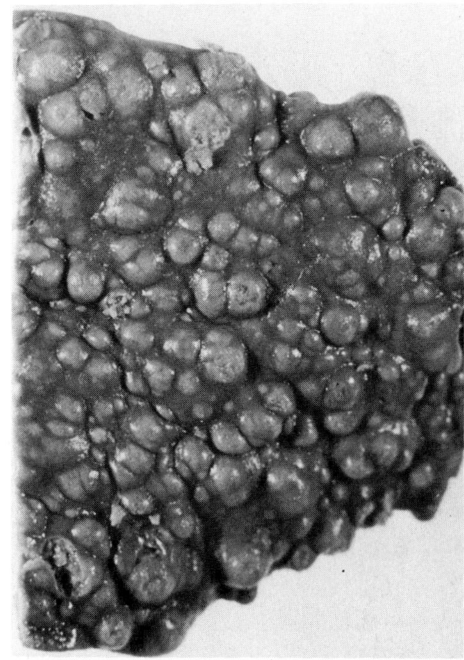

Figure 5–26. Nodular hyperplasia in a dog's liver.

Hypertrophy and hyperplasia are also used in the context of functional units in organs. Certain structures occur in fixed species-specified numbers; they can grow in size but their numbers are ***determinate.*** Hairs, feathers, villi and glands in the gut are examples. They may be replaced if lost, but their total population is fixed. Some structures can be neither replaced nor multiplied, such as neurons and striated muscle fibers. The ***functional units*** of the kidneys (nephrons) and of the lungs (alveoli) may increase by hypertrophy of the functional units through hyperplasia of individual cells, but new units are not formed.

Some normal organs never lose the ability to make new ***functional units,*** such as osteons, blood cells and endocrine cells. These are termed ***indeterminate units.*** Some of the most vital components of the body (heart, brain, kidneys, lungs) cannot produce new units. Since these organs work constantly, they cannot respond to functional demands by forming new units because the number of units might multiply in an uncontrolled manner. They appear to have given up the potential for hyperplasia of units in favor of the necessity for constant function. Those structures that may undergo hyperplasia are thought to be regulated by functional demands (Fig. 5–36).

Text continued on page 298

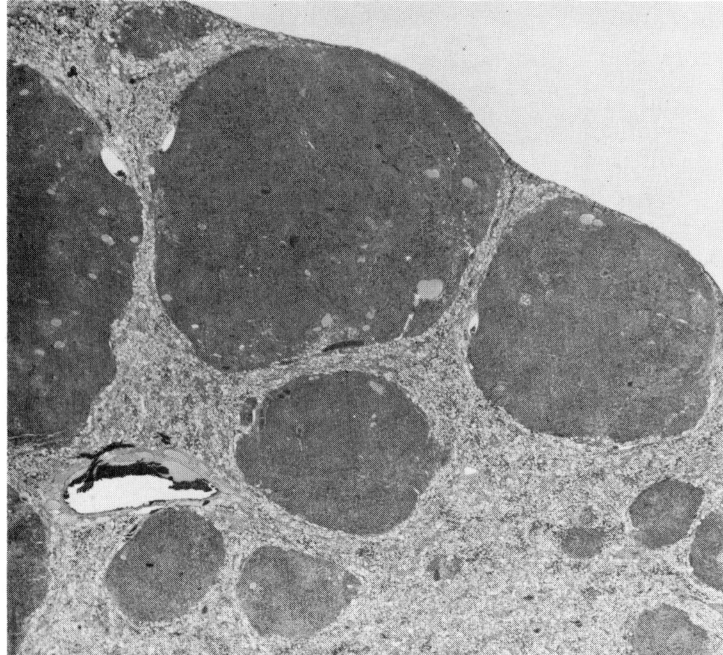

Figure 5–27. Lesion similar to that shown in Figure 5–26.

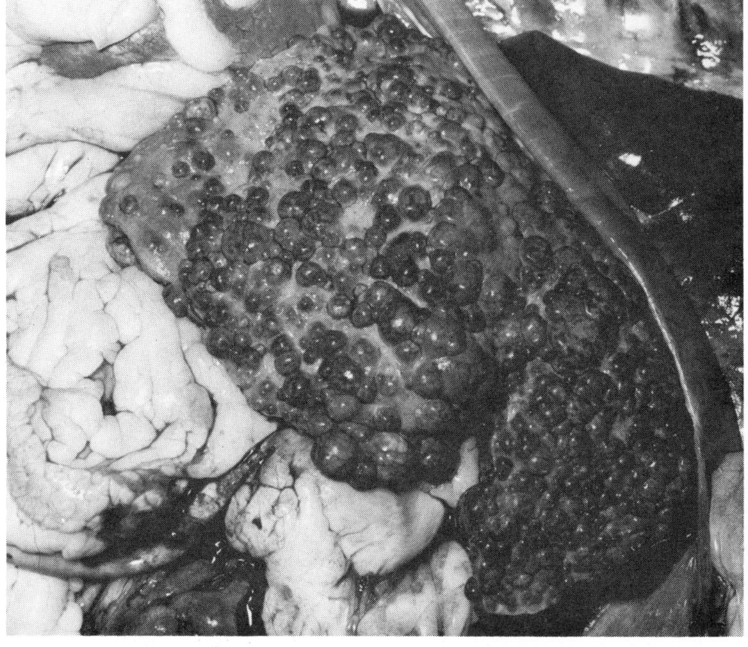

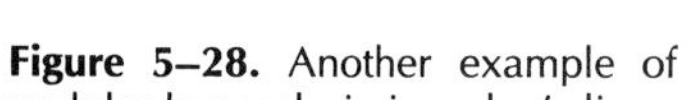

Figure 5–28. Another example of nodular hyperplasia in a dog's liver.

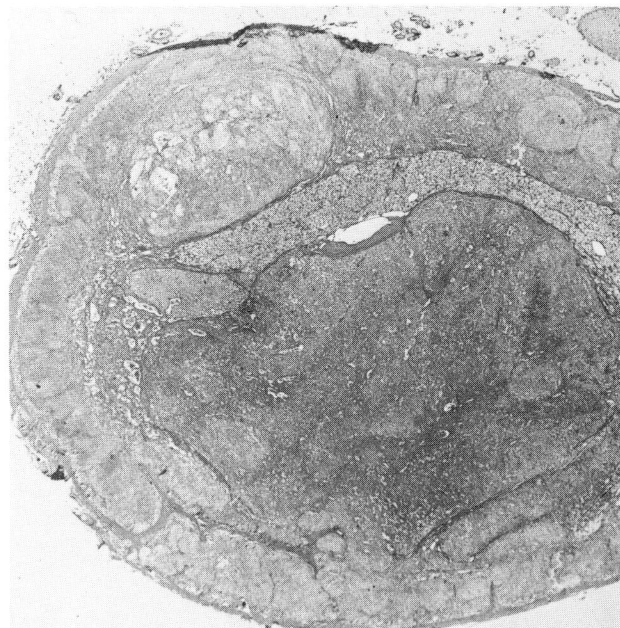

Figure 5–29. Nodular hyperplasia of the adrenal cortex in a cow. One large nodule fills most of the medulla.

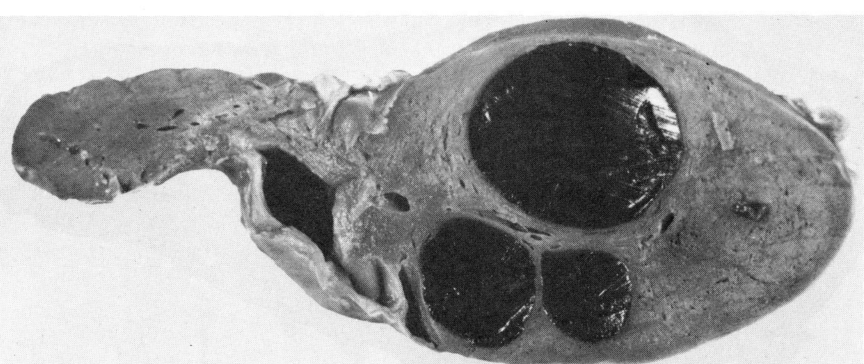

Figure 5–30. Hyperplasia in a dolphin's adrenal gland, in which the centers of some nodules contain fluid that is in part secretion and in part hemorrhage. This is a more extensive lesion than that shown in Figure 5–29. (Courtesy of J. R. Geraci.)

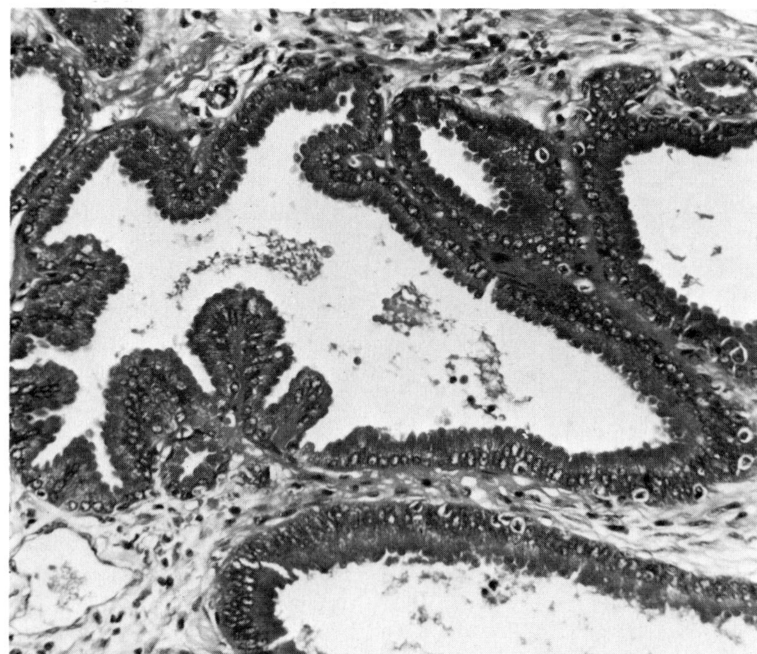

Figure 5–31. Hyperplasia of acinar epithelium in the prostate of a dog.

DYSPLASIA

Dysplasia refers to a microscopic lesion in which there is a loss of normal architectural orientation of cells or a loss in uniformity of individual cells or both. It usually is used with reference to epithelium. Dysplasia means an ***abnormally developed tissue*** and may refer to an anomaly, as in renal dysplasia. It may also refer to the organization of the tissue in an acquired growth change in areas in which the general architecture is recognizable but abnormalities exist either diffusely or focally. For example, the size of acinar units and the arrangement and appearance of cells within acini of a gland may vary from normal. ***Dysplastic cells vary in size, shape and staining characteristics.*** Within a multilayered epithelial lining, ***the arrangement of cells to each other*** may vary and the cells may develop an anaplastic appearance (Fig. 5–37). This example of dysplasia may be a form of hyperplasia and hypertrophy and could, depending on the location, be a preneoplastic lesion. Dysplasia is associated with chronic irritation and inflammation but may be due to nutritional disorders (Fig. 5–38). It is considered reversible if the etiological factor is withdrawn (Fig. 5–39). ***Dysplasia and hyperplasia may progress to a truly neoplastic appearance.*** If such a lesion has not broken through the basement membrane, it is called a ***carcinoma in situ,*** which is an intraepithelial tumor (Fig. 5–40).

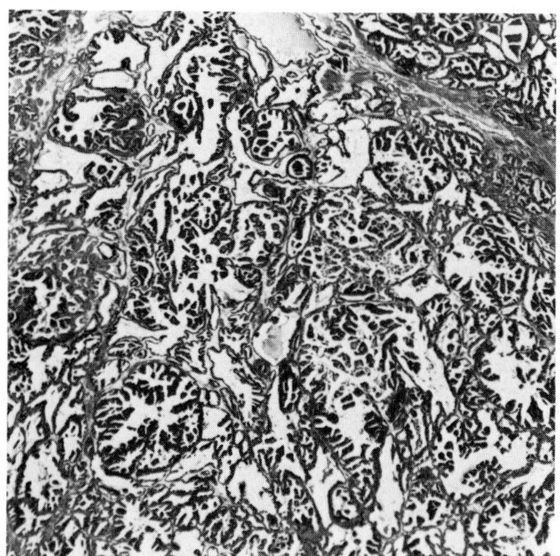

Figure 5–32. A view of hyperplasia of acinar epithelium in the prostate of a dog, shown at lower magnification than that in Figure 5–31.

Other terms used with reference to growth, usually of individual cells, include the following: ***euplasia,*** meaning normal growth; ***proplasia,*** meaning a slight in-

Text contiunued on page 303

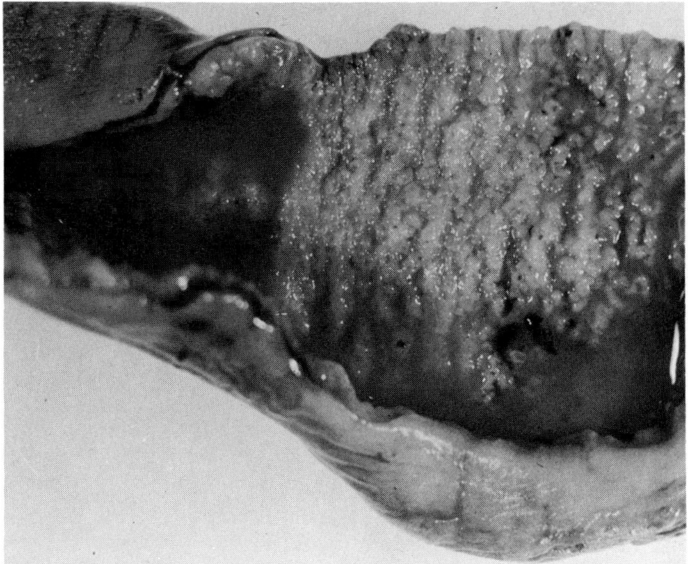

Figure 5–33. Cystic hyperplasia of the endometrium in a dog. This lesion often occurs with pyometra.

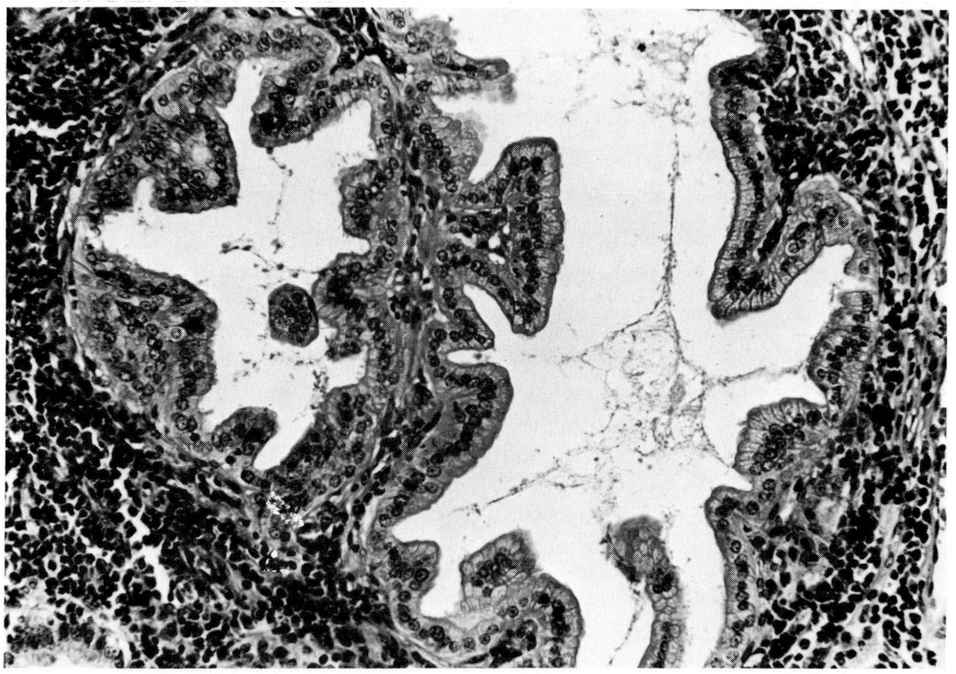

Figure 5–34. Microscopic view of cystic hyperplasia of a dog's endometrium. Note the chronic endometritis. The two lesions often occur together.

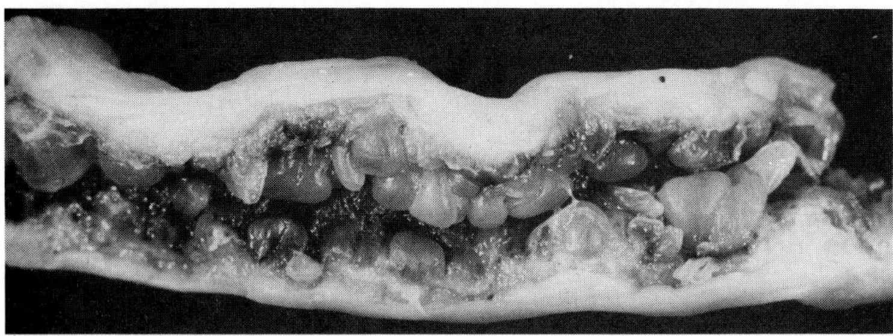

Figure 5–35. A more advanced case of canine cystic hyperplasia of the uterus with little evidence of inflammation. (Courtesy of J. Orr.)

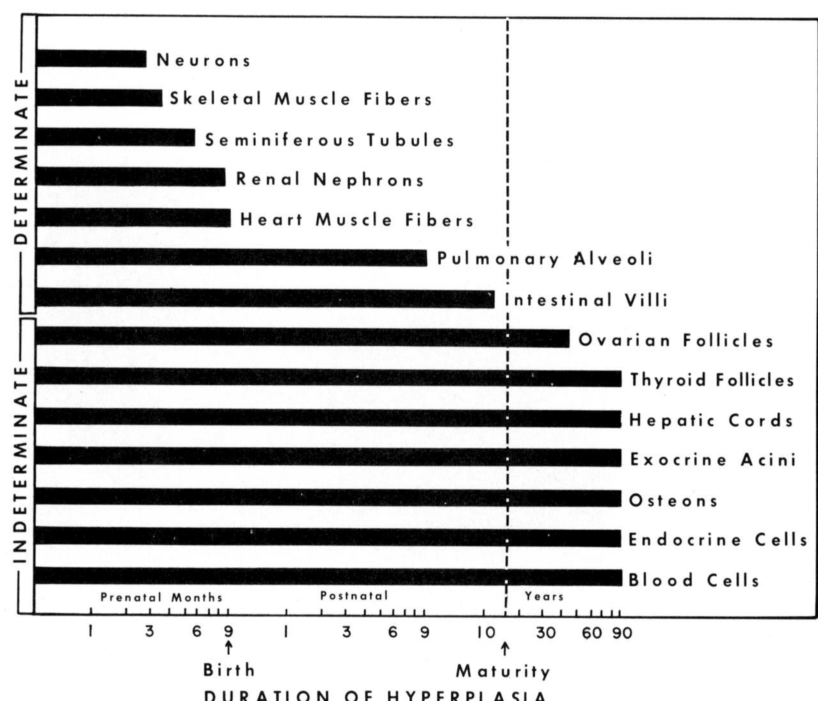

Figure 5–36. Duration of hyperplasia in various histological structures in humans. Organs in which substructures cease to multiply before maturity have determinate numbers of structural units and restricted capacities for growth beyond normal adult dimensions. Those that retain their hyperplastic abilities throughout life can grow potentially without limit and therefore have indeterminate numbers of structural units. (From Goss, R. J.: Hypertrophy versus hyperplasia. Science, *153*:1615–20, September 20, 1966. Copyright 1966 by the American Association for the Advancement of Science. Reprinted by permission.)

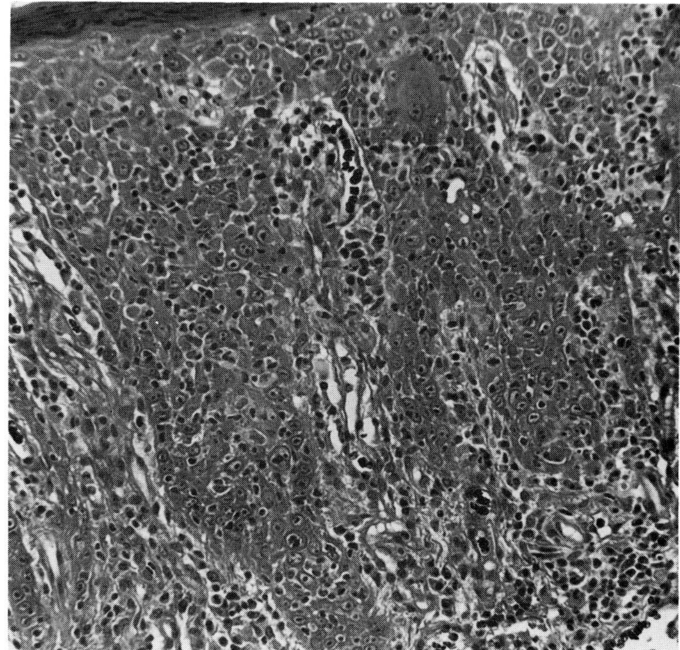

Figure 5–37. Hyperplasia and dysplasia in a dog's skin. Note the long rete pegs and disoriented relationship of the epithelial cells.

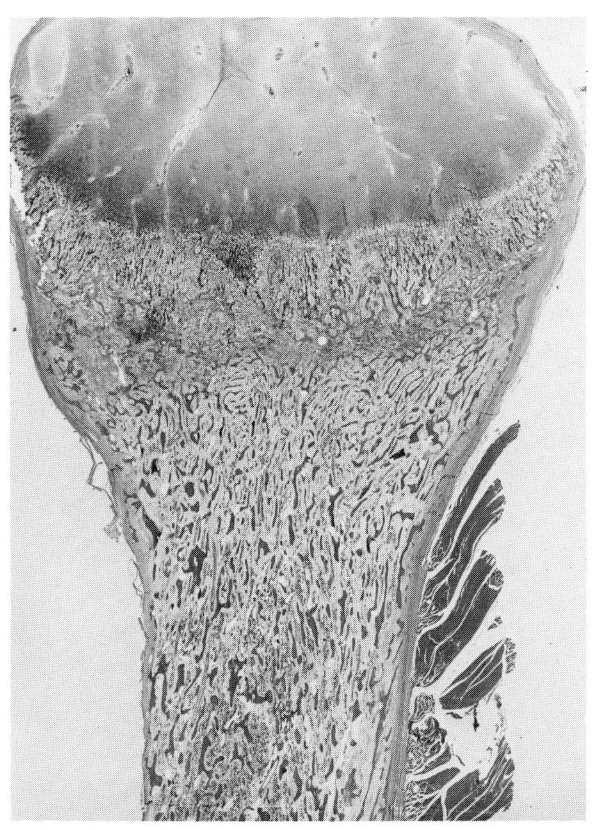

Figure 5–38. Costochondral junction in a pig's rib. Note the zone below the junction where there is abnormal orientation of bone spicules. The disorientation is caused by rickets, and the lesion could be called dysplasia. Dysplasias may be caused by nutritional disorders.

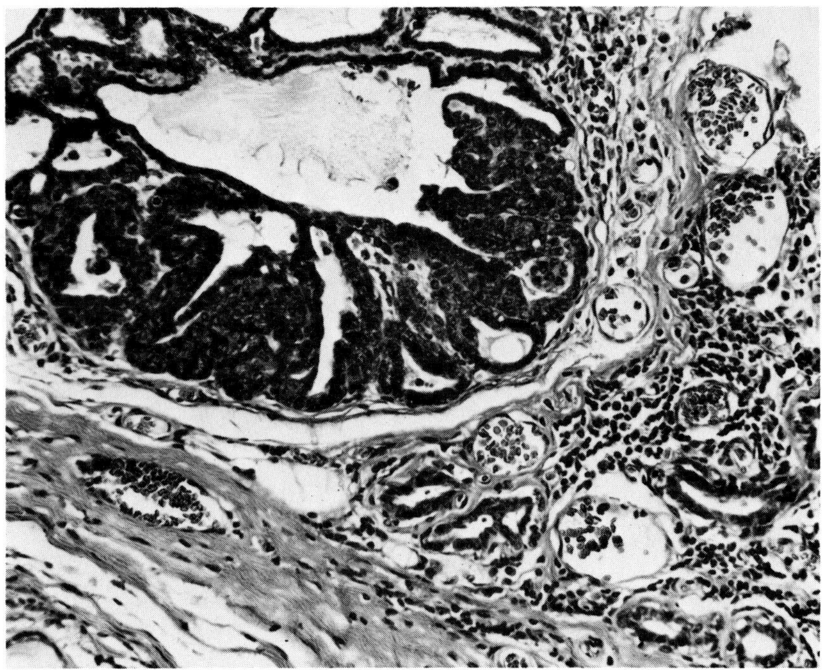

Figure 5–39. Dysplasia in a dog's mammary gland. Epithelium at the lower right is hyperplastic in some acini, and there is marked dysplasia and hyperplasia in the epithelium at the upper left.

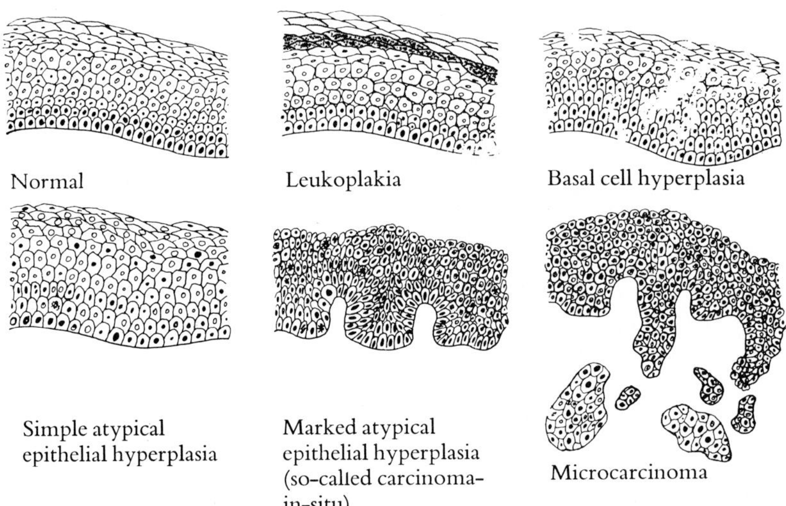

Figure 5–40. Diagram of changes in epithelium in the human cervix that indicates progression of abnormal growth from a squamous surface to hyperplasia and dysplasia, which might be called atypical hyperplasia or carcinoma *in situ,* and eventually to invasion into the submucosa. (From Sandritter, W.: Color Atlas and Textbook of Tissue and Cellular Pathology. 3rd ed. Chicago, Year Book Medical Publishers, Inc., 1969. Reprinted by permission.)

crease or stimulation of growth; and ***retroplasia,*** meaning decreased growth activity through injury or aging. ***Anaplasia*** refers to cells and tissues that are poorly differentiated; this concept will be mentioned later in discussion of neoplasia.

METAPLASIA

Metaplasia means the transformation of a fully differentiated normal adult tissue into a related type of adult tissue. The classic example in epithelial tissues is the transition from normal columnar epithelial lining to squamous epithelial lining that is named ***squamous metaplasia.*** Examples of the causes of such a change are chronic irritation as in bronchial epithelium, vitamin A deficiency in the urinary tract or salivary duct epithelium, chlorinated hydrocarbon toxicity in the genital tracts of sheep and cattle and estrogen toxicity in the urinary tract of mink. A few examples are included in Figures 5–41 through 5–44. The causes are variable and have species sensitivities. Glandular epithelium may have striking squamous metaplasia in healing lesions, such as necrotizing mastitis in cattle. ***Metaplasia is common in mesenchymal tissues*** and is best known as the change or conversion of fat or fibrous connective tissue to myxomatous connective tissue, cartilage or bone. The term applies to one step changes, cartilage to bone or fibrous to myxomatous connective tissue, as well as to the range of changes (Fig. 5–45). The microenvironment of the cells, in terms of availability of oxygen, pressure or tension, seems to influence which matrix products the cells will form, that is, collagen, myxoid, chondroid or osteoid. Nature's best example of metaplasia occurs in a normal callus of a healing bone fracture, particularly if some movement is possible (Figs. 5–46, 5–47 and 5–48). Islands of bone tissue may form in unexpected places and are called ***metaplastic bone.*** The spleen of an adult may convert much of its substance and resources to forming blood cells (extramedullary hematopoiesis) if the need arises; this is called ***myeloid metaplasia*** and may also occur in other organs. Metaplasia is considered ***reversible*** if the etiological factors are withdrawn. It may be a preneoplastic change in some instances, but there is marked variation between locations and species on this point. Metaplasia is very common in tumors.

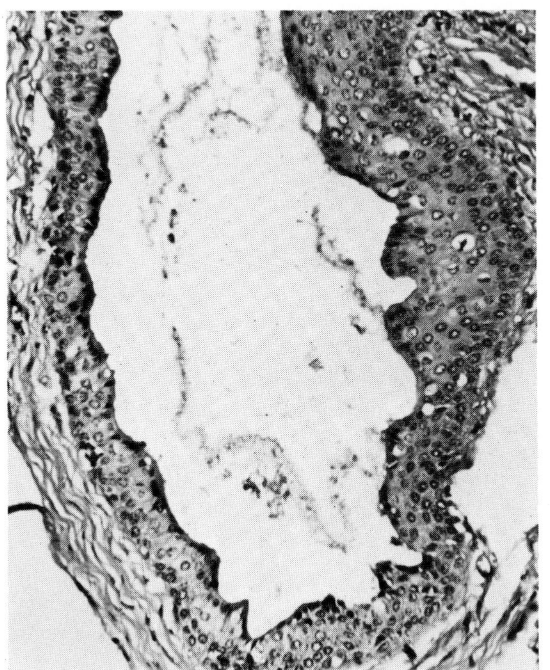

Figure 5–41. Squamous metaplasia in a duct in the salivary gland of a calf with vitamin A deficiency.

ANOMALIES OR MALFORMATIONS

The study of anomalies is called ***teratology.*** Anomalies and malformations are common and important aspects of disease. Detailed coverage of anomalies is not intended here, and ***emphasis will be on general features and terminology.*** References are provided for detail on ***some specific examples.*** The book by Willis (1958) discusses the principles of anomalies in various human tissues and organs.

Anomalies occur at any stage of development; major defects are lethal in embryonic life. Some defects may permit survival ***in utero*** but not postnatally. Some permit postnatal life but with marked impairment of normal existence that in animals leads to death from predation, starvation or euthanasia for economic reasons. Some defects allow relatively normal existence, and some are not recognized except at postmortem examination, where they are called incidental findings.

Text continued on page 306

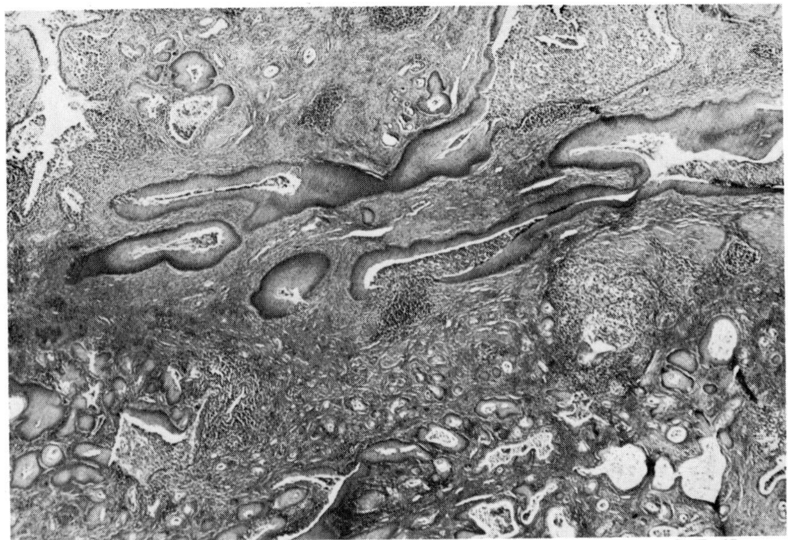

Figure 5–42

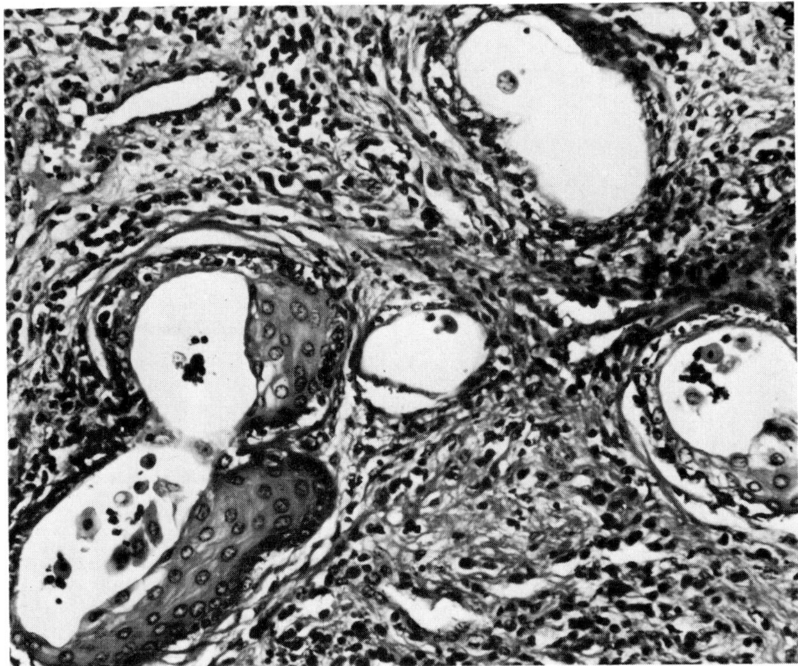

Figure 5–43

Figures 5–42 and 5–43. Squamous metaplasia in a dog's prostate gland. Chronic inflammation is also present.

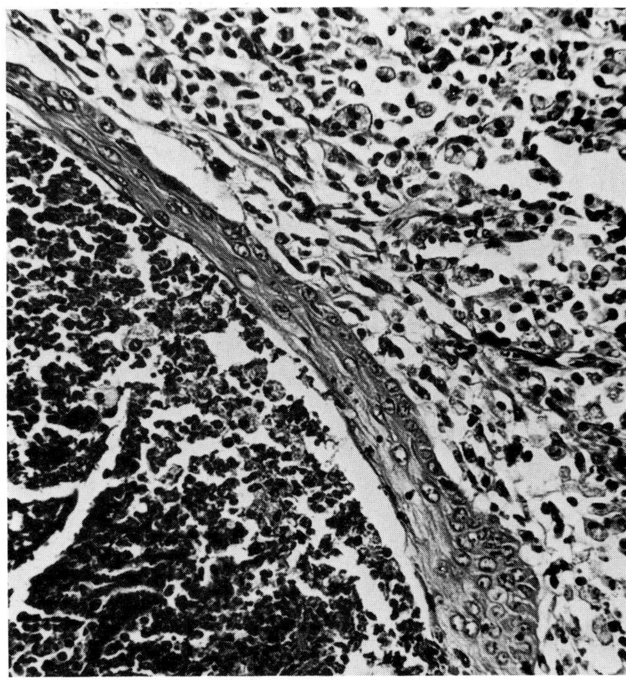

Figure 5–44. Squamous metaplasia in a duct in a mammary gland of a cow with chronic mastitis.

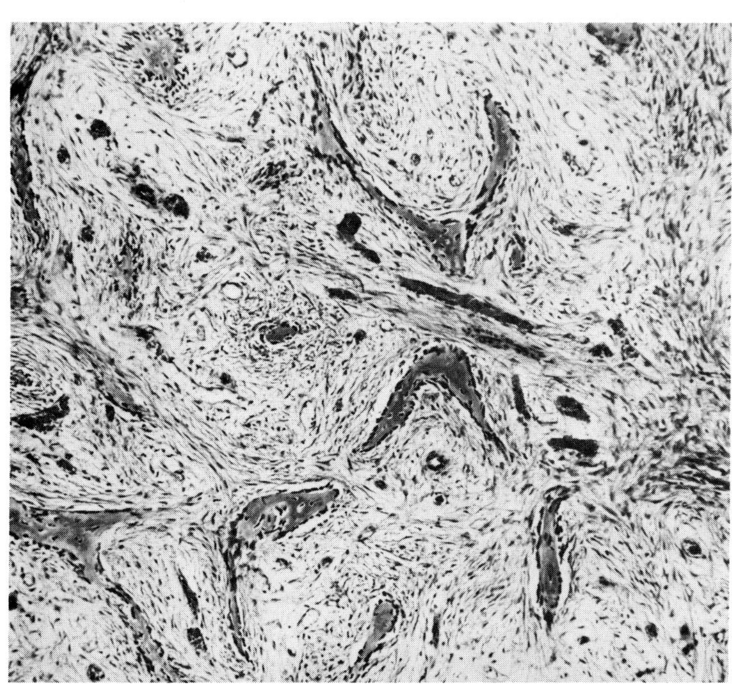

Figure 5–45. Fibrous metaplasia in the bone marrow of a mandible in a horse with nutritional secondary hyperparathyroidism.

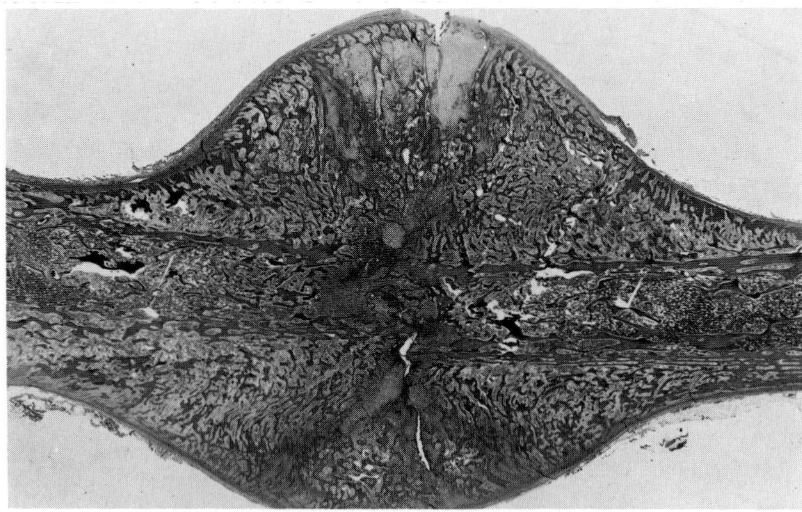

Figure 5–46. Callus in a fractured bone. The new bone and soft tissue of the callus have arisen from periosteal hyperplasia and metaplasia. Closer views are seen in Figure 5–47 and 5–48. Note the close proximity of cartilage, bone and fibrous tissue that are examples of metaplasia of connective tissue.

Defects in the newborn are ***congenital; that is, the individual is born with the defect, but this does not convey anything specific about etiological factors.***

The cause may be an ***inherited or genetic defect,*** exposure to an infectious disease or toxic compound, anoxia ***in utero*** or perhaps one of the many other presently unknown factors. ***There has been a tendency in the past to dismiss anomalies as "genetic" without differentiating between congenital and inherited.***

Most anomalies fall within the following general types (Table 5–1).

Agenesis, aplasia, atresia and hypoplasia are all anomalies and have been mentioned previously (Fig. 5–49). ***Developmental hypertrophy and hyperplasia*** of tissues or organs may sometimes occur. ***Failure of a part to close or coalesce*** (Figs. 5–50 and 5–51) may take place in a tissue, as in dysraphism, which is failure of the neural groove to close properly. Other examples are ventricular septal defects of the heart, in which the partitioning of the chambers is defective, and coloboma of the eye, in which the optic cup is malformed. Parts of tissue may have cystic spaces filled with fluid where normal parenchyma failed to develop. ***Vestigial structures*** may persist beyond when they should have disappeared (Figs. 5–52 and 5–53). Persistence of the thyroglossal duct, Rathke's pouch and mesonephric and paramesonephric tubular remnants are examples. ***Supernumerary or accessory organs*** may be present, such as polydactylia (excess digits) and accessory lung, adrenal cortex and parathyroid tissues. Organs may be located in abnormal places that are referred to as ***ectopic, aberrant or heterotopic. Hamartomas*** are improper mixtures of tissues, usually with excess of a part, and grossly may resemble tumors. Examples are the well-known nevi or moles in humans, as well as angiomas and some lipomas. ***Generalized defects*** in the development of the skeleton may occur, as in ***chondrodystrophy*** or dwarfism, and these are well known. There are many degrees and types of chondrodystrophy, however, and the expressions may be subtle. Many chondrodystrophic types of dogs

Text continued on page 310

TABLE 5–1. Principal Terms and Concepts Used to Describe Anomalies

1. Agenesis or aplasia
2. Hypoplasia
3. Developmental hyperplasia or hypertrophy
4. Failure of parts to coalesce or close
5. Failure of parts to separate or canalize
6. Persistence of vestigial structures
7. Supernumerary or accessory parts
8. Ectopic or heterotopic parts
9. Hamartoma
10. Generalized anomalies of skeletal development
11. Cellular and enzymic malformations
12. Neoplasms

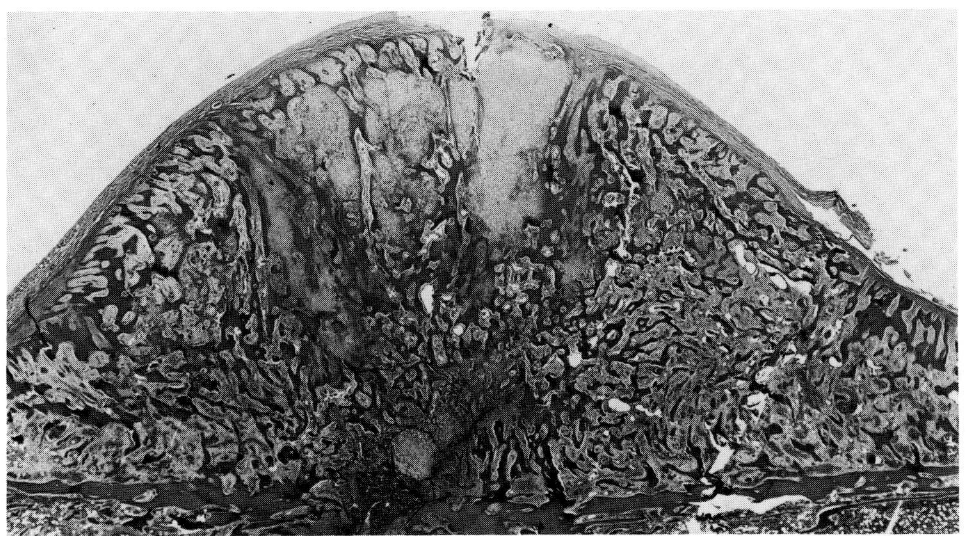

Figure 5–47

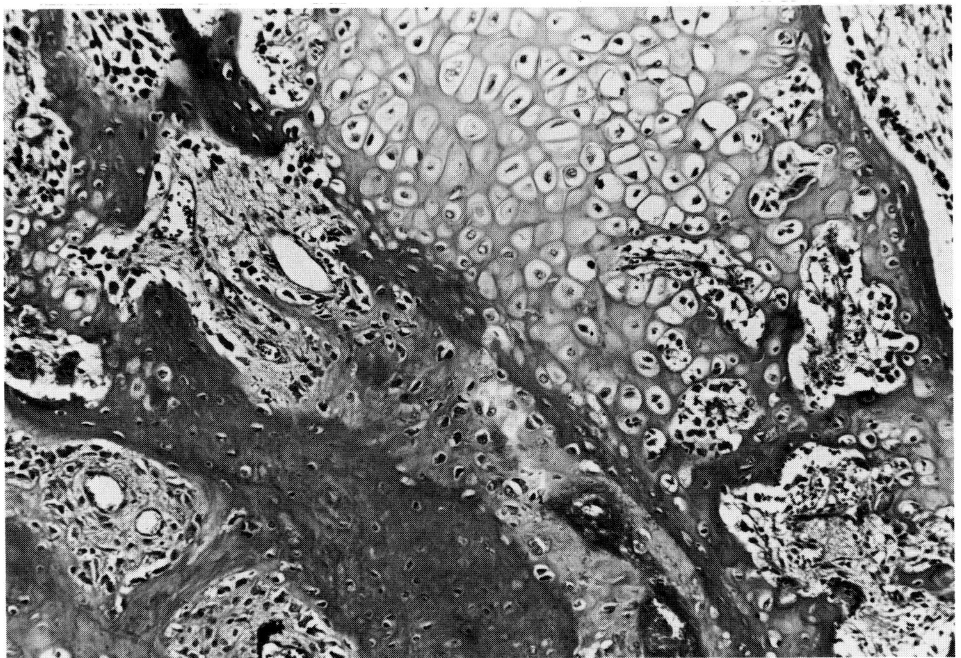

Figure 5–48

Figures 5–47 and 5–48. See the legend for Figure 5–46.

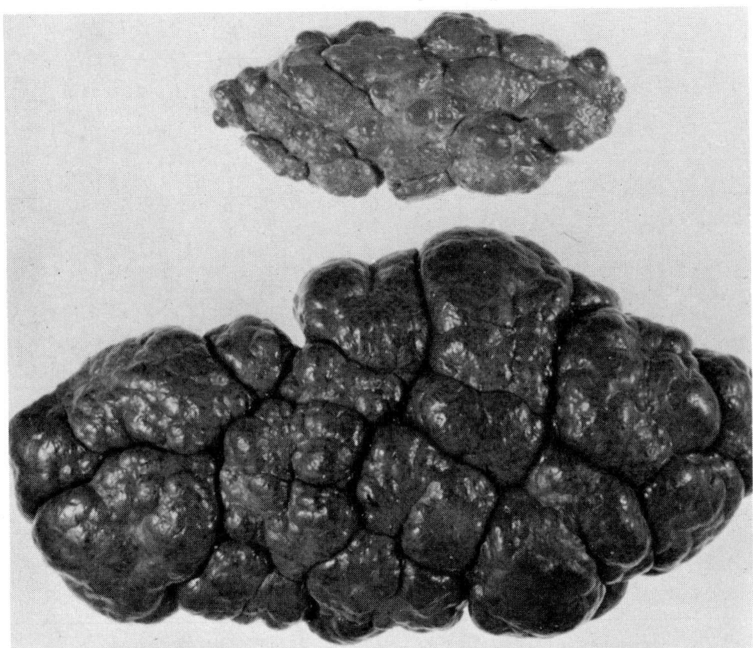

Figure 5–49. Renal hypoplasia and dysplasia in a cow. One kidney is very small, and the lobulation is noticeably abnormal (dysplasia) in the larger one.

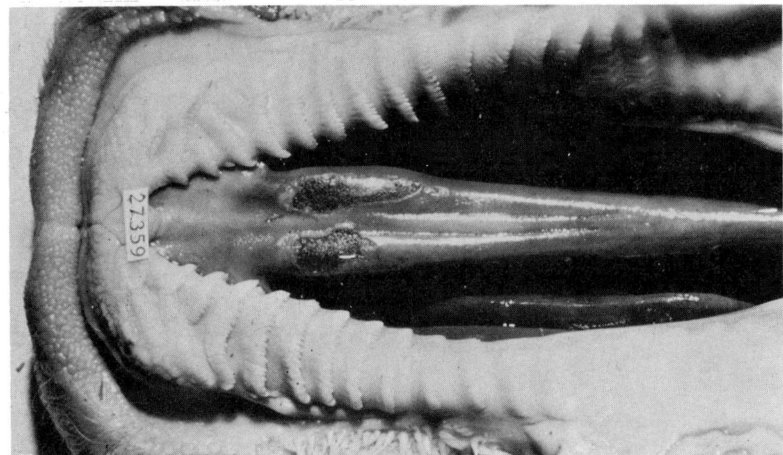

Figure 5–50. Cleft palate in a calf. The areas of necrosis on the nasal septum are probably because of irritation from food. This anomaly is used in laboratory animals in teratology studies of a variety of influences on the closure of the palate.

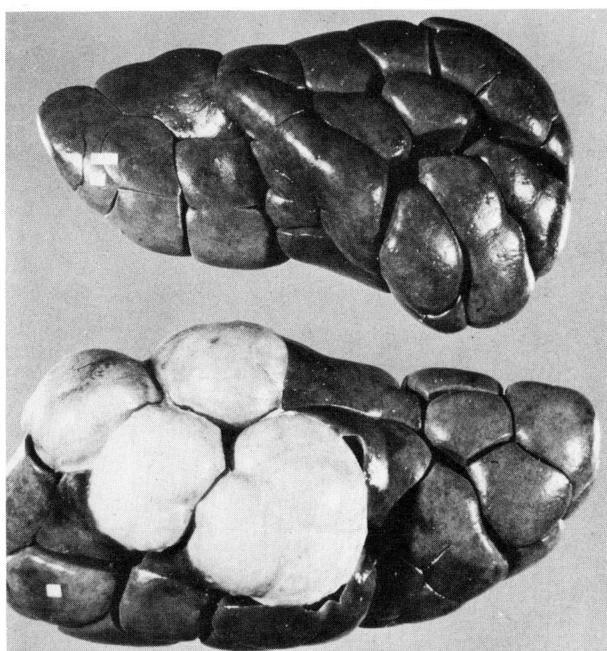

Figure 5–51. Bovine kidney. The white areas are distended with fluid and are called congenital cysts.

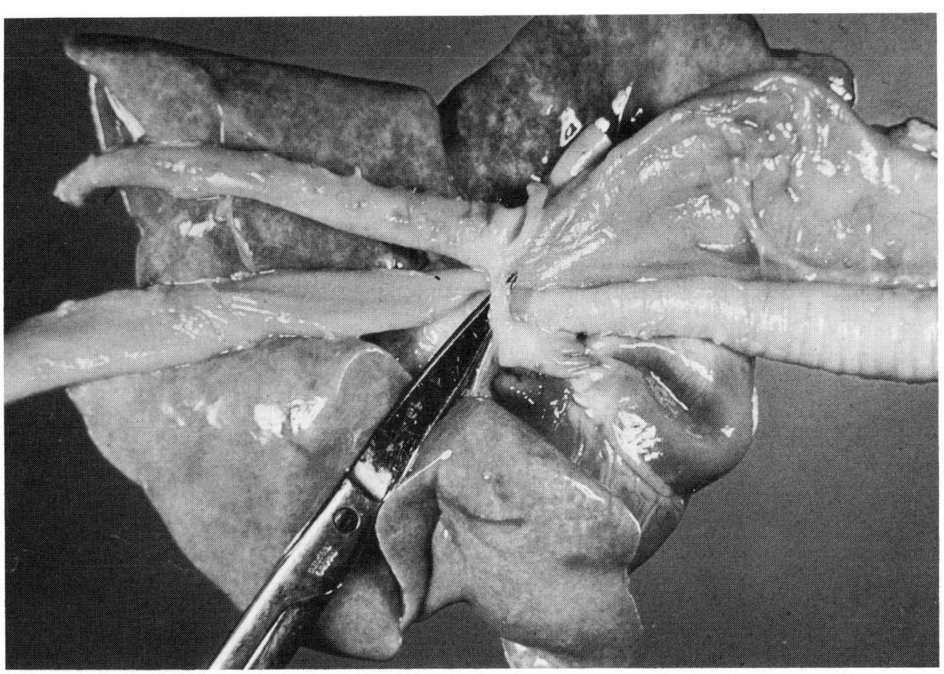

Figure 5–52. Persistent right aortic arch (at the point of the scissors) in a dog. Note that the esophagus is constricted at this point and is dilated anterior to the constriction.

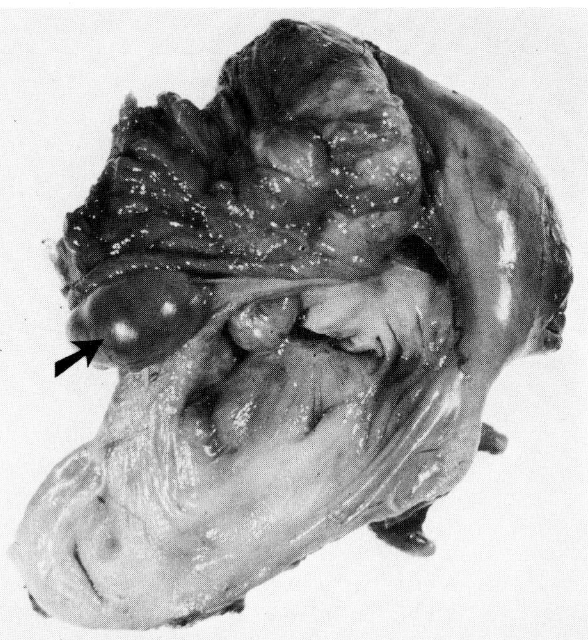

Figure 5–53. Equine ovary. Ovulation fossa is present near the middle to the right. The cystic structure in the fimbria (arrow) is the remnant of the end of the paramesonephric duct and is called the hydatid of Morgagni. These are common in horses but less so in other species.

have been developed into pure breeds, some of which have their main disease problems associated with being chondrodystrophics, as is the case with disc disease in dachshunds.

Some anomalies have unusual expressions and may not be primary lesions in the organ visibly affected. ***Arthrogryposis*** is a disease in which an animal is born with flexed, absolutely rigid limbs, but this is a primary problem not with bones or joints but rather with innervation of muscles because of dysraphism in the spinal cord.

The list of ***cellular or enzymatic defects*** is ever increasing. A key step in a metabolic chain or sequence may be blocked because the enzyme that controls the next step is congenitally absent or defective. For any major metabolic pathway, individuals are being identified that have a defect at some point in the chain, and different individuals have the problem at different points. Carbohydrate metabolism is one example of a process in which numerous congenital defects have been identified. The metabolism of porphyrins and the clotting cascade would be other examples. Lipid storage diseases of the brain are prominent examples of defective enzyme function.

The thalidomide problem highlighted the possibility of ***iatrogenic*** drug-induced anomalies and has had marked effects on the drug regulation structure and on safety testing. Recognition of virus-induced cerebellar hypoplasia in cats and cattle brought about revolutionary changes in thinking, even though it was known that a mother who had measles during pregnancy might have anomalous children and that the use of attenuated bluetongue or hog cholera vaccine in pregnant animals could cause anomalies. The association between Akabane virus with epizootic arthrogryposis and hydranencephaly in calves in Japan and Australia and an arthropod vector will stimulate a search for other such associations. The demonstration that cyclopia in lambs was due to ingestion of a weed, ***Veratrum californicum,*** by the dam between the 10th and 15th day of pregnancy was also a dramatic new development. These revelations have reduced the number of diseases that were attributed to genetic factors simply for lack of better understanding.

Wilson (1973) lists six general "principles" of teratology to describe the usual or typical, but not all, occurrences of anomalies (Table 5–2). Wilson's 1977 paper is a concise review and lists many ***specific teratogens*** of various types that affect animals and humans. Anomalies are also illustrated in Figures 2–121, 2–122 and 2–123.

TABLE 5–2. GENERAL PRINCIPLES OF TERATOLOGY

1. Susceptibility to teratogenesis depends on the genotype of the conceptus and the manner in which this interacts with adverse environmental factors
2. Susceptibility to teratogenesis varies with the developmental stage at the time of exposure to an adverse influence
3. Teratogenic agents act in specific ways (mechanisms) on developing cells and tissues to initiate sequences of abnormal developmental events (pathogenesis)
4. The access of adverse influences to developing tissues depends on the nature of the influence (agent)
5. The four manifestations of deviant development are death, malformation, growth retardation and functional deficit
6. Manifestations of deviant development increase in frequency and degree as dosage increases, from the no-effect to the totally lethal level

CYTOGENETICS

The discussion of anomalies invites discussion of ***cytogenetics and inheritance*** of anomalies.

Polygenic inheritance involves many characteristics of an individual. It may be defined as a physiological or pathological trait governed by the ***additive effect of many genes of small effect but conditioned by nongenetic environmental influences.*** Polygenic inherited diseases are expressed when a sufficient number of mutant genes are inherited; the severity of the disease varies according to the number of affected genes and the presence of predisposing factors. In humans, polygenic inheritance is considered to underlie such diseases as hypertension and diabetes.

Situations in which ***mutant genes of large effect*** occur are numerous and are expressed according to the laws of genetics as inherited autosomal dominant, autosomal recessive or sex-linked.

Another group of disorders relates to chromosomal aberrations and involves a ***change in number or morphological state of chromosomes,*** and thus a change in ***karyotype.*** Some of the changes in form and structure are illustrated in Figure 5–54. Abnormal numbers result from ***nondisjunction*** or ***anaphase lag*** in meiosis of germ cells or in mitosis in the zygote (Figs. 5–55 through 5–58).

Abnormalities in chromosomes tend to result in decreased viability and fertility, mental deficiency and structural abnormalities. A major anomaly is likely to be lethal to the gamete or to the zygote. Abnormalities in numbers do occur in normal individuals. The abnormalities in sex chromosomes seem to draw the most attention.

The paper by Jacobs indicates that over 50 per cent of spontaneous human abortions are associated with chromosomal abnormalities and that 10 per cent of all conceptions are chromosomally abnormal. It is hoped that this type of information will become available in veterinary medicine as well.

Each somatic cell contains homologous pairs of chromosomes (***diploid,*** 2N), one derived from each parent. The germ cells contain half this number (***haploid,*** N). Chromosomes are called autosomes when they include all except the one pair of sex chromosomes. An abnormal number of chromosomes is referred to as ***heteroploidy,*** and if these are exact multiples of the ***haploid*** number, the cells are called ***euploid*** and the condition is called ***euploidy.*** Abnormalities that do not involve exact multiples are called ***aneuploid.*** If three chromosomes occur instead of two, the condition is called ***trisomy;*** if only one occurs, it is ***monosomy.***

Mosaicism occurs when nondisjunction results in an abnormal number of chromosomes in an embryo (Fig. 5–57). The defect may have occurred in cell division shortly after fertilization, and the result may be two or more populations of cells with differing genotype, for example, XX and XXY. These defects can occur without clinical expression in some individuals, depending on which cell populations are affected. If the germinal cells are involved, the defect will probably be expressed, but it may not if other cell populations are involved. If two genotypes are present in one individual, one of which came from a twin via the placenta, the condition is called ***chimerism,*** of which the freemartin is an example. Defects in the sex chromosomes in humans are called ***gonadal dysgenesis,*** of which Turner's syndrome and Klinefelter's syndrome are examples.

Cytogenetics is being applied experimentally in animals to a considerable extent, particularly to explain basic biological abnormalities, such as freemartinism in cattle, but only to a limited extent in field problems, although research in this area is rapidly expanding.

Text continued on page 315

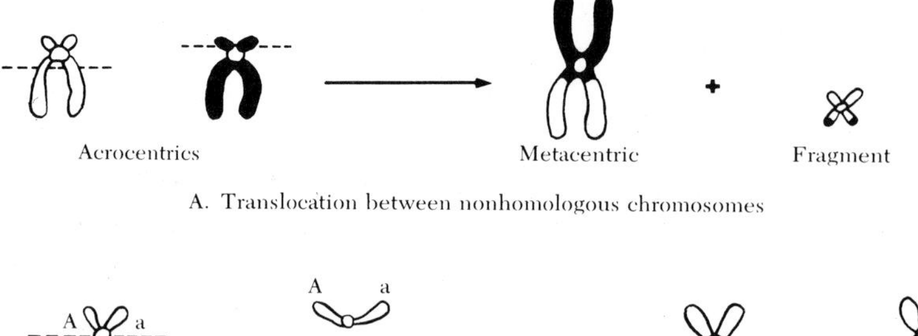

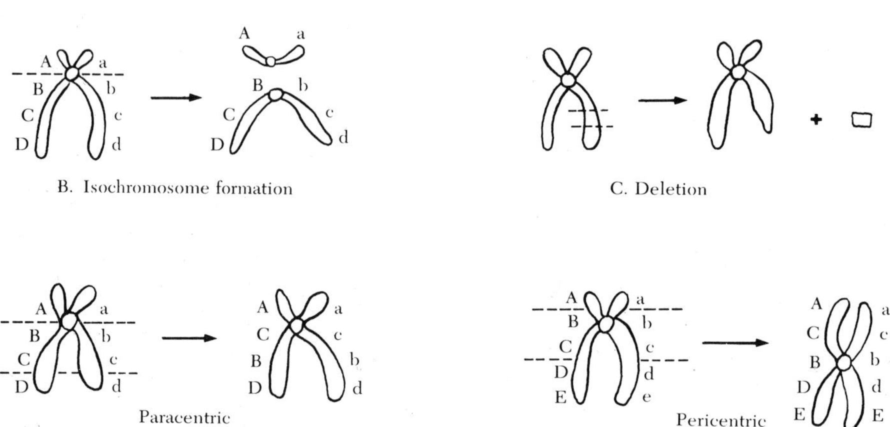

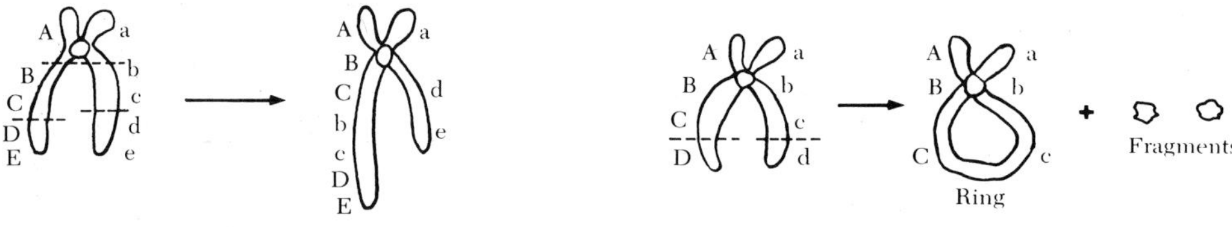

Figure 5–54. Types of chromosomal rearrangement. (From Robbins, S. L., and Angell, M.: Basic Pathology. 2nd ed. Philadelphia, W. B. Saunders Co., 1976.)

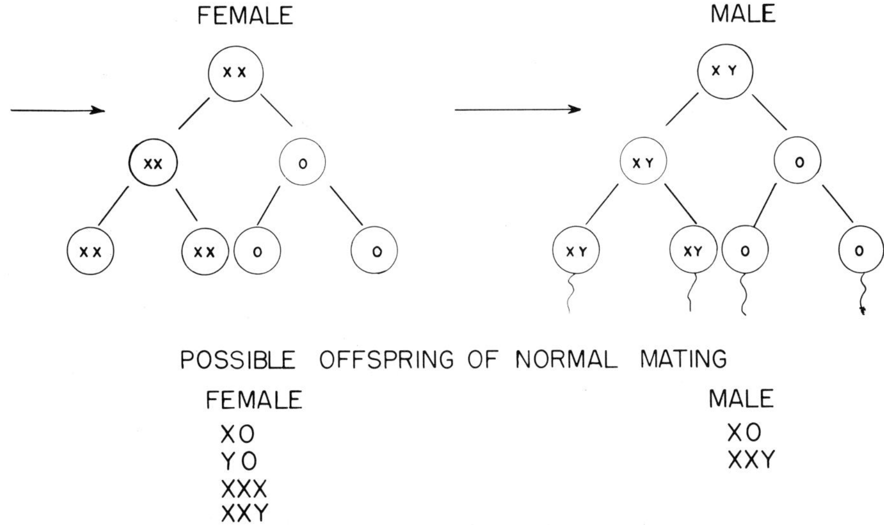

Figure 5–55. Nondisjunction at first meiotic division. Arrows indicate points of nondisjunction. Offspring listed under *Female* are those expected to result when nondisjunction occurs in the mother; those listed under *Male* are expected when nondisjunction occurs in the father. (From McKay, R. J.: Practical application of current knowledge concerning human chromosomes. Pediatr. Clin. North Am., *11*:172–182, 1964. Reprinted with permission.)

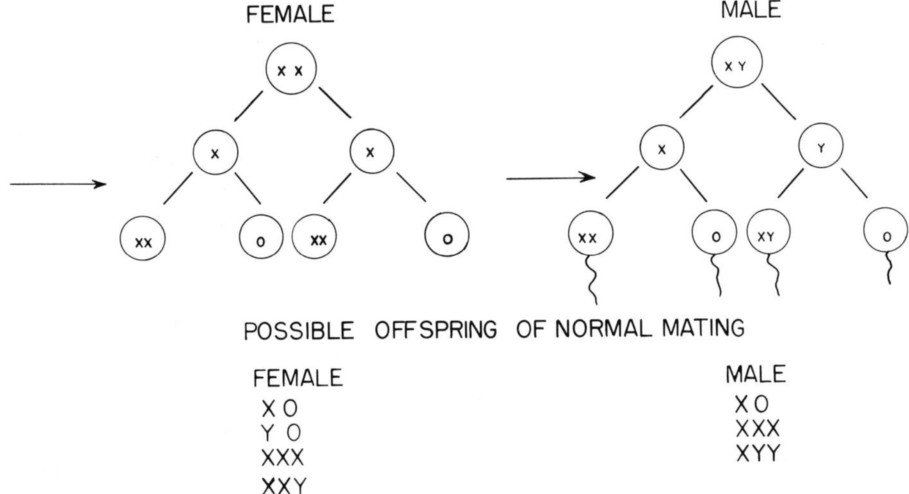

Figure 5–56. Nondisjunction at the second meiotic division. Arrows indicate points of nondisjunction. Offspring listed under *Female* are those expected to result when nondisjunction occurs in the mother; those under *Male* are expected when nondisjunction occurs in the father. (From McKay, R. J.: Practical application of current knowledge concerning human chromosomes. Pediatr. Clin. North Am., *11*:172–182, 1964. Reprinted with permission.)

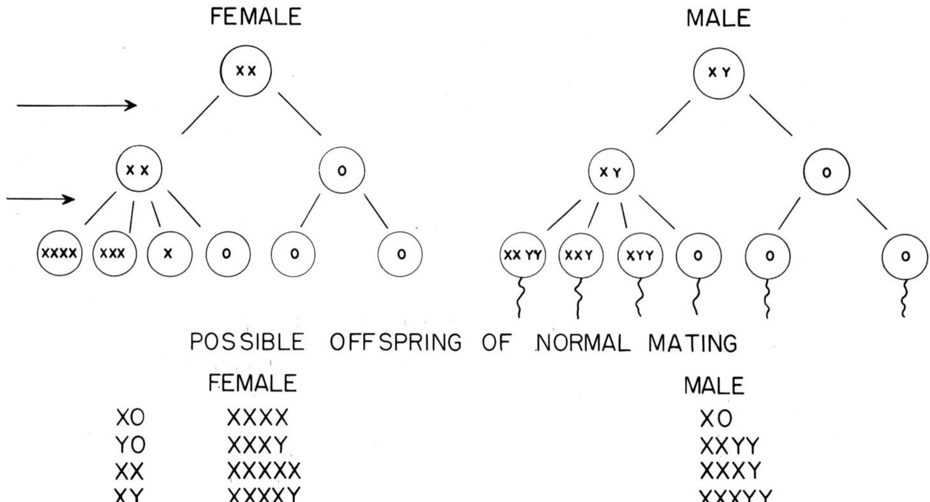

Figure 5–57. Nondisjunction at first and second meiotic divisions. Arrows indicate points of nondisjunction. Offspring listed under *Female* are those expected to result when nondisjunction occurs in the mother; those under *Male* are expected when nondisjunction occurs in the father. (From McKay, R. J.: Practical application of current knowledge concerning human chromosomes. Pediatr. Clin. North Am., *11*:172–182, 1964. Reprinted with permission.)

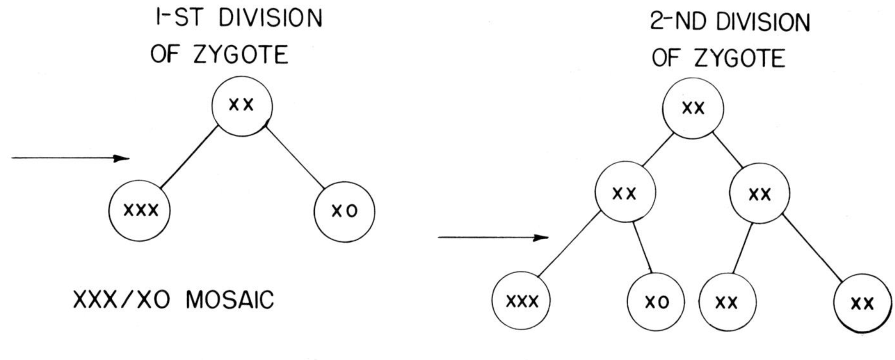

Figure 5–58. Mosaicism due to nondisjunction during either of first two divisions of zygote (fertilized ovum) of XX chromosome constitution. Arrows indicate points of nondisjunction. (From McKay, R. J.: Practical application of current knowledge concerning human chromosomes. Pediatr. Clin. North Am., *11*:172–182, 1964. Reprinted with permission)

AGING

A discussion of factors that influence growth invites comment on aging and the ***control of aging processes in tissues.*** There are several current concepts but no unifying one.

The ***cellular theory*** has several subdivisions. Some investigators believe that the cells' functional genetic program is the main influence and that it varies with age. Some cell cultures from embryos will multiply many more times than cells from the same tissue cultured at a later age. Others consider that mutations cause aging. Subtle damage to DNA may not be repaired, and the cell gradually becomes defective in its essential control systems and products. Another suggestion is that free radicals, from the environment or from within the cell, damage DNA and surface structures sufficiently to gradually but permanently alter the function of cells. The essence of these theories involves ***error in protein production*** that leads to changes in function and aging. The errors may occur by mutation, in transcription or in synthesis and lead to further self-perpetuating defects. This overall mechanism is termed ***"error catastrophe."***

The second main theory concerning aging is the ***immune theory.*** It is known that immune functions decrease with age, which in part accounts for autoimmune disease and cancer in older individuals. Opinion is divided as to whether these diseases compromise the immune system or whether the decrease in immunological functions predisposes to these diseases, but the latter receives the greatest acceptance. The T cells decline in functional activity, and this affects both humoral and cellular responses. It has been suggested that the time of involution of the thymus may be quite significant in terms of influence on the immune system and aging. Some regard loss of control of immunological tolerance as the main problem leading to autoimmunity and aging.

Other theories on aging relate to deficient response to hormones by tissue cells and to altered enzyme response of stimulated cells, perhaps by modification of receptor sites on cell membranes.

The life span of each species is characteristic and appears to correlate with the major functions, such as gestation, puberty, heart rate and metabolic rate, for that species. All animals tend to die of similar causes related to failure of the circulatory and immune systems, the latter relating to death from infection and cancer. Four causes of death may act in a programmed sequence to result in death of an individual; a genetically controlled biological clock acts on the endocrine system to cause deterioration of the circulatory and immune systems, which in turn decreases resistance to diseases listed as immediate causes of death. If species lived longer, more progeny would occur and inbreeding might increase and result in the expression of detrimental recessive genes that might eliminate the species in the long run. A fixed life span may increase the adaptability and, in the long run, viability of the species at the expense of the individual. Advances in medicine have not increased the life span of humans as a whole but have allowed more people to reach the limit of what appears to be a fixed life span.

SUGGESTIONS FOR FURTHER READING

General

Adler, C. P., et al.: Form and structure of cell nuclei in growing and hypertrophied human hearts. Beitr. Pathol., *161*:342–362, 1977.

Albert, D. M., et al.: Retinal neoplasia and dysplasia. I. Induction by feline leukemia virus. Invest. Ophthalmol. Vis. Sci., *16*:325–337, 1977.

Anversa, P., et al.: Morphometric study of myocardial hypertrophy induced by abdominal aortic stenosis. Lab. Invest., *40*:341–349, 1979.

Ashley, D. J., and Mostofi, F. K.: Renal agenesis and dysgenesis. J. Urol., *83*:211–230, 1960.

Baserga, R.: Cell growth. Beitr. Pathol., *152*:292–303, 1974.

Basrur, P. K.: Genetics in veterinary medicine. *In* Phillipson, A. T., and Hall, L. W. (eds.): Scientific Foundation of Veterinary Medicine. London, Heinemann Medical, 1981, pp. 393–413.

Bathija, A., et al.: Bone marrow adipose tissue: response to acute starvation. Am. J. Hematol., *6*:191–198, 1979.

Benirschke, K.: Cytogenetics. *In* Benirschke, K., et al. (eds.): Pathology of Laboratory Animals. New York, Springer-Verlag, 1978, pp. 1697–1747.

Bonikos, D. S., et al.: Bronchopulmonary dysplasia: the pulmonary pathologic sequel of necrotizing bronchiolitis and pulmonary fibrosis. Hum. Pathol., *7*:643–666, 1976.

Cameron, A. M., and Faulkin, L. J., Jr.: Hyperplastic and inflammatory nodules in the canine mammary gland. J. Natl. Cancer Inst., *47*:1277–1287, 1971.

Goodwin, R. F. W.: The concentration of blood sugar during starvation in the newborn calf and foal. J. Comp. Pathol., *67*:289–296, 1957.

Goss, R. J.: Hypertrophy versus hyperplasia. Science, *153*:1615–1620, 1966.

Hadlow, W. J.: Adrenal cortical atrophy in the dog. Report of three cases. Am. J. Pathol., *29*:353–361, 1953.

Helminen, H. J.: The cellular mechanisms of hormonally induced tissue atrophy. *In* Trump, B. J., and Arstila, A. U. (eds.): Pathobiology of Cell Membranes. New York, Academic Press, 1975. pp. 283–322.

Jacoby, R. O.: Transmissible ileal hyperplasia of hamsters. I. Histogenesis and immunocytochemistry. Am. J. Pathol., *91*:433–452, 1978.

Jones, T. C.: Hereditary diseases. *In* Benirschke, K., et al. (eds.): Pathology of Laboratory Animals. New York, Springer-Verlag, 1978, pp. 1981–2064.

Lucke, V. M., et al.: Chronic renal failure in young dogs—possible renal dysplasia. J. Small Anim. Pract., *21*:169–181, 1980.

McGavin, M. D., and Morill, J. L.: Scanning electron microscopy of ruminal papillae in calves fed various amounts and forms of roughage. Am. J. Vet. Res., *37*:497–508, 1976.

Neville, A. M.: The nodular adrenal. Invest. Cell Pathol., *1*:99–111, 1978.

Oksanen, A., and Osborne, H. G.: Fatty tissue in starved lambs. A quantitative and statistical study. Acta Vet. Scand., *13*:340–347, 1977.

O'Shea, J. D.: Squamous metaplasia of the canine prostate gland. Res. Vet. Sci., *4*:431–434, 1963.

Prentice, D. E., et al.: Pancreatic atrophy in young beagle dogs. Vet. Pathol., *17*:575–580, 1980.

Warner, M. R.: Age incidence and site distribution of mammary dysplasia in young beagle bitches. J. Natl. Cancer Inst., *57*:57–61, 1976.

Anomalies—General

Ajl, S., and Mori, J.: Birth defects: from here to eternity. Perspect. Biol. Med., *24*:302–334, 1981.

Barrow, M. V.: A brief history of teratology to the early 20th century. Teratology, *4*:119–130, 1971.

Benirschke, K.: Spontaneous chimerism in mammals: a critical review. Curr. Top. Pathol., *51*:1–61, 1970.

Bolande, R. P.: Developmental pathology: teaching monograph. Am. J. Pathol., *94*:627–683, 1979.

Carpenter, S. J., and Ferm, V. H.: Embryopathic effects of lead in the hamster—a morphologic analysis. Lab. Invest., *37*:369–385, 1977.

Carrig, C. B., et al.: Retinal dysplasia associated with skeletal abnormalities in Labrador Retrievers. J. Am. Vet. Med. Assoc., *170*:49–57, 1977.

Done, J. T.: Developmental disorders of the nervous system in animals. Adv. Vet. Sci. Comp. Med., *20*:69–114, 1976.

Ferm, V. H.: The teratological effects of metals on mammalian embryos. Adv. Teratology, *5*:51–76, 1972.

Foley, C. W., et al.: Abnormalities of Companion Animals: Analysis of Heritability. Ames, Iowa, Iowa State University Press, 1979.

Fraser, F. G.: The multifactorial/threshold concept—uses and misuses. Teratology, *14*:267–280, 1976.

Fraser, F. C.: Animal models for craniofacial deformities. *In* Melnick, M., and Bixler, D. (eds.): Etiology of Cleft Lip and Cleft Palate. New York, Alan R. Liss, 1980, pp. 1–23.

Greene, W. A., et al.: Sex-chromosome ratios in cattle and their relationship to reproductive development in freemartins. Cytogenet. Cell Genet., *18*:97–105, 1977.

Gruneburg, H.: The Pathology of Development. New York, John Wiley & Sons, 1963.

Hare, W. C. D., and Singh, E. L.: Cytogenetics in Animal Reproduction. New York, Unipub, 1981.

Harris, R. E.: Viral teratogenesis: a review with experimental and clinical perspectives. Am. J. Obstet. Gynecol., *119*:996–1008, 1974.

Jacobs, P. A.: Epidemiology of chromosome abnormalities in man. Am. J. Epidemiol., *105*:180–191, 1977.

Jolly, R. D., and Hartley, W. J.: Storage diseases of domestic animals. Aust. Vet. J., *53*:1–8, 1977.

Jolly, R. D.: Screening for genetic diseases. Principles and practice. Adv. Vet. Sci. Comp. Med., *25*:245–276, 1981.

Kaback, M. M.: Medical genetics: an overview. Pediatr. Clin. North Am., *25*:395–409, 1978.

Leipold, H. W.: Congenital defects in zoo and wild animals. *In* Montali, R., and Migaki, G. (eds.): Comparative Pathology of Zoo Animals. Washington, Smithsonian Institution Press, 1980, pp. 459–470.

Morison, J. E.: Foetal and Neonatal Pathology. Philadelphia, F. A. Davis, 1970.

Ohno, S.: Major regulatory genes for mammalian sexual development. Cell, *7*:315–321, 1976.

Priester, W. A., et al.: Congenital defects in domesticated animals: general considerations. Am. J. Vet. Res., *31*:1871–1879, 1970.

Priester, W. A., et al.: Congenital ocular defects in cattle, horses, cats, and dogs. J. Am. Vet. Med. Assoc., *160*:1504–1511, 1972.

Riddell, C.: Skeletal deformities in poultry. Adv. Vet. Sci. Comp. Med., *25*:277–310, 1981.

Rubin, A.: Handbook of Congenital Malformations. Philadelphia, W. B. Saunders Co., 1967.

Schardein, J. L.: Drugs as Teratogens. Cleveland, CRC Press, 1976.

Sillence, D. O., et al.: Morphologic studies in skeletal dysplasias. Am. J. Pathol., *96*:813–859, 1979.

Swatland, H. J.: Development disorders of skeletal muscle in cattle, pigs and sheep. Vet. Bull., *44*:179–202, 1974.

Tudor, D. C.: Congenital defects of poultry. World Poult. Sci. J., *35*:20–26, 1979.

Williams, R. B.: Trace elements and congenital abnormalities. Proc. Nutr. Soc., *36*:25–32, 1977.

Willis, R. A.: The Borderland of Embryology and Pathology. Philadelphia, F. A. Davis (Butterworth), 1958.

Wilson, J. G.: Present status of drugs as teratogens in man. Teratology, *7*:3–16, 1973.

Wilson, J. G.: Teratogenic effects of environmental chemicals. Fed. Proc., *36*:1698–1703, 1977.

Wilson, J. G., and Fraser, F. C.: Mechanisms and Pathogenesis. Handbook of Teratology, Vol. 2. New York, Plenum Press, 1977.

Wilson, J. G., and Warkany, J.: Teratology: Principles and Techniques. Chicago, University of Chicago Press, 1965.

Wilson, J. G., et al.: Developmental abnormalities. *In* Benirschke, et al. (eds.): Pathology of Laboratory Animals. New York, Springer-Verlag, 1978, pp. 1817–1946.

World Health Organization: Bibliography on congenital defects in animals. Supplement 1 to Volume 8, 1974–1981.

Anomalies—Cattle

Cho, D. Y., and Leipold, H. W.: Congenital defects of the bovine central nervous system. Vet. Bull., *47*:489–504, 1977.

Emmerson, M. A., and Hazel, L. N.: Radiographic demonstration of dwarf gene-carrier beef animals. J. Am. Vet. Med. Assoc., *128*:381–390, 1956.

Gledhill, B. L.: Inherited disorders causing infertility in the bull. J. Am. Vet. Med. Assoc., *162*:979–982, 1973.

Greene, H. J., et al.: Bovine congenital defects: arthrogryposis and associated defects in calves. Am. J. Vet. Res., *34*:887–891, 1973.

Greene, H. J., et al.: Bovine congenital skeletal defects. Zentralbl. Veterinaermed. [A]. *21*:789–796, 1974.

Hartley, W. J.: Pathology of congenital bovine epizootic arthrogryposis and hydranencephaly and its relationship to Akabane virus. Aust. Vet. J., *53*:319–325, 1977.

Inaba, Y.: Akabane virus: an epizootic congenital arthrogryposis-hydranencephaly syndrome in cattle, sheep and goats caused by Akabane virus. J. An. Res. Q., *25*:245–276, 1981.

Kemler, A. G., and Martin, J. E.: Incidence of congenital cardiac defects in bovine fetuses. Am. J. Vet. Res., *33*:249–251, 1972.

Lagerlof, N., and Boyd, H.: Ovarian hypoplasia and other abnormal conditions in the sexual organs of cattle of the Swedish Highland breed: results of postmortem examination of over 6,000 cows. Cornell Vet., *43*:64–79, 1953.

Leipold, H. W., et al.: Congenital defects in cattle. Nature, cause and effect. Adv. Vet. Sci. Comp. Med., *16*:103–150, 1972.

Nihleen, B., and Eriksson, K.: A hereditary lethal defect in calves—atresia ilei. Nord. Vet. Med., *10*:113–127, 1958.

Saunders. L. Z., and Fincher, M. G.: Hereditary multiple eye defects in grade Jersey calves. Cornell Vet., *41*:351–366, 1951.

Schleger, A. V., et al.: Histopathology of hypotrichosis in calves. Austr. J. Biol. Sci., *20*:661–688, 1967.

Scott, F. W., et al.: Virus induced congenital anomalies of the bovine fetus. I. Cerebellar degeneration (hypoplasia), ocular lesions and fetal mummification following experimental infection with bovine viral diarrhea–mucosal disease virus. Cornell Vet., *63*:536–560, 1973.

Shupe, J. L., et al.: Lupine, a cause of crooked calf disease. J. Am. Vet. Med. Assoc., *151*:198–203, 1967.

Thomson, R. G.: Congenital bronchial hypoplasia in calves. Pathol. Vet., *3*:89–109, 1966.

Thomson, R. G.: Failure of bone resorption in a calf. Pathol. Vet., *3*:234–246, 1966.

Anomalies—Sheep

Binns, W., et al.: A congenital cyclopian-type malformation in lambs induced by maternal ingestion of a range plant *Veratrum californicum*. Am. J. Vet. Res., *24*:1164–1175, 1968.

Dennis, S. M., and Leipold, H. W.: Ovine congenital defects. Vet. Bull., *49*:233–239, 1979.

Narita, M., et al.: The pathogenesis of congenital encephalopathies in sheep experimentally induced by Akabane virus. J. Comp. Pathol., *89*:229–239, 1979.

Anomalies—Swine

Bradley, R., and Wells, G. A. H.: Developmental muscle disorders in the pig. Vet. Annu., *18*:144–157, 1978.

Done, J. T.: Congenital nervous diseases of pigs: a review. Lab. Anim., *2*:207–217, 1968.

Flatla, J. L., et al.: Dermatosis vegetans in pigs; symptomatology and genetics. Zentralbl. Veterinaermed., *8*:25–42, 1961.

Huston, R., et al.: Congenital defects in pigs. Vet. Bull., *48*:645–675, 1978.

Thurley, D. C., and Done, J. T.: The histology of myofibrillar hypoplasia of newborn pigs. Zentralbl. Veterinaermed. [A], *16*:732–740, 1969.

Anomalies—Horse

Gerneke, W. H., and Coubrough, R. I.: Intersexuality in the horse. Onderstepoort J. Vet. Res., *37*:211–216, 1970.

Huston, R., et al.: Congenital defects in foals. J. Equine Med. Surg., *1*:146–161, 1977.

Anomalies—Dog

Barnett, K. C.: Comparative aspects of canine hereditary eye disease. Adv. Vet. Sci. Comp. Med., *20*:39–68, 1976.

Cheville, N. F.: The gray collie syndrome. J. Am. Vet. Med. Assoc., *152*:620–633, 1968.

Davies, A. P., et al.: Primary lymphedema in three dogs. J. Am. Vet. Med. Assoc., *174*:1316–1320, 1979.

Erickson, F., et al. Congenital defects in dogs. Can. Pract., *4*:4:54–61, *4*:5:52–61, *4*:6:40–53, 1977.

Fox, M. W.: Inherited structural and functional abnormalities in the dog. Can. Vet. J., *11*:5–12, 1970.

Gee, B. R., et al.: Segmental aplasia of the Mullerian duct system in a dog. Can. Vet. J., *18*:281–286, 1977.

Hayes, H. M., et al.: Canine congenital deafness: epidemiological study of 272 cases. J. Am. Anim. Hosp. Assoc., *17*:473–476, 1981.

Krook, L.: The pathology of renal cortical hypoplasia in the dog. Nord. Vet. Med., *9*:161–176, 1957.

Leipold, H. W.: Nature and causes of congenital defects of dogs. Surg. Clin. North Am., *8*:47–77, 1978.

Mair, I. W. S.: Hereditary deafness in the Dalmatian dog. Arch. Otolaryngol. *212*:1–14, 1976.

Patterson, D. F., and Medway, W.: Hereditary diseases of the dog. J. Am. Vet. Med. Assoc., *149*:1741–1754, 1966.

Patterson, D. F.: Congenital defects of the cardiovascular system in dogs: studies in comparative cardiology. Adv. Vet. Sci. Comp. Med., *20*:1–38, 1976.

Renshaw, H. W., and Davis, W. C.: Canine granulocytopathy syndrome. Am. J. Pathol., *95*:731–744, 1979.

Spurling, N. W.: Hereditary disorders of haemostasis in dogs: a critical review of the literature. Vet. Bull., *50*:151–173, 1980.

Wilson, J. W., et al.: Spina bifida in the dog. Vet. Pathol., *16*:165–179, 1979.

Anomalies—Cat

Bellhorn, R. W., et al.: Ocular colobomas in domestic cats. J. Am. Vet. Med. Assoc., *159*:1015–1021, 1971.

Bosher, S. K., and Hallpike, C. S.: Observations on the histological features, development and pathogenesis of the inner ear degeneration of the deaf white cat. Proc. R. Soc. (Biol.), *162*:147–170, 1965.

Chu, E. H. Y., et al.: Triploid-diploid chimerism in a male tortoiseshell cat. Cytogenet. Cell Genet., *3*:1–18, 1964.

DeForest, M. E., and Basrur, P. K.: Malformations and the manx syndrome in cats. Can. Vet. J., *20*:304–314, 1979.

Kilham, L., et al.: Cerebellar ataxia and its congenital transmission in cats by feline panleukopenia virus. J. Am. Vet. Med. Assoc., *158*:888–906, 1971.

Patterson, D. F., and Minor, R. R.: Hereditary fragility and hyperextensibility of the skin of cats: a defect in collagen fibrillogenesis. Lab. Invest., *37*:170–179, 1977.

Saperstein, G., et al.: Congenital defects in domesticated cats. Feline Pract., *6*:18–44, 1976.

Aging

Cutler, R. G.: Evolution of human longevity: a critical overview. Mech. Aging Dev., *9*:337–354, 1979.

Fries, J. F.: Aging, natural death and the compression of morbidity. New Engl. J. Med., *303*:130–135, 1980.

Getty, R.: Bibliography of canine gerontology and geriatrics. J. Am. Vet. Med. Assoc., *147*:38–46, 1965.

Grant, R. L.: Concepts of aging: an historical review. Perspect. Biol. Med., *6*:443–479, 1963.

Jones, M. L.: Lifespan in mammals. *In* Montali, R., and Migaki, G. (eds.): Comparative Pathology of Zoo Animals. Washington, D.C., Smithsonian Institution Press, 1980, pp. 495–509.

Makinodan, T., and Yunia, E. (eds.): Immunology and Aging. New York, Plenum Publishing Corp., 1977.

Martin, G. M.: Cellular aging—clonal senescence. A review (Part I). Am. J. Pathol., *89*:484–512, 1977.

Martin, G. M.: Cellular aging—postreplicative cells. A review (Part II). Am. J. Pathol., *89*:513–530, 1977.

Marx, J. L.: Aging research. I. Cellular theories of senescence. Science, *186*:1105–1107, 1974.

Timiras, P. S.: Biological perspectives on aging. Am. Sci., *66*:605–613, 1978.

Walford, R. L.: Immunologic Theory of Aging (II). Baltimore, Williams & Wilkins, 1969.

6
NEOPLASIA

Neoplasia occurs when a group of cells becomes free of normal growth control mechanisms, grows without regard for the normal structural and functional aspects of a tissue or an organ and, in a manner of speaking, becomes a rebellious autonomous state. The new growth often compromises the function of the organ in which it grows, or those nearby, by pressure or by replacement of normal functional tissue. The mechanisms that result in the new growth involve the ***fundamentals of biology in terms of growth control, aging, selection and survival of variants*** and eventually are the cause of death in a significant percentage of individuals within those species that normally survive well past maturity. Huge research efforts are attempting to unravel the mysteries of neoplasia mainly to prolong human life but also to gain comprehension of the mechanisms involved in the fundamentals of the neoplastic process.

DEFINITION

Oncology is the study of neoplasia, and this word is the basis of ***oncogenesis*** and ***oncogenic,*** which relate to the induction of neoplasia. The common term for a neoplasm is ***cancer,*** or ***tumor,*** and both of these tend to be used all-inclusively. In general it is not appreciated that cancer is a disease of animals as well as humans; it occurs in many species, from mammals to lower vertebrates and also in plants. Some species of domestic and laboratory animals have a high incidence of cancer and are often used to study basic oncogenic mechanisms in comparative medicine.

Many definitions of neoplasia may be found. Boyd (1970) states that "the term

The major emphasis here will be on the fundamentals of the neoplastic process, the causes, effects and consequences, and the general aspects of treatment, diagnosis and classification. An indication of the incidence in domestic animals is also included. Examples of specific neoplasms of domestic animals will be used to illustrate general points, but the purpose here is not to cover the special pathology of neoplasms but to deal with matters that might relate to all neoplasms.

neoplasia is restricted in pathology to tumor growth, a process which serves no useful purpose, which continues unchecked and which is not controlled by the laws of normal growth although undoubtedly controlled in ways that remain to be discovered." Robbins and co-workers (1981) state that "a neoplasm is best considered as a parasitic abnormal mass of cells which grows more or less progressively unless excised or controlled by therapeutic intervention." The most widely used and accepted definition is that by Willis (1967): "a tumor is an abnormal mass of tissue, the growth of which exceeds and is uncoordinated with that of the normal tissues and persists in the same excessive manner after cessation of the stimuli which evoked the change."

Let us examine Willis's definition more closely. The essential tissues of a tumor are ***cells of a specific kind derived from a single kind,*** and all classification and nomenclature are based on this fact. For example, a tumor of interstitial cells in a testicle is made of and is derived from Leydig cells even though connective tissue and blood vessels support the new growth of Leydig cells. A tumor may also develop from Sertoli cells or from seminiferous epithelium; each will look different and behave in a different manner in the host and many differ from species to species in behavior but not in basic structure. In another example, separate specific tumors may develop from connective tissue, smooth muscle, blood vessels or lymphocytes within the spleen. The amount and type of connective tissue stroma and the degree of vascularization may vary markedly in different kinds of tumors, but ***these components are supportive and are not neoplastic.*** The classification system that comes later will further expand on this point.

Proliferation of tumor cells usually results in a mass of abnormal tissue within an organ. Any clinical or pathological description that includes the statement that "there is an abnormal mass of tissue . . ." should prompt the observer to consider a tumor a possibility.

The mass may contain hemorrhage, necrosis or inflammation, depending upon its growth patterns and location, and these may hinder the recognition of the lesion as a neoplasm. It may grow in an uncoordinated fashion without regard for normal architecture and may massively ***infiltrate*** a tissue to destroy its normal function, or it may ***expand*** in a solitary mass so that pressure may compromise an important function. Normal tissues vary in their rate of cell turnover, and an all-inclusive statement about what is normal and what is excessive can not be made; however, the tumor cells multiply and persist beyond what is normal for the particular tissue and therefore appear as an abnormal mass of cells or tissue.

The excessive growth ***persists*** and tends to become ***autonomous.*** Some neoplasms grow at a consistent rate, others may stop or regress but most continue. The ***rate of growth is quite variable*** among different kinds of tumors, even among tumors of the same kind. It is usually not possible to determine the etiological factor or factors or when they influenced the tissue by examination of the tumor.

There are processes that at times result in considerable proliferation of tissue but are not neoplastic. How do they differ from neoplasia? ***Inflammatory lesions*** such as granulomas or abscesses may become large and persist for a prolonged period and disrupt function. Once the etiological factors have been overcome, however, the lesion will regress and cease to be progressive. ***Hyperplasia*** occurs in response to loss of tissue, increased functional demands or disturbed hormonal activity. It will regress if these stimuli are withdrawn and therefore is limited in amount and duration. If hyperplasia becomes excessive and independent of these stimuli, however, it may become neoplastic.

In summary, neoplasia is uncoordinated proliferation of tissue, independent of the structural and functional patterns of normal tissue, and is indefinitely progressive. Permanent cellular change, manifested as excessive proliferation, is transmitted to successive generations of cells.

CLASSIFICATION AND NOMENCLATURE

The terminology associated with tumors may become very complex, and an effort is required to keep it simple. The first contact may be forbidding and create a negative impression about tumor terminology. However, a slow, persistent, step-by-step approach will create understanding, and the words may then be used comfortably and accurately.

Histogenesis and Behavior

There are two bases of the classification of tumors, the first being ***histogenesis*** and the second being ***behavior.*** These two simple categories are the foundation for all classification and must be kept in mind even when the terminology appears complicated. ***Histogenesis is fundamental and primary*** in importance and can be specified in most instances. ***Behavior is secondary*** and may become arbitrary and subjective in interpretation.

Histogenetic classification means that the tumor must be named by the specific tissue or cell type ***from which it arose and of which it is composed. Tumors can develop from virtually any known cell type in the body.*** As mentioned previously, different kinds of tumors develop from Sertoli cells, Leydig cells and seminiferous epithelium even though they normally are very close together. The person identifying a tumor must, if at all possible, identify the tissue of origin because the ***biological behavior, treatment and prognosis*** may be quite different for different tumors, even for those arising from the same organ.

Usually, a tumor is first classified as either epithelial or mesenchymal. Difficulties may arise since some normal tissues are not easily placed into these broad categories, for example, melanocytes and ovarian stroma. Further problems may arise if a tumor is growing in such a manner that it does not resemble the parent tissue; it may even lack identification with any tissue near its location. Such tumors are said to be ***poorly differentiated*** or ***anaplastic.*** Also, ***metaplasia and hyperplasia may be mistaken for neoplasia,*** such as in exuberant granulation tissue or exostosis of new bone formation or in myeloid metaplasia.

Behavior is an assessment of whether the tumor is relatively harmless or a dangerous, life-threatening lesion. Tumors that are confined, slow-growing and noninvasive are called ***benign*** and carry the suffix ***oma.*** Tumors that are invasive, rapidly growing and dangerous are called ***malignant*** and carry the suffix ***sarcoma*** if derived from mesenchymal tissue or the suffix ***carcinoma*** if derived from epithelial tissue. In some instances, the use of carcinoma or sarcoma has been set aside because of common usage, and the words benign or malignant precede the name of the tumor. These situations will become apparent in time. The distinction between benign and malignant is often not easily made and, surprisingly, may vary considerably and subjectively among individual pathologists examining the same lesions. Some pathologists tend to be rather consistently "benign" and some "malignant" in their interpretation and diagnosis of tumors. The importance of an accurate assessment of behavior relates to the prognosis and treatment. Characteristic features of benign and malignant tumors are included in Table 6–1.

Kinds of Tumors

Table 6–2 outlines the ***classification terminology*** used for the more common tumors. Comments for purposes of general orientation on some aspects of the classification follow, with details coming later in special pathology.

Papillomas usually occur on skin and may have a variety of forms, from pedunculated to flat, smooth or villous. Warts are an example and occur in many species. ***Adenomas*** occur in glands and are common in dogs as circumanal gland adenoma, sebaceous gland adenoma and mammary gland adenoma; they also occur in adrenal and thyroid glands and in many other tissues. These lesions are often difficult to differentiate from nodular hyperplasia, and the distinction may be rather subjective.

A common group of epithelial tumors

TABLE 6–1. Characteristics of Benign and Malignant Tumors

	Benign Tumor	Malignant Tumor
1. Structure	usually well differentiated and typical of the tissue of origin	often imperfectly differentiated and atypical
2. Mode of growth	usually purely expansive and circumscribed	infiltrative as well as expansive, hence not strictly circumscribed
3. Rate of growth	usually slow, with scanty mitotic figures	may be rapid, with many mitotic figures
4. End of growth	may come to a standstill	rarely ceases growing
5. Metastasis	absent	frequently present
6. Clinical results	dangerous because of a. position b. accidental complications c. production of excess hormone	dangerous also because of progressive infiltrative growth and metastasis

TABLE 6–2. Classification of Some Tumors of Animals Based on Histogenesis and Behavior

Origin	Benign	Malignant
Epithelial		
nonglandular surface	papilloma	carcinoma
glandular surface	polyp	adenocarcinoma
glandular	adenoma	adenocarcinoma
Mesenchymal		
connective tissue	fibroma	fibrosarcoma
mucoid connective tissue	myxoma	myxosarcoma
fat	lipoma	liposarcoma
cartilage	chondroma	chondrosarcoma
bone	osteoma	osteosarcoma or osteogenic sarcoma
blood vessels	angioma or hemangioma	hemangiosarcoma
synovial lining	—	synovial sarcoma
meninges	meningioma	meningeal sarcoma
lymph vessels	lymphangioma	lymphangiosarcoma
smooth muscle	leiomyoma	leiomyosarcoma
striated muscle	rhabdomyoma	rhabdomyosarcoma
mast cell	mastocytoma	mast cell sarcoma
Hemopoietic		
lymphocytes	lymphoma	lymphosarcoma
plasma cells	—	myeloma
granulocytes	—	myelogenous leukemia
reticulum cells	—	reticulum cell sarcoma
Nervous		
astrocytes	astrocytoma	astrocytoma
oligodendroglia	oligodendroglioma	oligodendroglioma
ependyma	ependymoma	ependymoma
Schwann cell	neurofibroma	neurofibrosarcoma
nerve cells	neuroblastoma, ganglioneuroma	malignant neuroblastoma, malignant ganglioneuroma
chromaffin paraganglia (adrenal medulla)	pheochromocytoma	malignant pheochromocytoma
nonchromaffin paraganglia (carotid body and aortic body)	nonchromaffin paraganglioma	malignant nonchromaffin paraganglioma
Others		
melanocyte	melanoma	malignant melanoma
embryonic—kidney	nephroblastoma	malignant nephroblastoma
—gonad	teratoma	malignant teratoma

found in dogs is the ***basal cell*** group. These are derived from the basal layer of the squamous epithelium and can differentiate into tumors of any of the adenexa of the skin, such as sweat gland adenomas, sebaceous gland adenomas and hair follicle tumors (trichoepithelioma), or just proliferating ribbons of basal cells. Some may contain several or mixed components if they are not well differentiated. Also, some are locally invasive. Terminology for this group varies somewhat since some components fall between adenomas and carcinomas. Sometimes, they are designated as basal cell tumors—sebaceous gland–type or ribbon-type—without using the word adenoma or carcinoma.

Carcinomas should carry the name of the tissue of origin, for example, squamous cell carcinoma, transitional cell carcinoma, adrenal cortical carcinoma, hepatocellular carcinoma, pancreatic carcinoma, intestinal carcinoma, renal carcinoma, mammary carcinoma and uterine carcinoma. The prefix ***adeno*** is used when appropriate if glandular epithelium is involved. Some carcinomas induce much connective tissue growth and are called ***scirrhous carcinomas.*** Some adenocarcinomas grow in ***papillary*** form, and some result in retention of secretion, as in cystic hyperplasia, and lead to such terms as ***papillary cystadenocarcinoma.*** Descriptive terms such as "well differentiated" or "poorly differentiated" are also used.

Among the mesenchymal tumors, those of connective tissue, bone, blood vessels and smooth muscle are most common and some of the others are rare. Connective tissue tumors occur in many locations; fibromas are difficult to distinguish from scar tissue at times. Bone tumors are common in the extremities of large dogs. Hemangiomas are common in the skin of dogs.

Tumors of lymphocytes have been called various names, such as ***leukemia, leukosis, lymphoma, malignant lymphoma*** and ***lymphomatosis,*** but the proper term is ***lymphosarcoma*** if the tumor is malignant, and most are. These tumors are common in animals and have diffent morphological expressions in different species. The pattern in cattle is variable, and any combination of organ involvement may occur and include the lymph nodes, spleen, heart, uterus, kidneys, liver, nerves, thymus, intestines, stomach and others. Cats often have lesions in the anterior mediastinum and kidneys. A viral etiological factor has been confirmed in cats and chickens and is being investigated in other species; the distinction between T and B cell origin is also being investigated. Classification into the cell type—for example, lymphocyte, prolymphocyte or stem cell—of the tumor is significant because the prognosis and treatment may vary with each type.

A vaccine for prevention of one form of this disease in chickens is now used extensively. Perhaps lymphosarcoma in chickens will be a model for things to come in other species. For years, there were several "forms" of leukosis, as the disease is called in birds—neural, ocular, visceral, leukemic and bone. Investigation has revealed that there are two distinct diseases caused by two different viruses. A DNA virus causes Marek's disease. It occurs in young birds, is horizontally transmitted and can be prevented by vaccination. The other "forms" are caused by RNA viruses, are usually transmitted vertically and occur in older birds. Actually, research on these diseases of birds has set the pace for investigation of viral causes of tumors in animals.

Leukemia means that there are abnormal malignant cells present in the circulating blood, and it may occur in about half of the cases of ***lymphosarcoma,*** but this feature is more consistent in myelogenous leukemia. The red cells, eosinophils, neutrophils or megakaryocytes may be malignant in ***myelogenous leukemia,*** but usually it is the granulocytic group. Some proliferative, but not necessarily neoplastic, lesions in bone marrow are difficult to classify, and the use of such terms as ***reticuloendotheliosis*** and ***myeloproliferative disorder*** is proper when nonspecificity is advised.

Terminology for nervous tumors tends to name the tumor and to call it benign or malignant without a suffix. Most are locally invasive and therefore malignant. Tumors in tissues derived from neural crest tissue may have neuroendocrine functions.

Tumors of melanocytes are common in dogs and also in horses. Some do not produce melanin and are called ***amelanotic melanomas,*** which are usually highly malignant. ***Nephroblastomas*** are not common but occur in most species and may be malignant. Teratomas are unusual and tend to occur mostly in testes and ovaries.

In terminology, the separation of epithelial tumors from mesenchymal tumors is traditional, but there are examples of tumors that have mesenchymal and epithelial components. These are called ***mixed tumors*** and are best known in the mammary gland of dogs. The derivation of the epithelial components from acini and ducts is clear, but the derivation of the mesenchymal component has long caused controversy. It seems reasonably established now that the mesenchymal components originate from the myoepithelial cell, although controversy still exists. Not only mesenchymal differentiation but also the extremes of metaplasia occur within this component. Large areas of malignant fibrous tissue, cartilage or bone may be present along with malignant epithelial components. Separate carcinomas and sarcomas do arise in the mammary gland, but the true ***"mixed mammary tumor"*** is very common. As a matter of interest, mammary tumors in dogs are influenced by hormones, estrogens in particular, and the removal of the ovaries prior to the second estrous cycle has a marked sparing effect on the incidence of these tumors.

More than one tumor may occur in one individual, and examples have been recorded in which numerous separate unrelated tumors have been present in one animal.

Many of the kind of tumors listed in Table 6–2 will be illustrated in the remainder of the chapter as general points about neoplasia are made. Keep this in mind and look back at the table periodically to see where they fit.

STRUCTURE, APPEARANCE AND GROWTH

The normal ***gross description*** of any lesion includes ***location, color, size, shape, consistency and appearance of the cut surface.*** It is not possible to generalize about the appearance of tumors except in the phrase "there is an abnormal mass of cells or tissue." Tumors can occur anywhere in the body, but in each species, some are more common than others. With experience and knowledge, one learns to expect certain kinds of tumors in certain places in certain species, and this background assists in making one consider a tumor in a differential diagnosis.

Gross Features

Clinical examination may reveal whether the tumor is discrete, locally infiltrative but still relatively confined or spread extensively. Usually, the ***abnormal mass*** or ***greatly enlarged organ*** is easily visualized, but some tumors (for example, a lymphosarcoma in the liver) infiltrate diffusely throughout an organ and are not easily recognized. Tumors on a body surface may be ulcerated and may be suspect on the basis of a ***persistent nonhealing ulcerating lesion.*** Tumors may retain the ***color*** of the parent tissue, but usually there is a recognizable difference in color. ***Size and shape are quite variable.*** Some tumors will grow to a tremendous size, while others remain small, but both types may cause equal functional damage. ***Size is no indication of prognosis;*** a tiny tumor may be highly malignant and a huge one may be benign. Benign tumors tend to be discrete masses, which, in surgical jargon, are easily "shelled out." An ***infiltrative tumor*** may tie together several tissues; for example, growth of a thyroid carcinoma may infiltrate to such an extent that the skin and other structures are not freely moveable over the gland. The shape will depend on the mode of growth within a tissue. ***Consistency*** is variable, but the extremes from firmness to soft and mushy are striking. A scirrhous tumor may be so ***firm*** that the idea of a tumor may not arise. If ***necrosis*** is extensive within the tumor, it may be very ***soft*** in parts. The differences in consistency relate directly to the amount and type of stroma on the one hand and to necrosis on the other. The ***cut surface*** extends the information available from the outside and assists with an appreciation of infiltration, damage to normal tissue, pattern of growth or necrosis.

The main point in observing a lesion that may be a tumor is to describe the lesion and, in doing so, to differentiate it from other basic types of processes, such as inflammation or degeneration and necrosis. *Listen to the description and think about it; the answer is usually there.* Start out by trying to determine *if* the lesion is a tumor before deciding what type it might be.

Figures 6–1 through 6–32 illustrate various gross features of tumors and are used as examples to assist with ***recognition of a lesion as a tumor*** and to distinguish them from other lesions, such as inflammation.

These figures will assist in gaining familiarity with the names of tumors. When looking at the illustrations in this chapter, think about and observe what the growth of the tumor is doing to the normal structure and function of the affected organ and, in some instances, other organs nearby.

Text continued on page 340

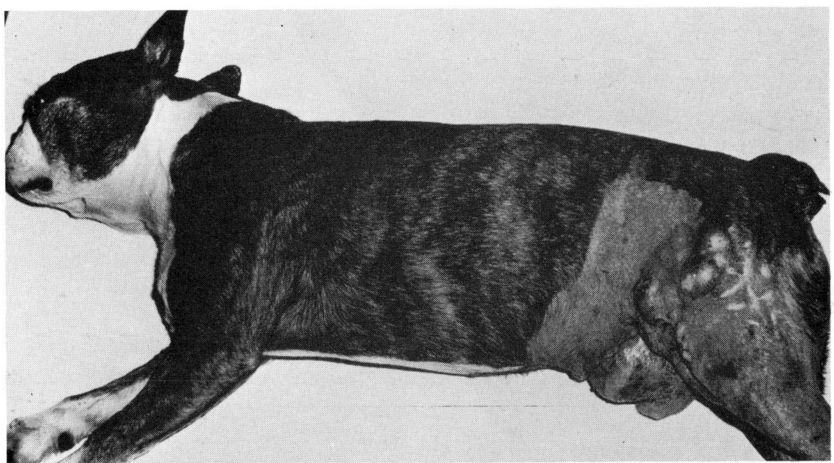

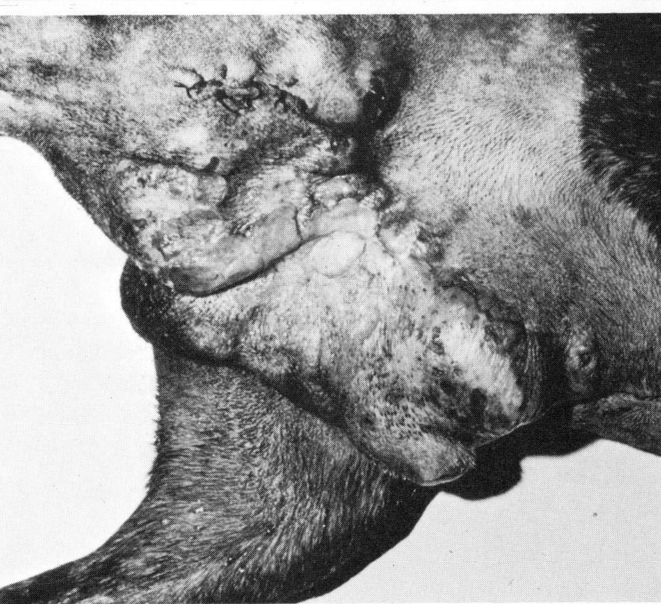

Figures 6–1 and 6–2. Mast cell tumor in the thigh region of a dog. Biopsy sites are visible. This tumor grew very rapidly.

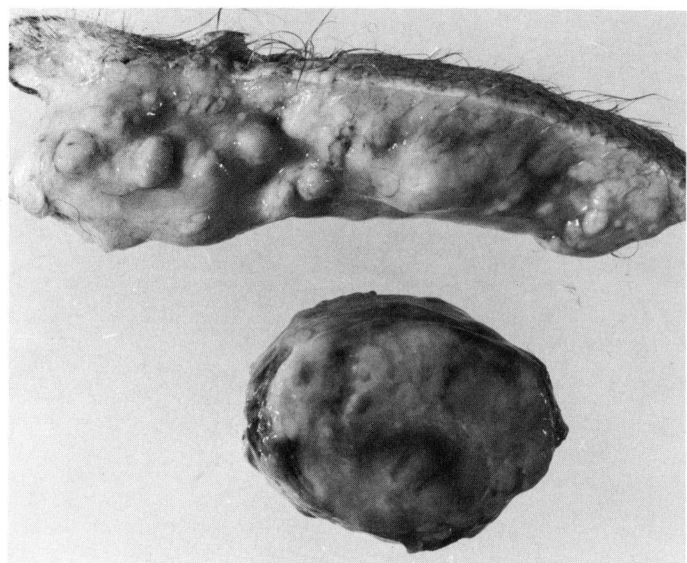

Figure 6–3. Mast cell tumor in a dog's skin and metastasis to a lymph node.

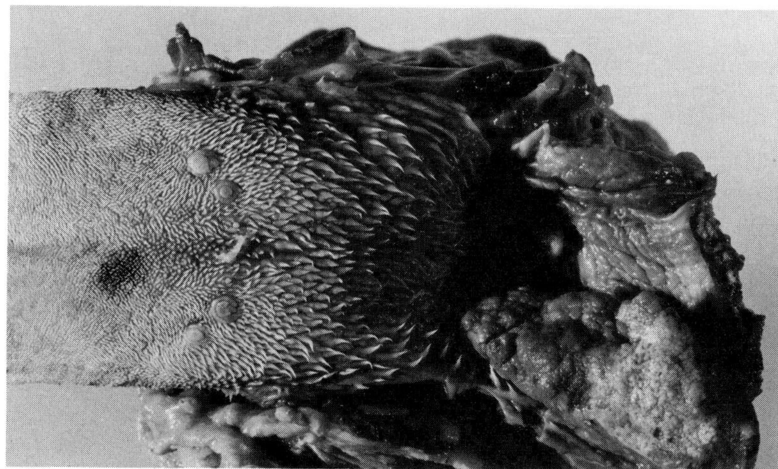

Figure 6–4. Squamous cell carcinoma in one tonsil in a dog (lower right). The mass was locally infiltrative in the upper neck region and a cross section of the main mass is shown in Figure 6–5. The trachea and esophagus are compressed at the top.

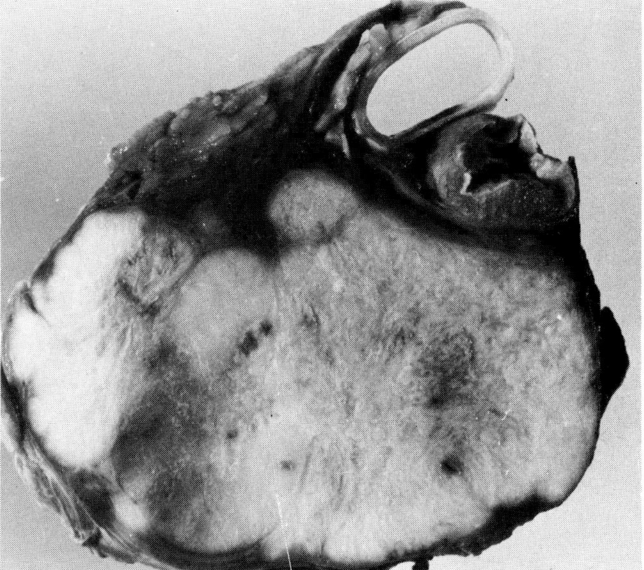

Figure 6–5. See the legend for Figure 6–4.

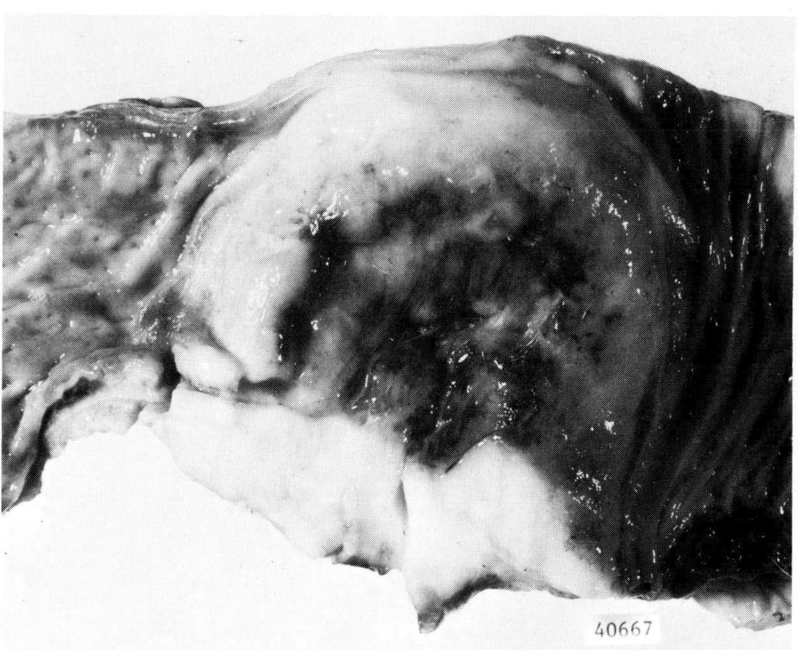

Figure 6–6. A discrete ulcerated mass of lymphosarcoma in the intestine of a dog. The cut surface is at the bottom.

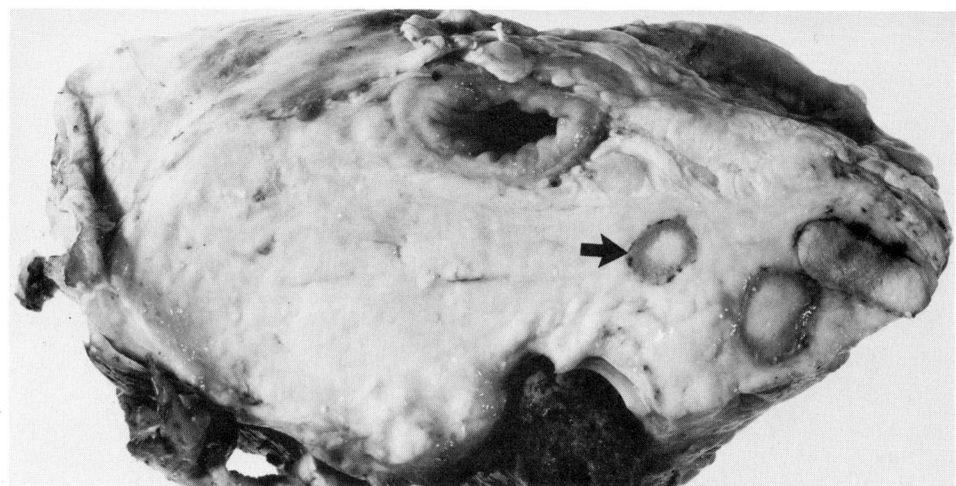

Figure 6–7. Mass of lymphosarcoma in the mesentery surrounding the intestine in a cow. This lesion may lead to intestinal obstruction. Note the area of necrosis to the right (arrow) within the tumor.

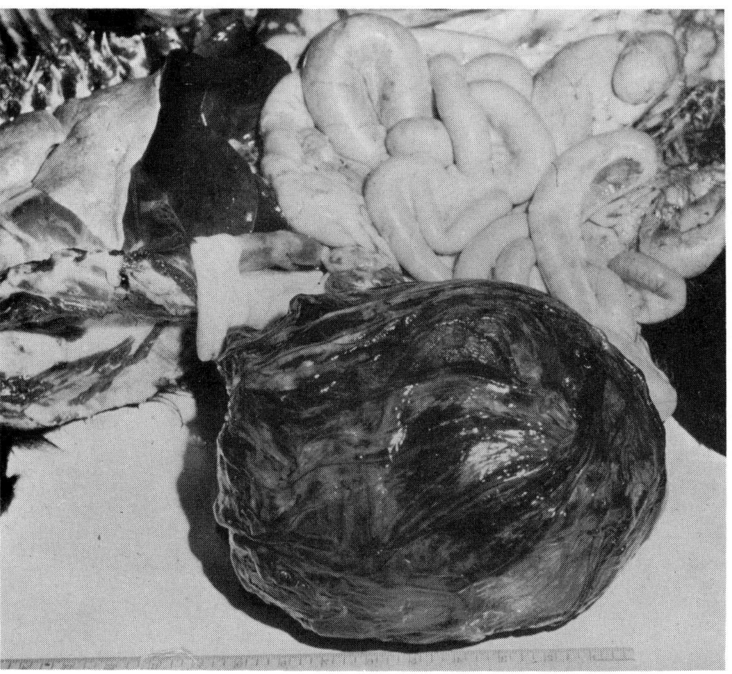

Figure 6–8. Large discrete mass of a hemangiosarcoma in the spleen of a dog. There was no metastasis. These often lead to sudden death from rupture and fatal hemorrhage into the abdomen.

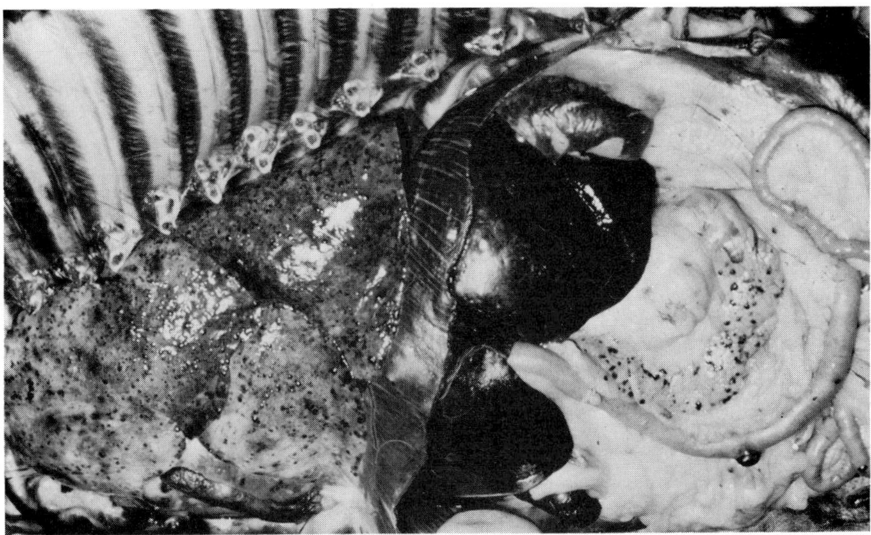

Figure 6–9. Hemangiosarcoma in a dog with extensive metastasis as small dark foci in the lung and abdomen. This lesion is often primary in the heart with subsequent metastasis, as shown here.

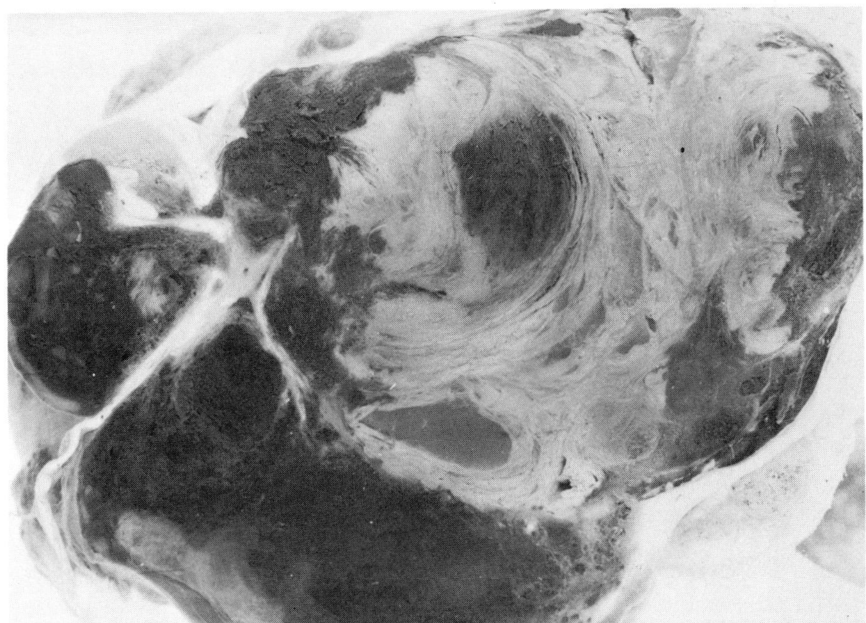

Figure 6–10. Cut surface of a splenic hemangiosarcoma. Large areas of thrombosis and hemorrhage are present. (Museum specimen.)

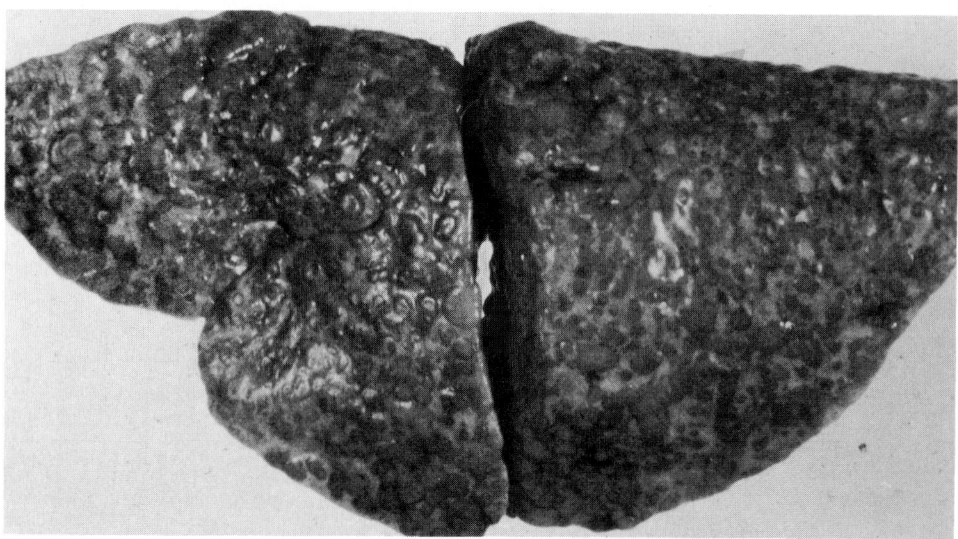

Figure 6–11. Multicentric nodules in a bronchiolar carcinoma in a dog's lung. These may be difficult to distinguish grossly from diffuse granulomatous pneumonia. (Museum specimen.)

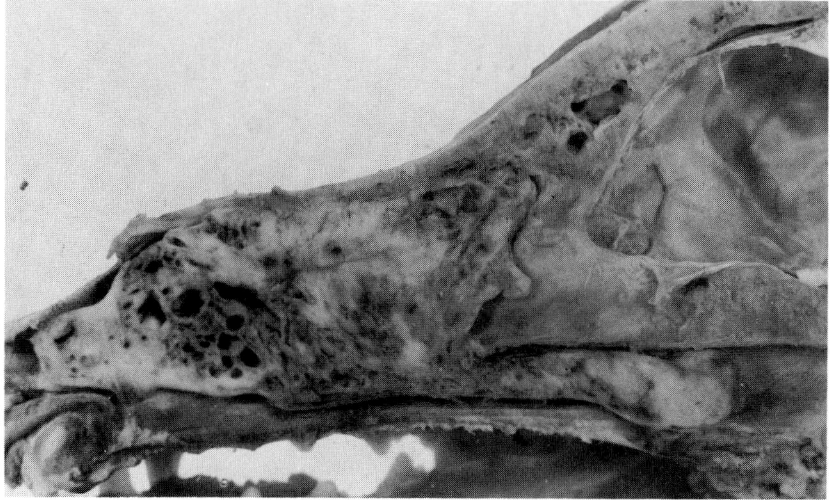

Figure 6–12. Nasal carcinoma in a dog. The tumor has disrupted the normal architecture of the turbinates and has filled the nasal passage. (Museum specimen.)

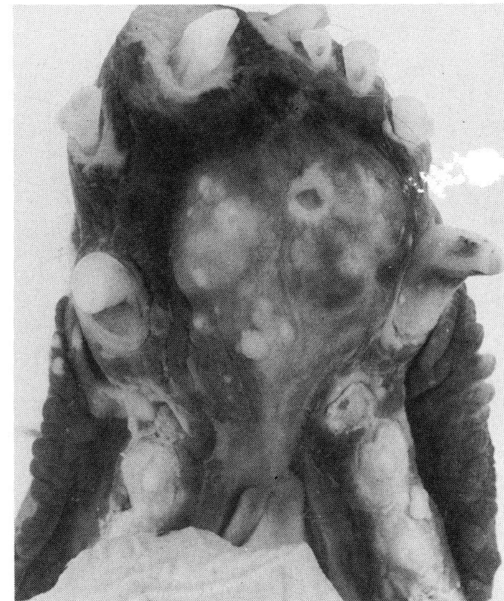

Figure 6–13. A melanoma in the oral cavity of a dog that has now disrupted the location of the teeth as well as the bone of the mandible. (Museum specimen.)

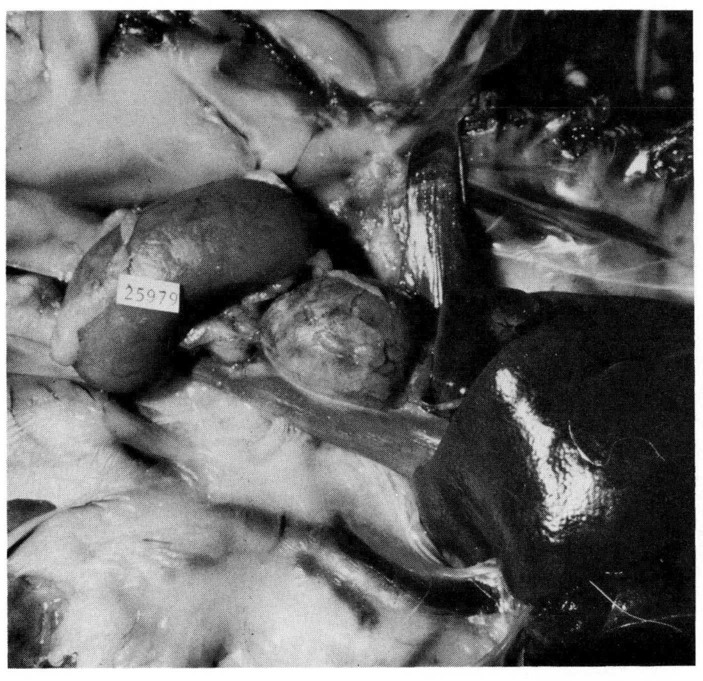

Figure 6–14. Posterior area of the abdominal cavity in a dog with an enlarged adrenal gland to the right of the kidney. This could be either a cortical or a medullary tumor of the adrenal gland, and the two may be difficult to differentiate.

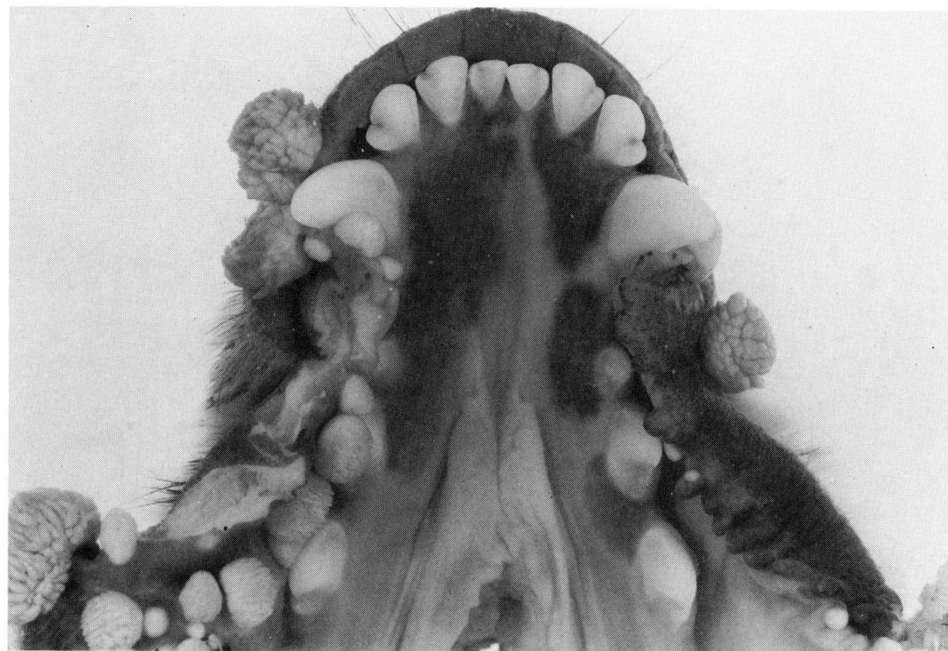

Figure 6–15. Oral papillomas or warts in a dog. These behave in a similar manner to infectious papillomas in other species.

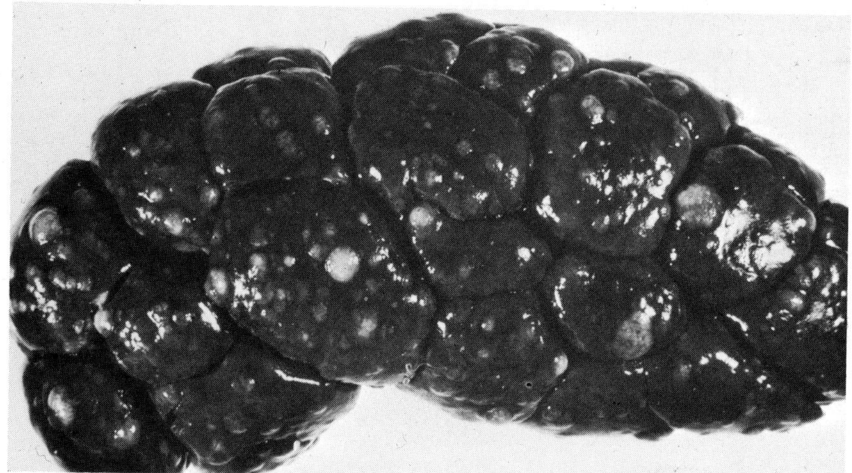

Figure 6–16. Multiple raised pale foci of lymphosarcoma in a bovine kidney.

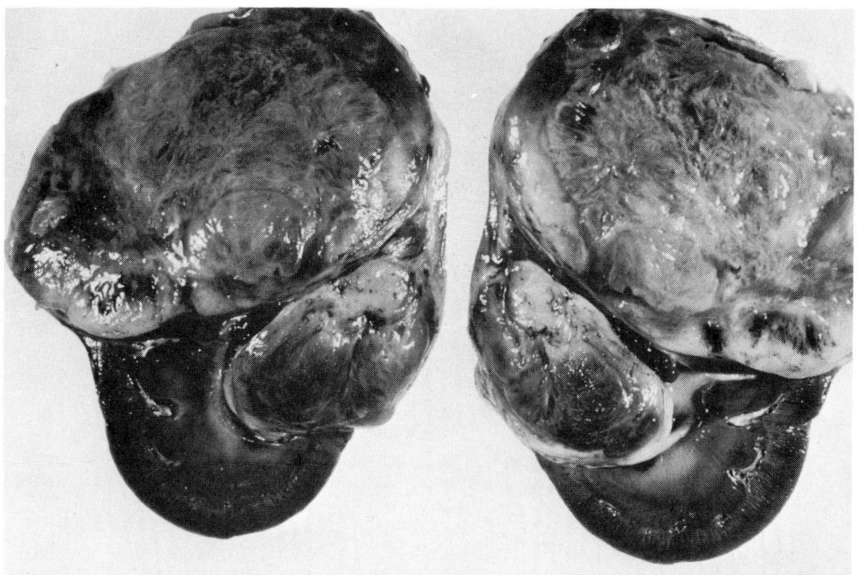

Figure 6–17. Extensive disruption and replacement of normal architecture of the kidney by a renal leiomyosarcoma in a dog.

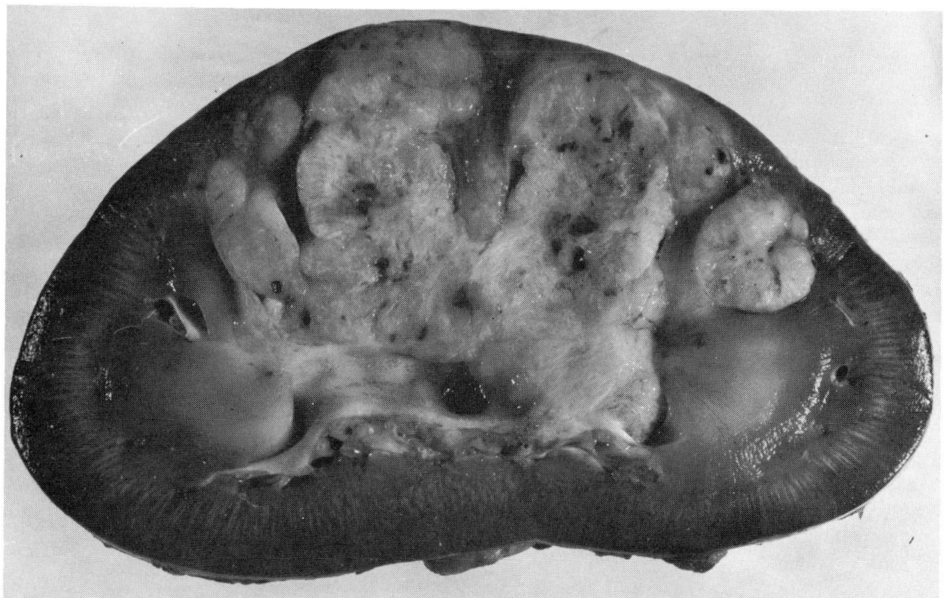

Figure 6–18. Intrarenal nonchromaffin paraganglioma in a dog. Note the replacement of renal tissue but the relatively small amount of compression of renal tissue by the tumor.

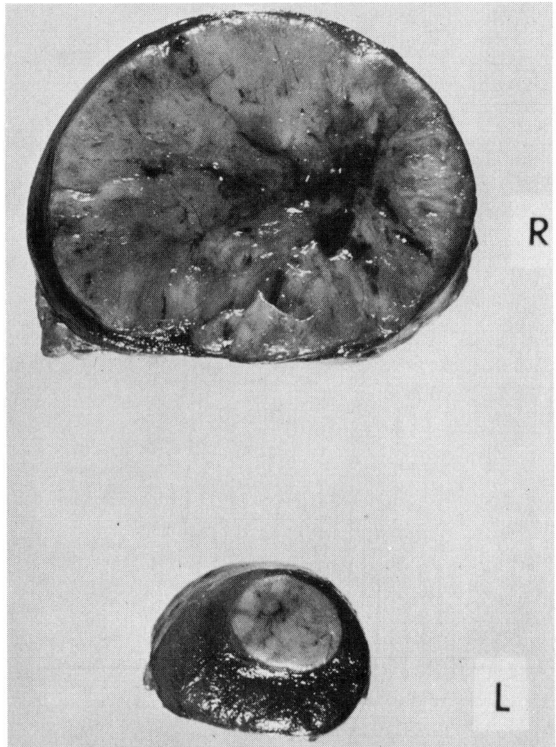

Figure 6–19. Thyroid glands of a horse. The left is about normal size but contains a white adenoma. The right gland is enlarged by a more extensive adenoma.

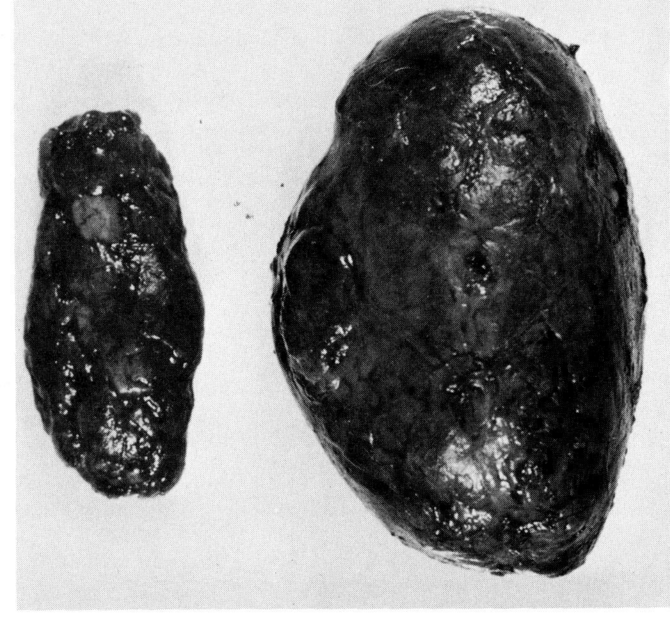

Figure 6–20. The canine thyroid gland on the left is slightly enlarged and has an uneven surface. The one on the right is considerably enlarged by an adenoma within the gland. Note that the tumor is not invasive and was easily removed from surrounding tissue.

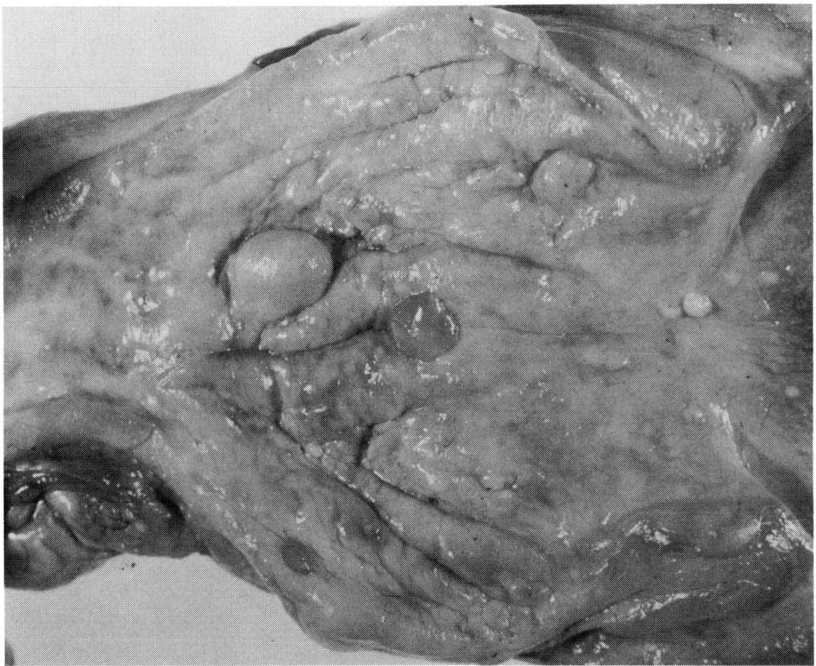

Figure 6–21. Thickened and nodular mucosal surface of the vagina of a dog. The lesions are multiple and partially confluent leiomyomas.

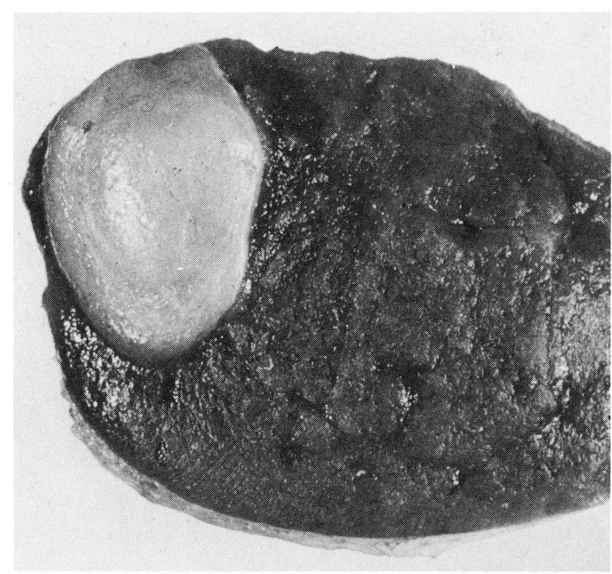

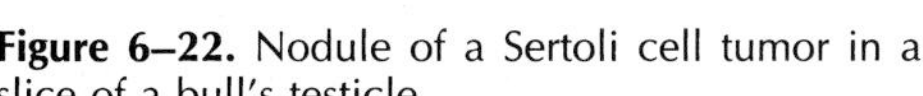

Figure 6–22. Nodule of a Sertoli cell tumor in a slice of a bull's testicle.

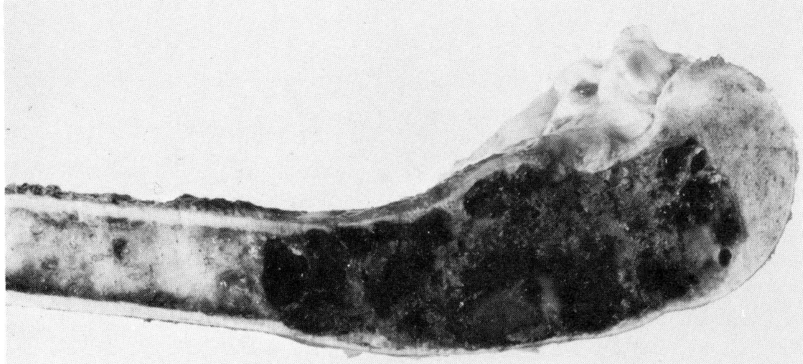

Figure 6–23. Osteogenic sarcoma in a dog. Note the disruption of architecture by the tumor. The weakened bone could lead to a pathological fracture.

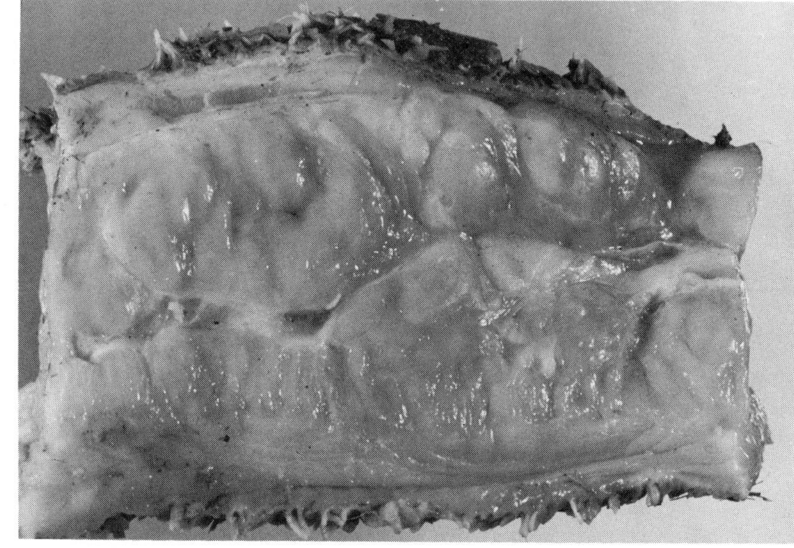

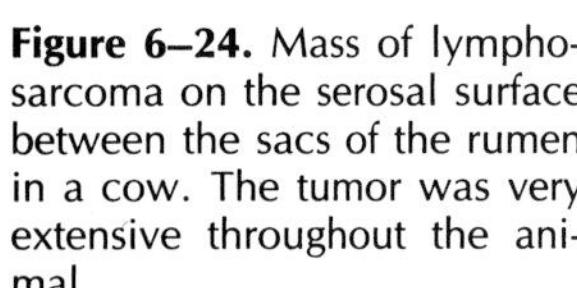

Figure 6–24. Mass of lymphosarcoma on the serosal surface between the sacs of the rumen in a cow. The tumor was very extensive throughout the animal.

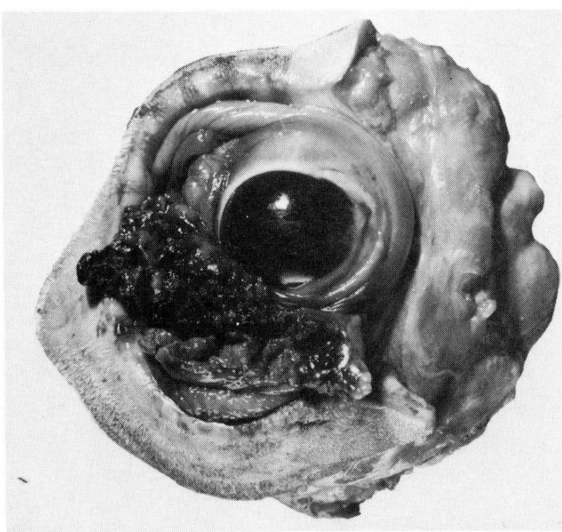

Figure 6–25. Squamous cell carcinoma of the conjunctiva in a cow. (Courtesy of C.A.V. Barker.)

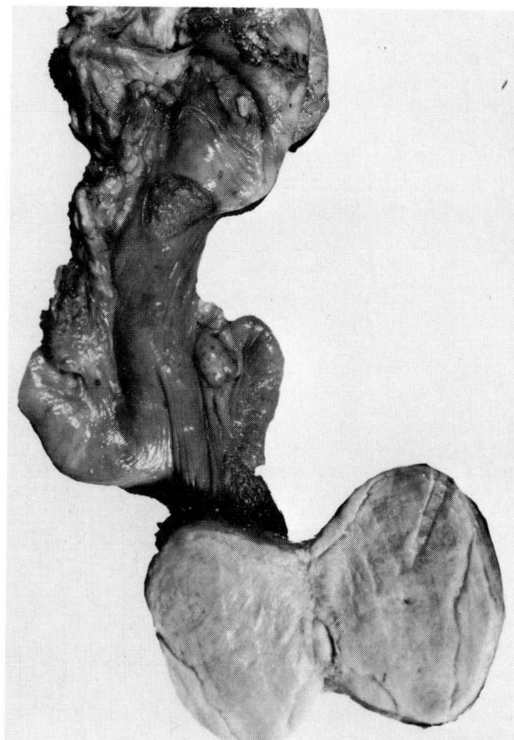

Figure 6–26. Cut surface of a large pendulous leiomyoma of a cow's uterus. (Courtesy of C.A.V. Barker.)

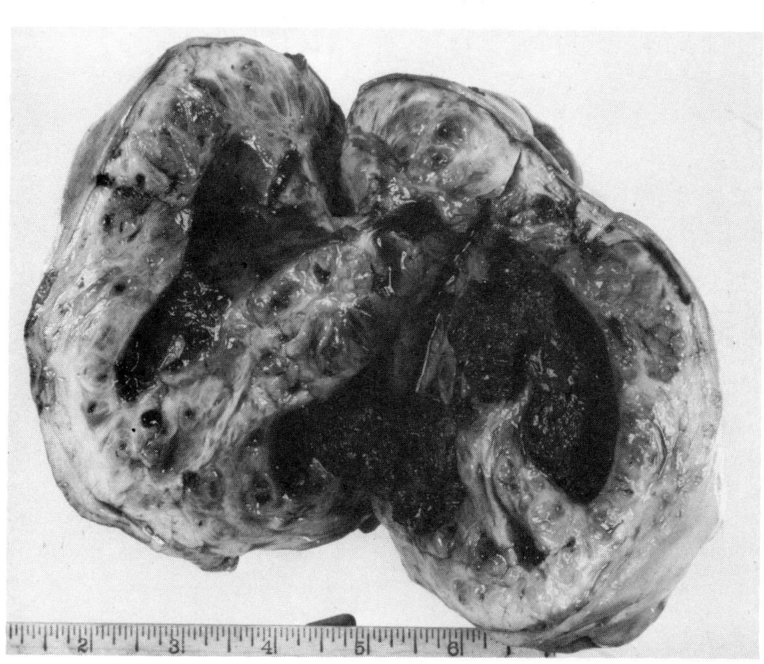

Figure 6–27. Granulosa cell tumor in the ovary of a cow. The center contains hemorrhage. (Courtesy of C.A.V. Barker.)

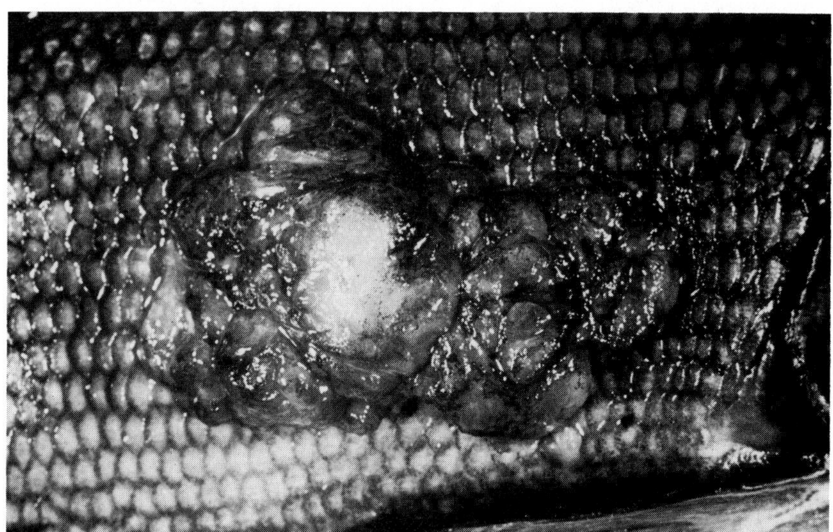

Figure 6–28. Fish with a lobulated tumor of the epidermis. (Courtesy of J. Bernstein.)

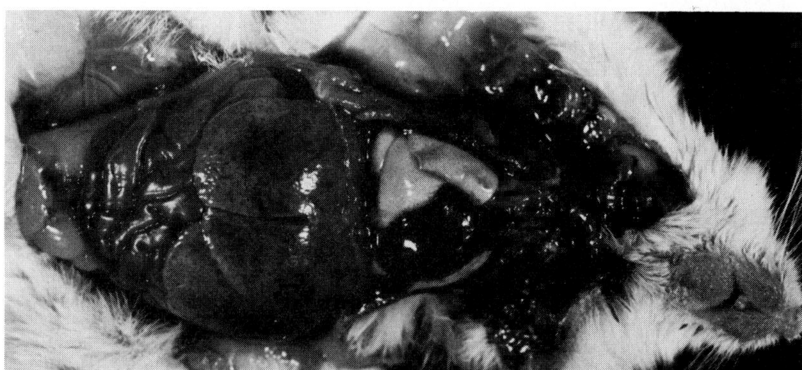

Figure 6–29. Mouse with greatly enlarged liver caused by lymphosarcoma. (Courtesy of B. Cross.)

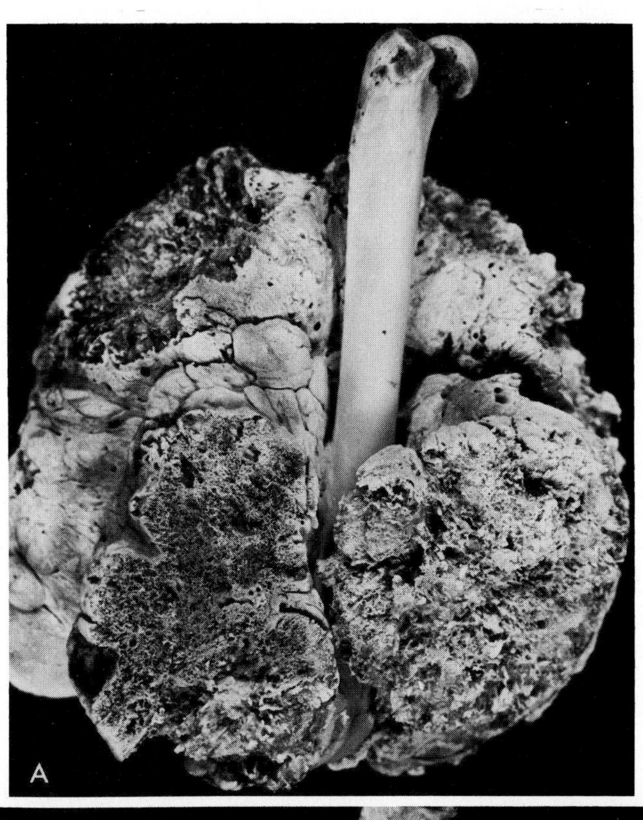

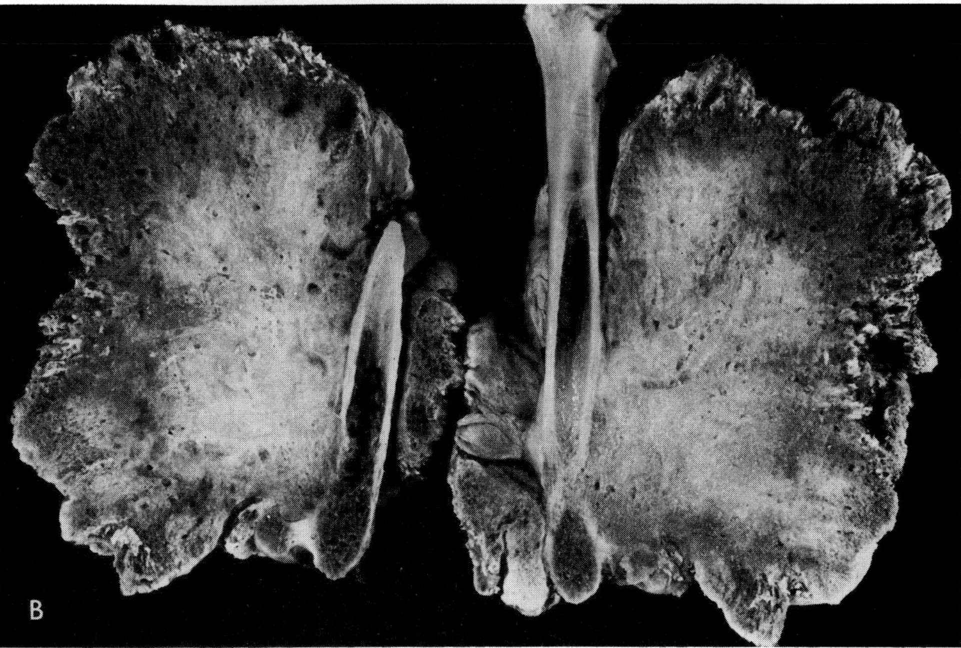

Figure 6–30. Large tumor mass of an osteogenic sarcoma from a cat. *A*, External surface, *B*, cut surface. (Courtesy of S. Friend.)

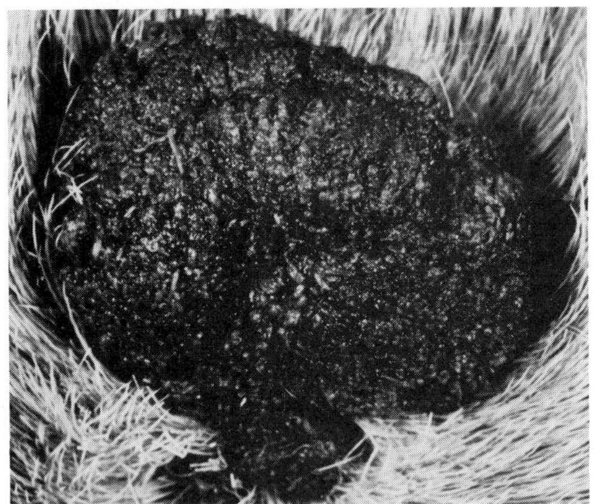

Figure 6–31. Papilloma in the skin of a white-tailed deer. (Courtesy of G. Wobeser.)

Microscopic Features

Microscopic patterns of growth are variable, but a few general patterns are useful for purposes of recognition and description. These refer particularly to carcinomas and to the pattern or amount of stroma.

The term ***sheets of cells*** is used to describe a monotonous pattern of masses of cells with similar appearance and very little apparent stromal support, just cell after cell after cell. Often, cytoplasmic borders are indistinct, which gives the impression of masses of nuclei. Examples of this pattern would be lymphosarcoma and seminoma (Figs. 6–33 through 6–37). ***Acinar arrangements*** are characterized by cells forming or attempting to form acinar units, as in a secretory gland like the thyroid or mammary gland (Figs. 6–38 and 6–39). ***Nests of cells*** are typical or endocrine tumors, in which a clump or nest of cells is surrounded by a narrow band of connective tissue stroma (Fig. 6–40). ***Palisading*** or ***trabecular*** patterns occur when cells line up in a picket fence–type arrangement along a strand of connective tissue, such as in the testicular interstitial cell tumor (Figs. 6–41 and 6–42). ***Tubular arrangements*** occur when single, double or finger-like projections of tumor cells invade surrounding tissue. Examples are basal cell tumors or anal gland tumors (Fig. 6–43).

When there is little apparent stroma, stromal arrangements may be described as ***scant,*** as in sheets of cells (Fig. 6–44) and as ***locular,*** as in the case of nests (Fig. 6–45). When the stroma is very dense and perhaps even predominating over actual tumor cells, the reaction is called ***scirrhous,*** and it is the dense stroma that accounts for the gross features of being hard and white (Fig. 6–46). Many carcinomas may have this scirrhous reaction, which is presumably induced by some secretion of the tumor cells (Fig. 6–47). Some tumors produce a substance that stimulates endothelial cells to proliferate.

The terminology for sarcomas is less specific and is usually composed to fit the pattern present in the tumor. Some of the terms used might be as follows: ***solid or loose arrangement, whorls, sheets, localized around blood vessels, spindly cells, "fleshy cells," well or poorly differentiated, monotonous or variable*** and so on (Figs. 6–48, 6–49 and 6–50).

Growth

The pattern of growth influences the type and extent of vascular supply, and these factors, combined with the rate of growth and opportunity for trauma, influence the extent to which ***hemorrhage*** occurs in tumors. Many tumors have considerable hemorrhage within them, and are known for this feature, for example, the testicular interstitial cell tumor and hemangiosarcoma in any location. A delicate blood supply or one with large sinusoidal-type vessels leads not only to hemorrhage but also to ***thrombosis and ischemic necrosis.***

Necrosis is prominent in many tumors, particularly in the center of a large mass, and the tissue becomes ***pale and soft.*** The surface of the tumor is often depressed and has a craterous appearance because of the loss of tissue from necrosis, as in a bile duct carcinoma. Large areas of necrosis may cause ***fever*** in a patient because of the release of pyrogens from the necrotic tissue. Also, there will be a degree of inflammatory reaction to the necrotic tissue and separation from viable tissue as a sequestrum.

The hemorrhage, necrosis and inflammation occurring with a tumor may create difficulties in recognition of the neoplasm or in differentiating the neoplasm from these other processes in both clinical and pathological examination.

Considerable ***variation in microscopic appearance*** may occur within a single tumor or between tumors of the same kind in a series. Usually, however, there are certain criteria or characteristics that indicate the

Text continued on page 351

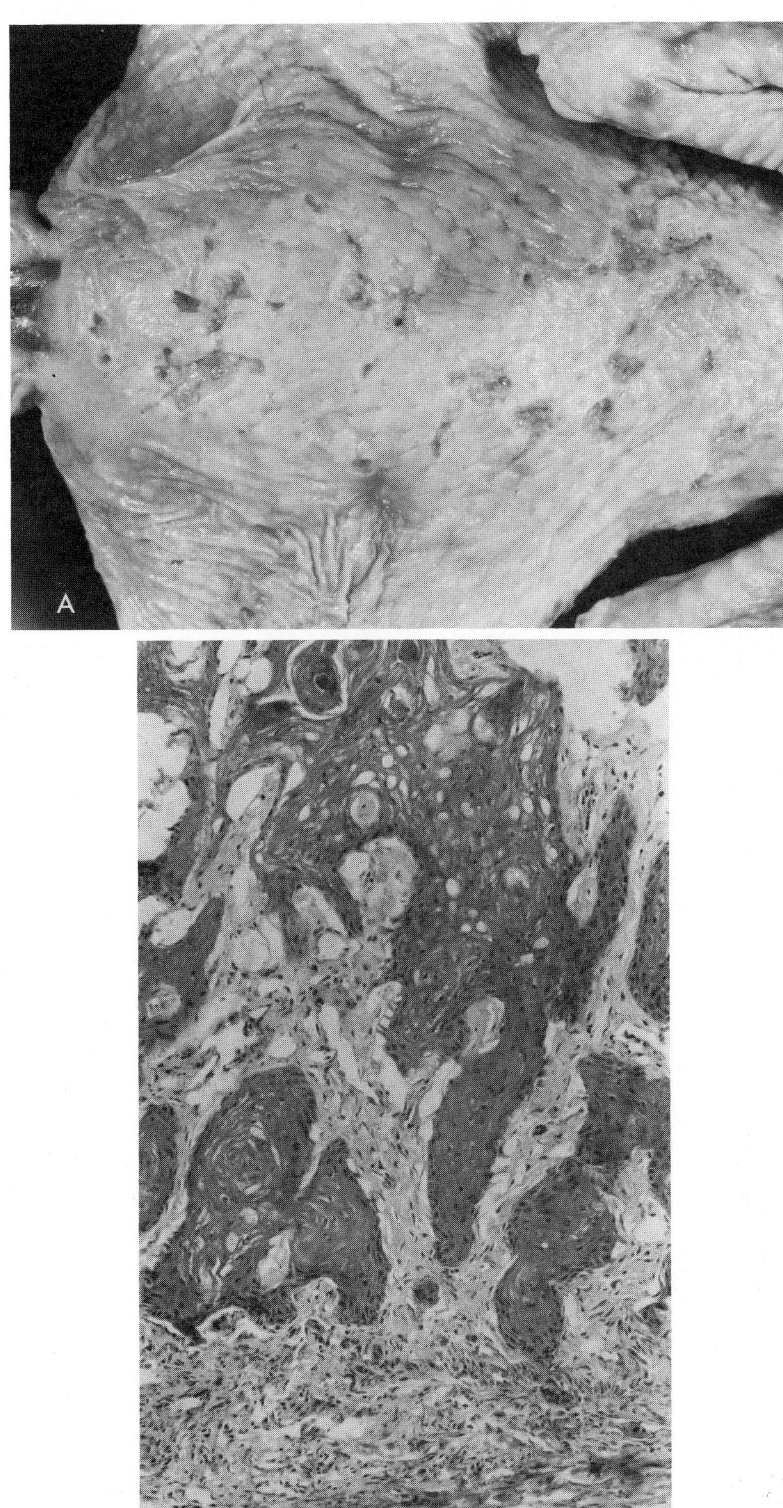

Figure 6–32. *A*, squamous cell carcinoma of the skin of a chicken. Note the irregular ulcerated lesions. *B*, Microscopic appearance of the invading squamous cells in the same lesion. (Courtesy of C. Riddell.)

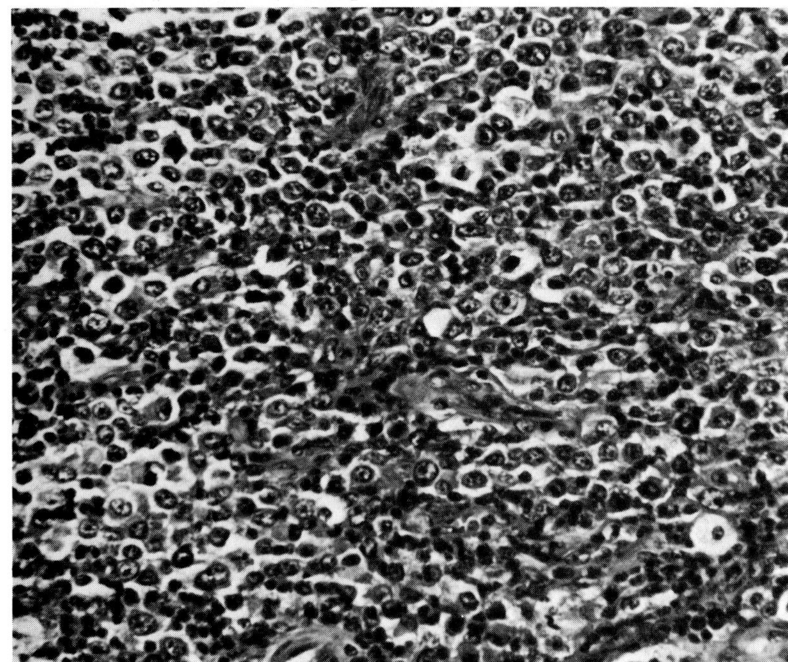

Figure 6–33. Masses of cells with little apparent tissue stroma in a mast cell tumor in a dog.

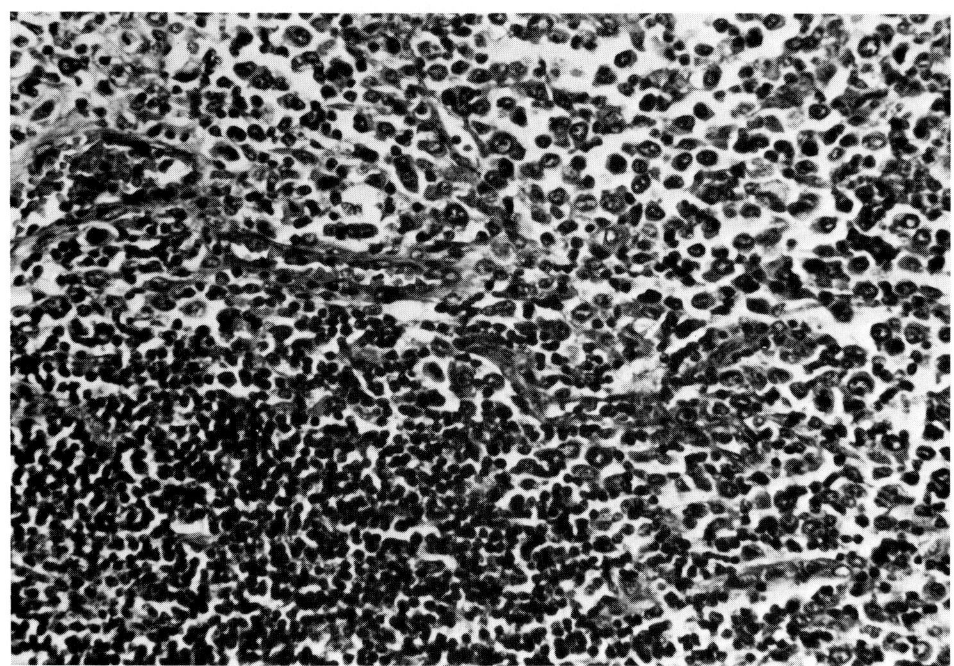

Figure 6–34. In the same tumor as shown in Figure 6–33, there are foci of lymphocytes (lower left), the significance of which will be mentioned later.

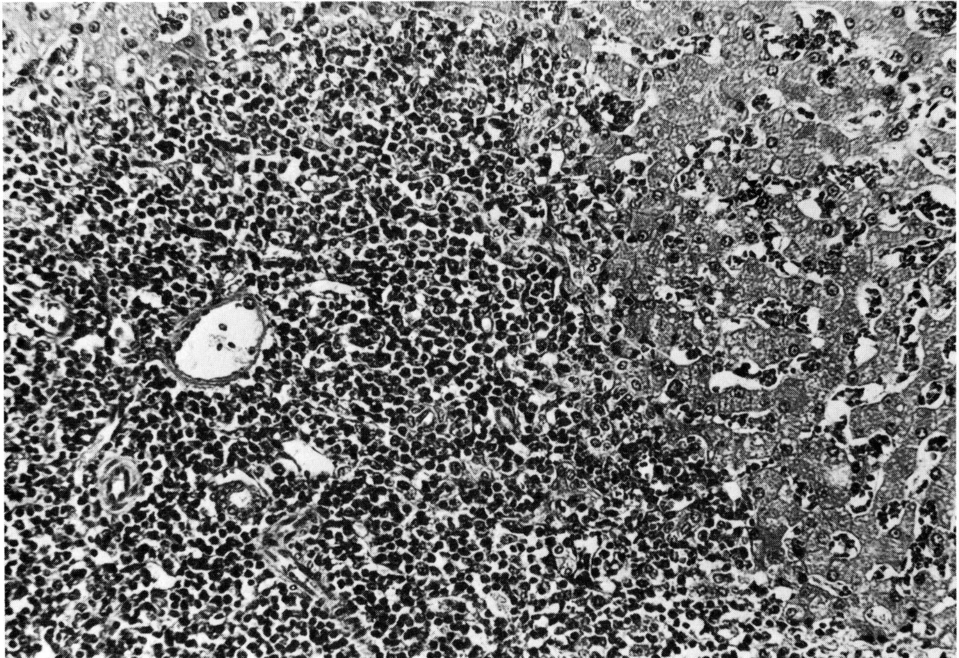

Figure 6–35. Masses of lymphocytes infiltrating the portal triads in a lymphosarcoma.

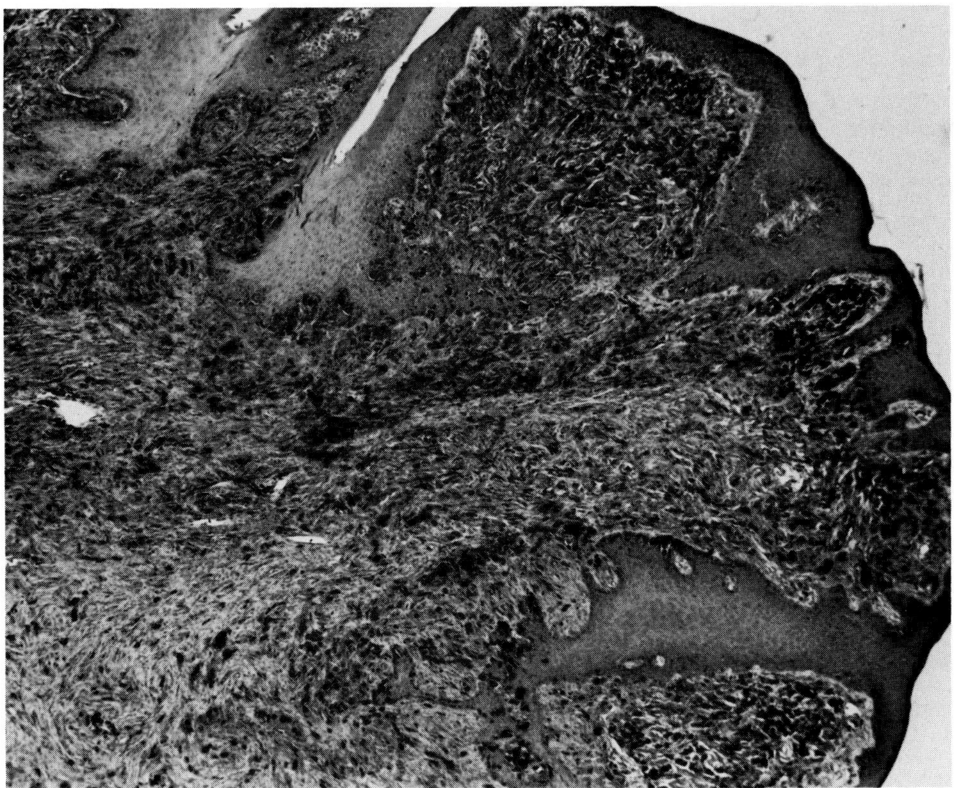

Figure 6–36. Malignant melanoma in oral mucosa of a dog. The cells are not arranged in any particular pattern, although they are in some melanomas.

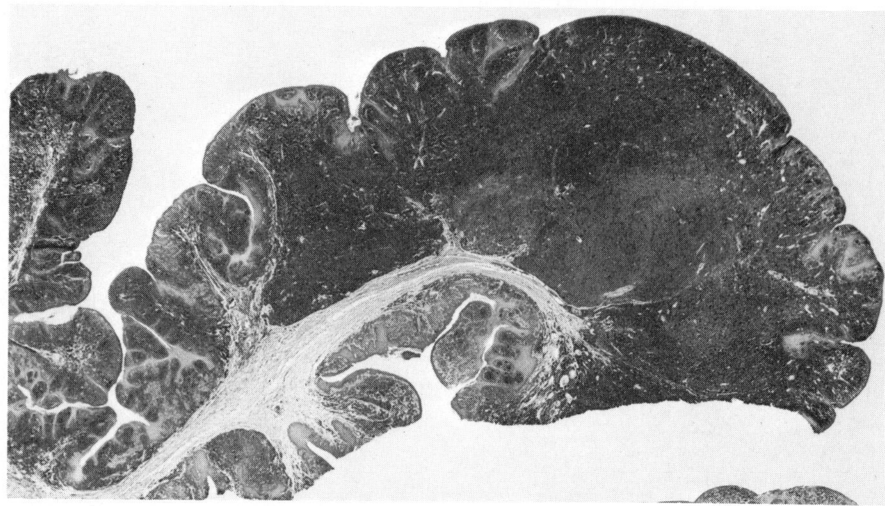

Figure 6–37. Lower power view of a tumor similar to that in Figure 6–36, providing an indication of the extent of growth in the tissue.

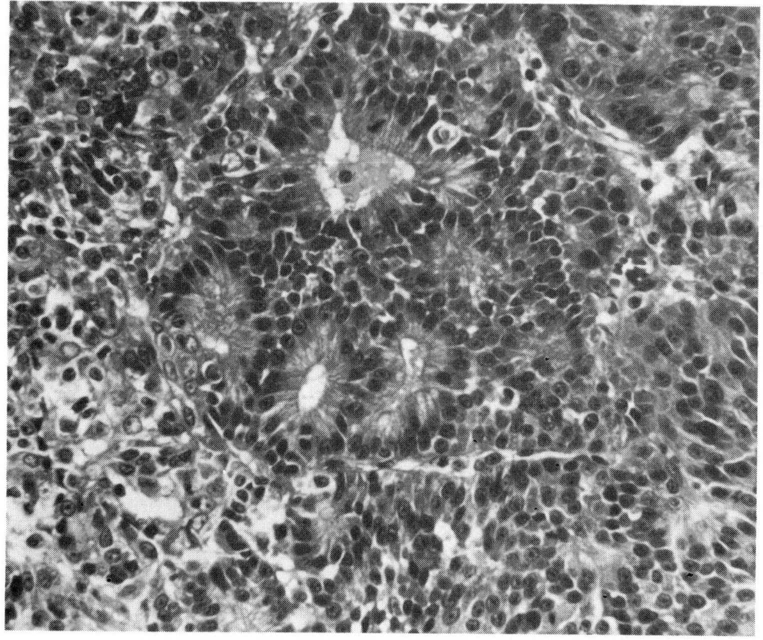

Figure 6–38. Acinar type of differentiation in part of a pancreatic adenocarcinoma in a cat. Note the columnar arrangement of cells around an apparent luminal space.

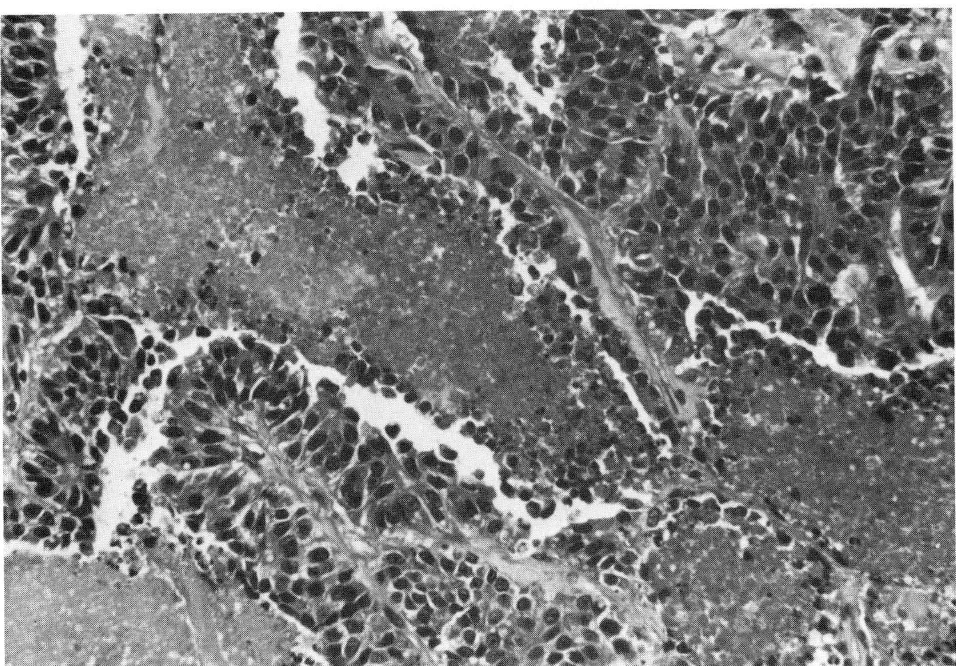

Figure 6–39. Another area of the same tumor shown in Figure 6–38. Large areas are lined by a type of glandular arrangement of epithelial cells, but necrosis of the cells occurs soon after they move away from the stromal blood supply.

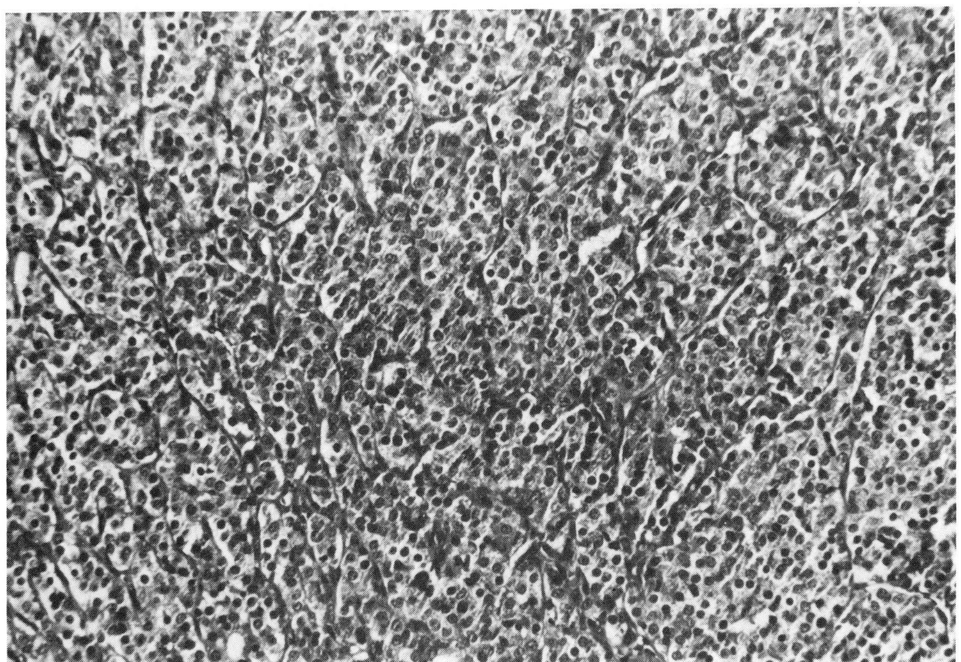

Figure 6–40. Nests and semitubular or acinar arrangements around delicate strands of stroma in a thyroid adenocarcinoma in a dog.

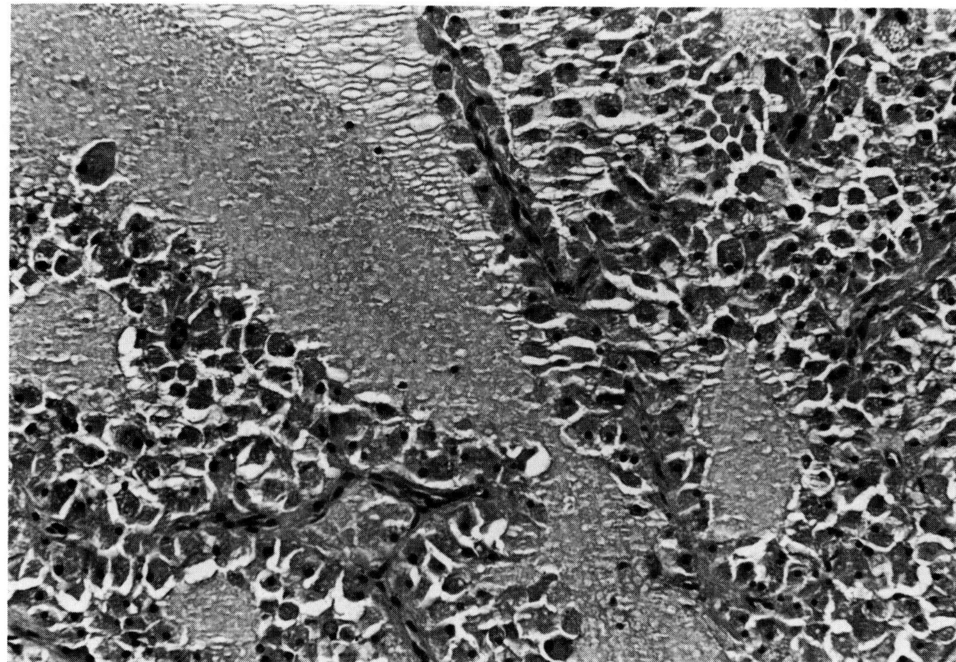

Figure 6–41. Testicular interstitial cell tumor in a dog, demonstrating palisading of cells along delicate trabecular strands of stroma. Some necrosis occurs as the cells move away from the band of stroma. Hemorrhage is common because of the thin trabeculae and long cords of cells.

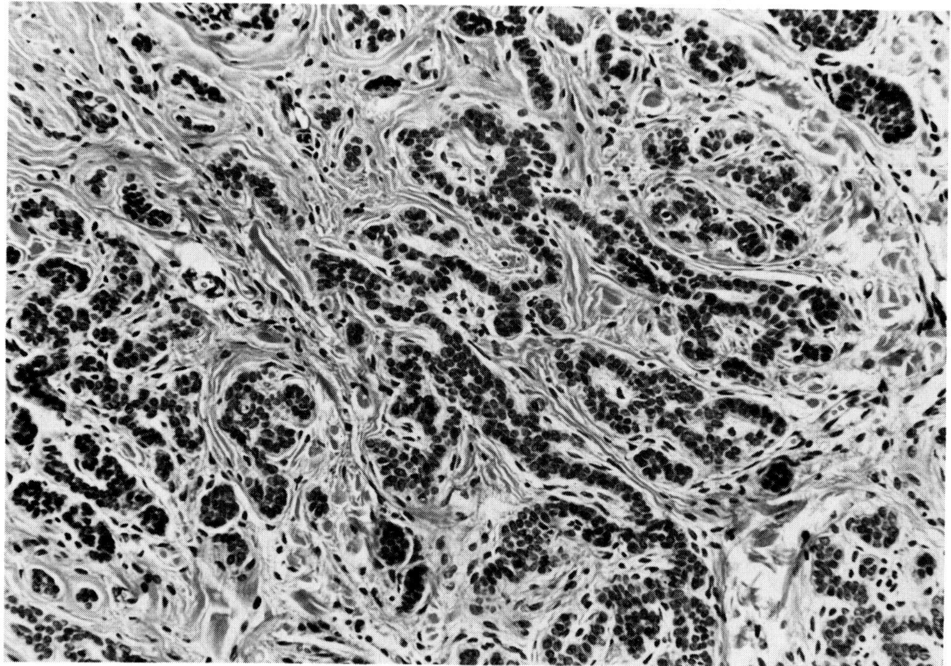

Figure 6–42. Trabecular ingrowth of a canine basal cell tumor in single or double columns of cells. This pattern is very characteristic of this tumor. Variations toward tubes and nests also occur, however (Fig. 6–43).

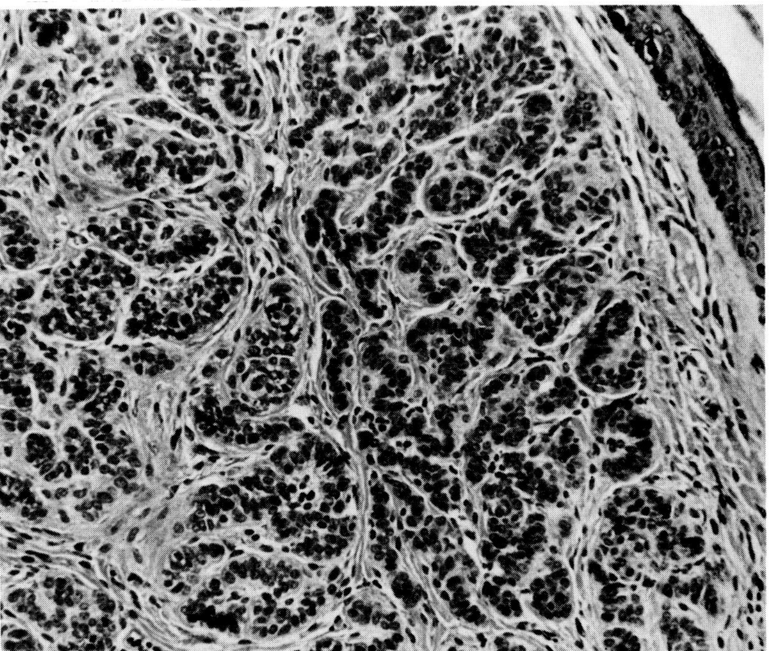

Figure 6–43. See the legend for Figure 6–42.

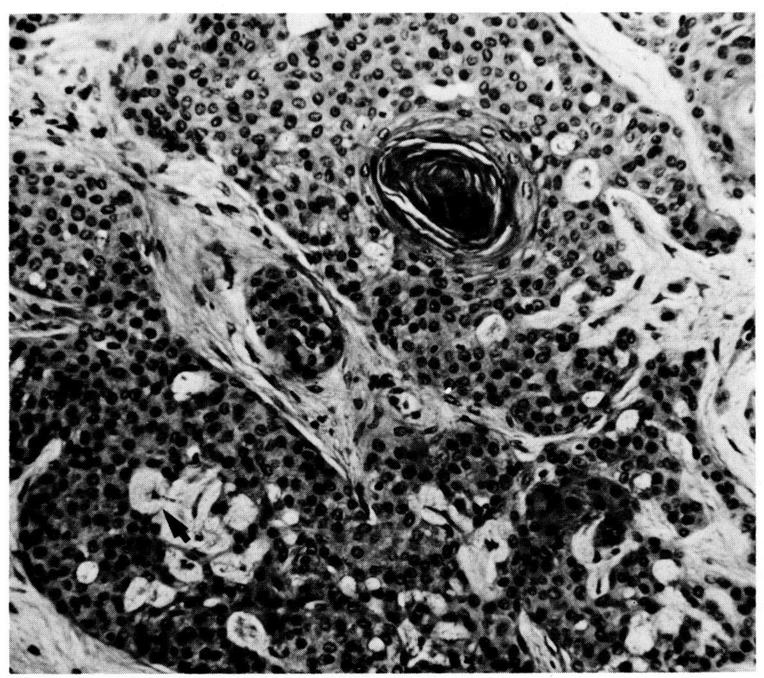

Figure 6–44. Basal cell tumor with nests of cells. The large pale cells (arrow) are differentiating toward sebaceous cells, and the circumscribed area containing keratin is differentiating toward hair follicle formation.

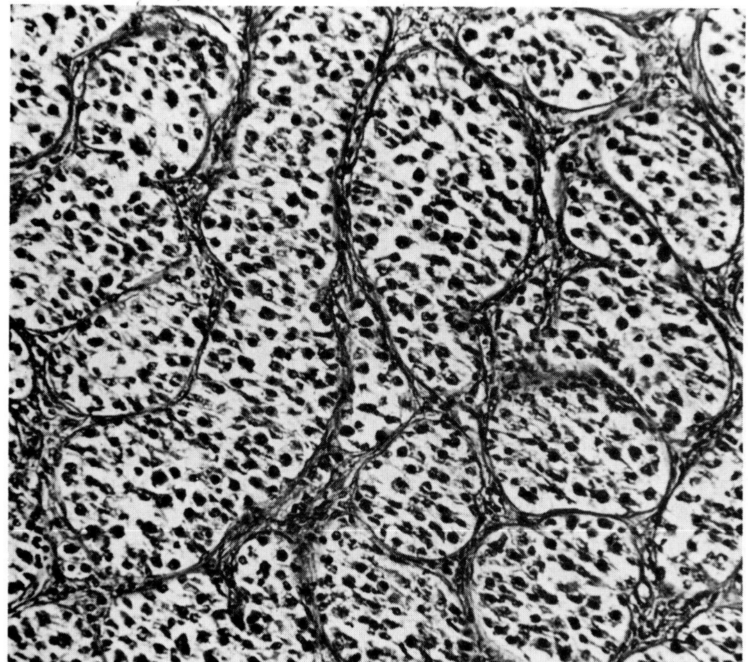

Figure 6–45. Definite tubular pattern within a Sertoli cell tumor in a dog.

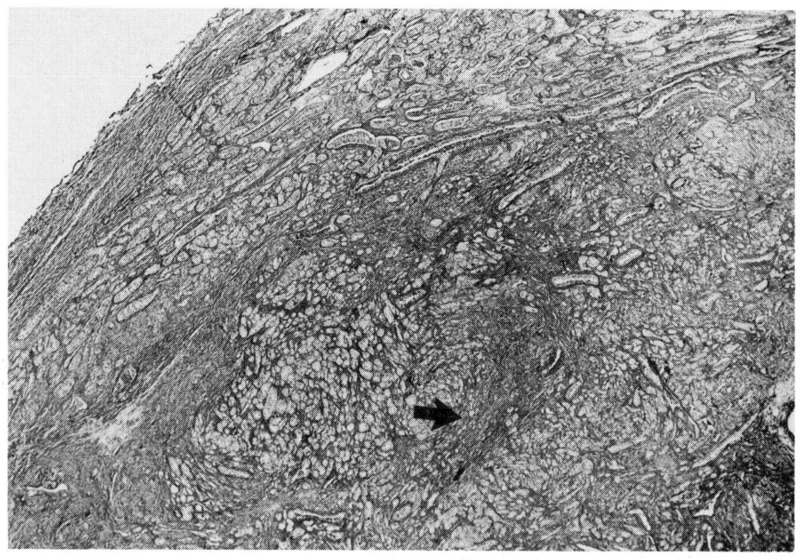

Figure 6–46. The overall pattern and variations of the same tumor as seen in Figure 6–45, as well as the more scirrhous areas (arrow).

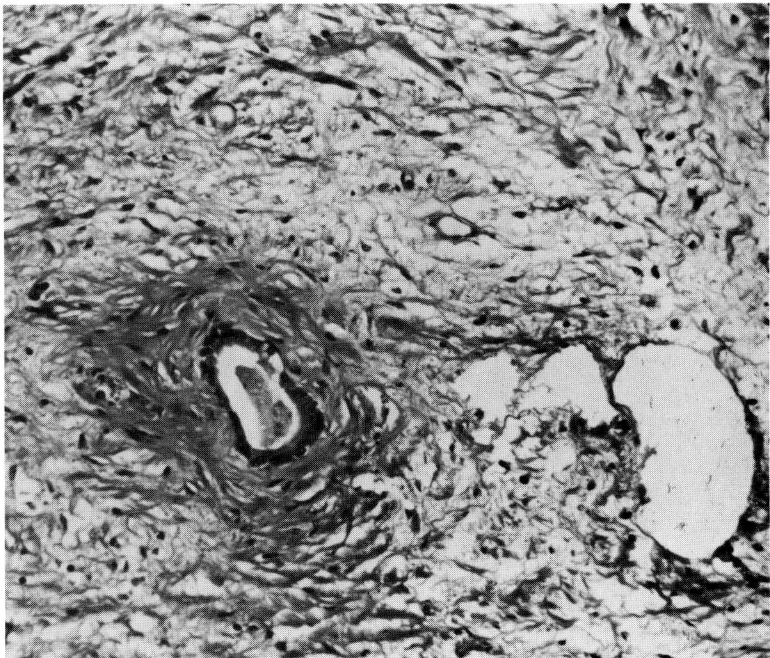

Figure 6–47. Scirrhous intestinal carcinoma in a sheep. This area is in the mesenteric fat some distance from the main site of the tumor. The epithelial cells in the acinus have induced a very extensive scirrhous reaction.

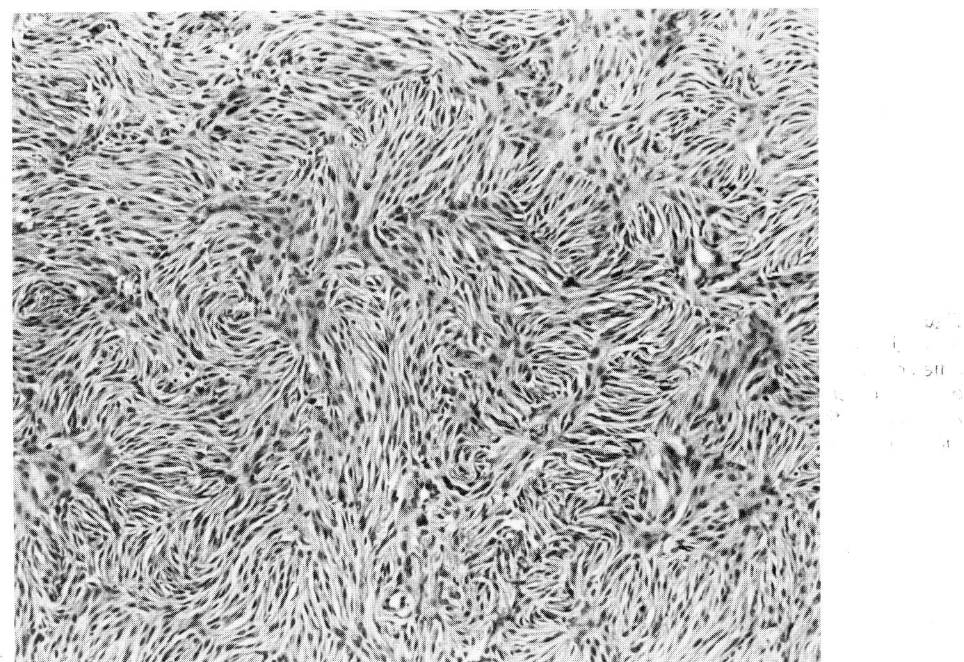

Figure 6–48. Very swirly arrangement of cells in a hemangiopericytoma. A closer view is seen in Figure 6–49. This general type of pattern occurs in some fibrosarcomas and neurofibromas and may make differential diagnosis a problem.

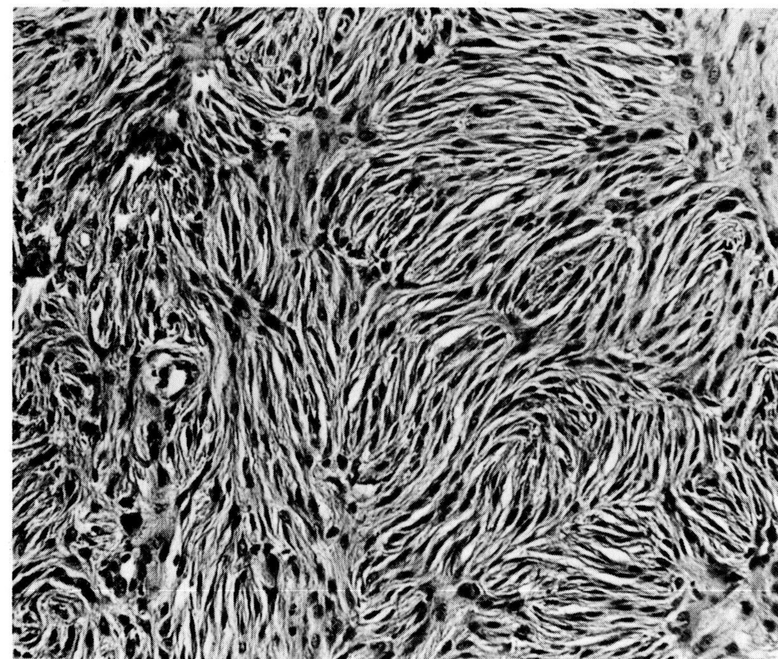

Figure 6–49. See the legend for Figure 6–48.

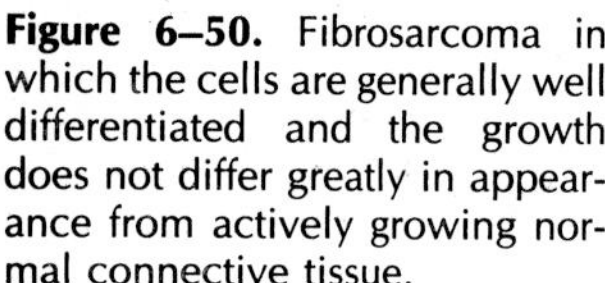

Figure 6–50. Fibrosarcoma in which the cells are generally well differentiated and the growth does not differ greatly in appearance from actively growing normal connective tissue.

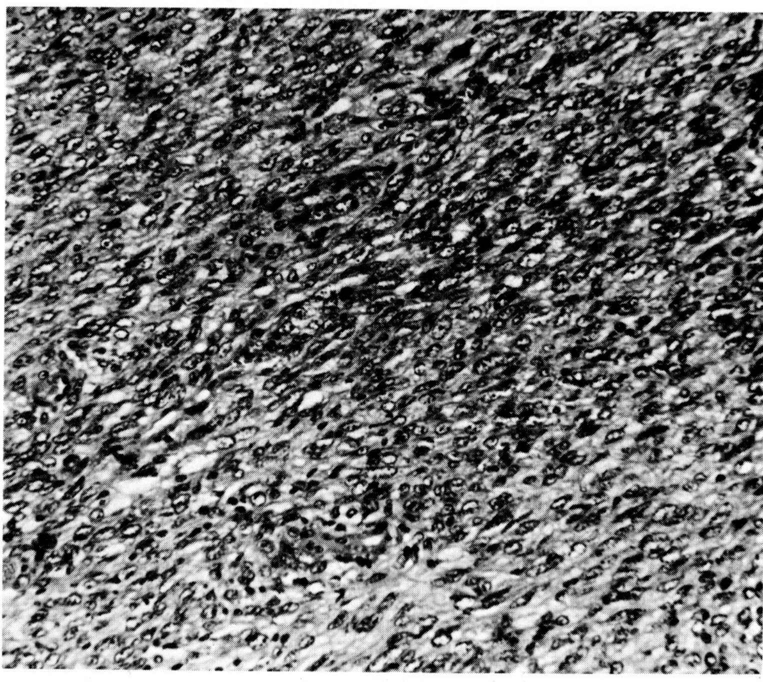

true identity of the tumor when it is examined by a pathologist. There are individual differences, but in a sense, "family characteristics" of specific kinds of tumors exist and are actually quite consistent. A tumor that grows in such a manner that either the cells or the pattern of growth is obviously similar to the parent tissue is called ***well differentiated.*** On the other hand, tumors that bear very little, if any, resemblance to the cells or architecture of the parent tissue are called ***poorly differentiated.*** Sometimes, both well-differentiated and poorly differentiated areas occur in the same tumor and add to the importance of examining several areas of the tumor. Marked lack of differentiation is called ***anaplasia.*** Anaplasia and evidence of invasion are highly significant characteristics of malignancy.

Metaplasia may be apparent to a minor or to a major degree within both mesenchymal and epithelial tumors. One osteogenic sarcoma may contain connective tissue, cartilage, immature bone and osteoid. An adenocarcinoma may contain squamous areas and adenomatous areas.

Some tumors are ***functionally active,*** particularly those of endocrine glands; even though the hormones produced may be biochemically abnormal, they may affect the appearance of the host or the functional response of the organs (Table 6–3). It is usually not possible to determine from the microscopic appearance of the tumor whether or not it is functional, and size is not necessarily related to function. Also, some tumors begin to make compounds that are completely foreign to the capabilities of the parent tissue. This may represent ***derepression of genetic coding*** in tumor cells that is repressed in the normal parent tissue. Examples of this feature are best known in human tumors, such as undifferentiated carcinomas in the lungs, which produce adrenocorticotrophic hormone. Recognition of such secretions is occurring in animals mainly by clinical features, rather than by assay. Some lymphosarcomas in animals produce a parathyroid hormone effect in terms of hypercalcium and resorption of bone.

The rate of growth and size of a tumor might be considered a function of the rate of multiplication of the cells composing the tumor. The relative number of mitotic figures was once considered to be indicative of the rate of growth, and the term ***mitotic index*** was commonly used. This index, however, or the more accurate measure of so-called ***doubling time*** (the time taken to

TABLE 6–3. Physiologically Active Tumor Cell Products and Their Effects in Animals

Tumor Cell Origin	Tumor	Active Tumor Product	Clinical Signs
Skin mast cells	Mast cell sarcoma	Protease, histamine, heparin and serotonin	Ulcers in gastrointestinal tract, histamine shock, increased blood coagulation time, bleeding tendencies
Thyroid gland	Thyroid adenomas	Thyroxine	Hyperthyroidism
Adrenal gland (chromaffin cells)	Pheochromocytoma	Adrenaline	Tachycardia, edema, cardiac hypertrophy
Pituitary gland	Basophilic adenoma	Adrenocorticotrophic hormone (ACTH)	Cushing's syndrome
Plasma cells	Myeloma	Immunoglobulins	Hyperviscosity syndrome, infection and bleeding diathesis
Kidney	Renal cell carcinoma	Erythropoietin	Polycythemia
Pancreas	Pancreatic islet cell adenocarcinomas	Insulin	Hypoglycemia
Ovary	Granulosa cell tumor	Estrogen	Mammary hyperplasia, prolonged estrus, cystic endometrial hyperplasia
Testicle	Sertoli cell tumor	Estrogen	Gynecomastia (feminizing syndrome), alopecia

(From Hardy, W. D., Jr.: Current concepts of canine and feline tumor. J. Am. Anim. Hosp. Assoc., *12*:295, 1976. Reprinted by permission.)

double the size of the tumor) by isotope labeling of dividing nuclei, ***does not reflect the resultant gross size of a tumor.*** A very significant factor influencing gross size is the degree of ***cell loss*** or necrosis of individual cells in the tumor. If all multiplying cells survived, the tumor would double its size in the theoretical time that it takes for all cells to divide, but most cells produced in a tumor die. The cause of the death of the cells is ***pressure, ischemia, anoxia, nutritive competition*** or ***abnormal mitosis.*** This fact is rather startling because there is a tendency to think that the visible mitotic index in a section of the tumor is indicative of its rate of growth. Actually, many tumors replicate cells at a rate slower than that of the parent tissue.

Cytology of Tumors

The cells making up neoplasms are abnormal cells, and the degree of abnormality usually reflects the degree of malignancy. ***Recognition of characteristics typical of neoplastic cells is highly significant in diagnosing a tumor,*** whether in a tissue section, blood smear or a smear of aspirated cells. One of the main functions of ***cytopathology*** is to determine whether a lesion is neoplastic, inflammatory, degenerative or hyperplastic. The use of cytopathology for this purpose is rapidly expanding and can be employed on an everyday basis in practice (see Appendix I).

Cells must be well preserved to be evaluated. In general, the uniformity of normal cells is replaced by ***irregularity, angularity and unpredictability*** in malignant cells. The following features are characteristic of malignant cells, particularly epithelial cells. ***Nuclear chromatin*** develops coarse clumped patterns with sharp edges, sharp angles and parachromatin clearing. ***Nuclear membranes*** develop variations in thickness as well as sharp, irregular, angled projections and very well-defined inner and outer surfaces. ***Nucleoli*** have irregular shapes with sharp projections and indentations with marked variation in size, shape and number. In general, ***multinucleation*** of cells is not a criterion of malignancy unless the nuclei vary markedly in size and shape. ***Abnormal mitosis*** is characteristic of malignancy. ***Abnormal karyotypes*** occur in many tumors but are not consistently present. Apparently, these abnormalities in karyotype develop after neoplasia begins and are not involved in initiation of cancer. Variation in karyotype occurs from all types of aneuploidy to all types of alterations of individual chromosomes. The changes tend to be consistent within the cells of a particular tumor.

Cytoplasmic changes typical of neoplasia are parallel cytoplasmic and nuclear membranes over extended distances and a small amount of cytoplasm around a large nucleus. Marked ***variability*** and ***irregularity*** of neighboring cells with evidence of crowding of nuclei are also characteristic features of neoplasia. These last features are indicative of cells that have lost control of contact inhibition and other growth control factors. ***Anaplasia*** refers to the lack of differentiation in a tumor. Poorly differentiated tumors are ***anaplastic.***

No single feature is specific for identification of a tumor cell. A simple method to gain an impression of nuclear size is to compare nuclei in a normal area of tissue with red blood cells and with the nuclei and red cells from an area where neoplasia is suspected. In general, the appearance of neoplastic cells indicates that the functions of the cell are directed toward ***replication*** rather than toward carrying out the normal physiological function or ***work*** normally required of the particular cell.

The changes just mentioned are best visualized in dried smears or wet-fixed in alcohol, in which shrinkage is minimal. Formalin-fixed cells or tissue sections undergo a considerable degree of shrinkage and cellular detail is reduced. Poor fixation or autolysis or a combination of the two compounds the problem and may eliminate the possibility of detecting neoplastic cells that are present.

Figures 6–51 through 60 illustrate cytological features of neoplasia in tissue sections. Many of these features would be more evident in individual cells in well-prepared smears or needle biopsy.

Spread of Tumors

Spread of tumors from the site of origin is characteristic of malignancy and important in prognosis.

The four main mechanisms for the spread

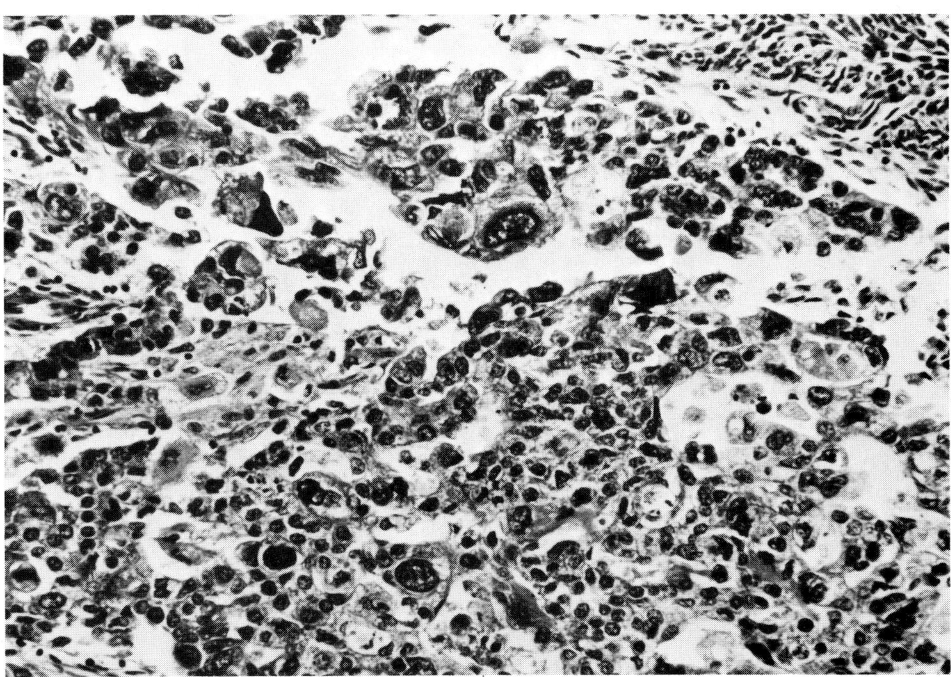

Figure 6–51. Uterine carcinoma. Look carefully at individual cells in this picture and those that follow for cellular detail of size and shape of nuclei and chromatin patterns. Similar cytological features of malignant growth are seen in Figure 6–52 from the same case.

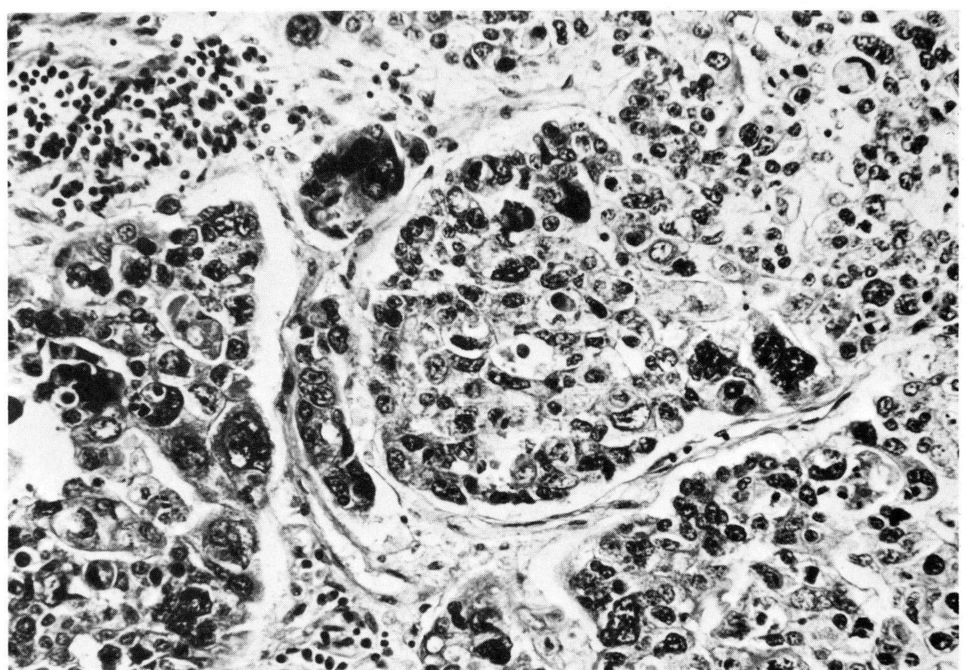

Figure 6–52. See the legend for Figure 6–51.

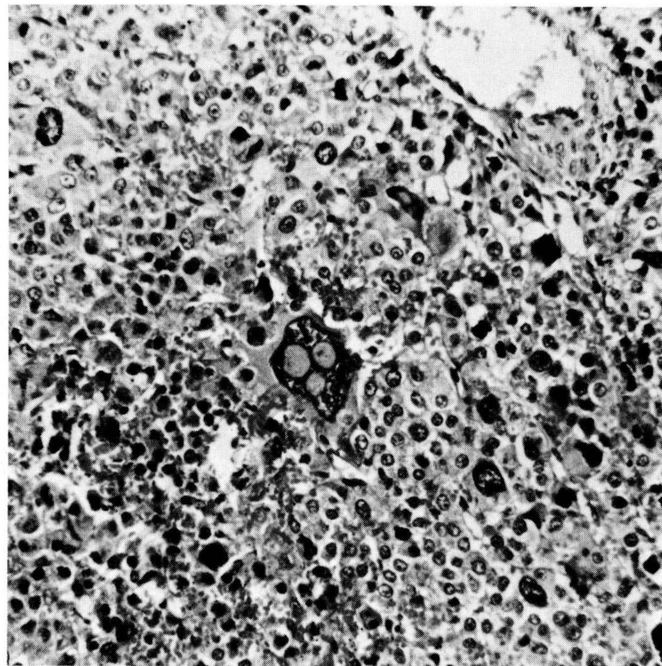

Figure 6–53. Nonchromaffin paraganglioma in a dog. Note the few very large nuclei characteristic of this tumor.

of tumors—infiltration, spreading via blood vessels, spreading via lymphatic vessels and implantation—are illustrated in Figure 6–61.

Spread may be by ***direct expansion and infiltration*** and depends on the invasive capabilities and properties of the tumor cells and the routes available. Spreading takes place by growth and multiplication of cells and may be likened to a ***root*** growing into soil. Some tumors are small and grow slowly but invade and infiltrate readily; others are large and grow rapidly but invade very little. All degrees of variation between these extremes occur. Direct spread may be by ***infiltration*** of tissue spaces between cells or by growth into the lymphatics or blood vessels.

Metastasis implies spread to another area not directly connected with the original site. Spread may be through ***lymphatic vessels*** to lymph nodes, which do not destroy tumor cells in the same manner as microorganisms. A tumor may completely replace the normal architecture of a node and move on to the next node in a drainage area. ***Invasion of blood vessels*** of all sizes may occur, and tumor cells may travel long distances by this route before lodging and forming a secondary growth or metastatic nodule. The two theories on the success of metastases are the ***soil*** theory and the ***mechanical*** theory. The soil theory states that a tumor must find "suitable soil" for its growth requirements before it will survive as a metastatic nodule, thus perhaps accounting for the favored sites of metastasis for some tumors. The mechanical theory states that the tumor will grow wherever it lands, and only mechanical factors and chance influence sites of metastases. There is no clear-cut choice between the two. Some tumors rarely metastasize, even though they may have invaded through the wall of a major vessel and protrude into the lumen. Metastasis to skeletal muscle is rare, even though it is a large component of the body mass, which perhaps is an unfavorable environment. Study of routes of metastasis has resulted in the discovery of some unusual flow patterns, shunts and anastomotic connections in the venous system to account for a site of metastasis. An example is spread of a tumor from the lower extremity to a vertebral body by reverse flow in vertebral veins because of sudden increased abdominal pressure.

Metastasis may also occur by spreading

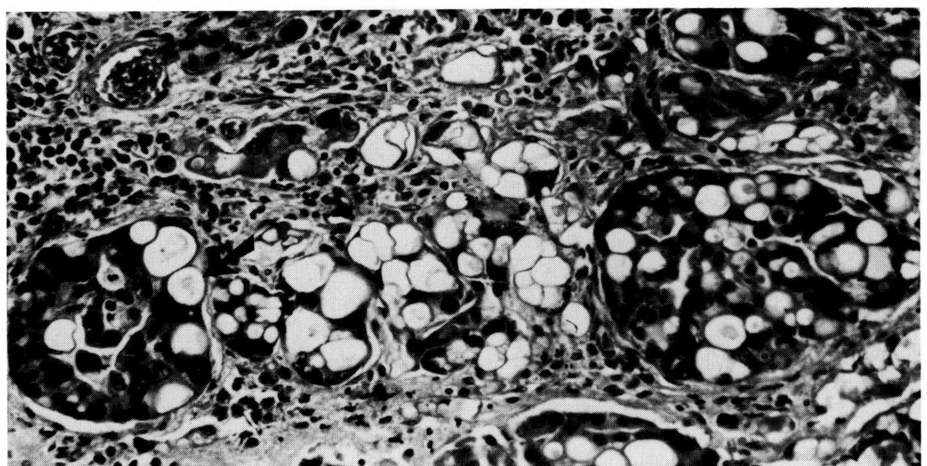

Figure 6–54

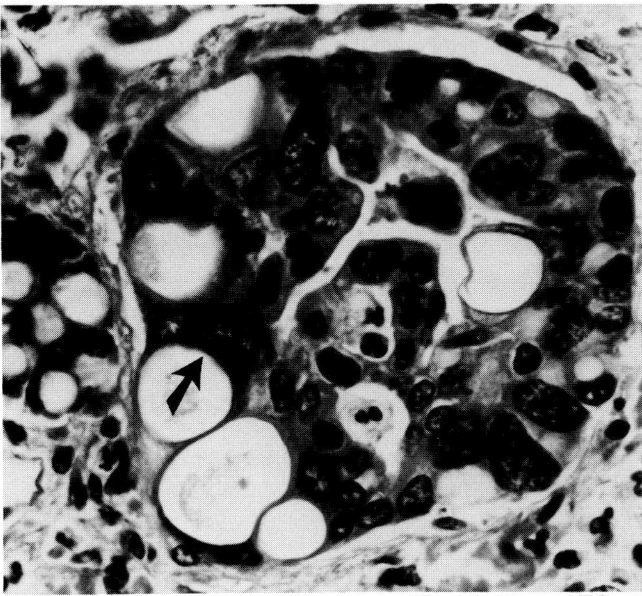

Figure 6–55

Figures 6–54 and 6–55. Transitional cell carcinoma in the bladder of a dog. Note the vacuolated cytoplasm of the cells, which contain lipid. These vacuoles push the nucleus aside (arrow) and the cells are called signet ring cells. These are characteristic of transitional cell carcinomas.

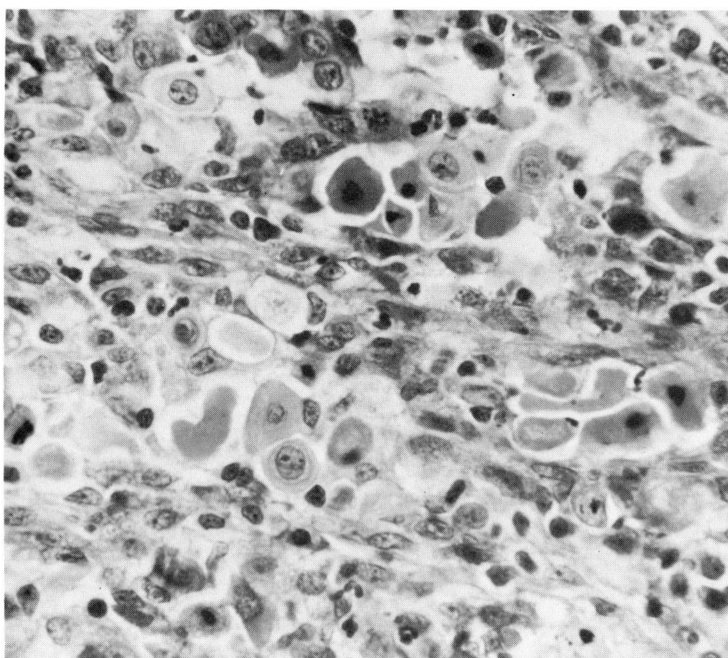

Figure 6–56. Squamous cell carcinoma of the tonsil. Note the large number of degenerate and necrotic cells in the tumor, i.e., pyknotic nuclei and dark cytoplasm.

through a body cavity, such as the abdomen or the thorax. Tumor cells usually seed down or ***implant*** on the peritoneum or pleura and form new nodules. Implantation in the abdomen usually results in ascites because the tumor cells are carried in fluid to the lymphatic drainage sites in the ventral diaphragm and grow into the lymphatic vessels, blocking them and preventing drainage from the abdomen. Some ovarian tumors in dogs typically cause ascites.

Figures 6–62 through 97 illustrate the means of growth, spread and metastasis in a variety of tumors.

The generalization that sarcomas travel via veins and that carcinomas travel via lymphatics does not apply in all tumors or species.

In general, the ability to metastasize involves one or a combination of the following properties of cells: ***decreased adhesiveness, loss of contact inhibition, increased mobility, increased contact guidance or synthesis of compounds that injure normal cells***. Experimental studies on the process of metastases have been carried out by injecting known numbers of malignant cells into blood vessels and following their survival. Thousands of cells may be required to produce a metastasis, but this varies with the tumor. ***Three steps*** are generally involved: release from the original site, transport and lodgement, and survival and growth at the new site. The presence of tumor cells in blood or in blood vessels does not imply that metastasis will occur. Experimentally, in an ideal system, metastasis requires several cells, and the events are represented in Figure 6–98. Formation of tumor emboli is a key requirement, as is thrombosis at the site of lodgement, after which the tumor cells go through a space in the vessel made by leukocytes. Tumor cells may reach lymphatic vessels and return to the blood stream to metastasize again. Anticoagulants reduce blood-borne metastasis by blocking the formation of the thrombus.

The ability to metastasize varies among groups of cells within a tumor. Other variable features within one tumor can be antigenic properties, immunogenicity, hormone receptors, pigment production, growth rates and susceptibility to drugs. Surface properties are highly significant. The metastatic process also varies among tumors and is usually a cascade effect involving several steps. ***Groups*** of cells are randomly selected for metastatic ability, providing a genotypic metastatic population. There may be transient metastatic compartments within a tumor. In addition, site-induced modulations occur, which may

Text continued on page 377

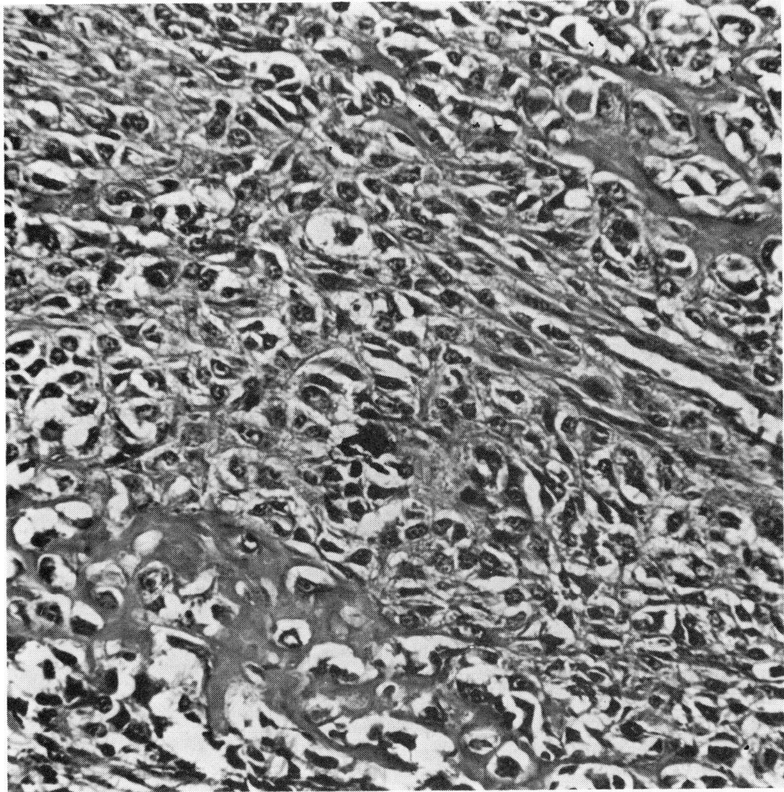

Figure 6–57

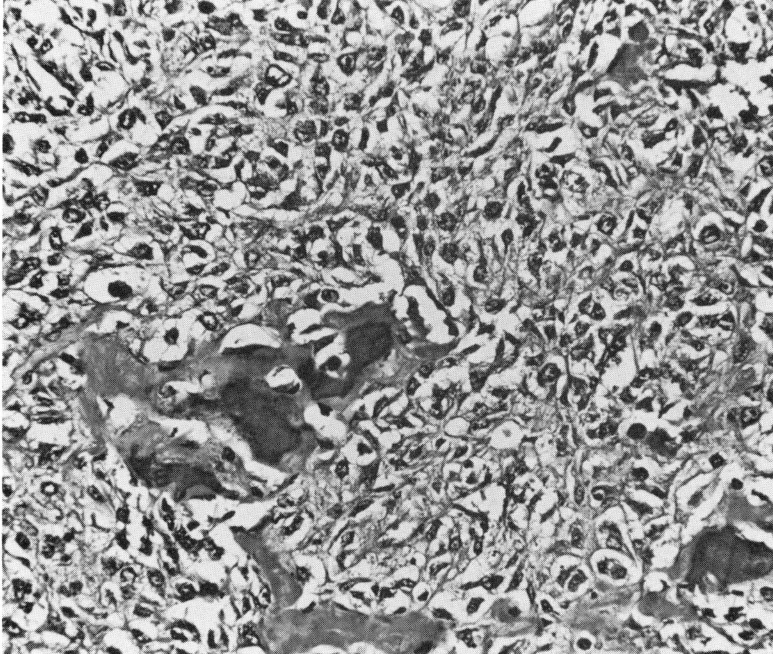

Figure 6–58

Figures 6–57 and 6–58. Osteogenic sarcoma with marked variation in size and shape of nuclei as well as chromatin patterns. Osteoid is present in Figure 6–57. In Figure 6–58, the osteoid is partially mineralized, as indicated by the dark areas of calcification within some of the osteoid. These two figures also indicate variations in differentiation.

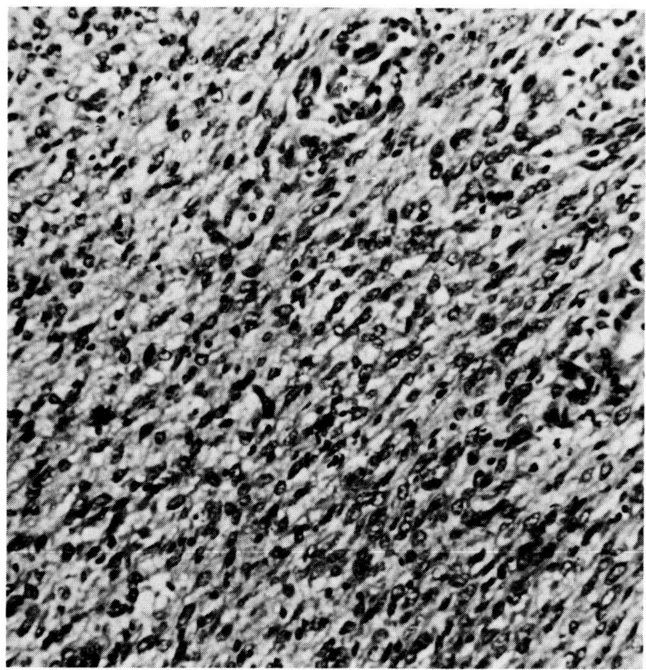

Figure 6–59

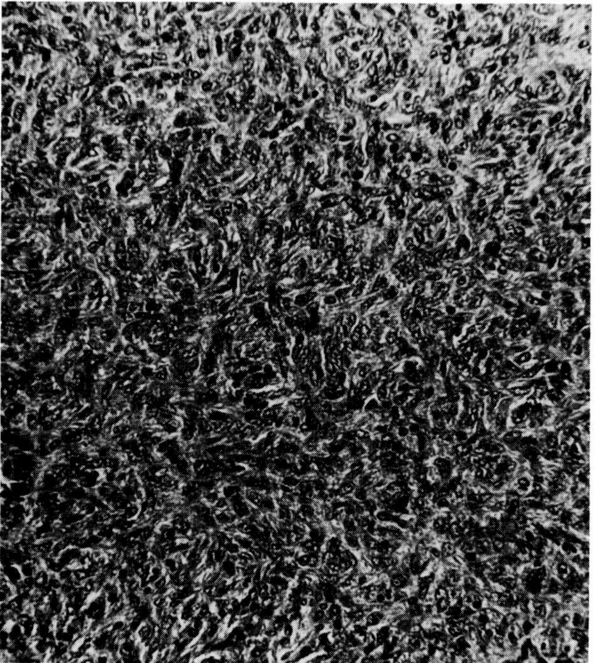

Figure 6–60

Figures 6–59 and 6–60. A fibrosarcoma in a dog, with variation in patterns of growth in different areas, as indicated by the variation between Figure 6–59 and Figure 6–60.

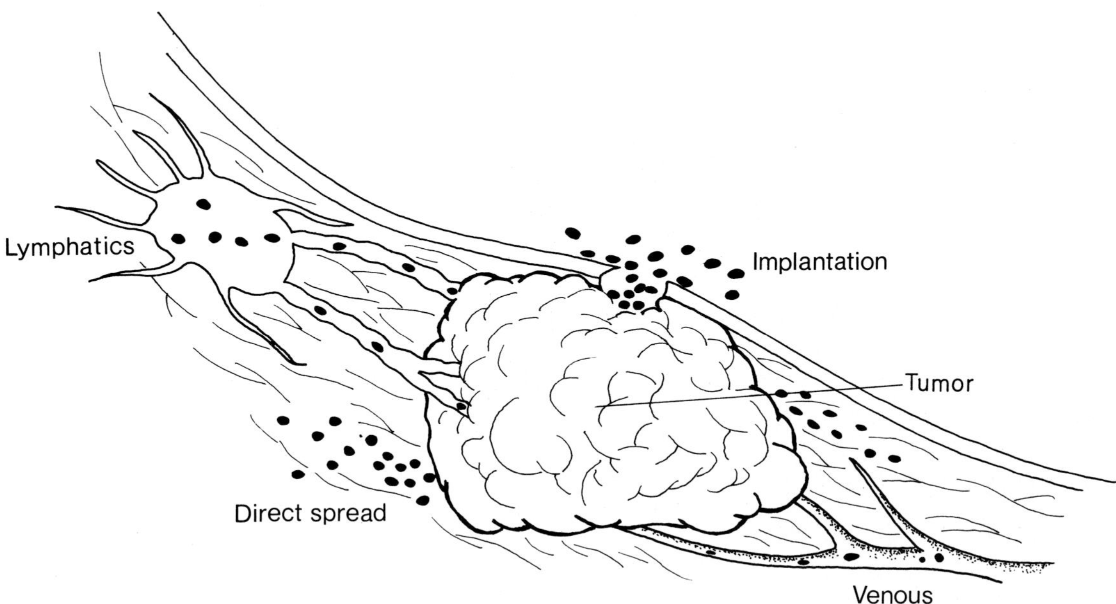

Figure 6–61. Four mechanisms of the dissemination of cancer cells. (From Boyd, W.: Textbook of Pathology. Philadelphia, Lea and Febiger, 1970. Reprinted by permission.)

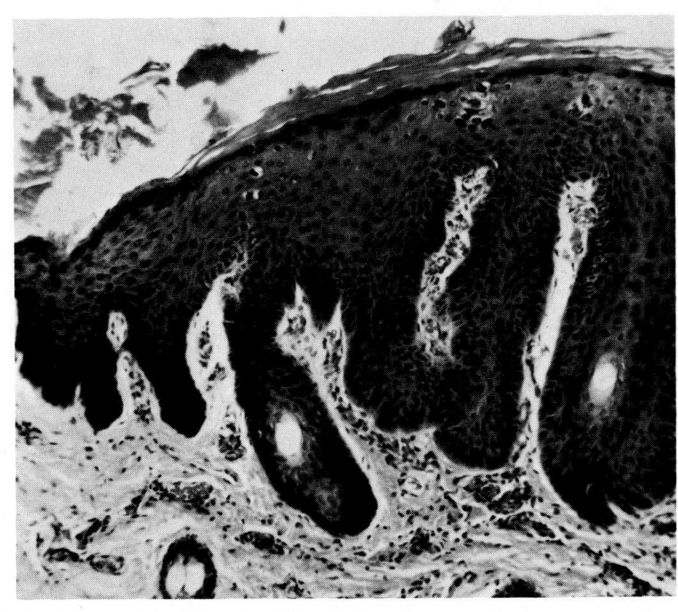

Figure 6–62. A papilloma in the skin of a horse. Epithelial hyperplasia is evident, and there is a degree of local infiltration but it seems confined and would not be considered as locally infiltrative, as in the case of the basal cell tumor (see Figs. 6–42 and 6–43).

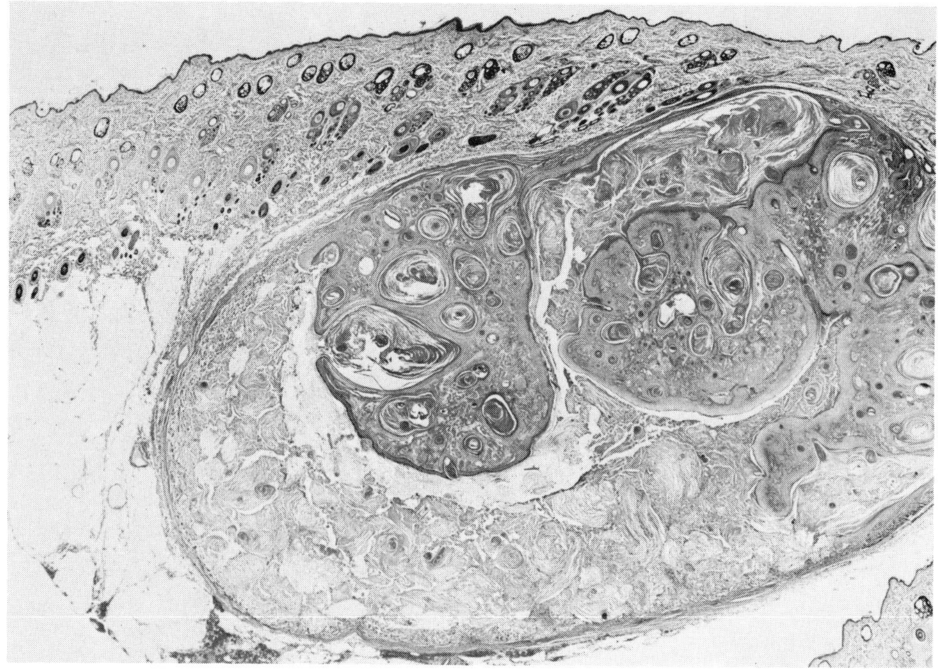

Figure 6–63. A benign trichoepithelioma in a dog's skin. The lesion is locally expansive but not infiltrative and could be removed easily and cleanly. The connective tissue around the edge of the tumor is from compression of existing stroma. Many benign tumors are situated in such a manner in tissue.

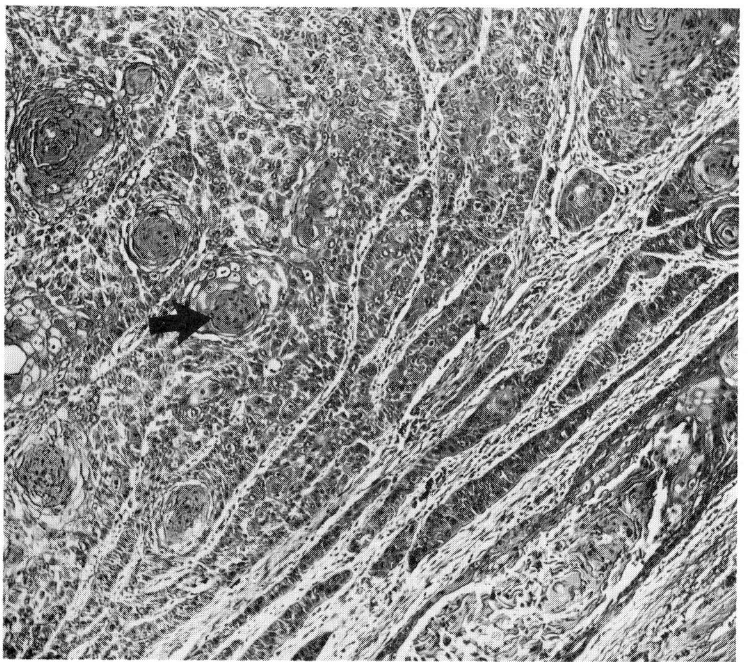

Figure 6–64. An infiltrative squamous cell carcinoma. Note the cords of cells and islands of keratinization (arrow) that are an indication of differentiation and are characteristic of this tumor.

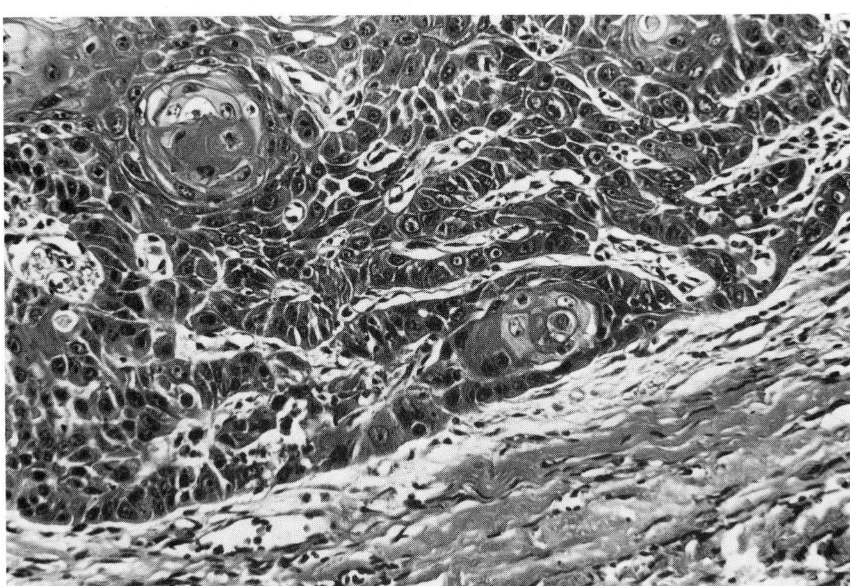

Figure 6–65. A closer view of infiltrative squamous cell carcinoma shown in Figure 6–64.

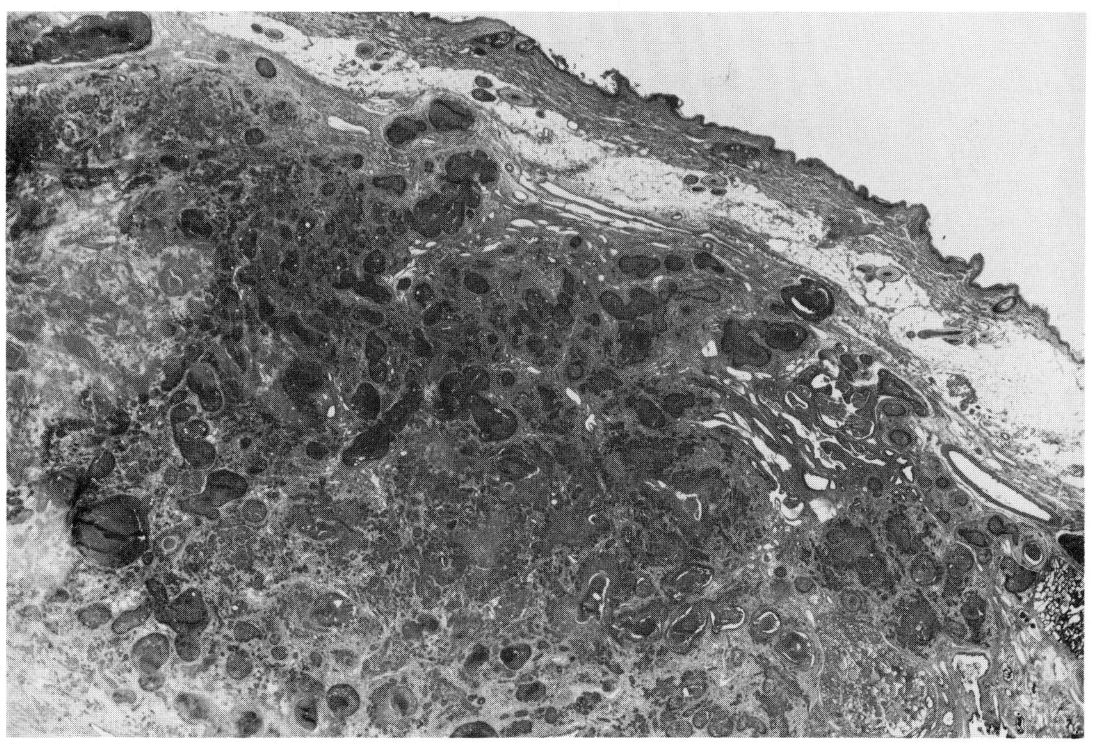

Figure 6–66. *See legend on following page*

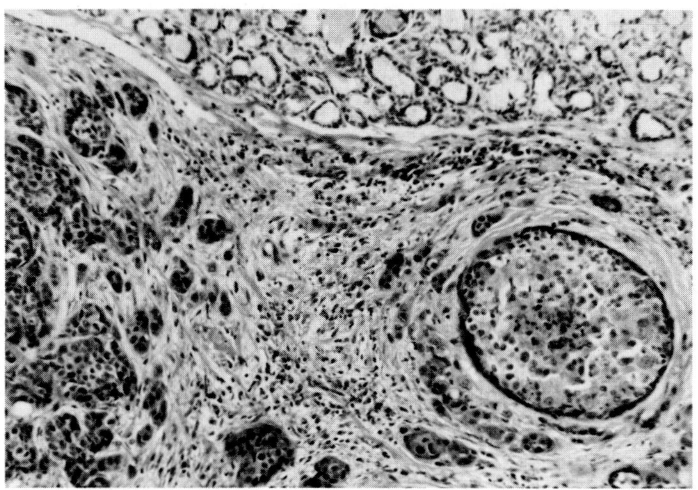

Figure 6–67

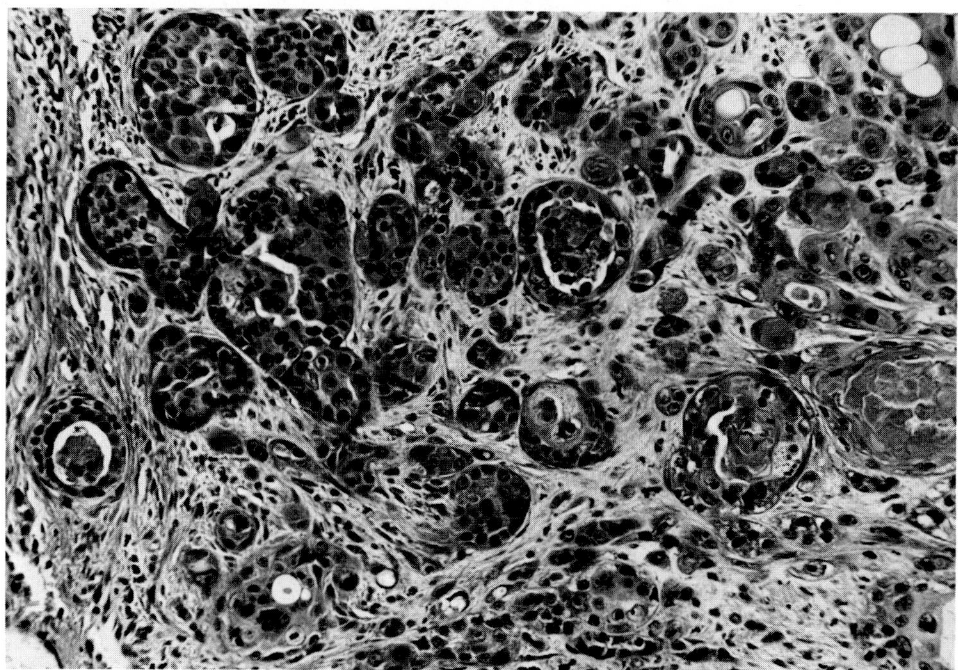

Figure 6–68

Figures 6–66, 6–67 and 6–68. Mammary carcinoma in a dog. Note the variation in epithelial growth in various areas from squamous to tubular and acinar. An area of necrosis is on the left. Some normal lobules are at the lower right. In Figure 6–67, a closer view of local infiltration near a normal lobule and possibly invasion into a vein (right) are shown. Variation in differentiation, as well as local infiltration, is further illustrated in the same tumor in Figure 6–68.

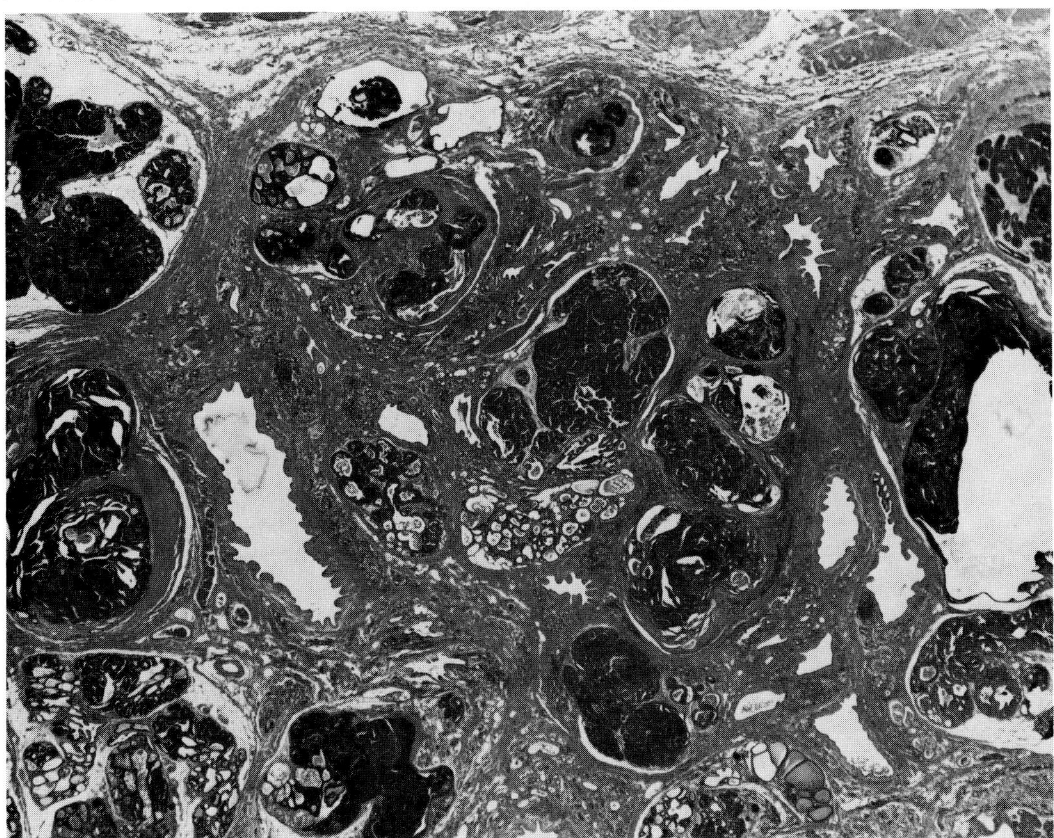

Figure 6–69

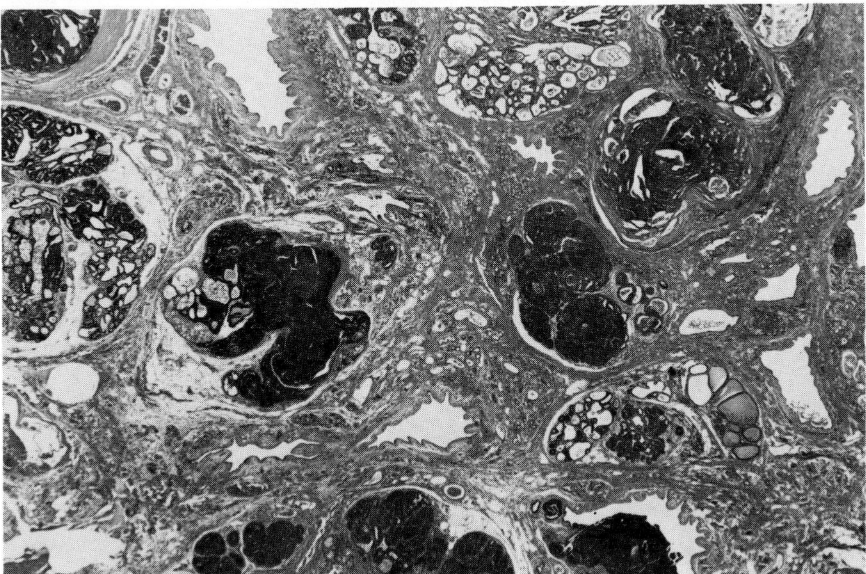

Figure 6–70

Figures 6–69 and 6–70. Mammary tumor in a dog, indicating variation in growth within the tumor. Dysplasia is evident in some lobules and acini. More detail is present in Figure 6–70. These pictures perhaps indicate that dysplasia and nodular hyperplasia can progress to a carcinoma and that such lesions arise in a multifocal pattern.

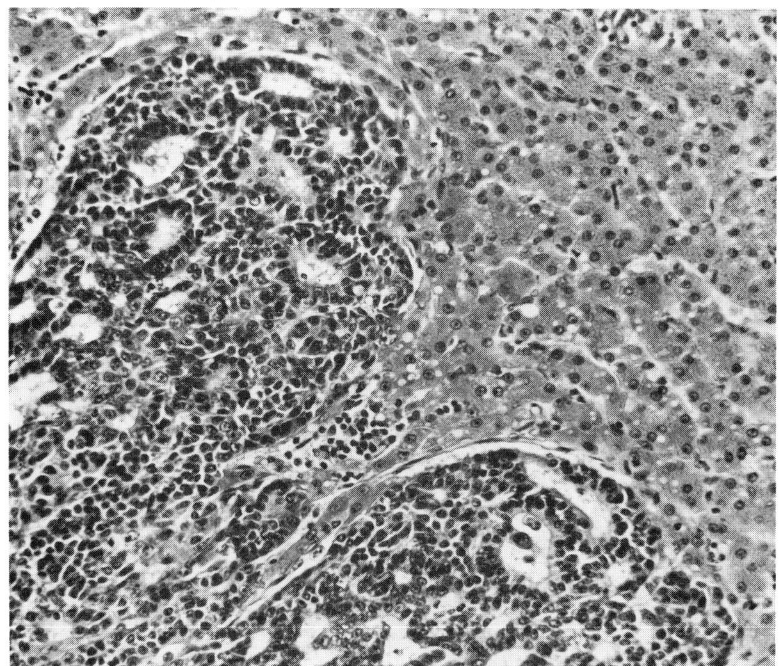

Figure 6–71. Expansion of bile duct carcinoma into the liver. Note the minimal evidence of compression or necrosis in the normal areas as the tumor expands.

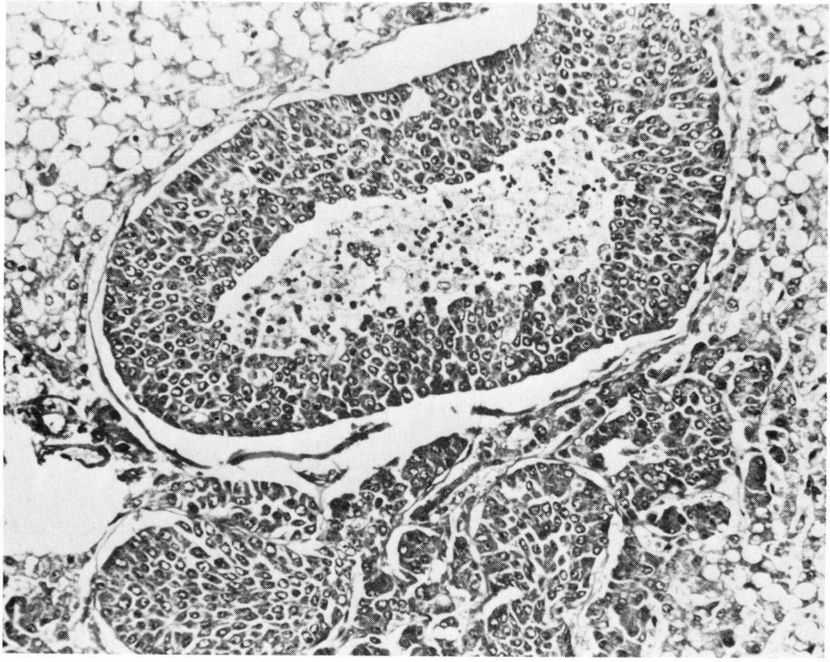

Figure 6–72. Bile duct carcinoma in a liver that is fatty. Necrosis of tumor cells has occurred in the central area of the larger nodule. Note the infiltration into liver parenchyma.

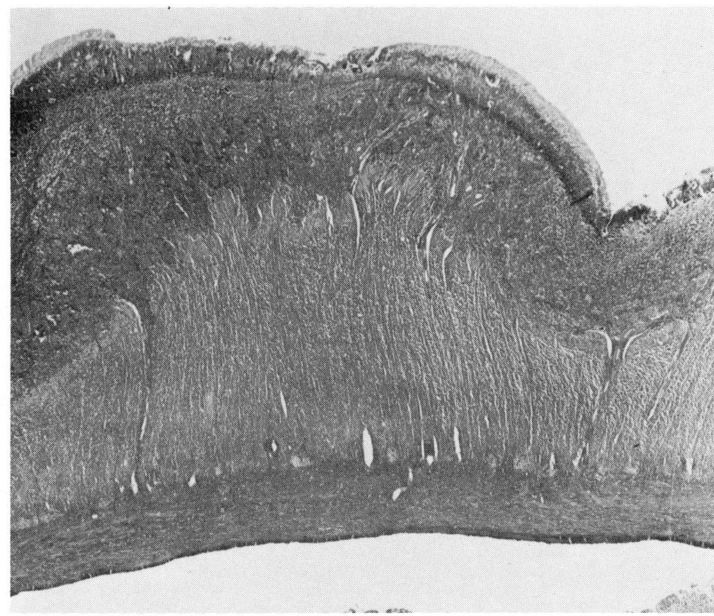

Figure 6–73

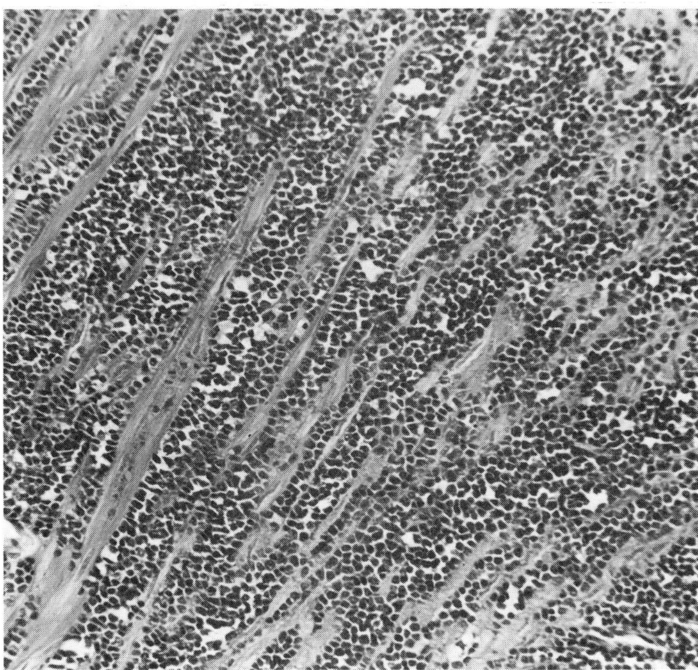

Figure 6–74

Figures 6–73 and 6–74. Massive infiltration with lymphocytes of all layers of a dog's intestine in lymphosarcoma. The amount of infiltration in the muscle layers is shown in Figure 6–74.

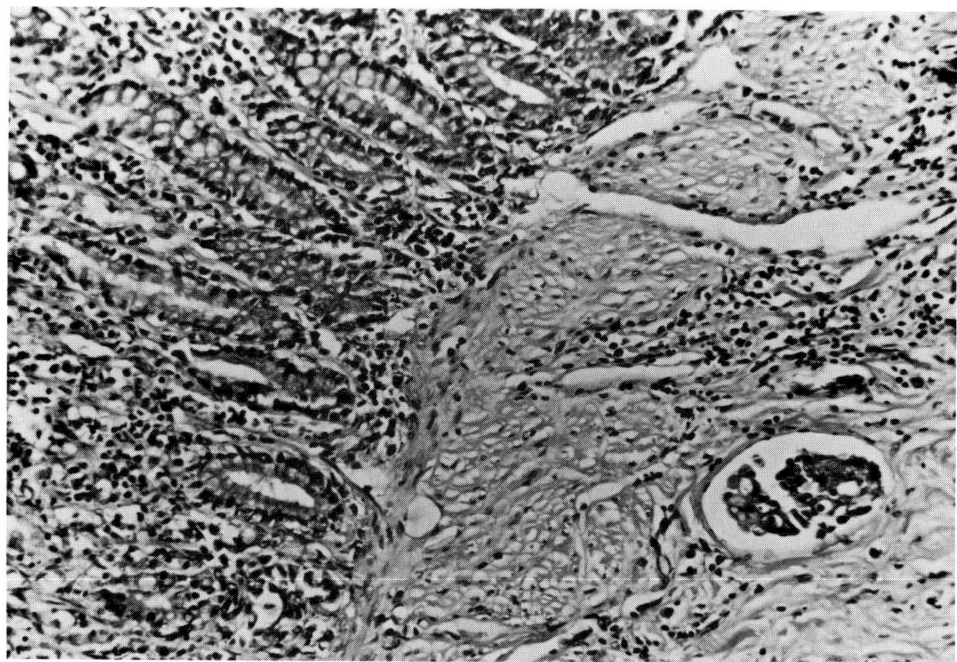

Figure 6–75

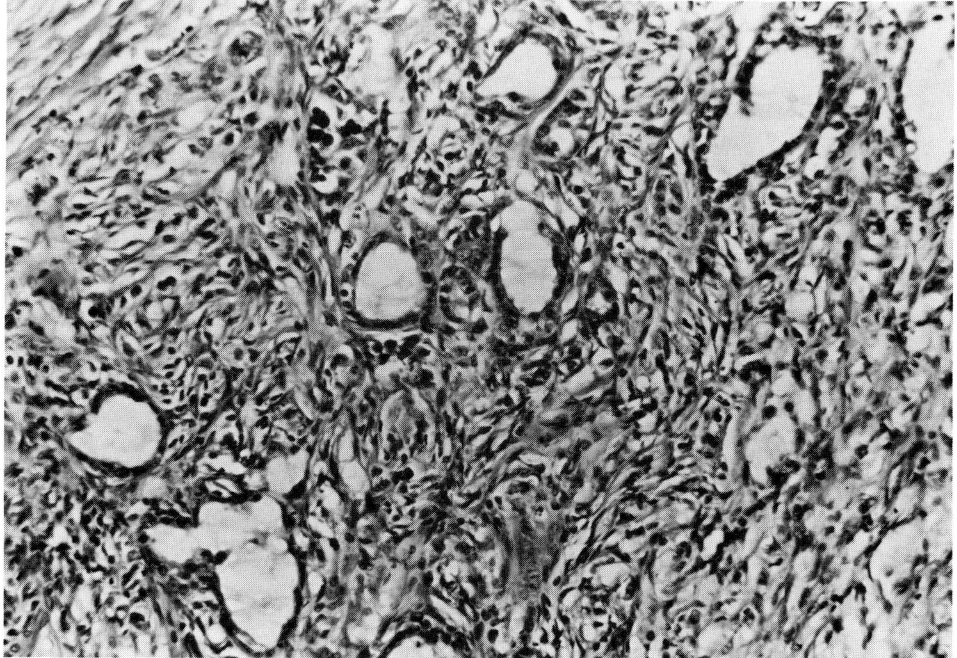

Figure 6–76

Figures 6–75 and 6–76. Intestinal carcinoma in a dog. Note the metastatic acinar arrangement in a lymphatic vessel below the mucosa in Figure 6–75, and several more in lymphatics spreading through the muscle layers toward the serosal surface in Figure 6–76.

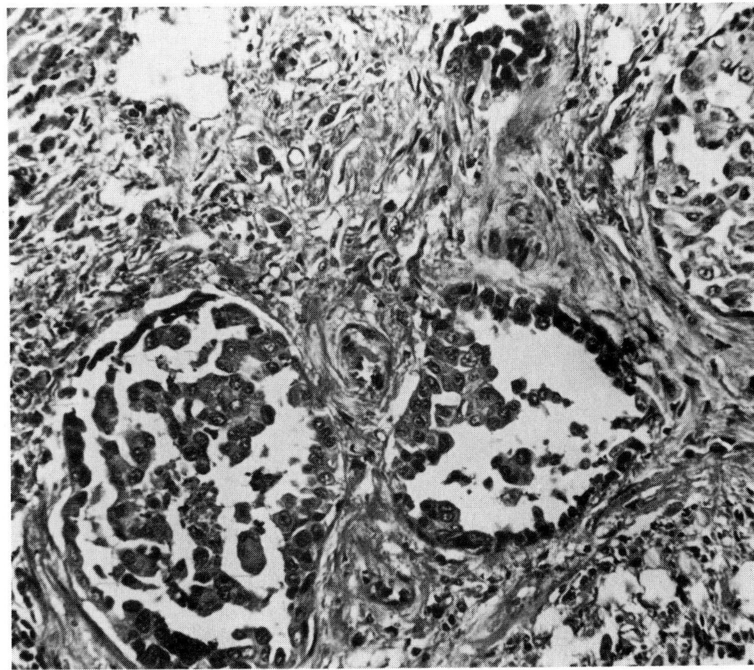

Figure 6–77. Mammary carcinoma in lymphatic vessels in the muscle layers of the abdominal wall toward the inguinal lymph nodes. Note the malignant cells lining the lymph vessel.

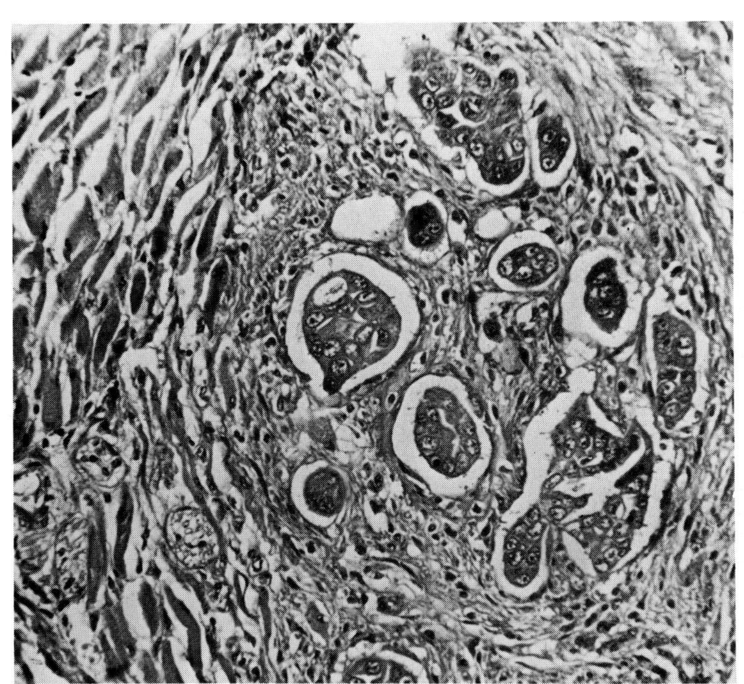

Figure 6–78. In another area of the lesion shown in Figure 6–77, there is somewhat of a scirrhous reaction around the lymphatics.

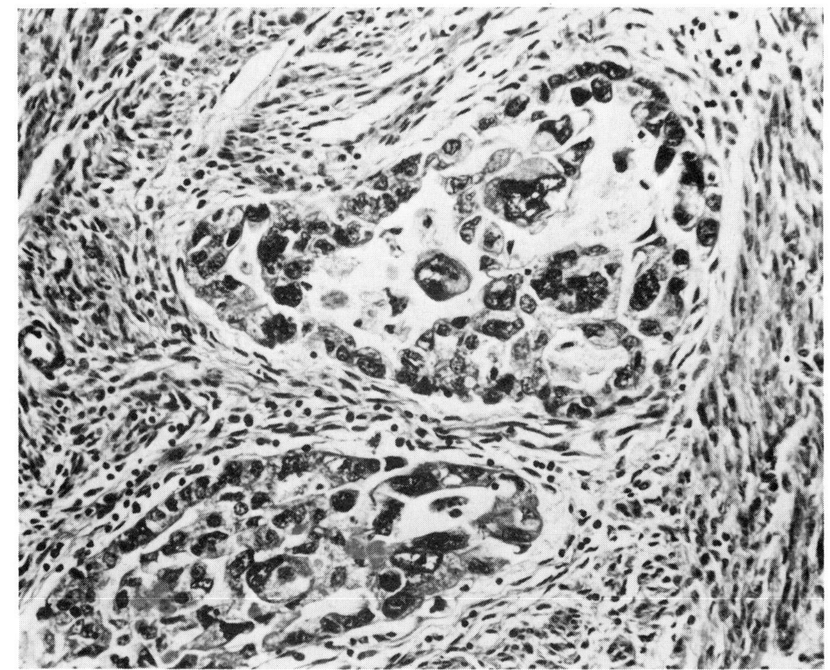

Figure 6–79. Highly malignant uterine carcinoma invading the muscle layers. Note the cytological features of the cells.

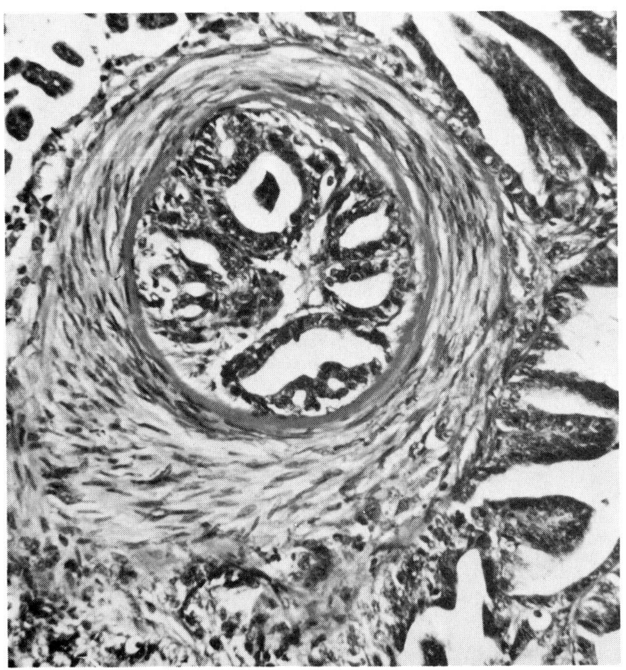

Figure 6–80. Pulmonary vessel containing a metastatic carcinoma of a glandular type. This could be a lung tumor leaving the lung or another tumor coming into the lung.

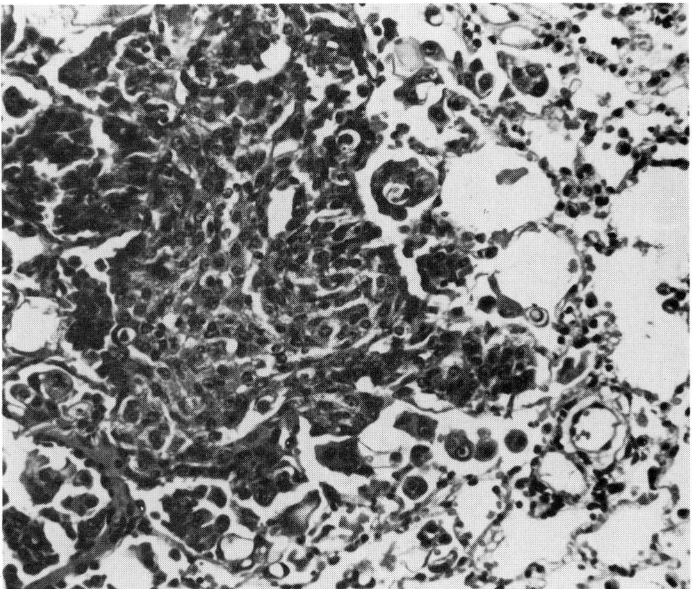

Figure 6–81. A metastatic focus has reached the lung via the blood stream and is now growing out into the surrounding lung tissue.

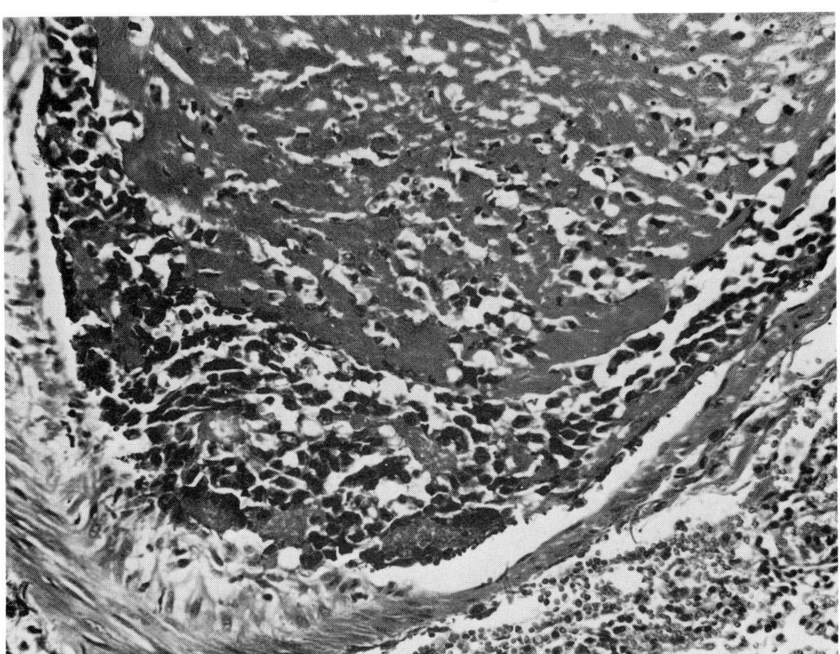

Figure 6–82. Metastatic fibrosarcoma cells in a pulmonary vessel. The cells are packed at one end and have produced a thrombus.

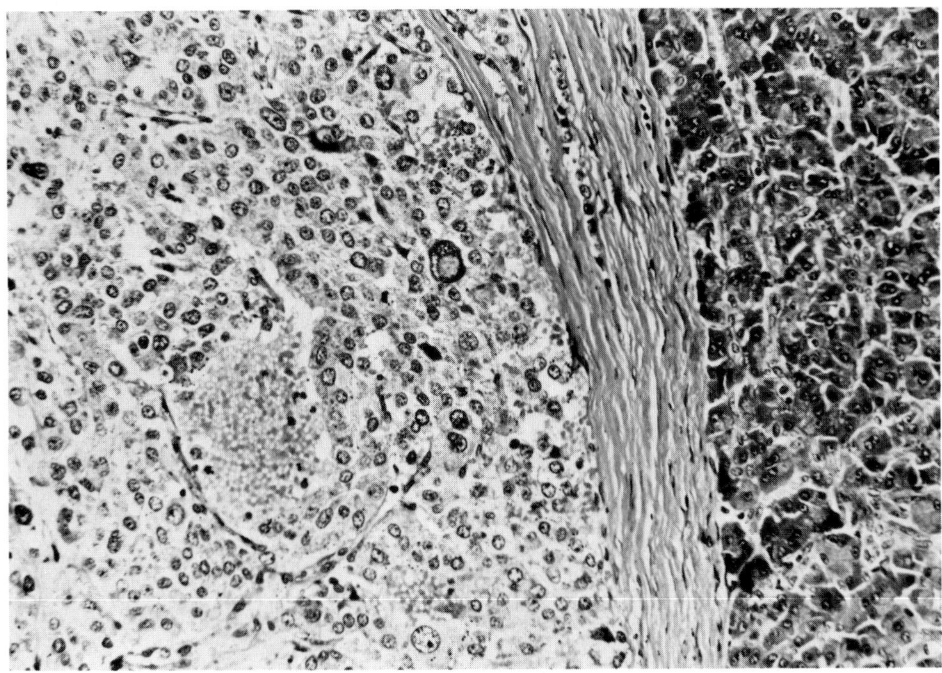

Figure 6–83. Metastatic nonchromaffin paraganglioma (left) in the pancreas (right) with a thick band of connective tissue between the two. Note the large nuclei in some cells which are characteristic of these tumors.

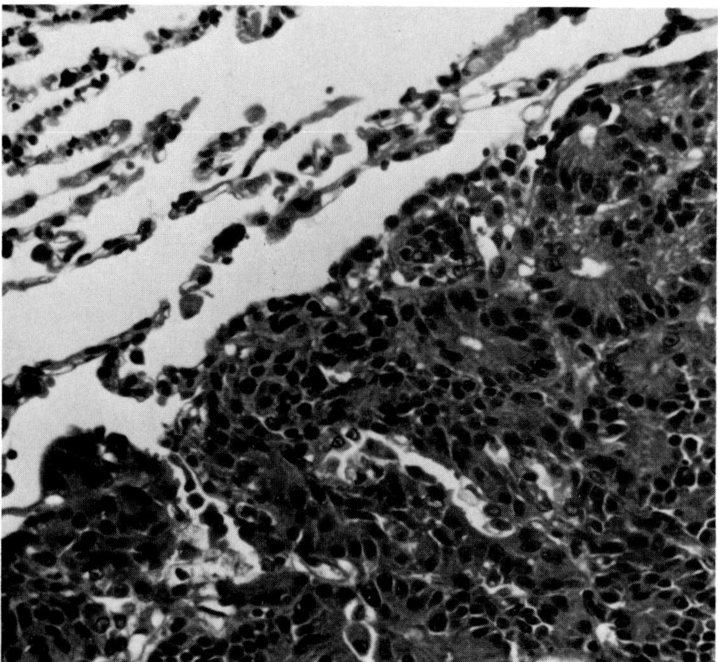

Figure 6–84. Metastatic pancreatic adenocarcinoma in the lung of a cat. There seems to be no inhibition to its growth.

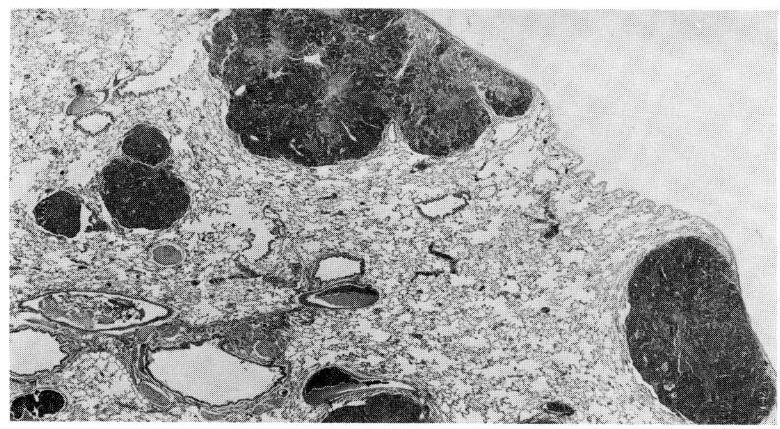

Figure 6–85. Same lesion as seen in Figure 6–84 viewed at a lower power.

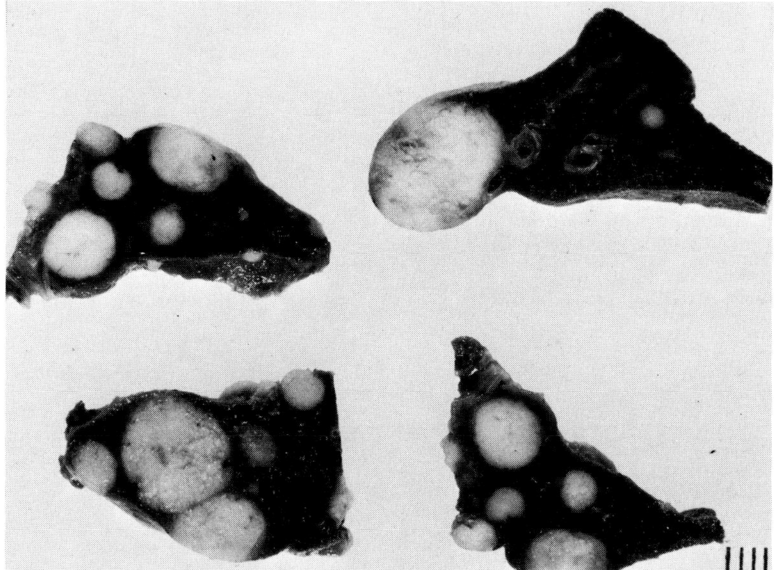

Figure 6–86. White nodules of metastatic tumor in cross sections of pieces of lung from the same cat as in Figures 6–84 and 6–85.

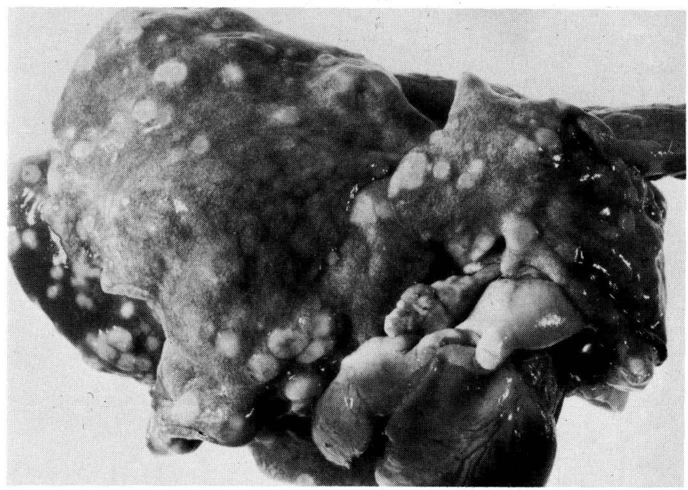

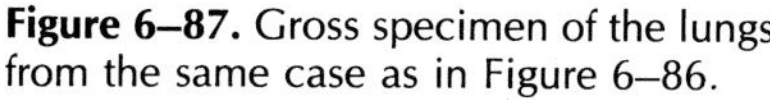

Figure 6–87. Gross specimen of the lungs from the same case as in Figure 6–86.

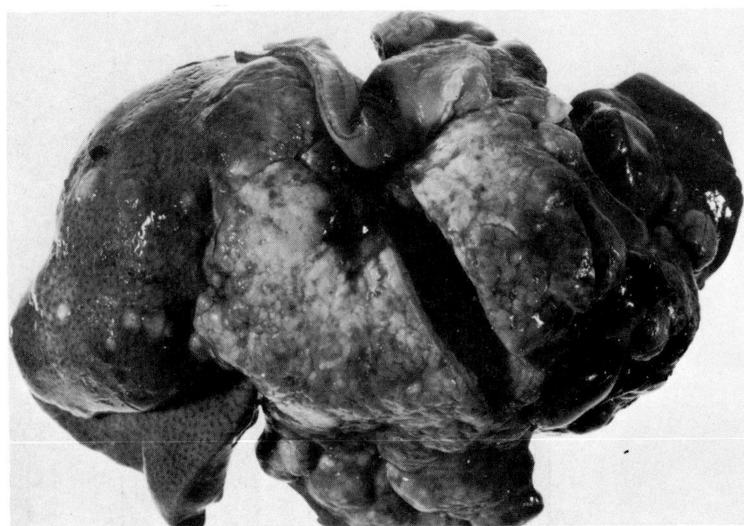

Figure 6–88. Metastasis to the liver from the same case as in Figure 6–87. Refer again to Figures 6–84 to 6–88.

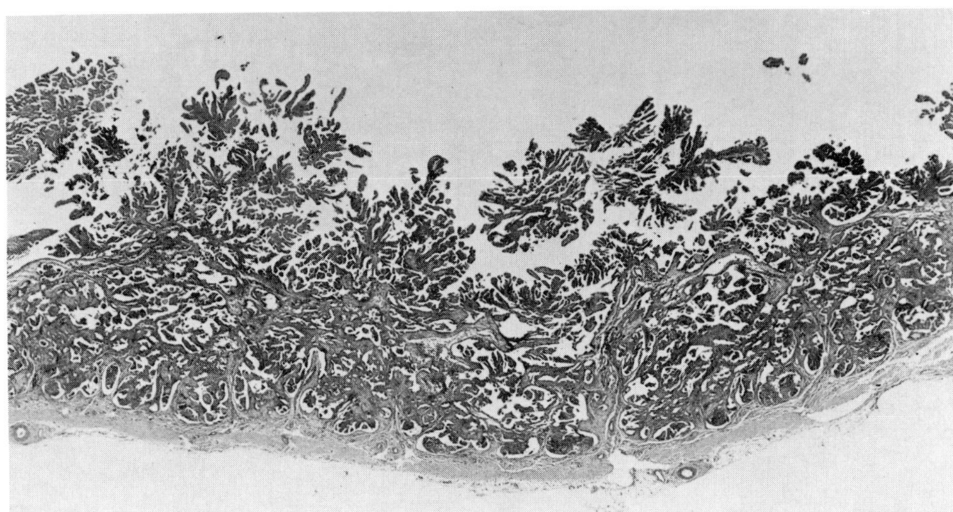

Figure 6–89. Papilliform growth of a mesothelioma. Pieces are easily detached to implant and form new growths.

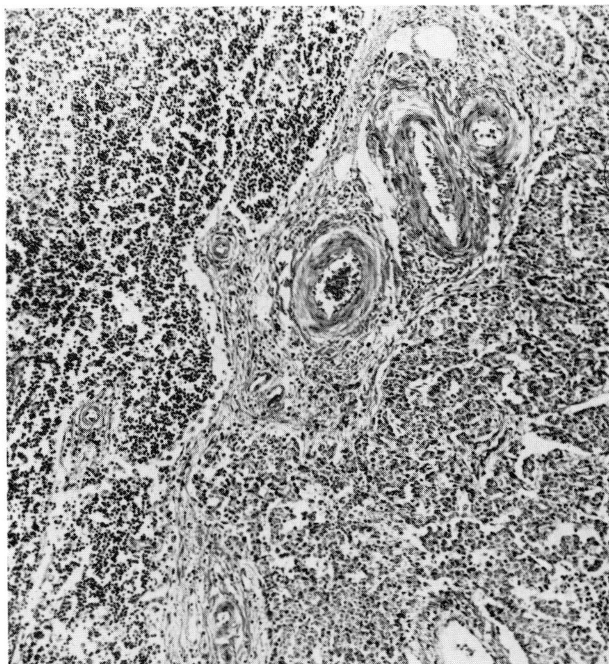

Figure 6–90. A metastatic carcinoma in a lymph node. The tumor cells are on the right.

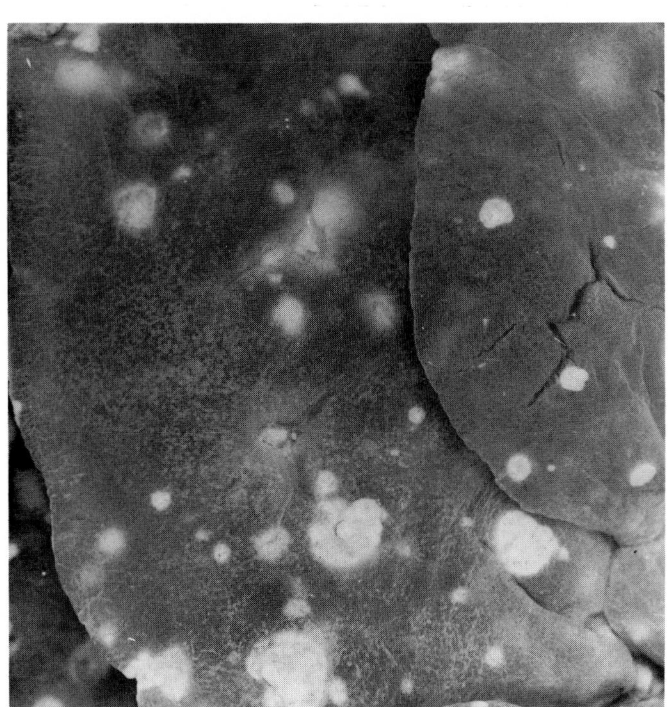

Figure 6–91. Metastatic tumor in a dog's lung. (Museum specimen.)

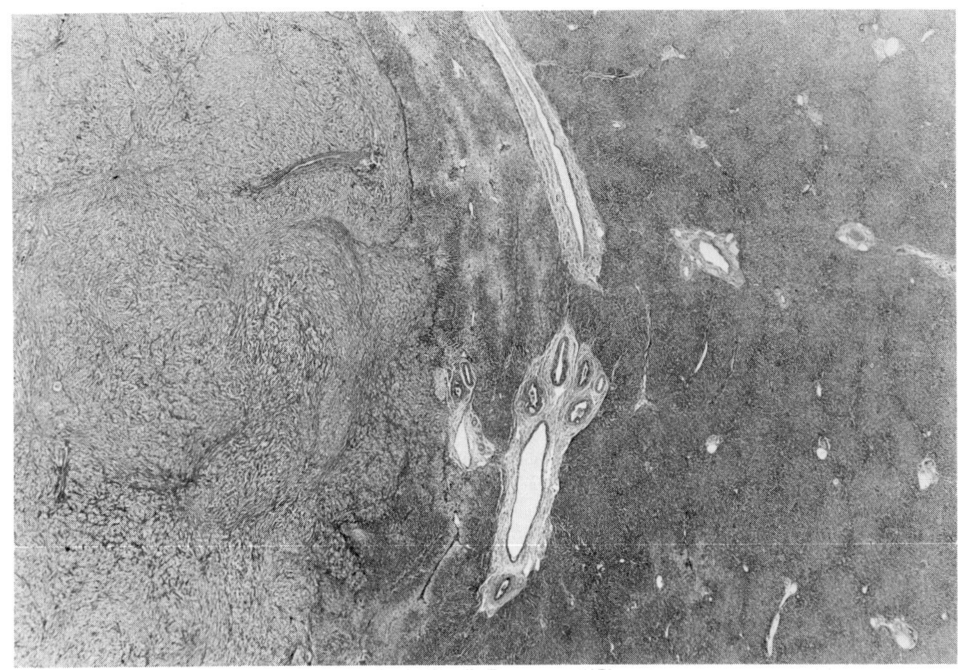

Figure 6–92. Metastatic nodule of an islet cell tumor (left) from the pancreas in the liver of a dog.

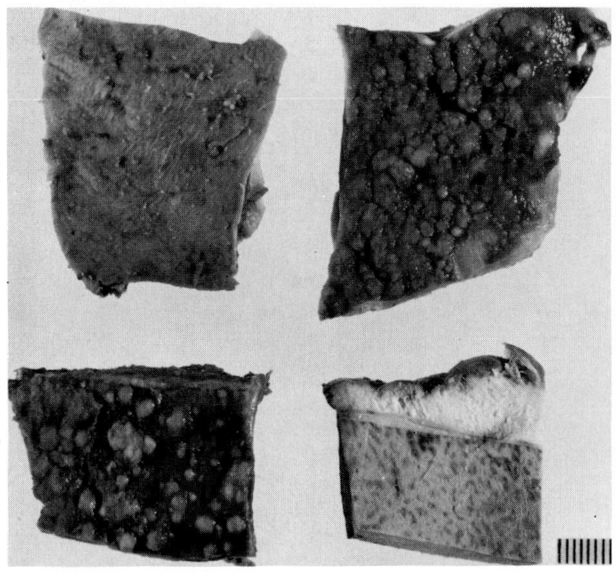

Figure 6–93. Implantation of a gastric carcinoma on the surface of pieces of viscera and peritoneum in the abdomen of a horse. At the lower right, the tumor is at the top on a cut surface of the liver.

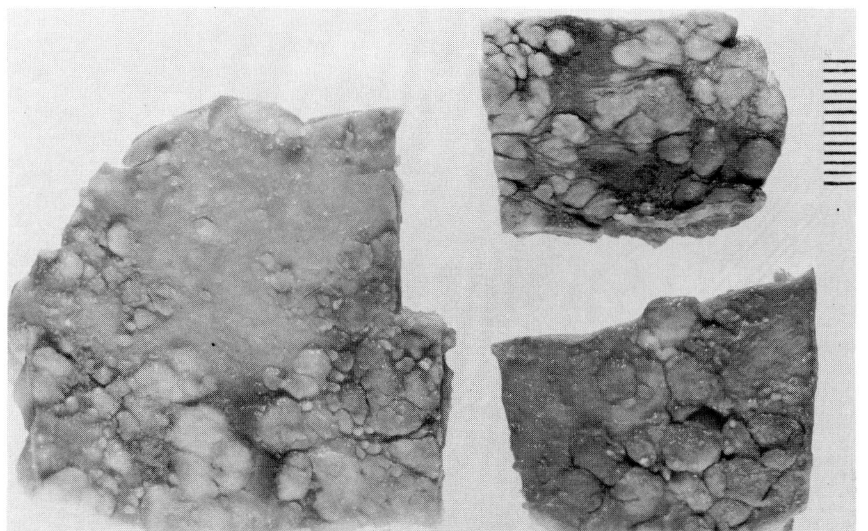

Figure 6–94. Closer view from the same case of a lesion similar to that shown in Figure 6–93.

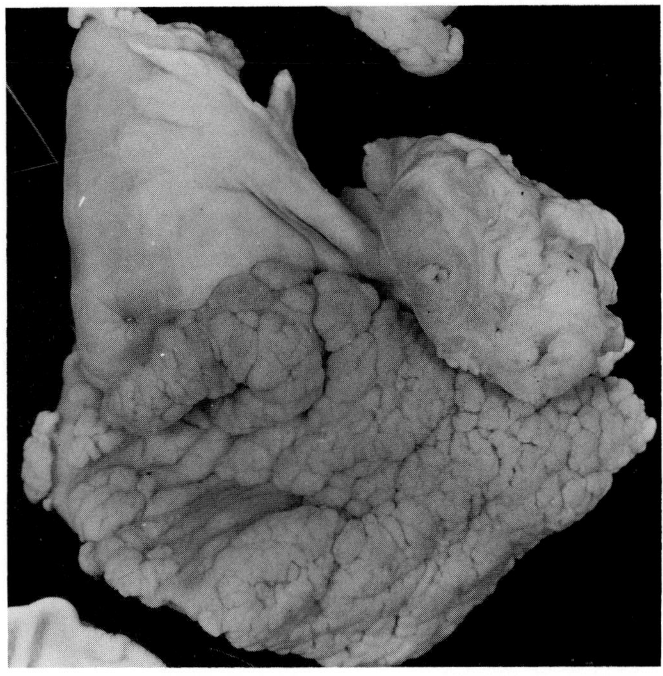

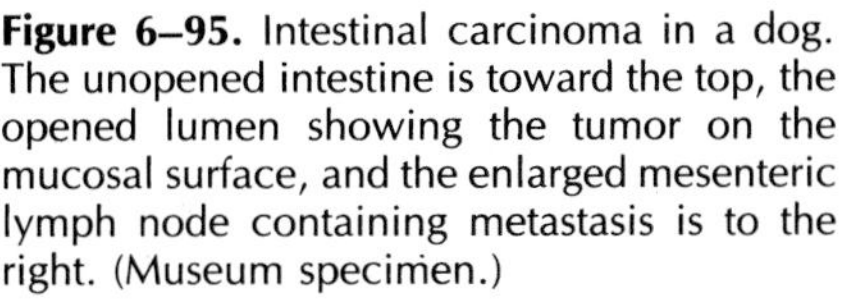

Figure 6–95. Intestinal carcinoma in a dog. The unopened intestine is toward the top, the opened lumen showing the tumor on the mucosal surface, and the enlarged mesenteric lymph node containing metastasis is to the right. (Museum specimen.)

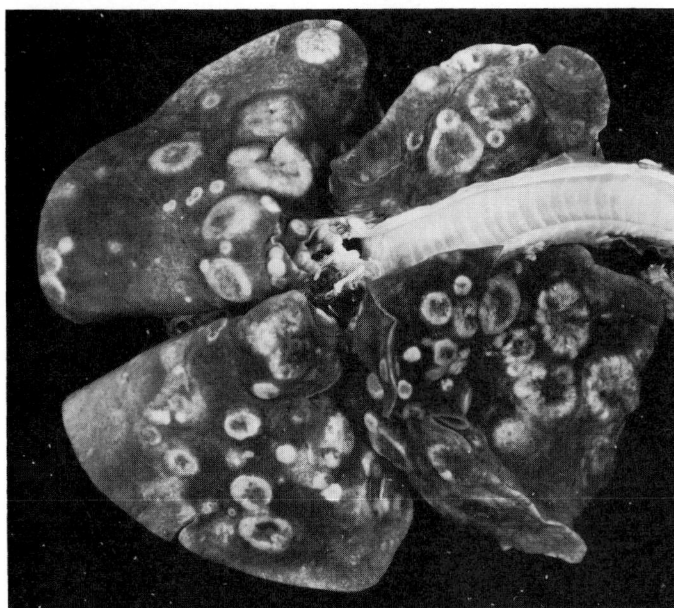

Figure 6–96. Metastatic thyroid gland carcinoma in a dog. Note the depressed umbilicate lesions. These usually indicate considerable necrosis within the tumor. (Courtesy of B. Schiefer.)

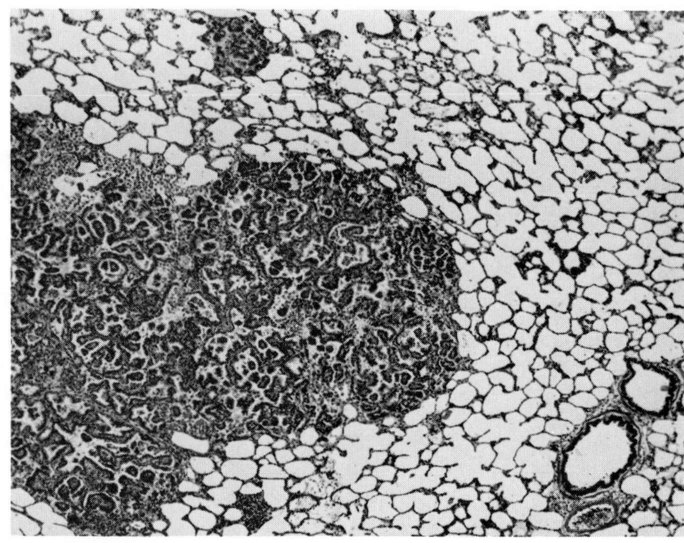

Figure 6–97. Bronchiolar carcinoma in the lung of a sheep with jaagsiekte. This is an infectious viral disease of sheep. Lesions are usually multifocal and can be very extensive throughout the lung.

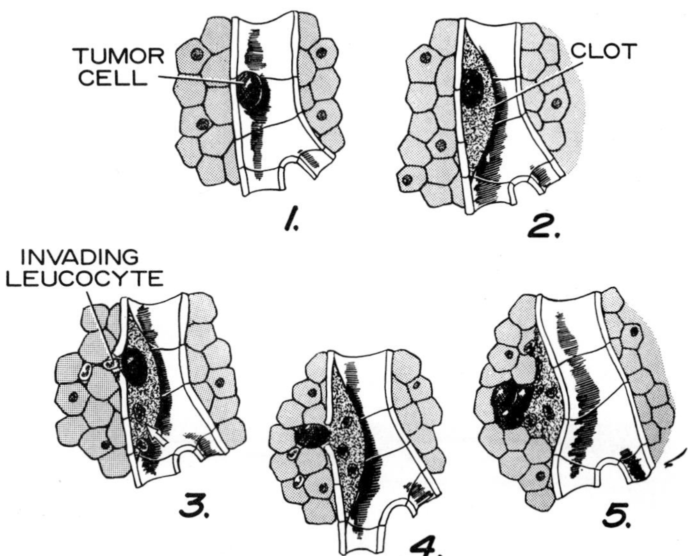

Figure 6–98. Diagrammatic summary showing the conversion of tumor cell embolus to a metastatic nodule associated with thrombosis and the progression through the vessel wall. (From Fisher, B., and Fisher, E. R.: Host factors influencing the development of metastases. Surg. Clin. North Am., *42*:335, 1962.)

further distinguish a metastatic group of cells. The cells in many tumors are genetically unstable, more so than normal tissue. Selective growth of a subpopulation continues in the "relentless emergence of new population with enhanced metastatic capacities" (see the references by Fidler). The metastatic process is very inefficient in that only a very few metastatic cells survive. Also individual tumors seem to have preferred metastatic sites, as demonstrated in rather consistent patterns of metastasis. In general, the heterogeneous nature of populations of cells within one tumor has not been considered sufficiently in treatment programs.

DIAGNOSIS AND PROGNOSIS OF TUMORS

The purpose of establishing an accurate diagnosis is to arrive at an accurate prognosis and to prescribe the best possible therapy. The pathologist must always keep these goals in mind when he undertakes a diagnosis, even though he may find himself more interested in the tumor than in the patient. Consider again that the identity of a tumor may be difficult to establish because of lack of differentiation and that each separate tumor has its own pattern of biological behavior; ***a specific accurate diagnosis is essential for the patient.***

The diagnosis involves ***the tumor and the patient***. An accurate complete gross description will often suggest that a particular lesion is a tumor and often indicates the type. The ***species*** of animal and its ***breed, age, sex, location*** and ***clinical history,*** including ***radiographic features*** when appropriate, contribute to a diagnosis. In time, familiarity with expected ***incidence*** and ***occurrence*** in particular species and breeds, together with ***characteristic locations*** and ***appearances*** of individual tumors, will add to an appreciation of this information's contribution to the diagnosis.

Too often, an accurate history or appropriate specimen from suspected cases of neoplasia is not submitted—to the disservice of the patient, the owner, the clinician and the profession.

Microscopic examination is essential, and often several areas of a tumor must be examined in order to identify it and, together with the clinical data, to establish whether or not malignancy is present. Examination of the edges of a tumor and the surrounding vessels, lymphatics and lymph nodes may also be required for evaluation of the prognosis, which implies that these tissues must be submitted for examination if an accurate prognosis is required. ***Needle biopsy, exfoliative cytology*** or ***direct contact impression smears*** may also be valuable in establishing a tentative diagnosis for initiation of immediate therapy in the clinic. Proper methods of selection, preservation and submission of specimens, with the clinical history and gross description, are highly significant for microscopic examination, as well as for a relationship between the clinician and the pathologist that is in the best interest of the patient and client. Although certain tumors carry a particular prognosis, the clinician may be in the best position to determine the prognosis after consideration of the patient, the history and the laboratory data.

Statistical data based on the behavior of large numbers of cases are very important in assessing the prognosis. These data involve a specific diagnosis and a determination of the extent or stage of the tumor and available therapy. In human medicine, the information is translated into ***five year survival rates***. For example, a carcinoma of the uterus might carry the following prognosis (using hypothetical figures): malignant, but still within the mucosa—80 per cent alive in five years; invading into the submucosa, 65 per cent; invading the serosa, 45 per cent; metastasis locally, 30 per cent; metastasis widely, 5 per cent.

For the most part, such information is lacking for animal tumors, but marked improvements are becoming visible, particularly with better record keeping and appreciation of the value of the information. Consistent information on a large scale is necessary. Brodey's work relating to the ***biological behavior of tumors in dogs*** has truly been pioneering in this area of veterinary medicine, because as a surgeon, he had a specific interest in the prognosis, the patient and the client. There has been a tendency in the past to only identify a tumor; however, by learning from the methods described in the literature on human tumors, much more information can be available for prognosis through long-term cooperative study of specific series of tumors by the clinician and pathologist. Knowledge of tumor behavior in the patient is essential and may differ from the impression gained from the histological evaluation. In general, a greater appreciation of the significance of the ***cytological features*** of tumors combined with a knowledge of the ***prognosis*** is likely to be very important in the future in veterinary medicine.

Histological grading of animal tumors has been useful for evaluation of prognosis in mammary tumors, mastocytoma and some others and is reviewed and discussed by Misdorp (1976). The points considered in grading are ***differentiation, nuclear pleomorphism, hyperchromatism*** and ***mitoses***. Each characteristic is evaluated on a 1 to 3 scale, and a total grade is determined. There is a strong correlation between grading and survival, with higher grades having shorter survival times than those of lower grades.

Clinical grading is more significant in the survival of the patient than histological grading for canine mammary tumors (Misdorp, 1976). Four stages are defined based on size, involvement of skin, and involvement of underlying tissues to arrive at a clinical grade. The mode of growth or invasiveness is the most important of many factors involved in evaluation of the prognosis; the others are listed and discussed in Misdorp's paper—histological grade, lymphatic permeation, location, treatment, regional lymph nodes, diameter and volume, and delay in opening. ***The importance of an accurate clinical assessment and history is therefore greater than or as great as histological examination and grading for assessment of prognosis.***

In national disease eradication programs, diagnosis of cancer on a massive scale may be required for the control of lymphosarcoma in cattle. Control programs now exist in some countries, but they are not yet based on ***accurate preclinical diagnosis*** in individual animals. Tests for the antigens of the etiological agents and the disease in individual cats and cattle are being developed.

From the standpoint of large scale diagnosis of cancer in populations of animals, it would be of interest at this point to consider the long-term diagnostic research objectives for human cancer at the National Cancer Institute in the United States. Diagnosis includes detection. Detection involves the process by which individuals with a high probability of having cancer are separated from the population by a screening device. These individuals are then studied by diagnostic methods to determine whether or not they have a cancer and, if so, where it is, what it is and its extent. These are required for a prognosis. Simple, precise methods are required in such a program.

The immediate goals are the development of a system that will identify 75 per cent of those in the population having a tumor (excluding skin tumors and leukemia) and the diagnosis of these early enough that ***90 per cent will be free of metastasis 10 years later***. The program involves examination of blood by immunological, chemical and cellular means and by ultrasonic, radiological and cytological examination of tissues. Specific organ programs associated with breast, lung, cervix, bowel and bladder tumors are planned.

Certain methods are advantageous in particular organs and for particular tumors. Automation of cytological examination will greatly expand the screening for tumors of the female genital tract and of the respiratory tract. Certain chemicals in the blood reflect products of specific tumors, whereas other compounds, such as increased levels of alpha fetoprotein antigen, may reflect the possibility of a range of different tumors. ***Alpha fetal globulin*** is produced by fetal hepatocytes but normally disappears late in fetal life. In certain cases of neoplastic disease, this substance is produced by the tumor cells and can be detected as an abnormal antigen in blood by immunological methods. This is useful in diagnosis and is best known in hepatocellular carcinomas. Apparently, this is a form of derepression of enzyme systems during specialization and maturation for which all cells are genetically coded. Another embryonic antigen is ***carcinoembryonic antigen***, which is widely used for cancer detection, particularly in respiratory and gastrointestinal tumors. It is normally made by intestinal epithelium in fetal life, appears in postnatal life in cases of tumors and in some other disease conditions and is not tumor-specific. It is, however, useful for large scale screening procedures.

The program is very energetic—but then so was putting a man on the moon.

Precancerous Lesions

Certain lesions in humans are known to ***precede and favor*** the development of a tumor in a ***statistically significant percentage of cases***. The lesion itself does not have neoplastic features, and the association has been arrived at by experience and by statistical results of the behavior of such lesions. The individual's age and sex and the site and type of lesion are essential in this kind of prediction, which is accurate on a statistical basis but not for individual cases. This information cannot be transposed from humans to animals and must be generated from case studies in animals.

Embryonic Tumors

Certain tumors are derived from and composed of embryonic tissues that have never reached postnatal differentiation. Although the tumor may reach clinical significance and may grow mainly in postnatal life, the tissue is truly in an embryonic stage. Examples are nephroblastoma and retinoblastoma. Some tumors have a suffix "blastoma" erroneously attached to their name because they are poorly differentiated and therefore have an embryonic appearance—for example, spongioblastoma of nervous tissue—but these are not truly embryonic tumors. The only one of significance in animals is the embryonal nephroma or nephroblastoma that occurs in several species at a low incidence and may be malignant.

Teratomas and Hamartomas

Teratomas are true tumors or neoplasms composed of ***multiple tissue of different kinds, foreign to the area in which they arise,*** and may be benign or malignant. They are not malformations and also differ from true mixed tumors, such as mixed mammary tumors, which contain tissues indigenous to the site of origin. Furthermore, the embryonic tumors do not qualify as teratomas since they are rarely mixed and are found at sites related to the parent tissue. Teratomas in animals are not common and have a strong association with the ***gonads***, particularly in horses. Many are found accidentally on microscopic examination, but some are large tumors. Most contain skin and derivatives of skin (including hair), nervous tissue and epithelium of glandular lining, or a type suggestive of bronchial or intestinal lining. Detailed examination will probably reveal ***tridermal***

composition, that is, tissues derived from ectoderm, endoderm and mesoderm, but the components have no orderly development or association.

Teratomas are considered by Willis as "arising from foci of plastic pluripotential embryonic tissue which escaped from the influence of the primary organizer during early embryonic development, this escape being in some way related to disturbances emanating from the invaginated organizing tissues of the primitive streak and so affecting median and para-median parts in close relationship to these tissues. The affected primordium, as it grows, differentiates in accordance with its own intrinsic labile determinations, producing a variety of tissues foreign to the part in which it grows." They may be dormant for years and then be activated.

Hamartomas are structures that are ***abnormal mixtures or amounts of tissue indigenous to their location***. They are considered anomalies and are ***not*** neoplasms but may be confused with neoplasms. Examples are angiomas and nevi and, in general, they are not common.

TREATMENT OF TUMORS

The methods of treatment are surgery, irradiation, chemotherapy and immunotherapy. Only surgery and irradiation have been used to any extent in animals, and there are recent reports on these subjects. Owen (1976) has reviewed the literature on treatment in animals and discusses methods used for many types of tumors. Because of the general interest in cancer, digression into methods of therapy in humans is appropriate here, since these methods may be used more commonly in animals in the future.

Surgical treatment is quite appropriate for small or localized tumors. For extreme tumors with metastasis, it soon becomes a matter of how much of the body can be removed and still sustain a reasonable life. Miller (1967) discusses such procedures as hemipelvectomy and hemicorporectomy (amputation between the lumbar vertebrae) but stresses that rehabilitation requires the stoicism of the patients, their will to live and to adjust to loss of certain functions and complete understanding of the patient and those involved later with the physical and economic care. He states that improved techniques in anesthesia and supportive therapy allow many radical operations with curative value that were not feasible a few years ago.

Brodey (1970) emphasized that ***treatment of any neoplasm is based on early accurate diagnosis, careful determination of the extent of the neoplastic process, a good understanding of its biological behavior and early adequate treatment***. He recognized that veterinary surgical literature on neoplasms dealt mainly with technique, contained little postsurgical follow-up information and consisted of retrospective studies that suffered from variation and inconsistency in the quality of clinical, radiographical and pathological observation, often carried out by many individuals over many years.

Irradiation and chemotherapy depend upon killing cells and act particularly during DNA synthesis and mitosis. The time interval of the ***cell cycle*** in a tumor thus becomes important in the timing of treatment, and for this reason it is useful to examine the cell cycle for a more detailed discussion of this point (Fig. 6–99). The cell cycle is not constant for a given tissue of a given animal but varies with conditions, such as age or hormonal stimulation. The cell cycle in tumor cells is not necessarily shorter than that in normal adult tissue. The length of the cell cycle does not depend on the size of the animal, and the length of the S phase varies in different tissues and different animals. G_1 may be absent and G_2 may vary. G_1 is the resting stage and requires RNA synthesis for progression to the next stage; it may last from 10 hours to many days. The S phase is initiated by a new protein that results in DNA synthesis and lasts six to eight hours. The subsequent stages follow a set temporal sequence of genetic transcription that is held in sequence by the dependency of one on the next. G_2 lasts from one to four hours, and mitosis, the M stage, lasts one hour and is followed by G_1. Mitosis occurs between G_2 and G_1.

The cell cycle for many individual tumors has been determined by radioisotope labeling. Therapeutic control of cell duplication occurs through ***interruption of the cell cycle. The rate of growth of a tumor depends on the length of the cell cycle, the number of***

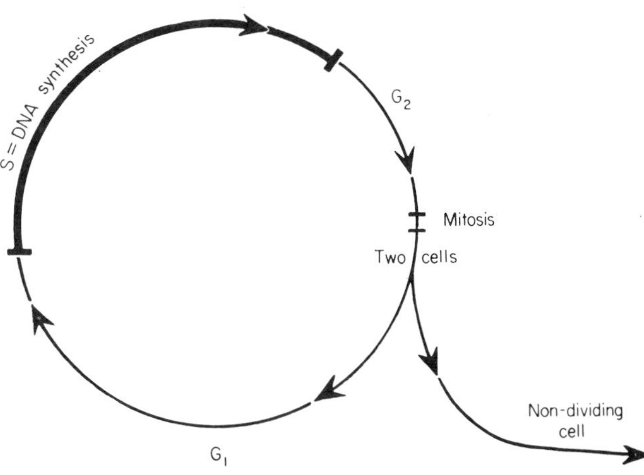

Figure 6–99. Diagram of the cell cycle. At completion of mitosis, the daughter cells may go through another cell cycle, divided into G_1 (the gap between mitosis and onset of DNA synthesis), S phase (the period during which DNA is replicated), G_2 (the gap between completion of DNA synthesis and mitosis) and mitosis again. Alternatively, one of the daughter cells may leave the cycle and become a nondividing cell, destined to die without dividing again. (From Baserga, R., and Wiebel, F.: The cell cycle in mammalian cells. *In* Richter, G. W., and Epstein, M. A. [eds.]: International Review of Experimental Pathology. Vol. 7. New York, Academic Press, 1969. Reprinted by permission.)

cells active in growth and the number lost by death. The cell cycle is often longer in a tumor than in the normal tissue and cannot be judged by the incidence of mitotic figures. Among different types of tumors there is a wide variation in the cell cycle and in the kinetics of duplication. Detailed information on the cell cycle in various tumors is required in order to improve the ***timing of therapy***, which depends on killing cells by interference with key steps in the cycle. This deficiency in knowledge probably accounts in part for lack of or reduced success in some forms of therapy. Even in rapidly progressive cancer, the cancer cells generally proliferate more slowly than some normal cells that replicate rapidly, such as intestinal epithelium and bone marrow. Therefore, these tissues are affected by therapy. Some cancer cells remain dormant for long periods and will not be susceptible to therapy during this time.

The response of tumors to ***irradiation*** depends on the quality of the irradiation source and its energy, on the total dose and its time of delivery, on associated sensitizing and protective agents and on the characteristics of the tissue irradiated. The objective is to deliver a dose lethal to the tumor without causing serious damage in the form of necrosis to the nearby tissues or organ containing the tumor. Problems arise from the variation of tumor sensitivity to this form of therapy, the difficulty in calculation of dosage and also the delivery to the specific site of the tumor. This method, however, is useful both for palliation and for cure in many human tumors, alone or in conjunction with other forms of therapy. ***Irradiation damages chromosomes and affects the ability of the cell to replicate.*** It may also cause cancer under some circumstances.

Chemotherapy used against tumors acts by interfering with the ability of the cell to divide. Unfortunately, it may act against all dividing cells and may cause serious problems in normal organs with a high rate of cellular renewal, such as bone marrow, lymphatic tissue and intestine, and by so doing could compound the problems of the patient considerably. The available drugs may be classified according to the type of compounds (as indicated in Table 6–4) and functional activity (Fig. 6–100). The action must relate to the stage of the cell cycle of the tumor cells, the number of cells at that stage and the rate of multiplication of the cells. ***The drugs bring about defects in mitosis or in DNA and RNA synthesis and function, or both.***

It has been established that chemotherapy is most useful if used heavily in ***young small tumors*** but is less useful in older larger tumors. Most tumors are recognized in an advanced state, and death results from metastasis. These factors limit the success of any form of therapy. In some cases, the metastatic site may be growing more rapidly than the primary site and be susceptible to a drug, whereas the original site may not. Therefore, surgical removal of the primary site with chemotherapy of the metastasis may be more beneficial.

Immunotherapy is the most recent and is based on certain premises. Tumor cells

TABLE 6–4. THE BIOLOGICAL EFFECT OF ANTICANCER AGENTS

Class of Compound	Molecular Basis	Cell Cycle Effect	Examples
A. Inhibitors of Nucleic Acid Biosynthesis			
Folic acid antagonists	Dihydrofolate reductase inhibitor-blocking nucleotide (thymidylate) synthesis	S phase	Methotrexate
Purine antagonists	Purine nucleotide inhibitor (conversion of inosinic acid to adenylic acid)	S phase	6-Mercaptopurine
Glutamine antagonists	Inhibit *de novo* purine synthesis	S phase	Azaserine
Pyrimidine synthesis inhibitors	Inhibit thymidylate synthetase and nucleotide (thymidylate) synthesis	S phase and possibly G_1 phase	5-Fluorouracil 5-Fluoro-2-deoxyuridine
Polynucleotide inhibitors	Inhibit DNA-dependent DNA polymerase	G_1, S phase	Cytosine arabinoside
	Inhibit nucleotide reduction	S phase	Hydroxyurea
B. The Antibiotics			
Inhibitor of protein synthesis	Prevent transfer of RNA information into polypeptides	G_1, S, G_2 phase	Puromycin
Inhibitor of RNA synthesis	Prevent DNA-dependent RNA synthesis	G_1, S, G_2 phase	Actinomycin D Mithramycin
	Intercalate with DNA and inhibit DNA-dependent RNA synthesis	G_2 phase	Daunomycin Adriamycin Streptonigrin
C. Plant Alkaloids			
Mitotic inhibitor	Prevent spindle formation and inhibit ribosomal RNA and protein synthesis	S phase	Vincristine Vinblastine
D. Alkylating Agents			
Inhibit DNA replication	Alkylate proteins and cross-link with DNA causing breaks	G_1, S, G_2 and possibly G_0 phase	Nitrogen mustard Cyclophosphamide Chlorambucil Busulfan Melphalan
E. Hydrazines			
Inhibit DNA replication and RNA synthesis	Prevent transmethylation of RNA and bind to DNA	G_1, S_1, G_2 phase	Procarbazine
F. Nitrosoureas			
Inhibit DNA replication	Probably cross-link with DNA and alkylate proteins	G_1, S, G_2, and possibly G_0 phase	BCNU CCNU Methyl-CCNU
G. Steroids			
Inhibit protein synthesis	Stimulate or inhibit production of specific forms of RNA	"Selective agent"	Adrenocortical hormones

(From Greenspan, E. M.: Clinical Cancer Chemotherapy. New York, Raven Press, 1975. Reprinted by permission.)

have antigens on their surface that differ from those on normal cells of the same tissue. The host can recognize these antigens and mount an effective immune response. Host responses can be manipulated to augment the effectiveness of the immune response. Reduction of the tumor load by cytotoxic therapy can create conditions favorable to immunological response.

Two of the methods used are active and passive immunization, both of which may be either specific or nonspecific. The ***specific active*** method involves immunization with either killed or attenuated vaccines of tumor cells, but many are irradiated or, more commonly, chemically treated. Spontaneous metastasis may be either facilitated or suppressed. ***Nonspecific active*** methods involve the use of bacterial vaccines or chemical compounds, or fractions of them, that produce nonspecific stimulation to the reticuloendothelial system and that augment humoral and cellular responses to unrelated antigens. Dosage and time point in the disease are important, and adverse reaction may occur with repeated usage. ***Specific adoptive*** methods involve injection of previously sensitized lymphocytes. In order to reduce graft versus host response, cell-free extracts of sensitized lymphocytes are used, one being transfer factor and another an RNA extract. ***Specific passive*** methods in-

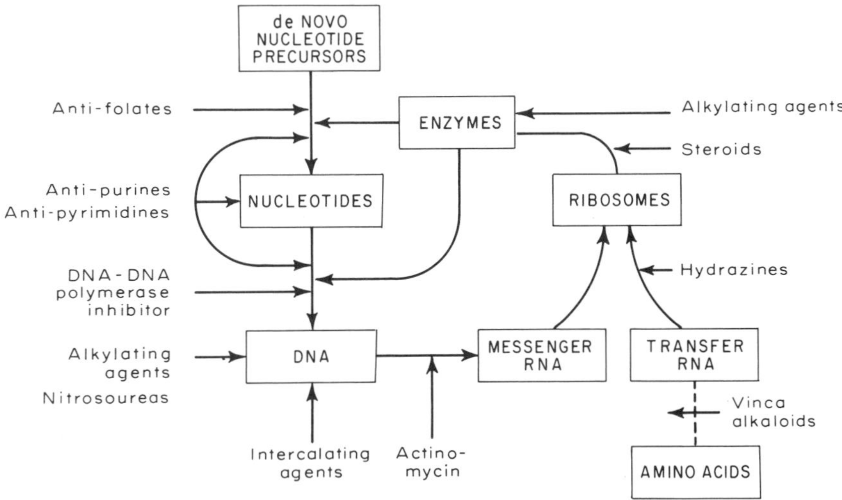

Figure 6–100. The sites of action of various chemotherapeutic agents for cancer. (From Greenspan, E. M. [ed.]: Clinical Cancer Chemotherapy, New York, Raven Press, 1975. Reprinted by permission.)

volve use of immune serum, but crossreactions and anaphylaxis may occur with repeated usage. ***Nonspecific passive*** methods use humoral substances, such as reagin or properdin. Evidence of regression in some cases using these methods offers encouragement for their use, but present lack of knowledge concerning the reactions involved requires some reservations about general usage.

The mechanisms that are active in antitumor immunity are presented in Figure 6–

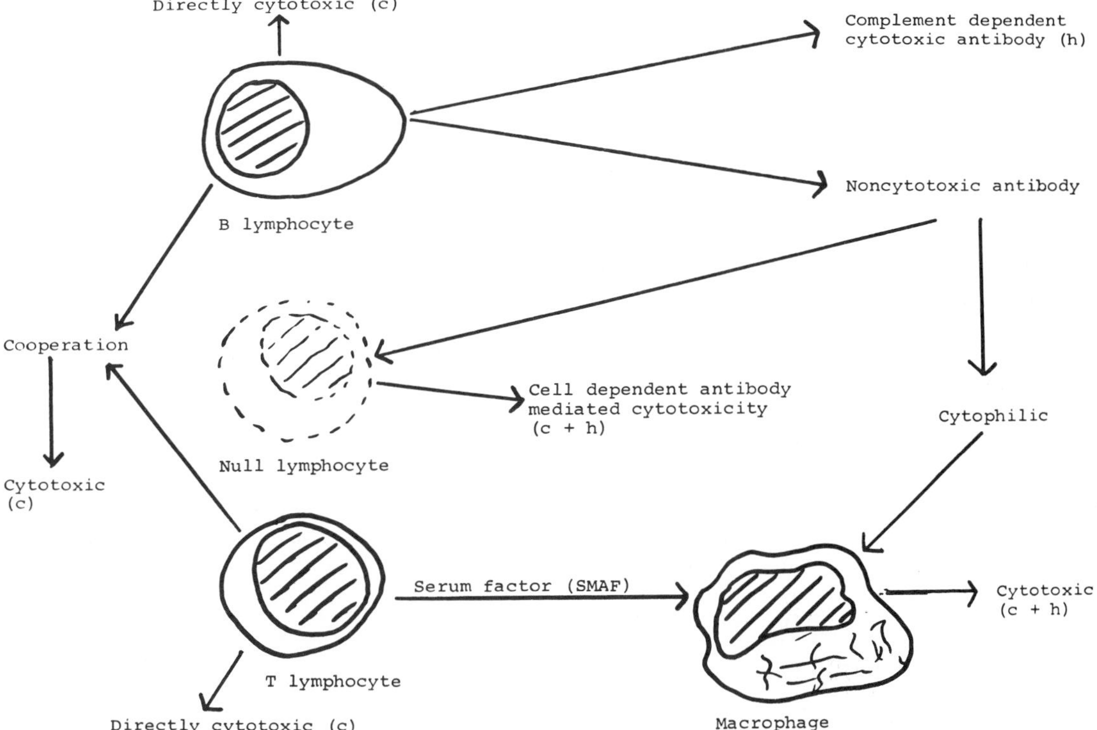

Figure 6–101. Presumed effector mechanisms of antitumor immunity; c = cellular mechanism, h = humoral mechanism. (From Proctor, J. B., Lewis, M. G., and Mansell, P. W.: Immunotherapy for cancer: an overview. Can. J. Surg., *19*:12, 1976. Reprinted by permission.)

101. Macrophages seem to be very important in destruction of tumor cells and thus in preventing growth of tumors. Immunosuppression, either genetic or iatrogenic, greatly increases the frequency of natural tumors in humans and of experimental tumors in animals.

The whole question of the relationship of the immune system to neoplasia is fascinating but very complex. Some sarcomas possess surface antigens that are distinguished from the normal transplantation antigens of the host. Lymphocytes can be sensitized to these tumor antigens and can be cytotoxic to sarcoma cells. Antibodies directed against sarcoma antigens can be blocked by the host; these antibodies can either block or enhance lymphocyte-mediated cytotoxicity. The lymphocyte–antibody–tumor cell interactions can have significant effects on tumor growth. The dynamics of these interactions can change during the course of the disease and be of prognostic value. ***Decreasing specific antibody levels tend to indicate that metastasis will soon occur.*** These methods have been used with human melanomas. Possibly, antibody levels suggest the presence of an infectious agent, particularly since antitumor antibody can be detected in the healthy relatives of some sarcoma patients.

Except for those forms of cancer that are curable by a single method, the most beneficial therapy will probably be a ***combination of irradiation, surgery, immunotherapy and chemotherapy.***

Cause of Death in Cancer Patients

Euthanasia is usually used for animals diagnosed as having advanced cancer. This procedure may change as methods of therapy become safer and are applied to animals. The cause of death in humans under heavy and often prolonged therapy for advanced cancer has been investigated in a group of patients who had many different types of tumors and were under considerable supportive therapy. Infection accounted for about one-third of the causes, particularly pulmonary disease and septicemia, mainly with gram-negative organisms. Metastasis accounted for 20 per cent, and hemorrhage accounted for about 12 per cent. Other causes were numerous and were small percentages of the total. ***Most forms of therapy result in immunosuppression, leukopenia and thrombocytopenia, all of which lead to complications.*** Many patients with cancer become ***cachectic*** and the term ***malignant cachexia*** is used. The usual causes are pain and impaired nutrition, which in large part are due to voluntary lack of food intake.

ETIOLOGY OF CANCER

The cells of a tumor are abnormal, as indicated previously. It follows that at some point they or their ancestors became abnormal and started down the neoplastic route. This section deals with ***what happened and how.*** The functions, and usually the genome, of the cells are changed, and some of these abnormal cells are allowed to persist and grow to eventually cause clinical disease and perhaps death. Many of the answers to obvious questions are unknown, but the research efforts applied to the questions fit new pieces to the puzzle rather rapidly.

Transformation

Transformation is the term used to indicate that a ***heritable change*** has occurred in cells; this process has been studied primarily in tissue cultures. It is necessary to extrapolate the results of these studies to infer what probably happens ***in vivo***, and there is no doubt that many of the data do apply. Cells grown in culture will replicate about 40 times and then apparently reach a natural age level and will not replicate further. Some cultures undergo a change that allows them to replicate indefinitely, however, and this culture is then called a ***cell line*** and the cells are said to be ***transformed.*** In a way, this change is considered to be preneoplastic, but transformation does ***not*** mean that the cells are neoplastic. Certain growth control mechanisms have changed, and, given further specific circumstances, neoplasia may be the end result. It is possible for cells to undergo transformation to malignancy in culture, and many cell lines of malignant cells have been established. There is considerable species variation in the ease with which tissues can be main-

TABLE 6–5. Properties of Normal Cells in Culture

1. The cells fail to grow from a small inoculum although cloning efficiency varies with different cells and media
2. The social behavior of the cells changes; there is loss of contact inhibition and polarization.
3. The mitotic potential decreases and will become zero
4. Cells lose their differential functions and become less able to perform work
5. Certain normal metabolic patterns change
6. Normal cells will not grow in liquid media or agar
7. The karyotype remains consistent
8. Tumors do not develop

tained in culture for long periods and also in the number of passages required before transformation occurs.

Consideration of the properties of normal cells grown in culture will provide insight into the meaning of transformation. The general points in Table 6–5 indicate the normal properties of cells in culture.

In transformation, there is a change in one or all of the characteristics listed in Table 6–5, and the changes may occur simultaneously or sequentially. Cells must be transformed to become a cell line. Cytologists make use of this property of cells to retain consistency in cell culture. This practice corresponds to the use of highly inbred strains of experimental animals to avoid genetic variation in experimental situations. Once it was appreciated that transformation was a type of preneoplastic change, oncologists studied the phenomenon in detail. Known carcinogens were soon shown to have the ability to transform certain cells and the mechanisms were investigated. ***It is now generally considered that carcinogens, the etiological agents of cancer, act by causing transformation of cells*** (Fig. 6–102). Usually, other factors must be present, or occur later, for the transformation of the cells to result in neoplasia.

Transformation means that specific genetic damage has occurred and certain features of fetal cells are "turned on." There

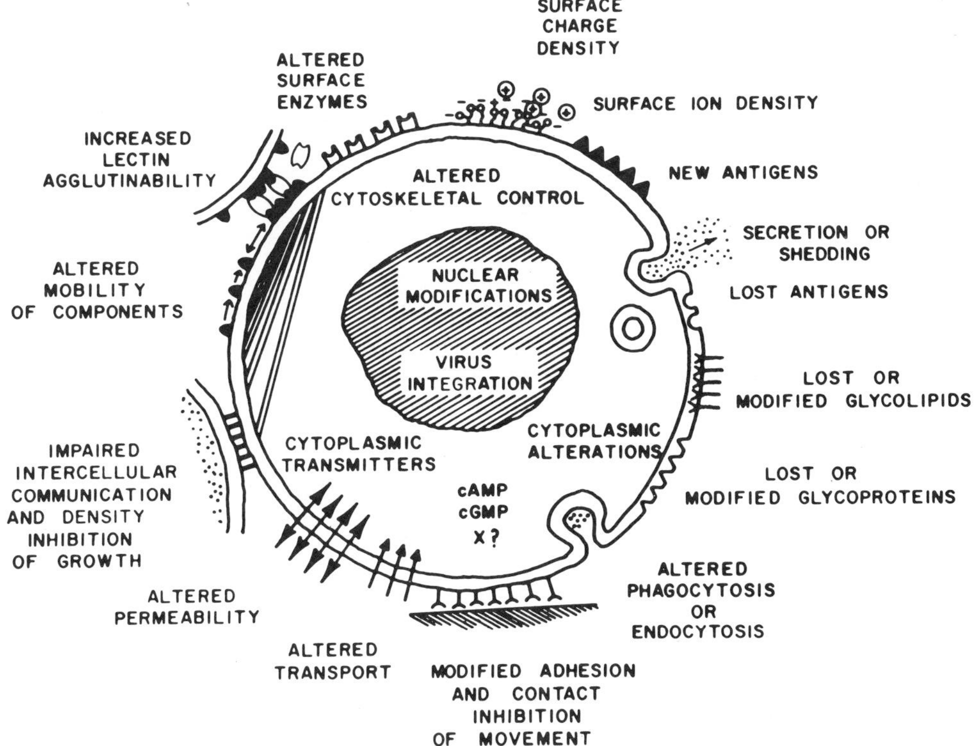

Figure 6–102. Several cell surface alterations found after neoplastic transformation are illustrated. See also Figure 6–108. (Reprinted, by permission, from Nicholson, G. L., and Poste, G.: The cancer cell: dynamic aspects and modifications in cell-surface organization. New Engl. J. Med., *295*:253–258, 1976.)

is a modulation of gene expression and a derepression of growth genes. Usually growth genes are derepressed only when regeneration or cell renewal is required. Differentiation results from selective activation and repression of genes. In transformation, there must be genomic reprogramming. Carcinogens may attack or alter certain specific genes more than others. Carcinogens induce epigenetic programmatic alterations, which eventually result in permanent change. Proliferative lesions may progress to a critical mass of altered transformed cells.

Carcinogens

The main etiological factors or carcinogens are categorized as ***irradiation, chemical agents*** and ***viruses,*** but there are a few others. Single uncomplicated trauma has not been implicated as a direct cause of cancer; however, ***trauma may act as a cocarcinogen*** and is known to increase the localization of metastatic lesions at the site of local trauma. The actions of carcinogens have been studied primarily in laboratory animals and cell cultures, and these data or their implications tend to be extrapolated to humans. This transfer may not be appropriate, considering species differences and genetic susceptibility, but the hazards of carcinogens are such that the information is sometimes used because of lack of better indicators for carcinogenesis in humans. Only the study of naturally occurring neoplasms will provide the answers concerning the precise role of "experimental carcinogens" in a natural setting. Circumstantial evidence, however, particularly occupational hazard, is compelling in some instances of association between known carcinogens and certain forms of cancer in humans. In fact, this evidence relating to occupational exposure was one of the main influences in the stimulus for research in cancer.

The causes of some naturally occurring tumors are listed in Table 6–6.

1. Irradiation. ***Irradiation*** probably influences oncogenesis by mutation effects and results in errors of genetic transcription. These errors may be corrected, but some may become permanently fixed. The following possibilities exist for the role of irradiation in tumor formation. Genetic changes that lead to loss of control of cell replication may be induced. Cellular aging may be accelerated with an increased incidence of spontaneous mutations and cancer. Oncogenic viruses may be activated. The environment of the cell may be altered, which influences the genetic expression of the cell. Selection of mutants may result from increasing the rate of proliferation of cells.

Evidence for the role of irradiation arises from increased incidence of cancer in radiologists prior to institution of proper safety controls, in radium and uranium miners, probably from inhalation, in survivors of atomic bomb blasts and in patients

TABLE 6–6. CAUSES OF NATURALLY OCCURRING NEOPLASMS

Organ	Tumor	Species	Agent Associated	Exposure
Liver	Hepatoma	Trout	Aflatoxin B_1	Contaminated feed
	Carcinoma	Rat	Taenia taeniaformis	Parasitic infection, liver
	Angiosarcoma	Man	Vinyl chloride gas	Aerosol, plastic industry
Kidney	Carcinoma	Frog	Herpesvirus	Infected water (via urine)
Bladder	Carcinoma	Cow	Bracken fern toxin	Feeding
	Carcinoma	Man	Azo dye (naphthaline)	Dye manufacture
Lung	Mesothelioma	Man	Asbestos	Asbestos industry
	Carcinoma	Man	Cigarette smoke	Smoking
Mammary gland	Adenocarcinoma	Mouse	Oncornavirus	Nursing (milk)
Esophagus	Sarcoma	Dog	Spirocirca lupi	Parasite localization
Rumen	Carcinoma	Cow	Plant toxin (?)	Feeding
Thyroid	Carcinoma	Man	Radiation (X rays)	Therapeutic radiation
Eye	Carcinoma	Cow	Radiation (solar)	Exposure to sun (UV)
Tongue	Carcinoma	Man	Radiation (radium)	Licking contaminated brushes (watch making)
Scrotum	Carcinoma	Man	Soot (benzpyrene)	Chimney sweeping

(From Cheville, N. F.: Cell Pathology. Ames, Iowa State Press, 1976. Reprinted by permission.)

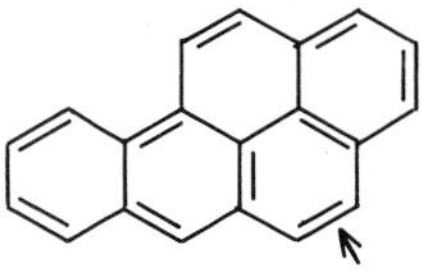

BENZO (a) PYRENE

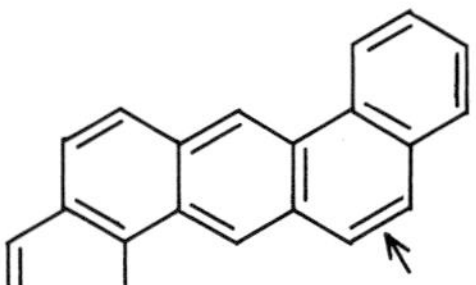

DIBENZ (a,i) ANTHRACENE

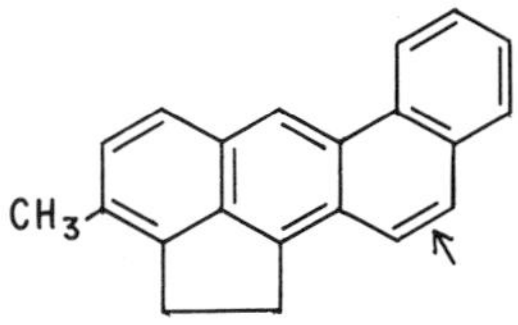

3-METHYLCHOLANTHRENE

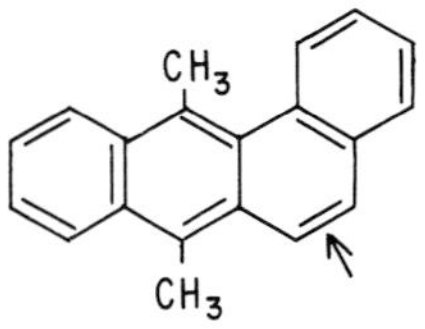

7, 12-DIMETHYLBENZ (a) ANTHRACENE

Figure 6–103. The four main carcinogenic polycyclic hydrocarbons (arrows point to the anthracenoid or K region). (Reprinted, by permission, from Ryser, H.: Chemical carcinogenesis. N. Engl. J. Med., *285*:721, 1971.)

who had received forms of therapy that used radiation before its oncogenic capabilities were appreciated.

2. Chemical Carcinogens. ***Chemical carcinogens*** are very numerous, but the best known are the polycylic aromatic hydrocarbons, alkylating agents, azo dyes and aromatic amines. A high incidence of scrotal squamous cell carcinoma in chimney sweeps, an observation recorded by Percival Potts in London 200 years ago, was an early association of an occupational hazard. In 1915, Japanese workers induced tumors on rabbits' ears by repeated painting with coal tars. This work was expanded in Britain by Kennaway's group and over many years this group established much of what is presently known about chemical carcinogenesis. An important observation made between 1940 and 1941 was that some chemicals do not act in the ***initiation*** stage of the tumor but rather act as ***promoters.*** This distinction was of great significance. The chemical formulas of common carcinogens are shown in Figures 6–103 and 6–104.

The five points summarized in Table 6–7

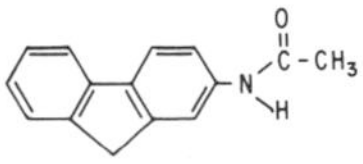

2-ACETAMINOFLUORENE (AAF)

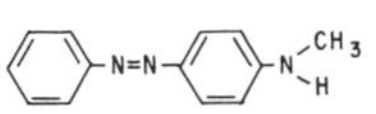

N-METHYL-4-AMINOAZOBENZENE (MAB)

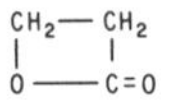

β-PROPIOLACTONE

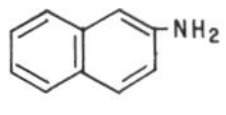

2-NAPHTHYLAMINE

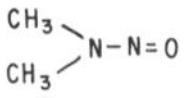

DIMETHYLNITROSAMINE

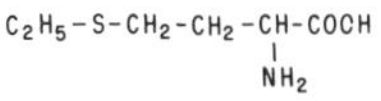

ETHIONINE

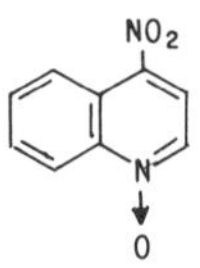

4-NITROQUINOLINE-1-OXIDE

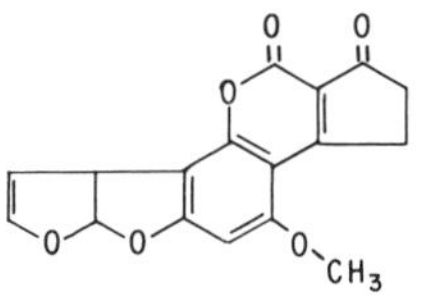

AFLATOXIN B_1

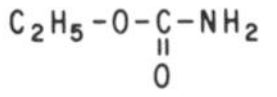

URETHAN

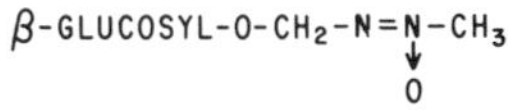

CYCASIN

Figure 6–104. Chemical formulas of some common carcinogens. All except aflatoxin and cycasin are synthetic compounds. AAF was developed as a potential insecticide. MAP and 2-naphthylamine were once used in the dye industry, as was butter yellow, the N-methyl derivative of MAB. B-propiolactone is an alkylating agent that does not require prior metabolic activation (Reprinted by permission from Ryser, H.: Chemical carcinogenesis. N. Engl. J. Med., *285*:721, 1971.)

TABLE 6–7. ESSENTIAL FEATURES OF CHEMICAL CARCINOGENESIS

1. The effects of carcinogens are dose-dependent, additive and irreversible
2. Carcinogenesis requires time
3. The cellular changes that trigger carcinogenesis are transmitted to daughter cells
4. Carcinogenesis can be influenced by factors that are not truly carcinogenic
5. Carcinogenesis requires cell proliferation

are the essential features of chemical carcinogenesis. Expansion of these points is presented in the paper by Ryser (1971), which is a remarkable distillation of a large amount of material in the literature.

The difference between initiation and promotion is exemplified in Figure 6–105. Croton oil is well known as an experimental promoter; but in general, promoters act as growth stimulants, and ***proliferation of cells,*** for whatever reason, ***is the essence of promotion.*** Hormones may be prominent as promoters. It is important to appreciate that long time periods may intervene between initiation and promotion under natural conditions. Using an appropriate combination of potent initiators, promoters and highly susceptible animals, however, the time intervals may be very short for experimental production of a tumor. Some environmental carcinogens are included in Table 6–8. ***A chemical carcinogen may induce different kinds of tumors in organs, depending upon the strain of animal, the dose and route of administration and the chemical used.*** The carcinogenic activity of some compounds can be predicted in strict experimental situations by knowledge of the chemical structure at the K region of hydrocarbons (Fig. 6–103).

Theories on how chemical carcinogenesis acts have involved consideration of (a) the deletion theory—a carcinogen causes the deletion or inactivation of a key growth control enzyme, (b) direct damage to DNA or perhaps RNA, which results in transcription into DNA, (c) activation of latent oncogenic viruses or (d) assistance with the selection of clones of initiated cells. The latter theory is gaining support. Nodules of cells induced by an initiator usually disappear, but some persist. Cells in such nodules have lesions on their surfaces, in microfilaments and in their endoplasmic reticulum and have undergone a metabolic conversion. They may be considered pre-

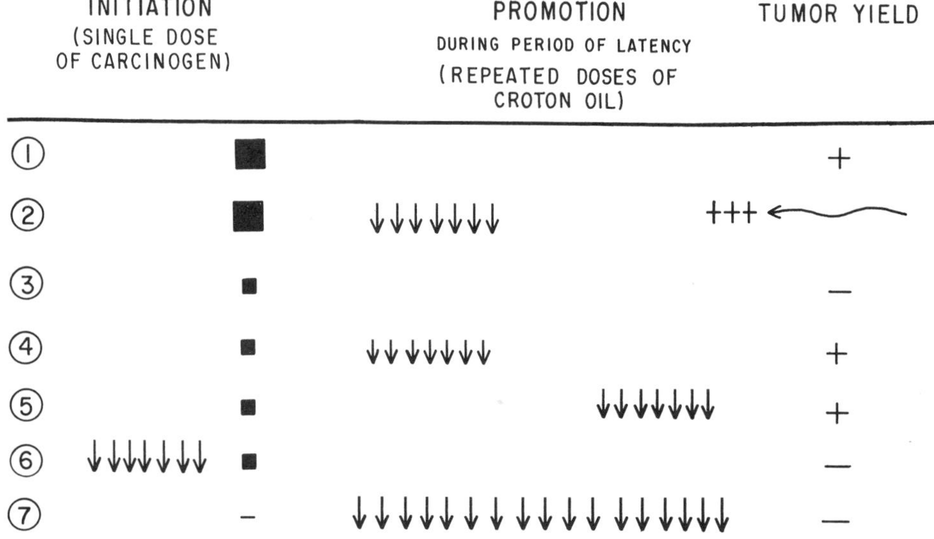

Figure 6–105. Distinction between initiation and promotion. Squares stand for single administrations of a carcinogen (e.g., methylcholanthrene) to the skin of a test animal. Vertical arrows represent administration of promoter (croton oil or phorbol ester, two to five applications per week) to the initiated skin. After initiation, promotion leads to a larger yield of tumors at an earlier time (lines 1 and 2). After a subcarcinogenic dose, promotion leads to the expression of an otherwise insufficient initiation (lines 3 and 4). Tumor yield is not decreased when the same promotion procedure is carried out later during the period of latency (line 5). Promotion, however, is ineffective when occurring more than three days before initiation (line 6) or the absence of initiation (line 7). (Reprinted, by permission, from Ryser, H.: Chemical carcinogenesis. N. Engl. J. Med., *285*:721, 1971.)

TABLE 6–8. Common Environmental Chemical Carcinogens

Carcinogen	Source	Tumors Induced	Susceptible Species
Aromatic amino, nitro and azo compounds (beta-naphthylamine, benzidine, alpha-naphthylamine)	Dyes	Urinary bladder	Human Dog
Coal tar derivatives (pitch, creosote, anthracene oil, asphalt)	Coal	Skin	Human Dog Mice
Petroleum and derivatives (benzene, vinyl chloride)	Automobile exhausts Waxes Carbon blacks Plastics	Skin Lung Larynx Leukemias Liver	Human Dog
Arsenicals	Mining Pesticides	Skin	Human Horse Cattle
Radioactive chemicals (Sr-90)	Medical use	Bone Lung Hematopoietic	Human Dog Cattle
Chlorinated hydrocarbons (DDT, carbon tetrachloride, chloroprene, aldrin, carbonates, choline, methionine)	Pesticides Herbicides Food additives	Lung Liver Leukemias	Human Dog Rats Trout

(From Hardy, W. D., Jr.: The etiology of canine and feline tumors. J. Am. Anim. Hosp. Assoc., *12*:313, 1976. Reprinted by permission.)

neoplastic. Initiators are electrophilic reactants with a strong positive charge and which react with DNA, RNA, and other cell constituents, particularly electron-rich sites. Initiators may act directly or may be a *procarcinogen,* which requires metabolism in the host to become an initiator. The "initiated" cells have acquired altered growth control mechanisms. Farber suggests three possible mechanisms for the change in these cells: (1) induction of a few initiated cells by an irreversible mechanism, (2) generation of a stimulus for repeated proliferation of cells, or (3) selective proliferation of only a very few cells in what might be referred to as a rare "mutation-like event," which can become "fixed" by proliferation and lead to atypical hyperplasia, dysplasia or carcinoma in situ. The latter mechanism is generally accepted. The whole process is considered to be chronic and multistaged and is dependent on many factors, including the general physiological state of the host at the time. The problems in the cell are apparently not just caused by miscoding lesions in DNA or a particular pattern of DNA repair. Most of the tests used on chemicals to assess their carcinogenic activity gauge damage to DNA or chromosomes and are measuring mutagenicity. However, not all mutagens are carcinogens.

The area of chemical carcinogenesis is and will be very much an issue of public discussion in the foreseeable future.

3. Viral Oncogenesis. ***Viral oncogenesis*** was observed before viruses were known when in 1908 a sarcoma of a chicken was passed to other birds in cell-free material, and a solid sarcoma was transferred in 1911 by Rous. These works attracted little attention until the 1930's and 1940's. Shope passed a fibroma in rabbits, and passage of Bittner's tumor through the mother's milk to young mice aroused great interest (Table 6–9). Since 1950, numerous viral agents have been demonstrated in infectious cancer, but usually in highly inbred strains of animals. A list of known DNA and RNA viral agents is included in Tables 6–10 and 6–11. Viral agents were suspected if tumors, called ***transplantable,*** could be passed with whole cells, and were confirmed if tumors, called ***transmissible,*** were passed with cell-free passage. Improved techniques have

TABLE 6–9. Milestone in Experimental Oncology

1838	Moller (Germany) demonstrates the celular nature of neoplasms by examining tumor tissue with light microscope.
1858	Leblanc (France) establishes that animal tumor has similar cellular composition.
1876	Novinsky (Russia) demonstrates transplantability of canine veneral tumor.
1903	Jensen (Denmark) inoculates suspension of mouse mammary gland tumor into mice, reproduces tumors, and passes them serially.
1908	Ellerman and Bang (Denmark) discover transmissibility of avian lymphoid tumors.
1910	Rous transmits sarcoma of chicken by cell-free suspensions.
1910	Clunet (France) produces tumors experimentally by X-radiation.
1912	Murphy shows that rat tumors will grow on chicken chorioallantoic membrane.
1914	Yamagiwa (Japan) proves carcinogenicity of coal tar by long-term application to skin of rabbits.
1924	Little and Strong develop inbred strains of mice for genetic analysis of tumors.
1932	Shope demonstrates viral nature of rabbit papilloma.
1933	Warburg shows high rate of anaerobic glycolysis in tumor cells.
1936	Lucke discovers virus-induced renal carcinoma of frog.
1936	Bittner discovers viral agent in milk causing mammary gland carcinoma of mice.
1943	Gross shows evidence for tumor-specific antigens by immunizing mice.
1947	Berenblum establishes two stages in chemical carcinogenesis: initiation and promotion.
1951	Gross isolates virus causing naturally occurring lymphoma in mice.
1962	Epstein and Barr isolate causal herpesvirus from Burkitt's lymphoma, shown later to cause infectious mononucleosis.
1964	Jarrett transmits lymphosarcoma to cats with retroviruses.
1969	Friedrich-Freksa shows early changes in liver chemical carcinogensis are multiple foci of cells with abnormal enzyme patterns.
1974	Brinster and Minz inoculate teratoma cells into normal mouse blastocysts to produce normal but mosaic mice (showing that tumor cells lose malignancy and differentiate normally).

(From Cheville, N. F.: Cell Pathology. Ames, Iowa State Press, 1983. Reprinted by permission.)

moved most transplantables to the transmissible category, and it seems only a matter of time before researchers identify the viral agent in a transmissible tumor.

Key factors in the progress of the study of viral oncogenesis have been (a) recognition of the ***carrier state*** of viruses and that other factors may influence the expression of a tumor caused by a virus, (b) recognition of the importance of the ***strain of animal*** in terms of susceptibility, which accounts for the genetic influence in so-called high or low incidence strains, and (c) recognition of ***age susceptibility*** as a factor, of which little was known until newborn animals were used in testing programs. The electron microscope had a great influence in terms of finding viruses in tumor cells, but it is another matter to demonstrate that the virus present is the one causing the tumor, particularly in natural cases.

Both RNA and DNA viruses may influence the development of cancer by causing transformation of cells.

DNA Viruses. The papova group are small DNA viruses including the ***pa***pillomavirus, ***po***lyomavirus and simian ***va***cuolating (SV-40) viruses. The papillomaviruses cause warts on the skin and on oral or genital mucosa. Polyoma occurs as an inapparent infection in adult mice but causes tumors when injected into newborn mice. This virus can cause many different kinds of tumors in a variety of tissues in mice and other rodents. SV-40 was discovered in kidney cell cultures from rhesus monkeys and causes sarcomas if injected into newborn hamsters. Polyoma and SV-40 may cause either productive infection with lysis of cells or transformation. Productive infection tends to occur in ***permissive cells of a natural host,*** whereas the permanent heritable change induced by ***transformation*** usually occurs in ***nonpermissive cells of an unnatural host.***

The steps in productive infection are illustrated in Figure 6–106 and are as follows:

1. Adsorption of the virus to the cell membrane and penetration.
2. Uncoating of viral DNA at the nuclear membrane.
3. Transcription of part of parenteral viral DNA in the nucleus to form early viral messenger RNA.
4. Translation of early messenger RNA into protein involved in viral DNA synthesis and in altering cell metabolism.
5. Replication of progeny viral DNA to form viral RNA.
6. Transcription of progeny viral DNA to form viral RNA.
7. Translation of late viral messenger RNA to form viral capsid and other protein.
8. Self-assembly of the virus in the cell nucleus.
9. Lysis of the cell.

In transformation (F and G in Figure 6–106) viral DNA, capsid protein and infectious virus are ***not*** produced. ***The cell is not lysed, but the viral genome is inserted into the host cell genome, is replicated with it and may later influence certain properties of the host cell in such a way as to induce***

TABLE 6–10. HOST RANGE AND ONCOGENICITY OF DNA ONCOGENIC VIRUSES

Virus Group	Representative Viruses	Oncogenicity in: Natural Host	Oncogenicity in: Experimental Host
Adenoviruses	Infectious canine hepatitis virus (ICH)	− (dog)	+ (hamster)
	Simian adenovirus	− (monkey)	+ (hamster)
	Bovine adenovirus	− (cow)	+ (hamster)
	Avian adenovirus	− (chicken)	+ (hamster)
Poxviruses	Yaba virus	+ (monkey & man)	+ (monkey)
	Tanapox virus	+ (monkey & man)	+ (rabbit)
	Myxoma virus	+ (rabbit)	+ (rabbit)
	Fibroma virus	+ (rabbit)	+ (rabbit)
Papovaviruses			
Papillomaviruses	Canine oral papilloma virus	+ (dog)	+ (dog)
	Equine papilloma virus	+ (horse)	+ (horse)
	Bovine papilloma virus	+ (cow)	+ (cow)
	Shope rabbit papilloma virus	+ (rabbit)	+ (rabbit)
Polyomaviruses	Polyoma virus	− (mouse)	+ (mice, rats, hamsters, rabbits)
	SV40	− (rhesus & cynomyologus monkeys)	+ (hamsters)
Herpesviruses	Marek's disease virus	+ (chicken)	+ (chicken)
	Herpes saimin	− (squirrel monkey)	+ (marmoset & others)
	Herpes ateles	− (spider monkey)	+ (marmoset & others)
	Lucke tumor virus	+ (leopard frog)	+ (leopard frog)

(From Hardy, W. D., Jr.: The etiology of canine and feline tumors. J. Am. Anim. Hosp. Assoc., *12*:313, 1976. Reprinted by permission.)

TABLE 6–11. HOST RANGE AND ONCOGENICITY OF ONCORNAVIRUSES

Representative Oncornaviruses	Oncogenicity in: Natural Host	Oncogenicity in: Experimental Host
Viper sarcoma virus	+ (viper snake)	−
Corn snake sarcoma virus	+ (corn snake)	−
Avian leukosis virus	+ (chicken)	+ (chicken)
Avian sarcoma virus	+ (chicken)	+ (dog, chicken, rat, mouse, rabbit, hamster, guinea pig, monkey, snake, tortoise)
Murine leukemia virus	+ (mouse)	+ (mouse, rat)
Murine sarcoma virus	+ (mouse)	+ (mouse, rat, hamster)
Murine osteosarcoma virus	+ (mouse)	+ (mouse)
Murine mammary tumor virus	+ (mouse)	+ (mouse)
Rat leukemia virus	+ (rat)	−
Guinea pig leukemia virus	+ (guinea pig)	+ (guinea pig)
Hamster leukemia virus	+ (hamster)	−
Hamster sarcoma virus	+ (hamster)	+ (hamster)
Feline leukemia virus	+ (cat)	+ (cat, dog)
Feline sarcoma virus	+ (cat)	+ (cat, dog, rat, rabbit, pig, sheep, monkey)
Bovine leukemia virus	+ (cow)	+ (sheep)
Simian sarcoma virus	+ (wooly monkey)	+ (monkeys)
Gibbon lymphoma virus	+ (gibbon ape)	+ (gibbon ape)
Mason-Pfizer monkey virus	+ (rhesus monkey)	−

(From Hardy, W. D., Jr.: The etiology of canine and feline tumors. J. Am. Anim. Hosp. Assoc., *12*:313, 1976. Reprinted by permission.)

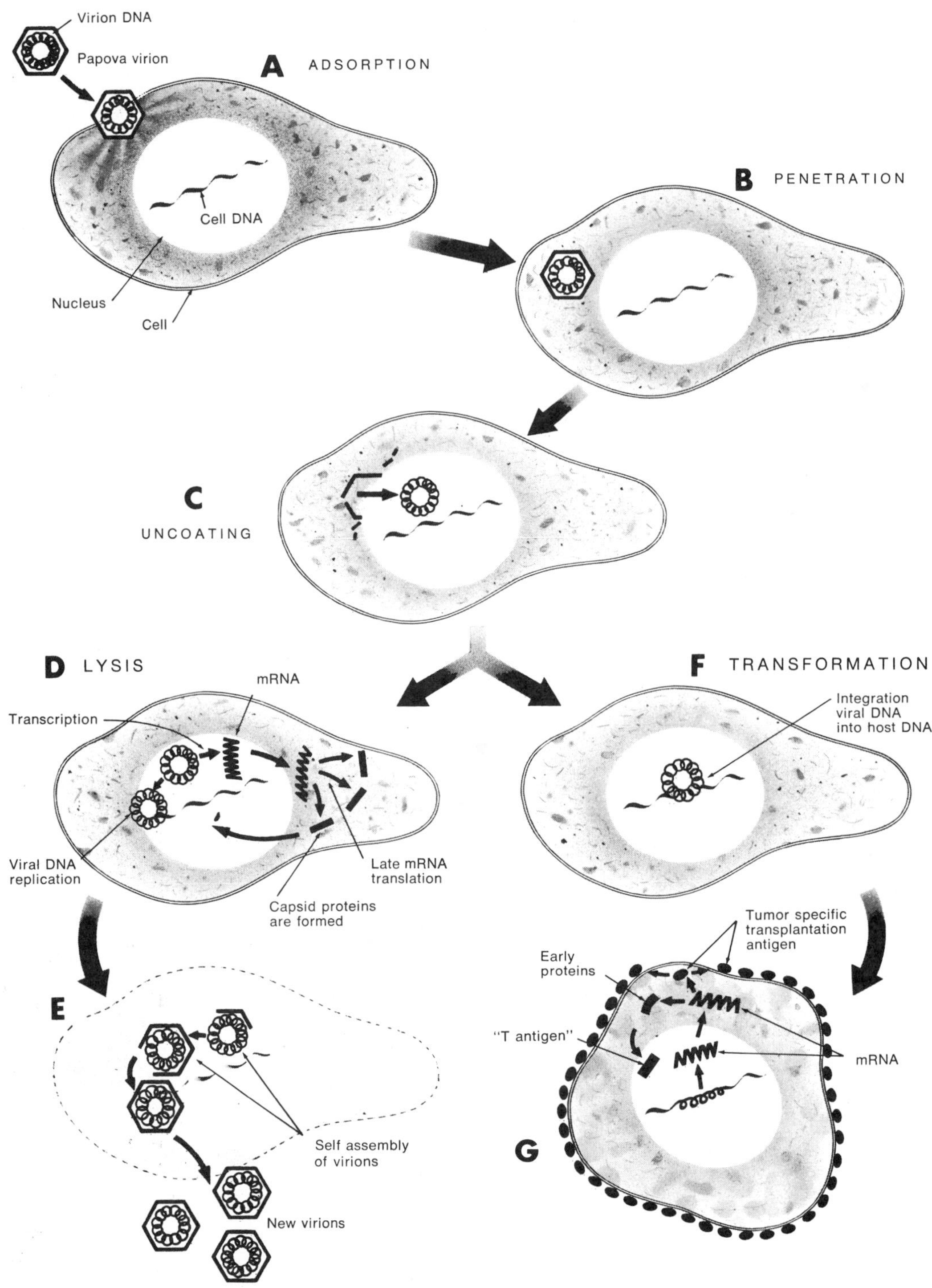

Figure 6–106. Schematic and tentative outline of interaction of papovavirus with cells. The end products are cellular lysis with production of new virus *(E)* or cellular cells transformed by virus-specific proteins *(G)*. (Reprinted, by permission, from Allan, D. W., and Cole, P.: Viruses and human cancer. N. Engl. J. Med., *286*:70–82, 1972.)

transformation. Transformation is accompanied by metabolic and chemical as well as physical changes in the cell and by a loss of certain cellular responses to growth control mechanisms.

Adenoviruses are not known to cause a natural tumor. There is an association between herpesviruses and cancer in humans, particularly uterine and cervical tumors; these viruses are also known to cause Burkitt's lymphoma, which occurs naturally in young Africans. The renal adenocarcinoma of frogs is of interest because the tumor grows in the summer but does not produce virus, whereas in the winter, tumor growth stops and the tumor cells produce virus. This is an example of ***temperature-dependent*** oncogenic herpesvirus. Marek's disease of poultry is caused by a herpesvirus, truly behaves as an infectious disease and can be prevented by vaccination, which, as mentioned previously, is perhaps a sign of things to come in other species. Poxviruses can induce fibromas in rabbits and squirrels.

RNA Viruses. RNA viruses have been demonstrated as the cause of some forms of leukemia or lymphosarcoma in animals and are known as ***leukoviruses*** or ***oncornaviruses.*** These viruses have remarkably consistent physical, chemical and oncogenic properties. Infection is usually vertical, which means congenital, but may also be horizontal, as exemplified by the feline leukemia virus. Infection with this virus may result in several different clinical syndromes including thymic atrophy, suppressed immunity, nonregenerative anemia, pancytopenia, glomerulonephritis, abortion, a wasting syndrome, myelofibrosis, and osteosclerosis. Lymphosarcoma is one of the most common expressions. Tumors of each cell type in the bone marrow may be caused by the virus. The infection appears to inhibit further development or maturation of the affected cell. For example, infected immature neutrophils would produce more immature neutrophils and not develop further. Actual expression of tumors occurs in a minority of infected animals. The main disease syndromes produced by the virus are usually summarized as lymphosarcoma, myeloid tumors or myeloproliferative disorders.

Feline sarcoma virus causes fibrosarcomas in cats and can infect tissues of many different species experimentally. This virus can not replicate, but can transform infected cells. Such viruses are called incomplete. Mainly the sarcoma virus is formed from genes supplied by the feline leukemia virus, but must have a host cell gene incorporated as well because the gene for replication is absent from its own genome. The feline leukemia virus has three genes for replication: "gag" for structural proteins, "pol" for reverse transcriptase and "env" for the viral envelope. The feline sarcoma virus has "gag" and "env," but not "pol." It picks up a "sarc" gene from the host cell genome, and thus can induce sarcomas. Animals infected with either virus produce antibody, which can be detected serologically. One of the antibodies is induced by a cell surface antigen and seems to be a reliable indicator of infection. It is called FOCMA, which is ***f***eline ***o***ncornavirus associated ***c***ell ***m***embrane ***a***ntigen. There is some concern about the public health aspects of having FOCMA-positive animals as pets.

The avian oncornaviruses also have multiple manifestations and are highly infectious. They can cause tumors of each of the myeloid cell types in addition to causing sarcomas of many tissues, such as lymph nodes, liver, kidney, ovary, pancreas, meninges, blood vessels, connective tissue and testes. There are several subgroups and strains of the virus.

In humans, there is a very strong association between a lymphosarcoma called Burkitt's lymphoma, which occurs in children particularly in central Africa, and the herpesvirus that causes infectious mononucleosis. Increasing evidence also suggests that Hodgkin's disease may be infectious.

Lymphosarcoma in animals is of great economic importance; its viral cause is also of great interest as a possible cause of a common type of cancer in many species, including humans. Prevention of Marek's disease by a vaccine is most impressive and excites the imagination about future possibilities. The disease in ***cattle*** is also of particular concern because some governments have instituted slaughter control programs to reduce the incidence, and there is much pressure from the livestock industry to control the disease. Specific and accurate diagnostic tests are required to identify "infected" animals. These tests are being used to some extent on ***cats and cattle.***

Lymphosarcoma has been identified as orginating from both T and B cell types in the same species, but apparent mixed types

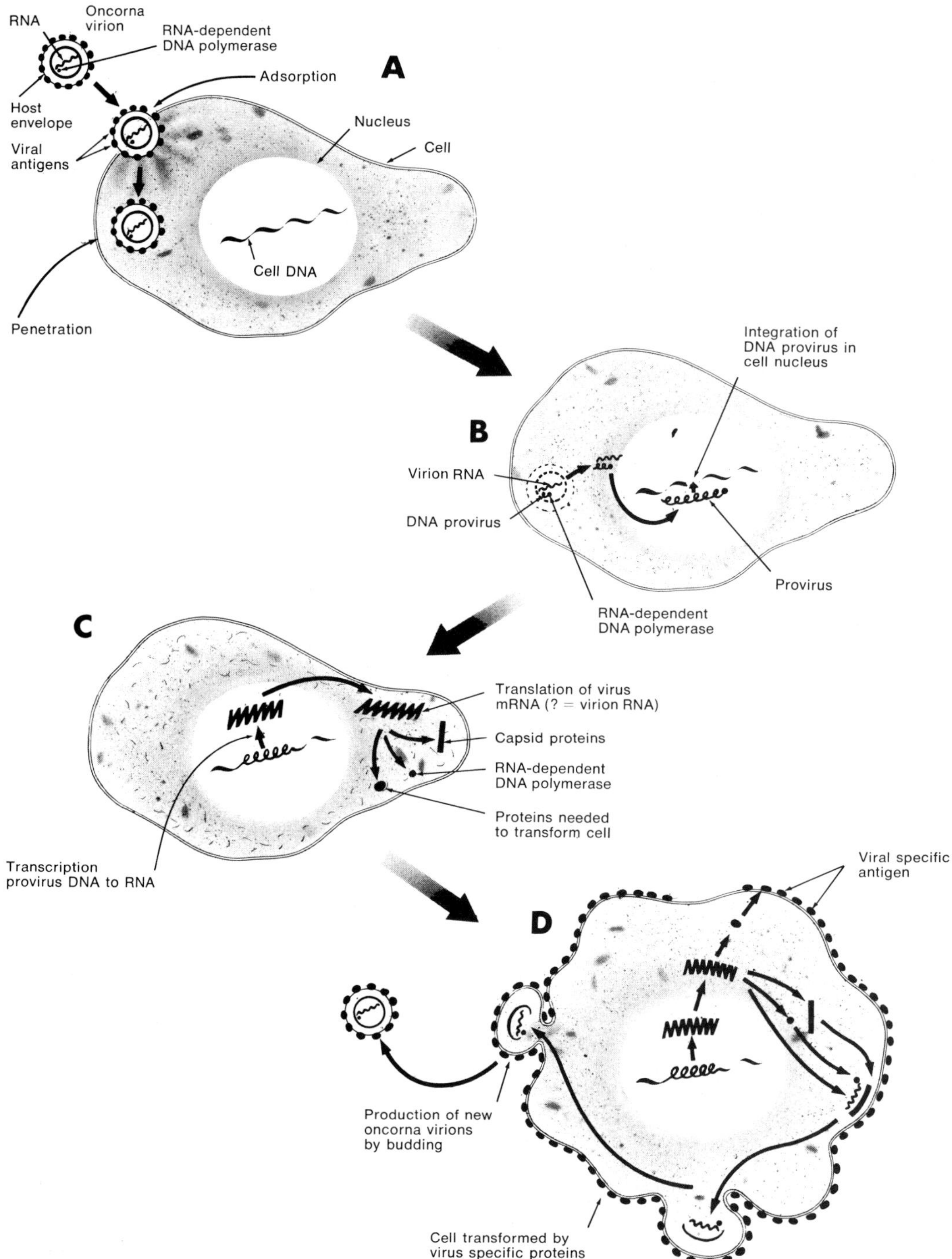

Figure 6–107. Schematic and tentative outline of interaction of oncornavirus with cells. After penetration *(A)* the virion RNA is transcribed to provirus *(B)*. Through transcription and translation, virus-specific proteins are formed *(C)*. The transformed cell produces oncorna virion by budding *(D)*. (Reprinted, by permission, from Allan, D. W. and Cole, P.: Viruses and human cancer. N. Engl. J. Med., *286*:70–82, 1972.)

occur as well. The induction of lymphosarcoma in sheep with the "bovine leukemia virus" has been reported.

The virus-cell interactions are demonstrated in Figure 6–107. All oncogenic RNA viruses contain a means by which viral RNA is transcribed into DNA of the host cell, and this process became well known as a great breakthrough in basic biology when the ability of RNA to transcribe for DNA was demonstrated. These viruses contain an enzyme that is an ***RNA-dependent DNA polymerase,*** also called reverse transcriptase. This enzyme uses the viral RNA genome to make a DNA copy of itself that is called ***provirus.*** The provirus serves as a template for virus production and is inserted into the genome of the cell.

In Figure 6–107, note that at ***A,*** the viral particle contains the RNA-dependent DNA polymerase and that at ***B,*** it causes the production of DNA provirus, which then enters the genome of the cell. At ***C,*** the provirus transcribes for viral RNA and results in replication of the virus, RNA-dependent DNA polymerase and new proteins that transform the cell. In contrast to the DNA oncogenic viruses, ***the cell is transformed and new virus is produced.*** In ***D,*** the virus is observed budding from the surface and at one point takes the shape of the letter "C" just before release from the cell surface, thus the term "C" particles.

Two theories have arisen to account for oncogenesis by RNA viruses. One is called the ***oncogene theory*** and proposes that a portion of the oncornavirus genome existing as the DNA provirus is part of the normal gene pool of all vertebrates and is passed vertically by the usual mechanisms of inheritance. This oncogene is normally ***repressed*** but may be ***depressed*** by carcinogens, irradiation or aging, all of which are accompanied by production of oncornaviruses and transformation in apparently uninfected cells. The other theory is called the ***protovirus theory*** and is based on the potential for genetic evolution in cells. It is proposed that transfer of information from DNA to RNA to DNA occurs in somatic cells. This could allow alteration among genes required for normal differentiation and could permit new genetic information to be encoded during the life of the individual. Disruption of this normal protovirus evolution with its frequent information transfers, which are quite susceptible to the influence of carcinogens, might result in transformation without formation of virus. These theories involve very basic biology and are the center of great research interest.

The complexity of disease associated with oncornaviruses is exemplified by the ***feline leukemia virus.*** There are several serotypes, and members of the group may cause ***different clinical syndromes,*** such as anemia, glomerulonephritis, enterocolitis, reproductive failure, a poorly defined lower motor neuron syndrome, various expressions of immunosuppression and the classic lymphosarcoma and myeloproliferative disorders. Future developments in the pathogenesis of these clinical expressions will probably reflect on associations of other agents in other species and similar clinical diseases.

Other Factors in Oncogenesis

Up to this point, the discussion has centered on how cells become transformed and the influence of carcinogens on this process. ***But how do these abnormal cells survive and result in a clinical neoplasm?*** They must be allowed to multiply many times and somehow elude the watchful eye of the immune system, which should recognize and destroy these abnormal cells. Apparently, the tumor antigens are poorly antigenic and may cause antibody production, which actually enhances growth. A scheme encompassing a host of carcinogens and related factors in a comprehensive overview is presented in Figure 6–108.

This figure may seem overwhelming at first, but taken in steps it is illuminating and worthy of detailed study.

Read the legend carefully. Note first the three steps of ***initiation, latent period*** and ***clinical tumor*** at the top. Next, on the left, all of the carcinogens separately or in combination act on the host tissue, which results in ***mutant cells*** with growth advantages ***(transformation)*** that survive and form clones. These may be acted on by

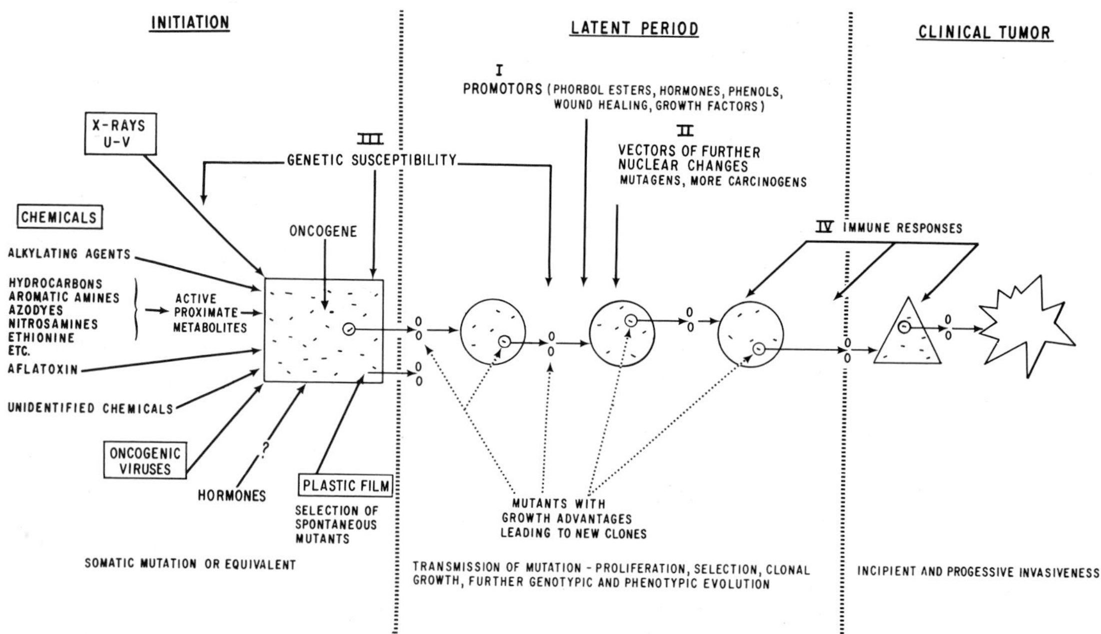

Figure 6–108. Schematic representation of carcinogenesis. The large square at the left represents the target organ subjected to initiators of carcinogenesis. The symbols in the square stand for random somatic mutations caused by carcinogenic exposures. One of them (circled) is singled out as having a growth advantage leading to cell division and clonal proliferation (first large circle). This process of selection and clonal proliferation is repeated several times to underline the dynamic character of carcinogenesis during the latent period (circles) and during the transition from clinical premalignancy (triangle) to clinical cancer (star). The major factors that initiate or influence carcinogenesis are indicated by plain arrows. Many groups of initiators are framed at the left. The variables that influence the course of carcinogenesis are identified by vertical arrows (I to IV). Hormones are considered to act mainly as promoters (Group 1), but a role as initiators of special kind is not excluded and is indicated with a question mark. For simplification, factors such as dose schedule, physical form and route of administration of carcinogens, diet, age and sex of subject and state of differentiation of target tissues have been omitted. The influence of species and strain is part of Group III. The presence in cells of an oncogene (oncogenic C virus) and its hypothetical role in carcinogenesis also fit under the heading of genetic susceptibility. It is postulated that the genetic makeup of a tissue plays a part in the activation of carcinogens and in the statistics of mutational events, as well as in the dynamics of the later stages. The biologic events occurring at the various stages of carcinogenesis are summarized at the bottoms of the three sections. (Reprinted, by permission, from Ryser, H.: Chemical carcinogenesis. N. Engl. J. Med., *285*:721–734, 1971.)

promoters and hormones, of which little has been mentioned so far, and *further selection* occurs. A key step is the ability to *evade the immune system.* At the end, there is clinical neoplasia. Probably, only a very few transformed cells make it through all the steps and result in clinical disease.

In summary, carcinogens result in somatic mutation that gives the cell an increased ability to grow and decreased contact inhibition, and this defect escapes repair. The mutation is transmitted to progeny cells and may be amplified or eliminated. These cellular changes result in hyperplasia, dysplasia and nodules of abnormal growth in the tissue. These may be influenced by promoters and environmental factors in further selective processes until the cells are emancipated from the restrictions of growth control and immune defense mechanisms. The cells become an autonomous invasive growth.

Having considered the agents, it is necessary to be reminded of host factors in neoplasia.

The many interactions of the ***host*** with the carcinogens are reminiscent of those interactions involved in the classic triangle in infectious disease—environment, host and agent. The paper by Weiss (1969) stresses the host-parasite relationship in neoplasia and takes this concept a step farther to consider the influence of ***emotional factors*** and their effect through hormonal changes on the immune system as related aspects in oncogenesis.

Genetic influences are striking in consideration of racial differences in the incidence of tumors (Table 6–12). Studies on races in quite different environments attempt to reveal whether racial factors really are influential; for example, the incidence of a particular tumor in Japanese living in Japan and in the United States (particularly Hawaii) may be compared. Having children—the earlier, the better—is protection against mammary gland tumors in human females, as is surgical or early menopause. Removal of the ovaries by age 35 reduces the incidence by 70 per cent. Ovariectomy in dogs is highly protective against mammary tumors if carried out before the first heat period and still protective if carried out before 2.5 years of age. Apparently, after this age, whether mammary tumors will occur has already been determined. In human females, investigation suggests that the natural estrogen profile of an individual (the ratio of estriol, estrone and estradiol) may be a factor, with estriol being protective and estrone conducive. The normal profile for these hormones is probably genetically determined.

INCIDENCE OF ANIMAL TUMORS

The biological behavior, diagnosis and treatment of individual tumors will be included in the study of special pathology, medicine and surgery. It is useful, however, to have an overall view of the general incidence of tumors in animals in order to become familiar with those that occur frequently and are important. Any survey varies according to the source of material, that is, surgery, slaughterhouse or necropsy, and only general indications, rather than precise figures, will be given here. These indications are drawn from many sources. The initiative and inspiration provided by some of the pioneers in animal oncology are commendable and set standards for work to follow. The detailed epidemiological approaches in recent literature, such as those by Dorn et al. (1968) and Schneider (1970), will be more prominent in the future. The staging of tumors for prognosis and the World Health Organization classification system are significant progressive steps.

Table 6–13 provides a general indication

TABLE 6–12. SCHEMATIC TABULATION OF THE RELATIVE FREQUENCIES OF SIX TYPES OF CANCER IN VARIOUS COUNTRIES

	Breast	Cervix	Esophagus	Stomach	Liver	Oral Cavity
Britain, Northern and Central Europe, and United States	+++++	+++	++	(+++)[1] +++++	±	+
Japan	+	++++	++	+++++	+++	++
China	++	+++	++++	+++	(+)[2] ++++	++
Philippines	+++	++	+	++	+++	++++
Sumatra:						
(*a*) Chinese	+	+	++	+++	++++	+
(*b*) Malayan	+	+++	±	+	+++++	+++
India	++[3]	+++++[3]	++	+	++	++++
South Africa (Bantu)	++	++++[4]	±	++	+++++	(+++)[5] +

[1]Lower incidence in Britain than in the rest of Europe or U.S.A.; highest in Sweden, Finland and Iceland.
[2]The high incidence refers to Southern China; the incidence is low in Northern China.
[3]Proportion of breast to uterine cancer in India varies according to communities (e.g., breast cancer is high among Parsees).
[4]Also unusually high incidence of cancer of uterine corpus.
[5]Relatively high incidence if carcinoma of maxillary antrum and of salivary glands is included.
(From Florey, H. W. [ed.]: General Pathology. 4th ed. Philadelphia, W. B. Saunders Co., 1970.)

TABLE 6–13. GENERAL INCIDENCE OF TUMORS IN DOMESTIC ANIMALS

	High	Moderate
Dog	basal cell tumors lymphoid and hemopoietic tumors mammary tumors mast cell tumor melanoma perianal adenoma sarcomas of skin testicular tumors	aortic body tumor hemangioma of skin hemangiopericytoma hepatic carcinoma intestinal carcinoma leiomyoma lipoma of skin nasal carcinoma neurofibroma oral carcinoma oral epulis osteosarcoma ovarian tumors pancreatic carcinoma papilloma of skin pulmonary carcinoma thyroid tumors transmissible venereal tumor
Cat	lymphoid and hemopoietic tumors	carcinoma of skin mammary tumors oral carcinoma osteosarcoma pancreatic carcinoma sarcoma of skin
Horse	sarcoid	carcinoma of conjunctiva carcinoma of penis lymphosarcoma melanoma nasal carcinomas ovarian tumors testicular tumors
Cattle	carcinoma of the eye lymphosarcoma	adrenal tumors carcinoma of skin fibroma of penis hepatic carcinoma leiomyoma melanoma mesothelioma neurofibroma ovarian tumors pulmonary tumors sarcoma of skin warts
Sheep		adrenal tumors carcinoma of the eye carcinoma of skin hepatic carcinoma intestinal carcinoma lymphosarcoma ovarian tumors renal tumors thyroid tumors
Pig		lymphosarcoma melanoma nephroblastoma

of the incidence of tumors. The tumors in each category are not given in any particular order, and many other tumors of low incidence are not listed. Some are listed by specific tumor and others are listed by organ, implying two or three different kinds in that organ. Benign and malignant tumors are generally grouped under one name. ***The incidence of tumors in dogs is higher than in all other species by far.*** Some canine tumors of low incidence would rank higher in total incidence than some tumors of high incidence in sheep, for example. These relationships must be kept in mind when studying Table 6–13.

There is a danger in putting together such a table since oncology experts argue at some length about the incidence of specific tumors and species comparisons. The purpose here is only to provide a simple overview.

The overall incidence in sheep and pigs is very low. To some extent the incidence reflects the age to which the animals usually live, which in livestock is usually determined by the age of slaughter for food production. Suggestions for further readings regarding the incidence of tumors in other species, including laboratory animals and exotic species, are listed at the end of this chapter. The book by Theilen and Madewell (1979) is a good source of information on incidence rates as well as on many other aspects of cancer in animals.

Any scientist working in biology should have some knowledge of the principles involved in oncology. More particularly, owners of animals expect veterinarians to be knowledgeable about cancer in order to answer their questions. This point has been emphasized by the spread of oncogenic viruses in cats and cattle and the concern of animal owners when they hear of this. If either a pet or its owner has cancer, questions may arise regarding the relationship of the one in the animal to the one in the human or the reverse. The owner is quite right in expecting the veterinarian to answer these questions.

Knowledge of carcinogenesis assists in assessing the sometimes dramatic revelations in the news about carcinogens and may in time assist the objectivity of legislators and scientists in development of policies regarding control of carcinogens and the use of public funds for research in cancer.

SUGGESTIONS FOR FURTHER READING

General Aspects

Armstrong, D., et al.: Infectious complications of neoplastic disease. Med. Clin. North Am., *55*:729–745, 1971.

Baserga, R.: The cell cycle. New Engl. J. Med., *304*:453–459, 1981.

Berlin, N. I.: Diagnostic research plans of the National Cancer Institute. Bull. Int. Pathol., *15*:19–25, 1974.

Boyd, W.: A Textbook of Pathology. 8th Ed. Philadelphia, Lea & Febiger, 1970.

Christopherson, W. M.: Dysplasia, carcinoma in situ, and microinvasive carcinoma of the uterine cervix. Hum. Pathol., *8*:489–501, 1977.

Cooper, E. H.: The biology of cell death in tumours. Cell Tissue Kinet., *6*:87–95, 1973.

Cullen, J. W., et al.: Cancer: The Behavioral Dimensions. New York, Raven Press, 1976.

DiPaolo, J. A., and Papescu, N. C.: Relationship of chromosome changes to neoplastic cell transformation. Am. J. Pathol., *85*:709–726, 1976.

Essex, M., and Grant, C. K.: Tumor immunology in domestic animals. Adv. Vet. Sci. Comp. Med., *23*:183–228, 1979.

Feline Oncology (14 papers). J. Am. Anim. Hosp. Assoc., *16*:889–1039, 1981.

Folkman, J.: The vascularization of tumors. Sci. Am., *234*:59–73, 1976.

Gelfant, S.: A new concept of tissue and tumor cell proliferation. Cancer Res., *37*:3845–3862, 1977.

Handleman, S. L., et al.: The cytology of spontaneous neoplastic transformation in culture. *In* Vitro, *13*:526–536, 1977.

Hardy, W. D.: General concepts of canine and feline tumors. J. Am. Anim. Hosp. Assoc., *12*:295–306, 1976.

Hibbs, J. B., et al.: The macrophage as an antineoplastic surveillance cell: biological perspectives. J. Reticuloendothel. Soc., *24*:549–570, 1978.

Huntington, R. W., and Huntington, R. W., III. Classification of neoplasms: a critical appraisal. Perspect. Biol. Med., *20*:215–222, 1977.

International Histological Classification of Tumours of Domestic Animals. Bull. WHO, *50*:1–142, 1974.

Kaiser, H. E. (ed.): Neoplasms—Comparative Pathology of Growth in Animals, Plants, and Man. Baltimore, Williams & Wilkins, 1981.

Klasterksy, J., et al.: Causes of death in patients with cancer. Eur. J. Cancer, *8*:149–154, 1972.

MacPherson, I.: The characteristics of animal cells transformed *in vitro*. Adv. Cancer Res., *13*:169–215, 1970.

Misdorp, W.: Histological classification and further characterization of tumors in domestic animals. Adv. Vet. Sci. Comp. Med., *20*:191–221, 1976.
Moulton, J. E.: Tumors in Domestic Animals. 2nd Ed. Berkeley, University of California Press, 1978.
Murray, J., and Murray, A.: Toward a nutritional concept of host resistance to malignancy and intracellular infection. Persp. Biol. Med., *24*:290–301, 1981.
Norgaard-Pedersen, B.: Human alpha-fetoprotein. A review of recent methodological and clinical studies. Scand. J. Immunol., Suppl. 4:5–45, 1976.
Owen, L. N., and Steel, G. G.: The growth and cell population kinetics of spontaneous tumours in domestic animals. Br. J. Cancer, *23*:493–509, 1969.
Owen, L. N.: TNM Classification of Tumors in Domestic Animals. Geneva, World Health Organization, 1980, pp. 1–53.
Pitot, H. C.: The natural history of neoplasia. Am. J. Pathol., *89*:402–412, 1977.
Pitot, H. C.: The stability of events in the natural history of neoplasia. Am. J. Pathol., *89*:703–716, 1977.
Richards, V.: On the nature of cancer. Oncology, *21*:4–28, 1967.
Robbins, S. L., Angell, M., and Kumar, V.: Basic Pathology. 3rd Ed. Philadelphia, W. B. Saunders Co., 1981.
Scott, R. E., and Florine, D. L.: Cell cycle models for the aberrant coupling of growth arrest and differentiation in hyperplasia, metaplasia and neoplasia. Am. J. Pathol., *107*:342–348, 1982.
Singer, C., et al.: Bacteremia and fungemia complicating neoplastic disease. Am. J. Med., *62*:731–732, 1977.
Synderman, R., and Pike, M. C.: Macrophage migratory dysfunction in cancer. Am. J. Pathol., *88*:727–740, 1977.
Spriggs, A. I.: History of cytodiagnosis. J. Clin. Pathol., *30*:1091–1102, 1977.
Theilen, G. H., and Madewell, B. R.: Veterinary Cancer Medicine. Philadelphia, Lea & Febiger, 1979.
Triolo, V. A.: Nineteenth century foundations of cancer research advances in tumor pathology, nomenclature, and theories of oncogenesis. Cancer Res., *25*:75–106, 1965.
Weber, G.: Enzymology of cancer cells. N. Engl. J. Med., *296*:486–493, 541–551, 1977.
Weijer, K., et al.: Feline malignant mammary tumors. I. Morphology and biology: some comparisons with human and canine mammary carcinomas. J. Natl. Cancer Inst., *49*:1697–1701, 1972.
Willis, R. A.: Pathology of Tumours. Philadelphia, F. A. Davis (Butterworth), 1948.
Willis, R. A.: The Spread of Tumours in the Human Body. Philadelphia, F. A. Davis (Butterworth), 1952.

Metastasis

Bross, I. D. J.: The biostatistical and biological basis for a cascade theory of human metastasis. *In* Grundman, E. (ed.): Metastatic Tumor Growth. Stuttgart, Gustav Fischer, 1980.
Carr, J. I., et al.: Lymphatic metastasis: invasion of lymphatic vessels and efflux of tumour cells in the afferent popliteal lymph as seen in the walker rat carcinoma. J. Pathol., *132*:287–305, 1980.
Carter, R. L.: Metastatic potential of malignant tumours. Invest. Cell. Pathol., *1*:275–286, 1978.
Fidler, I. J.: Tumor heterogeneity and the biology of cancer invasion and metastasis. Cancer Res., *38*:2651–2660, 1978.
Fidler, I. J., and Hart, I. R.: Biological diversity in metastatic neoplasms: origins and implications. Science, *217*:998–1002, 1982.
Fidler, I. J.: The biological diversity of cancer metastasis. Hosp. Pract., July, pp. 57–64, 1982.
Mareel, M. M.: Recent aspects of tumor invasiveness. Int. Rev. Exp. Pathol., *22*:65–129, 1980.
Marx, J. L.: Tumors: a mixed bag of cells. Science, *215*:275–277, 1982.
Onuigbo, W. I. B.: A history of hematogenous metastasis. Cancer Res., *30*:2821–2826, 1970.
Poste, G., and Fidler, I. J.: The pathogenesis of cancer metastasis. Nature, *283*:139–146, 1980.
Weiss, L.: Dynamic aspects of cancer cell populations in metastasis. Am. J. Pathol., *97*:601–608, 1979.

Etiology

Allen, D. W., and Cole, P.: Viruses and human cancer. N. Engl. J. Med., *286*:70–82, 1972.
American Institute of Nutrition Symposium: Nutrition and cancer. Fed. Proc., *35*:1307–1338, 1976.
Anderson, D.: An appraisal of the current state of mutagenicity testing. J. Soc. Cosmet. Chem., *29*:207–223, 1978.
Arley, N., and Eker, R.: Mechanisms of carcinogenesis. Adv. Biol. Med. Phys., *8*:375–436, 1962.
Beard, J. W.: Biology of avian oncornaviruses. *In* Klein, G. (ed.): Viral Oncology. New York, Raven Press, 1980, pp. 55–87.
Becker, F. F.: Recent concepts of initiation and promotion in carcinogenesis. Am. J. Pathol., *105*:3–9, 1981.
Brent, R. L.: Radiation teratogenesis. Teratology, *21*:281–298, 1980.
Burny, A., et al.: RNA oncogenic viruses: a very short overview. Vet. Microbiol., *1*:103–120, 1976.
Chapman, A. J., and Race, G. J.: Trauma and cancer: a survey of recent literature. J. Forensic Sci., *14*:167–176, 1969.
Chrisp, C. E., and Fisher, G. L.: Mutagenicity of airborne particles. Mut. Res., *76*:143–164, 1980.
Clayson, D. B.: Nutrition and experimental carcinogensis: a review. Cancer Res., *35*:3292–3300, 1975.
Farber, E.: Chemical carcinogenesis. N. Engl. J. Med., *305*:1379–1389, 1981.
Farber, E.: The sequential analysis of cancer induction with chemicals. Acta Pathol., *31*:1–11, 1981.
Ferrer, J. V., et al.: Diagnosis of bovine leukemia virus infection: evaluation of serologic and hematologic tests by a direct infectivity detection assay. Am. J. Vet. Res., *38*:1977–1981, 1977.
Hamilton, J. M.: Comparative aspects of mammary tumors. Adv. Cancer Res., *19*:1–45, 1974.
Hardy, W. D.: The etiology of canine and feline tumors. J. Am. Anim. Hosp. Assoc., *12*:313–334, 1976.
Hardy, W., et al.: The epidemiology of the feline leukemia virus (FeLV). Cancer, *39*:1850–1855, 1977.
Heidelberger, C.: Chemical carcinogenesis. Cancer, *40*:430–433, 1977.
Karpas, A.: Viruses and leukemia. Am. Sci., *70*:277–285, 1982.
Klein, G. (ed.): Viral Oncology. New York, Raven Press, 1980.
Lancaster, W. D., and Olson, C.: Animal papillomaviruses. Microbiol. Rev., *46*:191–207, 1982.

Madewell, B. R.: Neoplasms in domestic animals: a review of experimental and spontaneous carcinogenesis. Yale J. Biol. Med., *54*:111–125, 1981.

Miller, E. C.: Some perspectives on chemical carcinogenesis in humans and experimental animals. Cancer Res., *38*:1479–1496, 1978.

Nazerian, K.: Marek's disease: a herpesvirus-induced maligant lymphoma of the chicken. *In* Klein, G., (ed.): Viral Oncology. New York, Raven Press, 1980, pp. 665–684.

Newberne, P. M., and McConnell, R. G.: Nutrient deficiencies in cancer causation. J. Environ. Pathol. Tox., *3*:323–356, 1980.

Novick, M., et al.: Burn scar carcinoma: a review and analysis of 46 cases. J. Trauma, *17*:809–817, 1977.

Ogawa, K., et al.: Sequential analysis of hepatic carcinogenesis. A comparative study of the ultrastructure of preneoplastic malignant, prenatal, postnatal, and regenerating liver. Lab. Invest., *41*:22–35, 1979.

Olson, C., and Baumgartner, L. E.: Pathology of lymphosarcoma in sheep induced with bovine leukemia virus. Cancer Res., *36*:2365–2373, 1976.

Pitot, H. C.: Carcinogenesis and aging—two related phenomena? Am. J. Pathol., *87*:444–472, 1977.

Purtilo, D. T., et al.: Genetics of neoplasia—impact of ecogenetics on oncogenesis. A review. Am. J. Pathol., *91*:609–681, 1978.

Rigdon, R. H.: Trauma and Cancer (Pathology for the Lawyer). Springfield, Illinois, Charles C Thomas, 1975.

Rous, P.: A transmissible avian neoplasm[1] (sarcoma of the fowl). J. Exp. Med., *12*:696–705, 1910.

Rous, P.: The virus tumors and the tumor problem. Am. J. Cancer, *28*:233–272, 1936.

Rubin, H.: Is somatic mutation the major mechanism of malignant transformation? J. Natl. Cancer Inst., *64*:995–1000, 1980.

Ryser, H. J. P.: Chemical carcinogenesis. N. Engl. J. Med., *285*:721–734, 1971.

Saffciotte, J. K. W.: Occupational carcinogenesis. Ann. N. Y. Acad. Sci., *271*:1–516, 1976.

Selkirk, J. K.: Chemical carcinogenesis: a brief overview of the mechanism of action of polycyclic hydrocarbons, aromatic amines, nitrosamines, and aflatoxins. *In* Slaga, T. J. (ed.): Carcinogenesis. Vol. 5: Modifiers of Chemical Carcinogenesis. New York, Raven Press, 1980, pp. 1-31.

Strong, L. C.: Genetic etiology of cancer. Cancer, *40*:438–444, 1977.

Temin, H. M.: Viral oncogenes. Cold Spring Harbor Symp. Quant. Biol., *44*:1–7, 1980.

Ts'o, P. O. P.: Some aspects of the basic mechanisms of chemical carcinogenesis. J. Toxicol. Environ. Health, *2*:1305–1315, 1977.

Ulrich, R. L.: Interactions of radiation and chemical carcinogens. *In* Slaga, T. J. (ed.): Carcinogenesis. Vol. 5: Modifiers of Chemical Carcinogenesis. New York, Raven Press, 1980, pp. 169–184.

Visek, W. J., et al.: Nutrition and experimental carcinogenesis. Cornell Vet., *68*:3–39, 1978.

Weiss, D. W.: Immunological parameters of the host-parasite relationship in neoplasia. Ann. N. Y. Acad. Sci., *164*:431–448, 1969.

Weiss, R. A.: Viral mechanisms of carcinogenesis. *In* Bartsch, H., and Armstrong, B. (eds.): Host Factors In Carcinogenesis. Lyon, I.A.R.C. Scientific Publications, No. 39, 1982, pp. 307–316.

Wheelock, E. F., and Robinson, M. K.: Endogenous control of the neoplastic process. Lab. Invest., *48*:120–139, 1983.

Wynder, E. L.: Dietary habits and cancer epidemiology. Cancer, *43*:1955–1961, 1979.

General Incidence of Tumors

Anderson, L. J., et al.: A British abattoir survey of tumours in cattle, sheep and pigs. Vet. Rec., *84*:547–551, 1969.

Anderson, L. J., and Sandison, A. T.: Tumours of connective tissues in cattle, sheep and pigs. J. Pathol., *98*:253–263, 1969.

Blair, A., and Hayes, H. M.: Cancer and other causes of death among U.S. veterinarians, 1966–1977. Int. J. Cancer, *25*:181–185, 1980.

Bostock, D. E., and Owen, L. N.: Neoplasia in the Cat, Dog and Horse. London, Wolfe Publishing Ltd., 1975.

Brodey, R. S.: Canine and feline neoplasia. Adv. Vet. Sci. Comp. Med., *14*:309–354, 1970.

Burmester, B. R., and Purchase, H. G.: The history of avian medicine in the United States. V. Insights into avian tumor virus research. Avian Dis., *3*:1–29, 1979.

Cotchin, E.: Neoplasms of the Domesticated Mammals. Farnham Royal, England, Commonwealth Agriculture Bureaux, 1956.

Cotchin, E.: Neoplasia in the cat. Vet. Rec., *69*:425–434, 1957.

Cotchin, E.: A general survey of tumours in the horse. Equine Vet. J., *9*:16–21, 1977.

Doll, R.: The epidemiology of cancer. Cancer, *45*:2475–2485, 1980.

Dorn, C. R., et al.: Survey of animal neoplasms in Alameda and Contra Costa Counties, California. II. Cancer morbidity in dogs and cats from Alameda County. J. Natl. Cancer Inst., *40*:307–318, 1968.

Fisher, L. F., and Olander, H. J.: Spontaneous neoplasms of pigs—a study of 31 cases. J. Comp. Pathol., *88*:505–517, 1978.

Harshbarger, J. C.: Neoplasms in zoo poikilotherms emphasizing cases in the registry of tumors of lower animals. *In* Montali, R. J., and Migaki, G. (eds.): Comparative Pathology of Zoo Animals. Washington, Smithsonian Institution Press, 1980, pp. 585–591.

Hayes, H. M.: The comparative epidemiology of selected neoplasms between dogs, cats and humans. A review. Eur. J. Cancer, *14*:1299–1308, 1978.

Jackson, C.: Incidence and pathology of tumors of domesticated animals in South Africa. Onderstepoort J. Vet. Res., *6*:3–460, 1936.

MacVean, D. W., et al.: Frequency of canine and feline tumors in a defined population. Vet. Pathol., *15*:700–715, 1978.

McCrea, C. T., and Head, K. W.: Sheep tumours in North-East Yorkshire. I. Prevalence on seven moorland farms. Br. Vet. J., *134*:454–461, 1978.

Meier, H., and Hoag, W.: Epizootiology of cancer in animals. Ann. N.Y. Acad. Sci., *108*:617–1325, 1963.

Migaki, G.: Naturally occurring neoplastic diseases. VIII. Cow, horse, pig, sheep and goat. *In* Melby, E. C., and Altman, N. H. (eds.): CRC Handbook of Laboratory Animal Science. Cleveland, CRC Press, Inc., 1976, pp. 289–307.

Misdorp, W.: Tumors in newborn animals. Pathol. Vet., *2*:328–343, 1965.

Monlux, A. W., et al.: A survey of tumors occurring in cattle, sheep, and swine. Am. J. Vet. Res., *17*:646–677, 1956.

Mulligan, R. M.: Neoplasms of the Dog. Baltimore, Williams & Wilkins, 1949.

Murray, M.: Neoplasms of domestic animals in East Africa. Br. Vet. J., *124*:514–524, 1968.
Nielsen, S. W.: Canine and feline neoplasia. *In* Melby, E. C., and Altman, N. H. (eds.): CRC Handbook of Laboratory Animal Science. Vol. 3. Cleveland, CRC Press, Inc., 1976, pp. 892–943.
Priester, W. A., et al.: Nine simultaneous primary tumors in a boxer dog. J. Am. Vet. Med. Assoc., *170*:823–826, 1977.
Schamber, G. J., et al.: Neoplasms in calves *(Bos taurus)*. Vet. Pathol., *19*:629–637, 1982.
Schneider, R.: Comparison of age, sex, and incidence rates in human and canine breast cancer. Cancer, *26*:419–426, 1970.
Sundberg, J. P., et al.: Neoplasms of equidae. J. Am. Vet. Med. Assoc., *170*:150–152, 1977.
Vitovec, J.: Statistical data on 370 cattle tumors collected over the years 1964–1973 in South Bohemia. Zentralbl. Veterinaermed. [A], *23*:445–453, 1976.
World Health Organization: Eighteenth supplement to the bibliography in comparative oncology. Geneva, World Health Organization, September, 1981.
Zdeb, M. S.: The probability of developing cancer. Am. J. Epidemiol., *106*:6–16, 1977.

Cardiovascular Tumors

Mills, J. H. L., and Nielsen, S. W.: Canine hemangiopericytomas—a survey of 200 tumours. J. Small Anim. Pract., *8*:599–604, 1967.
Oksanen, A.: Haemangiosarcoma in dogs. J. Comp. Pathol., *88*:585–595, 1978.
Stambaugh, J. E., et al.: Lymphangioma in four dogs. J. Am. Vet. Med. Assoc., *173*:759–761, 1978.
Turk, J. R., et al.: Cystic lymphangioma in a colt. J. Am. Vet. Med. Assoc., *174*:1228–1230, 1979.

Integumentary Tumors

Barron, C. N.: The comparative pathology of neoplasms of the eyelids and conjunctiva with special reference to those of epithelial origin. Acta Dermatol. Venereol. (Stockholm) (Suppl.), *42*:1–100, 1962.
Bostock, D. E.: The prognosis in cats bearing squamous cell carcinoma. J. Small Anim. Pract., *13*:119–125, 1972.
Bostock, D. E.: The prognosis following surgical removal of mastocytomas in dogs. J. Small Anim. Pract., *14*:27–40, 1973.
Bostock, D. E., and Dye, M. T.: Prognosis after surgical excision of canine fibrous connective tissue sarcomas. Vet. Pathol., *17*:581–588, 1980.
Brown, N. O., et al.: Soft tissue sarcomas in the cat. J. Am. Vet. Med. Assoc., *173*:744–749, 1978.
Cockerell, G. L., and Saulson, D. O.: Patterns of lymphoid infiltrate in the canine cutaneous histiocytoma. J. Comp. Pathol., *89*:193–203, 1979.
Cotchin, E.: Melanotic tumours in dogs. J. Comp. Pathol., *65*:115–129, 1955.
Duncan, J. R., and Prasse, K. W.: Cytology of canine cutaneous round cell tumors—mast cell tumor, histiocytoma, lymphosarcoma and transmissible venereal tumor. Vet. Pathol., *16*:673–679, 1979.
Hamir, A. N. J., et al.: An immunopathological study of bovine ocular squamous cell carcinoma. J. Comp. Pathol., *90*:535–549, 1980.
Hayes, H. M., and G. P. Wilson: Hormone-dependent neoplasms of the canine perianal gland. Cancer Res., *37*:2068–2071, 1978.
Hottendorf, G. H., and Nielsen, S. W.: Pathologic survey of 300 extirpated canine mastocytomas. Zentralbl. Veterinaermed. [A], *14*:272–281, 1967.
Hottendorf, G. H., and Nielsen, S. W.: Canine mastocytoma—a review of clinical aspects. J. Am. Vet. Med. Assoc., *154*:917–924, 1969.
Huck, R. A.: Bovine papillomatosis. Vet. Bull., *35*:475–478, 1965.
Kopecky, K. E., et al.: Biological effect of ultraviolet radiation on cattle: bovine ocular squamous cell carcinoma. Am. J. Vet. Res., *40*:1783–1788, 1979.
Kraft, I., and Frese, K.: Histological studies on canine pigmented moles: the comparative pathology of the naevus problem. J. Comp. Pathol., *86*:143–155, 1976.
Ladds, P. W., and Entwistle, K. W.: Observations on squamous cell carcinomas of sheep in Queensland, Australia. Br. J. Cancer, *35*:110–114, 1977.
McGovern, V. J.: Epidemiological aspects of melanoma: a review. Pathology, *9*:233–241, 1977.
Nielsen, S. W., and Aftosmis, J.: Canine perianal gland tumors. J. Am. Vet. Med. Assoc., *144*:127–135, 1964.
Nielsen, S. W., and Cole, C. R.: Cutaneous epithelial neoplasms of the dog—a report of 153 cases. Am. J. Vet. Res., *21*:931–948, 1960.
Spradbrow, P. B., and Hoffmann, D.: Bovine ocular squamous cell carcinoma. Vet. Bull., *50*:449–459, 1980.
Turnquest, R. U.: Dermal squamous cell carcinoma in young chickens. Am. J. Vet. Res., *40*:1628–1633, 1979.

Digestive Tract Tumors

Brodey, R. S., and Cohen, D.: An epizootiologic and clinicopathologic study of 95 cases of gastrointestinal neoplasms in the dog. *In* Proceedings of the 1964 Annual Meeting of the American Veterinary Medical Association, pp. 167–179.
Carakostas, M. C., et al.: Malignant foregut carcinoid tumor in a domestic cat. Vet. Pathol., *16*:607–609, 1979.
Dubielzig, R. R., et al.: The nomenclature of periodontal epulides in dogs. Vet. Pathol., *16*:209–214, 1979.
Gorlin, R. J., et al.: The oral and pharyngeal pathology of domestic animals. A study of 487 cases. Am. J. Vet. Res., *20*:1032–1061, 1959.
Gorlin, R. J., et al.: Odontogenic tumors in man and animals: pathologic classification and clinical behavior. A review. Ann. N.Y. Acad. Sci., *108*:722–771, 1963.
Hayden, D. W., and Nielsen, S. W.: Canine alimentary neoplasia. Zentralbl. Veterinaermed. [A], *20*:1–22, 1973.
Koestner, A., and Buerger, L.: Primary neoplasms of the salivary glands in animals compared to similar tumors in man. Pathol. Vet., *2*:201–226, 1965.
Krook, L., and Kenney, R. M.: Central nervous system lesions in dogs with metastasizing islet cell carcinoma. Cornell Vet., *52*:385–415, 1962.
Lingeman, C. H., and Garner, F. M.: Comparative study of intestinal adenocarcinomas of animals and man. J. Natl. Cancer Inst., *48*:325–346, 1972.
Patnaik, A. K.: Feline intestinal adenocarcinoma. A clinicopathologic study of 22 cases. Vet. Pathol., *13*:1–10, 1976.
Patnaik, A. K., et al.: Canine gastric adenocarcinoma. Vet. Pathol., *15*:600–607, 1978.
Plowright, W.: Malignant neoplasia of the oesophagus

and rumen of cattle in Kenya. J. Comp. Pathol., *65*:108–114, 1955.

Ridgway, R. L., and Suter, P. F.: Clinical and radiographic signs in primary and metastatic esophageal neoplasms of the dog. J. Am. Vet. Med. Assoc., *174*:700–704, 1979.

Ross, A. D.: Small intestinal carcinoma in sheep. Aust. Vet. J., *56*:25–28, 1980.

Seibold, H. R., et al.: Observations on the possible relation of malignant esophageal tumors and *Spirocerca lupi* lesions in the dog. Am. J. Vet. Res., *16*:5–14, 1955.

Seiler, R. J.: Colorectal polyps of the dog: a clinicopathologic study of 17 cases. J. Am. Vet. Med. Assoc., *174*:72–75, 1979.

Simpson, B. H., and Jolly, R. D.: Carcinoma of the small intestine in sheep. J. Pathol., *112*:83–92, 1974.

Todoroff, R. J., and Brodey, R. S.: Oral and pharyngeal neoplasia in the dog. A retrospective survey of 361 cases. J. Am. Vet. Med. Assoc., *175*:567–571, 1979.

Turk, M. A. M., et al.: Nonhematopoietic gastrointestinal neoplasia in cats: a retrospective study of 44 cases. Vet. Pathol., *18*:614–620, 1981.

Vitovec, J.: Carcinomas of the intestine in cattle and pigs. Zentralbl. Veterinaermed. [A], *24*:413–421, 1977.

Hepatic Tumors

Anderson, W. A., et al.: Epithelial tumors of the bovine gallbladder. A report of eighteen cases. Am. J. Vet. Res., *19*:58–65, 1958.

Anderson, N. V., and Johnson, K. H.: Pancreatic carcinoma in the dog. J. Am. Vet. Med. Assoc., *150*:286–295, 1967.

Patnaik, A. K., et al.: Canine hepatic neoplasms: a clinicopathologic study. Vet. Pathol., *17*:533–564, 1980.

Patnaik, A. K., et al.: Canine bile duct carcinoma. Vet. Pathol., *18*:439–444, 1981.

Patnaik, A. K., et al.: Canine hepatic carcinoids. Vet. Pathol., *18*:445–453, 1981.

Patnaik, A. K., et al.: Canine hepatocellular carcinoma. Vet. Pathol., *18*:427–438, 1981.

Rowlatt, U.: Spontaneous epithelial tumors of the pancreas of mammals. Br. J. Cancer, *21*:82–107, 1967.

Trigo, F. J., et al.: The pathology of liver tumors in the dog. J. Comp. Pathol., *92*:21–39, 1982.

Male Genital Tract Tumors

Brodey, R. S., and Martin, J. E.: Sertoli cell neoplasms in the dog. The clinicopathological and endocrinological findings in thirty-seven dogs. J. Am. Vet. Med. Assoc., *133*:249–257, 1958.

Bomhard, D. von, et al.: The ultrastructure of testicular tumors in the dog. I. Germinal cells and seminomas. J. Comp. Pathol., *88*:49–57, 1978.

Bomhard, D. von, et al.: The ultrastructure of testicular tumors in the dog. II. Leydig cells and Leydig cell tumors. J. Comp. Pathol., *88*:59–65, 1978.

Bomhard, D. von, et al.: The ultrastructure of testicular tumors in the dog. III. Sertoli cells and Sertoli cell tumors and general conclusions. J. Comp. Pathol., *88*:67–73, 1978.

Cotchin, E.: Testicular neoplasms in dogs. J. Comp. Pathol., *70*:232–248, 1960.

Dow, C.: Testicular tumors in the dog. J. Comp. Pathol., *72*:247–265, 1962.

Reif, J. S., and Brodey, R. S.: The relationship between cryptorchidism and canine testicular neoplasia. J. Am. Vet. Med. Assoc., *155*:2005–2010, 1969.

Reif, J. S., et al.: A cohort study of canine testicular neoplasia. J. Am. Vet. Med. Assoc., *175*:719–723, 1979.

Stick, J. A.: Teratoma and cyst formation of the equine cryptorchid testicle. J. Am. Vet. Med. Assoc., *176*:211–214, 1980.

Weaver, A. D.: Fifteen cases of prostatic carcinoma in the dog. Vet. Rec., *109*:71–74, 1981.

Willis, R. A., and Rudduck, H. B.:Testicular teratomas in horses. J. Pathol., *55*:165–171, 1943.

Female Genital Tract and Mammary Gland Tumors

Anderson, L. J., and Sandison, A. T.: Tumors of the female genitalia in cattle, sheep and pigs found in a British abattoir survey. J. Comp. Pathol., *79*:53–63, 1969.

Brodey, R. S., et al.: The relationship of estrous irregularity, pseudopregnancy, and pregnancy to the development of canine mammary neoplasms. J. Am. Vet. Med. Assoc., *149*:1047–1049, 1966.

Brodey, R. S., and Roszel, J. F.: Neoplasms of the canine uterus, vagina, and vulva: a clinicopathologic survey of 90 cases. J. Am. Vet. Med. Assoc., *151*:1294–1307, 1967.

Burdin, M. L.: Squamous-cell carcinoma of the vulva of cattle in Kenya. Res. Vet. Sci., *5*:497–505, 1964.

Cotchin, E.: Canine ovarian neoplasms. Res. Vet. Sci., *2*:133–142, 1961.

Cotchin, E.: Spontaneous uterine cancer in animals. Br. J. Cancer, *18*:209–227, 1964.

Dorn, C. R., and Schneider, R.: Inbreeding and canine mammary cancer: a retrospective study. J. Natl. Cancer Inst., *57*:545–548, 1976.

Else, R. W., and Hannant, D.: Some epidemiological aspects of mammary neoplasia in the bitch. Vet. Rec., *104*:296–304, 1979.

Fidler, I. J., et al.: The biological behavior of canine mammary neoplasms. J. Am. Vet. Med. Assoc., *151*:1311–1318, 1967.

Fidler, I. J., and Brodey, R. S.: A necropsy study of canine malignant mammary neoplasms. J. Am. Vet. Med. Assoc., *151*:710–715, 1967.

Giles, R. C., et al.: Mammary nodules in beagle dogs administered investigational oral contraceptive steroids. J. Natl. Cancer Inst., *60*:1351–1364, 1978.

Graf, K. J., and El Etreby, M. F.: Endocrinology of reproduction in the female beagle dog and its significance in mammary gland tumorgenesis. Acta Endocrinol., *90*(Suppl. 222):1–34, 1979.

Hayden, D. W., and Nielsen, S. W.: Feline mammary tumours. J. Small Anim. Pract., *12*:687–697, 1971.

Misdorp, W.: Histologic classification and further characterization of tumors in domestic animals. Adv. Vet. Sci. Comp. Med., *20*:191–221, 1976.

Misdorp, W., and Hart, A. A. M.: Canine mammary cancer. I. Prognosis. J. Small Anim. Pract., *20*:385–394, 1979.

Misdorp, W., and Hart, A. A. M.: Canine mammary cancer. II. Therapy and causes of death. J. Small Anim. Pract., *20*:395–404, 1979.

Monlux, A. W., et al.: Adenocarcinoma of the uterus of the cow—differentiation of its pulmonary metastases from primary lung tumors. Am. J. Vet. Res., *17*:45–73, 1956.

Monlux, A. W., et al.: Classification of epithelial canine mammary tumors in a defined population. Vet. Pathol., *14*:194–217, 1977.

Owen, L. N.: A comparative study of canine and human breast cancer. Invest. Cell Pathol., *2*:257–275, 1979.

Pulley, L. T.: Ultrastructural and histochemical demonstration of myoepithelium in mixed tumors of the canine mammary gland. Am. J. Vet. Res., *34*:1513–1522, 1973.

Schneider, R., et al.: Factors influencing canine mammary cancer development and postsurgical survival. J. Natl. Cancer Inst., *43*:1249–1261, 1969.

Stabenfeldt, G. H., et al.: Clinical findings, pathological changes and endocrinological secretory patterns in mares with ovarian tumors. J. Reprod. Fertil. (Suppl.) *27*:277–285, 1979.

Weijer, K., et al.: Feline malignant mammary tumors. I. Morphology and biology: some comparisons with human and canine mammary carcinomas. J. Natl. Cancer Inst., *49*:1697–1704, 1972.

Weijer, K.: Feline mammary tumors and dysplasias. A multidisciplinary study of feline mammary tumors and dysplasias. Some comparisons with human and canine mammary tumours and dysplasias. Thesis, Amsterdam, 1979.

Hemopoietic Tumors

Anderson, L. J., and Jarrett, W. F. H.: Lymphosarcoma (leukemia) in cattle, sheep and pigs in Great Britain. Cancer, *22*:398–405, 1968.

Dorn, C. R., et al.: Epizootiologic characteristics of canine and feline leukemia and lymphoma. Am. J. Vet. Res., *28*:993–1001, 1967.

Ferrer, J. F.: Bovine lymphosarcoma. Adv. Vet. Sci. Comp. Med., *24*:1–68, 1980.

Fraser, C. J., et al.: Acute granulocytic leukemia in cats. J. Am. Vet. Med. Assoc., *165*:355–359, 1974.

Gilmore, C. E., et al.: Reticuloendotheliosis, a myeloproliferative disorder of cats: a comparison with lymphocytic leukemia. Pathol. Vet., *1*:161–183, 1964.

Hadlow, W. J.: High prevalence of thymoma in the dairy goat. Vet. Pathol., *15*:153–169, 1978.

Holmberg, C. A., et al.: Feline malignant lymphomas: comparison of morphologic and immunologic characteristics. Am. J. Vet. Res., *37*:1455–1460, 1976.

Holzworth, J.: Leukemia and related neoplasms in the cat. I. Lymphoid malignancies. J. Am. Vet. Med. Assoc., *136*:47–69, 1960.

Johnstone, A. C., and Manktelow, B. W.: The pathology of spontaneously occurring malignant lymphoma in sheep. Vet. Pathol., *15*:301–312, 1978.

Nazerian, K.: Marek's disease: a herpesvirus-induced malignant lymphoma of the chicken. *In* Klein, G. (ed.): Viral Oncology. New York, Raven Press, 1980, pp. 665–682.

Nielsen, S. W.: Spontaneous hematopoietic neoplasms of the domestic cat. Natl. Cancer Inst. Monogr., *32*:73–94, 1969.

Olson, C., and Driscoll, D. M.: Bovine leukosis: investigation of risk for man. J. Am. Vet. Med. Assoc., *173*:1470–1472, 1978.

Squire, R. A.: Hematopoietic tumors of domestic animals. Cornell Vet., *54*:97–150, 1964.

Squire, R. A.: Spontaneous hematopoietic tumors of dogs. Natl. Cancer Inst. Monogr., *32*:97–116, 1969.

Squire, R. A., et al.: Clinical and pathologic study of canine lymphoma: clinical staging, cell classification and therapy. J. Natl. Cancer Inst., *51*:565–574, 1973.

Valli, V. E., et al.: Histocytology of lymphoid tumors in the dog, cat and cow. Vet. Pathol., *18*:494–512, 1981.

Endocrine Tumors

Capen, C. C., et al.: Neoplasms in the adenohypophysis of dogs. A clinical and pathologic study. Pathol. Vet., *4*:301–325, 1967.

Howard, E. B., and Neilsen, S. W.: Pheochromocytomas associated with hypertensive lesions in dogs. J. Am. Vet. Med. Assoc., *147*:245–252, 1965.

Jubb, K. V., and McEntee, K.: Tumors of the nonchromaffin paraganglia in dogs. Cancer, *10*:89–99, 1957.

Jubb, K. V., and McEntee, K.: The relationship of ultimobranchial remnants and derivatives to tumors of the thyroid gland in cattle. Cornell Vet., *49*:41–69, 1959.

Leav, I., et al.: Adenomas and carcinomas of the canine and feline thyroid. Am. J. Pathol., *83*:61–122, 1976.

Patnaik, A. K., et al.: Canine medullary carcinoma of the thyroid. Vet. Pathol., *15*:590–599, 1978.

Sandison, A. T., and Anderson, L. J.: Tumours of the endocrine glands in cattle, sheep and pigs found in a British abattoir survey. J. Comp. Pathol., *78*:435–444, 1968.

Siegel, E. T., et al.: Functional adrenocortical carcinoma in a dog. J. Am. Vet. Med. Assoc., *150*:760–766, 1967.

Vitovec, J.: Epithelial thyroid tumors in cows. Vet. Pathol., *13*:401–408, 1976.

Yates, W. D. G., et al.: Chemoreceptor tumors diagnosed at the Western College of Veterinary Medicine, 1967–1979. Can. Vet. J., *21*:124–129, 1980.

Urinary Tract Tumors

Baskin, G. B., and De Paoli, A.: Primary renal neoplasms of the dog. Vet. Pathol., *14*:591–605, 1977.

Migaki, G., et al.: Prevalence of embryonal nephroma in slaughtered swine. J. Am. Vet. Med. Assoc., *159*:441–442, 1971.

Mugera, G. M., et al.: The pathology of urinary bladder tumours in Kenya Zebu cattle. J. Comp. Pathol., *79*:251–254, 1969.

Osborne, C. A., et al.: Neoplasms of the canine and feline urinary bladder: incidence, etiologic factors, occurrence and pathologic features. Am. J. Vet. Res., *29*:2041–2055, 1968.

Pamukcu, A. M.: Tumors of the urinary bladder in cattle and water buffalo affected with enzootic bovine hematuria. Zentralbl. Veterinaermed., *4*:185–197, 1957.

Sandison, A. T., and Anderson, L. J.: Tumors of the kidney in cattle, sheep and pigs. Cancer, *21*:727–742, 1968.

Respiratory Tract Tumors

Anderson, L. J., and Sandison, A. T.: Pulmonary tumours found in a British abattoir survey: primary carcinomas in cattle and secondary neoplasms in cattle, sheep and pigs. Br. J. Cancer, *22*:47–57, 1968.

Confer, A. W., and De Paoli, A.: Primary neoplasms of the nasal cavity, paranasal sinuses and nasopharynx in the dog. Vet. Pathol., *15*:18–30, 1978.

McKinnon, A. O., et al.: Enzootic nasal adenocarcinoma of sheep in Canada. Can. Vet. J., *23*:88–94, 1982.

Migaki, G., et al.: Primary pulmonary tumors of epithelial origin in cattle. Am. J. Vet. Res., *35*:1397–1400, 1974.

Moulton, J. E., et al.: Classification of lung carcinomas in the dog and cat. Vet. Pathol., *18*:513–528, 1981.

Nielsen, S. W., and Horava, A.: Primary pulmonary tumors of the dog. A report of sixteen cases. Am. J. Vet. Res., *21*:813–830, 1960.

Thrall, D. E., and Goldschmidt, M. H.: Mesothelioma in the dog: six case reports. J. Am. Vet. Radiol. Soc., *19*:107–115, 1978.

Central Nervous System Tumors

Canfield, P.: A light microscopic study of bovine peripheral nerve sheath tumours. Vet. Pathol., *15*:283–291, 1978.

Hayes, K. C., and Schiefer, B.: Primary tumors in the CNS of carnivores. Pathol. Vet., *6*:94–116, 1969.

Koestner, A., and Zeman, W.: Primary reticuloses of the central nervous system in dogs. Am. J. Vet. Res., *23*:381–383, 1962.

Luginbuhl, H., et al.: Spontaneous neoplasms of the nervous system in animals. *In* Krayenbuehl, H. (ed.): Progress in Neurological Surgery. Vol. 2. White Plains, New York, Albert J. Phiebig (S. Karger), 1968, pp. 85–164.

Luttgen, P. J., et al.: A retrospective study of twenty-nine spinal tumors in the dog and cat. J. Small Anim. Pract., *21*:213–226, 1980.

Nafe, L. A.: Meningiomas in cats: a retrospective clinical study of 36 cases. J. Am. Vet. Med. Assoc., *174*:1224–1227, 1979.

Russo, M. E.: Primary reticulosis of the central nervous system in dogs. J. Am. Vet. Med. Assoc., *174*:492–500, 1979.

Saunders, L. Z., and Barron, C. N.: Primary pigmented intraocular tumors in animals. Cancer Res., *18*:234–245, 1958.

Bone Tumors

Brodey, R. S.: The use of naturally occurring cancer in domestic animals for research with human cancer: general considerations and a review of canine skeletal osteosarcoma. Yale J. Biol. Med., *52*:345–361, 1979.

Dubielzig, R. R., et al.: Bone sarcomas associated with multifocal medullary bone infarction in dogs. J. Am. Vet. Med. Assoc., *179*:64–68, 1981.

Goedegebuure, S. A.: Secondary bone tumours in the dog. Vet. Pathol., *16*:520–529, 1979.

Jacobson, S. A.: The Comparative Pathology of the Tumors of Bone. Springfield, Illinois, Charles C Thomas, 1971.

Madewell, B. R., and Pool, R.: Neoplasms of joints and related structures. Vet. Clin. North Am., *8*:511–521, 1978.

Misdorp, W., and Hart, A. A. M.: Some prognostic and epidemiologic factors in canine osteosarcoma. J. Natl. Cancer Inst., *62*:537–545, 1979.

Tumors in Nondomestic Species

Appleby, E. C.: Tumours in captive wild animals: some observations and comparisons. Acta Zool. Pathol., Antverp., *48*:77–92, 1969.

Billips, L. H., and Harshbarger, J. C.: Naturally occurring neoplastic diseases. XII. Reptiles. *In* Melby, E. C., and Altman, N. H. (eds.): CRC Handbook of Laboratory Animal Science. Vol. 3. Cleveland, CRC Press, Inc., 1976, pp. 343–356.

Cockrill, W. R.: Pathology of the Cetacea—a veterinary study on whales. Br. Vet. J., *116*:133–144, 175–190, 1960.

Dawe, C. J. (ed.): Tumors in aquatic animals. *In* Progress in Experimental Tumor Research. Vol. 20. Basel, S. Karger, 1976, pp. 1–438.

Griesemer, R. C.: Naturally occurring neoplastic diseases. IX. Nonhuman primates. *In* Melby, E. C., and Altman, N. H. (eds.): CRC Handbook of Laboratory Animal Science. Vol. 3. Cleveland, CRC Press, Inc., 1976, pp. 309–323.

Griner, L. A.: Malignant leukemic lymphoma in two harbor seals *(Phoca vitulina geronimensis)*. Am. J. Vet. Res., *32*:827–830, 1971.

Harshbarger, J. C.: Neoplasms in zoo poikilotherms emphasizing cases in the registry of tumors in lower animals. *In* Montali, R. J., and Migaki, G. (eds.): The Comparative Pathology of Zoo Animals. Washington, Smithsonian Institution Press, 1980, pp. 585–591.

Jakowski, R. M., and Helmboldt, C. F.: Naturally occurring neoplastic diseases. X. Domestic fowl. *In* Melby, E. C., and Altman, N. H. (eds.): CRC Handbook of Laboratory Animal Science. Vol. 3. Cleveland, CRC Press, Inc., 1976, pp. 325–342.

Jones, S. R.: Naturally occurring neoplastic diseases. I. Mouse. *In* Melby, E. C., and Altman, N. H. (eds.): CRC Handbook of Laboratory Animal Science. Vol. 3. Cleveland, CRC Press, Inc., 1976, pp. 221–225.

Jones, S. R.: Naturally occurring neoplastic diseases. II. Rat. *In* Melby, E. C., and Altman, N. H. (eds.): CRC Handbook of Laboratory Animal Science. Vol. 3. Cleveland, CRC Press, Inc., 1976, pp. 227–251.

Landy, R.: A review of neoplasia in marine mammals (pinnipedia and cetacea). *In* Montali, R. J., and Migaki, G. (eds.): Comparative Pathology of Zoo Animals. Washington, Smithsonian Institution Press, 1980, pp. 579–584.

Mawdesley-Thomas, L. E.: Neoplasia in fish—bibliography. J. Fish. Biol., *1*:187–207, 1969.

Mawdesley-Thomas, L. E.: Neoplasia in fish: A review. Curr. Topics Comp. Pathol., *1*:87–170, 1971.

Mawdesley-Thomas, L. E.: Neoplasia in fish. *In* Ribelin, W. E., and Migaki, G. (eds.): The Pathology of Fishes. Madison, University of Wisconsin Press, 1975, pp. 805–870.

McClure, H.: Neoplastic diseases in nonhuman primates: literature review and observations in an autopsy series of 2,176 animals. *In* Montali, R. J., and Migaki, G. (eds.): Comparative Pathology of Zoo Animal Symposium, 1978. Washington, Smithsonian Institution Press, 1980, pp. 549–565.

Montali, R. J.: An overview of tumors in zoo animals. *In* Montali, R. J., and Migaki, G. (eds.): Comparative Pathology of Zoo Animals. Washington, Smithsonian Institution Press, 1980, pp. 531–542.

Rigdon, R. H., and Leibovitz, L.: Spontaneous-occurring tumors in the duck: review of the literature and report of three cases. Avian Dis., *14*:431–444, 1970.

Robinson, F. R.: Naturally occurring neoplastic diseases. III. Hamster. *In* Melby, E. C., and Altman, N. H. (eds.): CRC Handbook of Laboratory Animal Science. Vol. 3. Cleveland, CRC Press, Inc., 1976, pp. 253–270.

Robinson, F. R.: Naturally occurring neoplastic diseases. V. Guinea pig. *In* Melby, E. C., and Altman, N. H. (eds.): CRC Handbook of Laboratory Animal Science. Vol. 3. Cleveland, CRC Press, Inc., 1976, pp. 275–278.

Stedham, M. A.: Naturally occurring neoplastic diseases. VI. Rabbit. *In* Melby, E. C., and Altman, N. H. (eds.): CRC Handbook of Laboratory Animal Science. Vol. 3. Cleveland, CRC Press, Inc., 1976, pp. 279–285.

Stolk, A.: Some tumours in whales. II. Proc. K. Ned. Akad., *56*:301–408, 1953.

Squire, R. A., et al.: Tumors. *In* Benirschke, K., Garner, F. M., and Jones, T. C. (eds.): Pathology of Laboratory Animals. New York, Springer-Verlag, 1978, pp. 1051–1283.

Ulys, C. J., and Best, P. B.: Pathology of lesions observed in whales flensed at Saldanha Bay, South Africa. J. Comp. Pathol., *76*:407–412, 1966.

Van Kampen, K. R.: Lymphosarcoma in the rabbit. A case report and general review. Cornell Vet., *58*:121–128, 1968.

7

HOST–PARASITE RELATIONSHIPS

The preceding chapters contained details of lesions and pathogenetic mechanisms; this chapter attempts to put the overall aspects of disease and how agents and circumstances result in disease in a simplified perspective. Many of the points have been mentioned or implied previously but in a somewhat different context. The parasite in the term "host-parasite" refers to any disease-producing infectious agent. Only a few examples are provided; the general points will come up again in many other contexts in the study of disease.

The concept of the host-parasite relationship has changed markedly over the last century from the time when almost the entire emphasis in infectious disease was placed on the parasite. The Henle-Koch postulates were carved in stone for decades, and every student memorized the essence of the content: "the parasite occurs in every case of the disease in question and under circumstances which can account for the pathological changes and clinical course of the disease; it occurs in no other disease as a fortuitous or nonpathogenic parasite; after being fully isolated from the body and repeatedly grown in pure culture, it can induce the disease anew" (Evans, 1976). Evans' paper puts causation of disease in an up-to-date perspective that, although quite general, seems to fit the circumstances of multiple agents, environment and host factors in relation to many diseases of animals. today (Table 7–1). ***The content and tone of Table 7–1 indicate a marked contrast to the Henle-Koch postulates.***

The great epidemics or *epizootics* of highly infectious diseases still occur, but government and international agencies now keep these to a minimum by means of massive vaccination schemes, or in the case of animals by massive slaughter programs, and by controlling movement into and out of the affected area. Economic factors and protection of markets prevail in animal agriculture. The greatest economic losses under modern husbandry conditions now occur from *enzootic* diseases or from those diseases triggered by environmental changes or stresses.

FACTORS INFLUENTIAL IN INFECTIOUS DISEASE

Microorganisms and parasites may coexist with a host by living in or on the host,

TABLE 7–1. Criteria for Causation: A Unified Concept

1. ***Prevalence*** of the disease should be significantly higher in those exposed to the putative cause than in cases with controls not so exposed[a]
2. ***Exposure*** to the putative cause should be present more commonly in those with the disease than in controls without the disease when all risk factors are held constant
3. ***Incidence*** of the disease should be significantly higher in those exposed to the putative cause than in those not so exposed as shown in prospective studies
4. ***Temporally,*** the disease should *follow* exposure to the putative agent with a distribution of incubation periods on a bell shaped curve
5. ***A spectrum*** of host responses should follow exposure to the putative agent along a logical biological gradient from mild to severe
6. ***A measurable host response*** following exposure to the putative cause should ***regularly appear*** in those lacking this before exposure (i.e., antibody, cancer cells) or should ***increase*** in magnitude if present before exposure; this pattern should not occur in persons so exposed
7. ***Experimental reproduction*** of the disease should occur in higher incidence in animals or man appropriately exposed to the putative cause than in those not so exposed; this exposure may be deliberate in volunteers, experimentally induced in the laboratory, or demonstrated in a controlled regulation of natural exposure
8. ***Elimination or modification*** of the putative cause or of the vector carrying it should decrease the disease (control of polluted water or smoke or removal of the specific agent)
9. ***Prevention or modification*** of the host's response on exposure to the putative cause should decrease or eliminate the disease (immunization, drug to lower cholesterol, specific lymphocyte transfer factor in cancer)
10. The whole thing should make biological and epidemiological sense

[a]The putative cause may exist in the external environment or in a defect in host response.
(From Evans, A. S.: Causation and disease: the Henle-Koch postulates revisited. Yale J. Biol. Med., *49*:175–195, 1976. Reprinted by permission.)

which is called ***symbiosis,*** meaning living together. There are three categories of symbiosis. ***Mutualism*** means that the two live together without disadvantage to either, and most examples of this occur in lower animals. ***Commensalism*** is a situation in which there is advantage to one partner but no real disadvantage to the other. ***Parasitism*** results when one partner damages the other during their coexistence and induces disease in the member generally considered to be the host. The disease may be clinical or subclinical. Only a very few symbiotic relationships are parasitic and of these, only a few of the parasites live intracellularly.

The parasite is attracted to its environment by the ***ability to exploit a food supply.*** Many factors must be recognized in this relationship with reference to the parasite. It must ***gain entry to the host, not be destroyed and not destroy a vital function of the host.*** It must ***multiply, be released and be able to get to the next host or cell.*** Deficiencies in any of these arrangements mean that the parasite might not survive and encourage its continued adaptation and evolution.

Infectious disease results from the interaction of an *infectious agent* with the *host* in its particular *environment.* Each of these parts will be discussed separately, but their interaction must always be kept in mind.

The Host

The host might be wise in the long run to accommodate the parasite, particularly if it is quite damaging, and therefore it would protect itself from the parasite both from a long-term evolutionary standpoint and from a short-term standpoint. The host's primary protective factor is ***resistance,*** of which there are four types: genetic, age, immune and nutritional.

Genetic resistance, sometimes called ***natural resistance,*** means that the agent may ***enter the host but not become established or even if it does become established, causes no ill effects.*** The basic reason for the induction of lesions in the host relates to the foreignness of the constituents of the agent. In general terms, if the proteins of the etiological agents are compatible with those of the host, they do not injure the host and do not cause a host immune response that might be harmful to the agent or the host's tissues. For example, the larvae of the nematode ***Pneumostrongylus tenuis*** may migrate through the neural tissue of the brain of the white-tailed deer but cause no lesions, whereas the same parasite migrating in the brain of a moose causes chronic encephalitis and extensive lesions.

Also, ***the agent may not be able to survive or replicate in the host,*** or ***the agent may enter and replicate but not cause disease.***

The range of host susceptibility to agents varies considerably. For example, rabies virus causes disease in most mammalian hosts; either the virus itself creates incompatibility in the host so that the ensuing attempt to overcome the virus causes lesions, disease and death, or the host's defenses react in such a way as to cause lesions, disease and death. Hog cholera virus causes disease in pigs but not in most other species.

Age resistance means that a particular agent may infect a young animal and cause lesions but be harmless or less harmful in an older animal of the same species, and the reverse may also occur. This effect must relate at least in part to compatibility of the agent and the host, which presumably implies ***variations with age in the environment of functional morphology in the host tissues.*** Many agents are involved strictly with neonatal disease and others are involved with disease in adults. Examples will become well known with the study of medicine and special pathology.

Immune resistance is usually acquired through previous natural exposure to an agent or through immunization, but it may be partly natural. If the host has immune resistance, ***the agent or its products will be overcome*** before a foothold can be secured or will be ***confined.*** In many diseases, immune resistance is highly effective in prevention, but there are many common and serious diseases for which effective immunogens have not been found.

Sometimes ***severe lesions*** may develop in the immunized or partially immunized animal, and although the agent is overcome or confined, the struggle may be quite damaging to host tissues. In some instances, the immune response is effective but ***does not deliver enough protection soon enough.*** For example, in a group of dogs with experimentally induced distemper, by 10 days some will have a high antibody titer with only mild illness, others will have moderately high titers with serious clinical disease that may be fatal and still others will have low titers with severe clinical disease that will be fatal. In virus diarrhea, which is usually a subclinical disease, a small percentage of cattle seem ***unable to adequately respond immunologically*** and develop a chronic progressive illness. Others develop severe acute clinical disease and almost invariably die. With this disease, three clearcut clinical responses result from the same agent. Most of the reasons relate to the susceptibility of the host in terms of immune resistance. An additional aspect of immune mechanisms relates to the thymus. In some disease states in young animals, the thymus is much smaller than in a normal animal of the same age. This may well relate to a specific deficiency in cellular immunity but also seems to be an indication of a weak immune response in general. The state of the thymus should be noted at postmortem examination so that, in time, accurate interpretations and correlations may be made concerning its contribution to the cause of death. Numerous examples of ***immunological deficiency*** are being found in association with specific diseases, a good example being adenoviral pneumonia in Arabian foals.

Variations in microorganism ***virulence*** in relation to ***immune resistance*** have been demonstrated by using vaccines in which ***avirulent*** live organisms of a severe pathogen seem ideal for immunization. Some viruses can be passed in tissue culture for several hundred passages, and at some point—at 60 passages, for example—the virus will be a good immunogen and avirulent in its natural host, but it would not be a good immunogen at 100 passages. The same vaccine strain, however, may be passed several times in its natural host and become highly virulent again. Such changes have been demonstrated with distemper virus. This is an example of ***artificial alteration of virulence and of the response of the host; similar processes occur in nature on***

an evolutionary basis. Each infectious disease has a somewhat different story with regard to immune resistance.

Nutritional resistance implies that an animal in good nutritional condition is more resistant to disease than one in poor condition. This seems logical but is difficult to substantiate. In some experimental work, specific deficiencies have made animals ***more*** susceptible to a particular infection, but ***there is no consistent pattern.*** Variation occurs among the effects of ***different specific nutrient deficiencies*** in ***different species*** and with ***different infectious agents.*** The end result is inconclusive. It seems clear that overnutrition, that is, overfeeding or exaggerated intake of proteins or vitamins, is ***not*** more advantageous for prevention of infectious disease than the required optimum. If intake of vitamins and amino acids does exceed normal requirements for growth and reproduction, however, antibody responses and phagocytosis are better, so that a maximum response by the host is possible. Exceptions occur. Distemper virus was given to three groups of dogs: the first group was obese and had a very high caloric intake, the second group had a moderately high caloric intake and the third group had a low caloric intake. The incidence of paralytic distemper in the three groups was 87 per cent, 74 per cent and 31 per cent, respectively. As was mentioned, ***generalizations about nutrition and resistance to infection are difficult to substantiate.***

The Agent

The influential factors for the agent are virulence, tropism, and the ability to multiply, spread and persist in the host.

Virulence implies the ability to invade and cause lesions, with greater degrees of virulence being associated with more destructive lesions and more serious consequences for the host. Some virulent agents cause massive physical damage while others cause fatal consequences rapidly and subtly; for example, tuberculosis as compared to botulism. The destructive agent may cause death of cells ***by its own presence or secretions,*** or the destruction may in large part be caused ***by the reaction of the host to the agent*** via the immune response. Virulence, as judged by lesions and illness, may not be entirely the property of the agent. Some agents carry tools such as enzymes that help them gain entry to tissues and remain there, or they may secrete potent toxic substances that damage the host, and these are related to virulence. The potential for genetic change by the agent may allow it to remain virulent and to stay a step ahead of the host in terms of their reaching genetic compatibility.

Tropism is an advantage to the agent and may allow it to strike at a vital site, as in a case of rabies, for example, or to accumulate in unusual proportions because of a particular local environment in a tissue. An environment may be preferred because of a ***biochemical preference*** or the availability of a particular substrate, but the precise biochemical explanation usually remains unknown. It is known in at least one case, and that is brucellosis. The placenta contains a high level of erythritol, a 4-carbon sugar that has a marked stimulatory effect on the growth of the organism. The organism, however, kills cells by its growth, and this eventually leads to serious problems for the host and for the fetus. As the pathogenesis of various diseases becomes clearer, there will be further specific examples of tissue tropisms and agents. In the past, agents were considered to have tropism for the tissue in which lesions were found, but it is now known that the agent may have really preferred to live elsewhere and that the lesions were somewhat incidental as far as the agent was concerned. ***The pathogenesis of very few diseases has been clarified.***

An infectious agent must ***survive*** to cause disease. ***Persistence*** in the host may often be accomplished best by maintaining an intracellular existence, except for periodic disruptive excursions outside. The location inside the cell provides protection from the immune response of the host, and if the agent can live there without killing the cell, it may survive for long periods. Salmonellosis is an example of this. The ease with which an agent can survive ***outside*** the host under natural conditions is also significant in terms of its ability to cause disease. Rabies virus does not survive well outside, but the virus of foot and mouth disease may persist in the environment for some time, as will the spores of some of the clostridial species and the anthrax bacillus. ***The ease with which an infectious agent spreads*** from animal to animal will often determine the extent of a disease problem, particularly in a closed environment. Temperature and humidity factors relate to properties of aerosolization and aerosol stability and therefore to spread. The recent studies on the natural spread of foot and mouth disease virus by aerosol for 40 to 60 miles have been most illuminating with respect to the spread of disease.

The *response* of the host to an agent with some degree of virulence will be disease or illness that may be clinical, subclinical or latent.

Clinical disease as a result of infection results from abnormal functional and morphological changes in constituents of the body that upset homeostasis and cause pain, discomfort or mental stress and that result in the individual's not feeling well or being sick. In the case of an animal, these are reflected in behavioral changes called ***clinical signs,*** such as not eating, lying down too much, diarrhea and heavy respiration, all of which will catch the attention of an owner or attendant. Clinical disease from infection may be ***acute*** or ***chronic.*** The chronic state may begin and remain chronic or may develop from an acute state.

The discovery of ***subclinical disease*** may depend on the extent to which the animals are observed, how detailed the clinical examination is, or the number and type of laboratory tests carried out. These may be used to determine whether or not disease is present when the animal's rate of growth or milk production falls below optimum. This term applies to such conditions as mastitis, enzootic pneumonia and marginal nutritional deficiencies. ***The animals do not show obvious signs of clinical illness, but rate of growth or production is reduced.***

A step beyond the subclinical state is the ***latent infection,*** or the so-called inapparent carrier state, in which an individual harbors and excretes a known pathogen but has no clinical evidence of the disease. Examples of agents that may be carried are salmonellae and the herpesviruses. Infection is persistent, and in some cases it is most difficult to determine whether or not the individual is a carrier. The individual carrier may have an acute attack of disease or may spread agents to susceptible hosts without overt signs of disease. This means of spread is significant in hosts of the same species and also among species that are very different. Some hosts are inapparent carriers of agents highly fatal to other species. For example, the wildebeest carries the virus of malignant catarrhal fever with no ill effects, but the virus is highly fatal to cattle.

Subclinical or latent infection may cause clinical disease after variations occur in environmental conditions or immune status of the host.

The Environment

The factors that are perhaps of greatest importance in initiating or influencing disease are ***environmental,*** particularly among domestic animals for which intensive husbandry practices are followed. ***These factors may change subclinical or latent infection into acute or chronic disease.*** For example, dust and ammonia in poultry houses increase the incidence of air sac disease. Ammonia from dirty cages has a marked synergistic effect on the incidence of chronic respiratory disease caused by ***Mycoplasma pulmonis*** in rats. Sudden changes in feed plus weaning may induce a rapid change in the intestinal flora in pigs, resulting in coliform gastroenteritis or gut edema. Weaning and shipping steers may change the normal nasal bacterial flora with the result that it becomes an important factor in the pathogenesis of shipping fever. Crowding of calves or pigs plus unsatisfactory temperature and humidity may increase the incidence and severity of enzootic pneumonia.

In contrast to Koch's postulates, the agents that cause disease in some of these situations are members of the ***normal flora*** or are truly inapparent infections until the environmental influences precipitate a state of disease.

Many of these adverse environmental influences are well recognized, but the problem in animal disease is *how to prevent them and retain an economically profitable production unit.* This is one of the major problems facing the animal industry. Antibiotics and vaccines cannot replace good management.

PATHOGENESIS OF DISEASE CAUSED BY VARIOUS AGENTS

Next is a discussion relating to some of the mechanisms by which disease-producing agents gain access and cause disease relative to some general mechanisms. The text will be very general and the references will provide details. The book by Mims (1982) and the symposium on microbial pathogenicity in man and animals edited by Smith and Pearce (1972) are recommended for further reading.

Bacteria

Acute bacterial disease usually results from a rapid accumulation of organisms that have gained entry through the skin or through the digestive, respiratory or urogenital tract. Species of bacteria vary as to the number of organisms required to produce disease. ***Pasteurella haemolytica*** in sheep and ***Actinobacillus equuli*** in horses need to be present in tremendous numbers to cause illness and death, whereas only a few ***Clostridium tetani*** are required. Disease may result from the necrosis of cells, the response of the host in overcoming the agent, the toxins produced by the organism acting directly on tissue cells or the effect of the organism on the blood, such as initiation of sludging or disseminated intravascular coagulation. The effect will vary with the agent and the site and extent of the lesion in particular tissues and organs.

Chronic bacterial disease occurs when the agent persists in the host for long periods and causes localized lesions that result from what is more or less a stand-off between the host and the agent. Disease may result from space-occupying lesions in the form of granulomatous inflammation or large abscesses but with some systemic effects. Some agents persist on mucosal surfaces as irritants and are not easily overcome or removed.

The main requirements for ***pathogenicity*** of an agent relate to its ability to (1) enter the host by surviving on and penetrating mucous membranes, (2) multiply ***in vivo,*** (3) inhibit or avoid stimulation of the host's defense mechanisms and (4) damage the host. ***Virulence refers to the degree of pathogenicity.*** Often, agents lose pathogenicity in culture and are thus not the same organisms as those that grew in the host.

Agents may require specific host factors in order to replicate, and different factors may be required for each step of replication. Some bacteria produce compounds with the general name of ***aggressins*** that help the organism break down the host's defense, for example, by impairing phagocytosis, but that are not directly toxic. The host might be damaged more by its immune response to an antigen of the organism than by a toxin secreted by the organism.

Bacteria may produce disease by ***attaching*** to an epithelial surface and secreting toxins (enterotoxigenic ***Escherichia coli***), by invading the epithelial cells and destroying them (***Shigella***) or by invading the lamina propria in order to disseminate from there (***Salmonella***). There may be competition between pathogens and normal flora, and disease may not occur unless the normal flora is markedly altered, as in the coliform enteritis that develops in weanling pigs when sudden changes in feed occur. The replacement time of small intestine epithelium in pigs one day old is about nine to ten days; in pigs three weeks old, the replacement time is two to four days. The ***E. coli*** may remain attached for longer periods in the young and therefore have more time to produce toxins before being carried away. The toxins interfere with fluid dynamics across the epithelium. Cholera organisms cause disease in this manner also. ***Clostridium perfringens*** secretes potent ***toxins.*** Usually, a situation that allows the organism to multiply in large quantities must develop, and then there is enough toxin to cause disease. A sudden change to rich feed provides the opportunity to cause Type D enterotoxemia in sheep.

Many bacteria that cause disease are components of the normal flora, particularly those on mucous membranes. The mechanisms that induce such species of bacteria to become pathogens are not well understood, but one important aspect is the ability to attach by "adhesins" to epithelial cells. Bacteria and host cell must have the proper "hook-up" by receptors for the bacteria to survive and grow on a cell surface. Normal flora survives in this manner and pathogens require such an attachment in order to cause disease. Diseases of the urinary, respiratory and intestinal tract are often caused by organisms that increase in numbers and have the appropriate adhesins. Factors that suddenly alter flora in the intestine often relate to sudden changes in feed, resulting in massive growth of a particular species of bacteria because it was preferentially nourished by the dietary change. Examples are *E. coli* in postweaned pigs, grain overload in cattle and enterotoxemia in sheep. Stress or viral infection or antibiotic therapy may seriously alter flora by influencing adhesin formation on organisms.

The bacterial control mechanisms of the immune system are becoming identified in that some organisms are controlled by cellular immunity alone, such as *Listeria monocytogenes*, or by antitoxin antibody such as in tetanus; but in general the specific mechanisms for particular organisms are not well defined.

Bacteria that cause purulent lesions tend not to enter cells and are controlled mainly by opsonizing antibodies. Bacteria that cause granulomatous lesions are able to survive within phagocytes and are controlled primarily by cellular immune mechanisms.

Anaerobic infections are common, but definition of their etiology is difficult for technical reasons. These infections usually occur in anoxic tissue, or necrotic tissue or tissue previously infected with aerobic bacteria or viruses. The anaerobes are usually part of normal flora, and numerous species may be involved in the same lesion. Clues to their presence may be much necrosis, foul smell, gas production in the lesion, failure to culture aerobes, failure of some antibiotics to control the infection and smears containing many different kinds of bacteria.*

*The following figures illustrate lesions which are or probably are caused by bacteria:

Chapter 2: Figures 2–84, 2–91, 2–92, 2–93, 2–97, 2–98, 2–100, 2–108, 2–109, 2–110, 2–111, 2–116.

Chapter 3: Figures 3–13, 3–20, 3–29, 3–31, 3–39, 3–48, 3–55, 3–70, 3–71.

Chapter 4: Figures 4–24, 4–29, 4–31, 4–32, 4–33, 4–34, 4–35, 4–36, 4–37, 4–38, 4–43, 4–47, 4–48, 4–49, 4–51, 4–54, 4–55, 4–56, 4–57, 4–58, 4–59, 4–61, 4–62, 4–63, 4–64, 4–65, 4–66, 4–67, 4–68, 4–69, 4–70, 4–71, 4–72, 4–73, 4–74, 4–75, 4–76, 4–86, 4–87, 4–88, 4–91, 4–92, 4–96, 4–98, 4–99, 4–100, 4–102, 4–108, 4–155, 4–156, 4–159.

Chapter 5: Figure 5–33.

Viruses

Viruses cause disease (1) by cytolysis, (2) by maintaining a steady state with the host or (3) by integrating into the genome of the host. The disease may be localized or generalized, depending on both the attributes of the virus to spread and its virulence. Viruses need not break down defense barriers, but can multiply right in the cells making up certain defense barriers. The interaction of the virus with the host cell requires exquisite specificity of binding sites by both. Examples of susceptibility and resistance in inbred strains of laboratory animals illustrate the specificity. Antibody may protect by blocking adherence, or may allow adsorption, but not penetration, or may agglutinate the virus or coat infected cells and cause them to be lysed or phagocytosed.

Cytolytic effects arise from destruction of the host cell following maturation of the virus intracellularly and the release of infectious virus into the environment to infect and destroy more cells. Some viruses cause production of compounds toxic to the cell in which they are growing. Viruses may cause release or activation of lysosomal enzymes that may cause lesions. Thus, the lesions are virus-induced morphological changes or metabolically induced functional changes. The immune response to the viral agent may cause morphological and functional lesions that damage the tissue in which the virus grows and result in more lesions and clinical disease. The agent and the lesions may remain localized or may become generalized. Infectious bovine rhinotracheitis is an example of an agent that can be highly destructive in one or several tissues.

The ***steady state*** type of infections are typical of those **RNA** viral infections in which the host cell may survive and continue to produce virus by budding. In some diseases, lack of compatibility between host and virus may result in considerable necrosis of cells as well, or the lesions may develop from the host's immune response to the agent. Virus may also be spread from cell to cell without being released into the environment of the host, and therefore, persistent killing of cells continues in spite of the efforts of interferon.

Acute viral infections often result in leukopenia and do so in part by causing necrosis in lymphoid follicles. One cause of the necrosis may be direct cytolytic effects from replication of the virus or from toxicity. Another cause may be the influence of endogenous corticosteroids released as a result of severe clinical illness. The leukopenia may last a short time or a long time and may impair the immune response of the host. Necrosis in lymph follicles may also be caused by antigenic stimulation and the activity of the lymphocytes in the immune response.

Integrated infections are characteristic of the oncogenic viruses discussed earlier. A relatively new term used in viral disease is ***slow virus infection.*** Incubation occurs over months or years, and the disease is chronic and usually fatal. The virus either remains hidden by integration or is masked by antibody. Examples of these diseases are visna and scrapie of sheep and Aleutian mink disease; the elucidation of the pathogenesis of such diseases will be followed with great interest.

The initial effect of a virus takes place within the cell, where it induces ***cytopathic changes*** by altering the form and function of membranes and organelles either selectively or nonspecifically. The virus takes over protein production for itself at the expense of the cell. Masses of new virus may accumulate in the cell, sometimes in the form of inclusion bodies. Abnormal fluid control by the damaged cell membranes leads to swelling of the cell and of many organelles. At some stages, autophagy may be prominent in an effort to dispose of injured cell constituents or abnormal products induced by the virus. These may develop the appearance of inclusion bodies at some stages of infection. Viral damage to cell membrance is the most direct means of inducing cell death.

There are some examples that suggest that viral infection is not haphazard and that the cells have ***specific receptors*** allowing the virus to attach and then gain entry to the cell. The host responds to virus infection with phagocytosis of virus and virus-infected cells, production of interferon, humoral antibody and cellular immunity. ***Persistent infection may lead to immune-complex disease.*** Altered immune response may lead to widespread viral infection or long-term persisting infection leading to chronic progressive disease.

A few examples of ***specific tissue affinities*** for viral diseases in the intestine may serve as samples of the information that may be forthcoming with other viruses and tissues. Cells lining the epithelium of the intestinal wall are produced in the crypts and mature as they move to the top of the villus. The replacement time of the cells is two to four days, except in very young individuals, for which the time is eight to ten days. Replication of cells is controlled by chalones from the villi through a feedback mechanism to the crypts. Which lesions develop depends on which area of the epithelium is attacked. The coronavirus of transmissible gastroenteritis (TGE) in pigs attacks all villous epi-

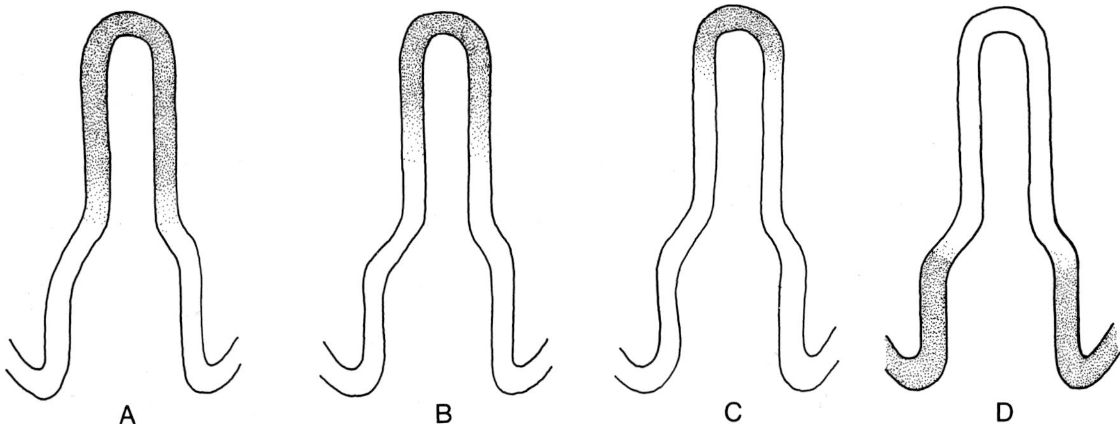

Figure 7–1. Variation in the site of action of viral agents in the intestine. *A,* The virus of transmissible gastroenteritis of pigs; *B,* the rotavirus of enteritis in calves; *C,* the rotavirus of epidemic diarrhea of mice; *D,* the panleukopenia virus in cats.

thelia, the rotavirus of calf diarrhea strikes the upper half of the villus, the rotavirus of epidemic diarrhea of mice attacks the tip of the villus and the parvovirus of panleukopenia of cats strikes the crypt epithelium (Fig. 7–1).

The lesion of TGE is villous atrophy. Virus destroys epithelial cells, and the villus is shortened to the point that the cells available do not cover the villus; however, the villus eventually returns to normal as regeneration of cells occurs. In newborn animals, the disease is fatal because the epithelial replacement time is nine to ten days and the animal cannot replace the epithelium quickly enough to maintain vital functions. Much virus can build up in the cells because of the longer replacement time. Animals three weeks old and over may become quite ill but usually recover. This is an example of age resistance, which in this case is related to the development of the intestinal epithelium. Panleukopenia is often fatal because the cells in the crypts are not able to replace those on the villi that move off. The lesion that results can be very destructive to large areas of the intestine, and regeneration is markedly impaired by the virus.

Resistance to and recovery from viral disease depends on a complex interaction of virus and host mechanisms in which species, age and prior immune status of the host are as critical as the size of inoculum, strain of virus and portal of entry.

Many specific ultrastructural lesions are illustrated in Cheville's *Cytopathology of Viral Diseases* (1975).*

Parasites

Parasitic agents generally cause disease by local destruction of cells or tissue, by their effects on the blood circulation, by their effects as space-occupying lesions or by nutritive competition.

Local destruction is exemplified by intestinal coccidiosis or by migrating nematodes. Strongylus infection in horses is an example of a situation in which part of the life cycle inadvertently results in thrombosis of major vessels and infarction of parts of the gut, which may be fatal. Some of the bloodborne protozoa cause clinical disease through microthrombi, sludging and degrees of disseminated intravascular coagulation. Tapeworm cysts may take up much space in a vital area or nematodes may obstruct a lumen or an orifice. Some of the intestinal parasites suck blood or reduce the growth of the animal by partaking of limited food supplies.

In general, ***the damage caused is a function of numbers of organisms*** and whether or not they expose themselves or become exposed to the immune response of the host. Virulence factors and immune response are not as well known in parasitic diseases as in bacterial and viral diseases, and the ability of some parasites to survive and take up considerable space with minimal response by the host is surprising. Perhaps parasites are "better parasites" than some other agents because they tend to look after their own interests and survival without killing the host and losing their homes.

Some of the means by which they cause disease are discussed here. Trichinella is an example of a parasite that takes over a cell within a host and does not kill it but ***converts the functions of the cell entirely to its own purposes.*** The occupied muscle cell undergoes complete internal reorganization, the muscle fibrils disappear and the functions of the cell are directed toward production of cysts. The cell is transformed in such a way that a new, highly differentiated host cell–parasite relationship results. ***Immune-complex disease*** may be highly significant in malaria, trypanosomiasis and schistosomiasis. ***Cell-mediated immunity*** is a major factor in the development of parasitic granulomas. Immune mechanisms trigger the release of ***histamine*** in the intestinal mucosa and may result in rapid expulsion of intestinal nematodes. ***Blood loss*** is likely to be the cause of death in hookworm infection or coccidiosis. In ***Haemonchus*** infections, blood loss is likely to be the cause of death if the disease is acute, but iron deficiency may become the limiting factor in less acute disease.

---

*The following figures illustrate lesions caused by viruses:

Chapter 2: Figures 2–24, 2–25, 2–26, 2–27, 2–28, 2–29, 2–30, 2–31, 2–32, 2–33, 2–34, 2–72, 2–73, 2–90, 2–94, 2–99, 2–102.

Chapter 4: Figures 4–13, 4–14, 4–44, 4–45, 4–46, 4–104, 4–129, 4–130.

Chapter 5: Figures 5–2, 5–10.

Chapter 6: Figures 6–7, 6–15, 6–16, 6–24, 6–31, 6–97.

The ***mechanisms*** by which many resident intestinal parasites produce disease are ***surprisingly unclear.*** It is sometimes assumed that villous atrophy and malabsorption or nutritive competition may be the mechanisms, but there is little firm evidence to substantiate these suggestions. In some instances, loss of differentiation of absorbing cells or loss of protein into the gut has been documented, but the factors leading to or responsible for anorexia are not clear. There is considerable information concerning local factors that are available and required by the parasite to hatch or exsheath. ***These are usually locally confined biochemical and physiological circumstances that account for the site and host specificity of the parasite.*** The setting in motion of certain stages of gastrointestinal parasitic infection by physiological or endocrinological influences at parturition or lactation with the spring rise phenomenon is an example of an activation influence.

An important phenomenon in parasitic infections is arrested development of larvae because of the immune status of the host or because of seasonal or climatic changes, which is called hypobiosis. Release of these controls, which is poorly understood, can result in sudden heavy exposure to infection.

Ostertagia infection has received much study in terms of pathogenesis and illustrates how the parasite affects gastric function. Third-stage larvae enter the gastric mucosal glands, where they develop into adults and then emerge. The development may take 10 days or up to six months. The lesions develop as the parasite emerges and are due to hyperplasia of glandular epithelial cells together with loss of differentiation of the acid-producing parietal cells throughout the mucosa. The pH rises, pepsinogen is not converted to pepsin, bacteria increase and the mucosa becomes permeable owing to breakdown of cell junctions. Indications of the permeability change are the increase in plasma pepsinogen levels and the leakage of plasma proteins into the lumen. These changes lead to diarrhea, anorexia and weight loss.

Parasitic infection usually results from one of the following factors: increase in infecting masses, altered susceptibility of existing animals, introduction of susceptible animals into an infected area, or introduction of new vectors.

Some lesions caused by parasites are illustrated in Figures 7–2 through 7–17.*

---

*The following figures also illustrate lesions caused by parasites:

Chapter 2: Figures 2–37, 2–55, 2–62, 2–96, 2–104, 2–105.

Chapter 3: Figures 3–11, 3–63, 3–64.

Chapter 4: Figures 4–52, 4–83, 4–93.

Chapter 5: Figure 5–17.

Text continued on page 424

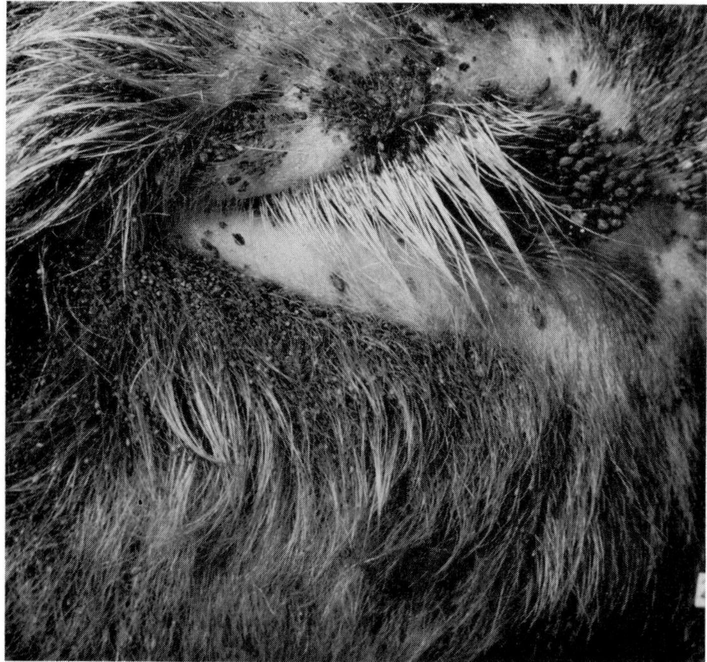

Figure 7–2. A calf with a very heavy infestation of lice around the eyes and over much of the skin surface. The mechanism by which lice cause clinical illness is not clear but, in the case of sucking lice, illness is not entirely due to anemia.

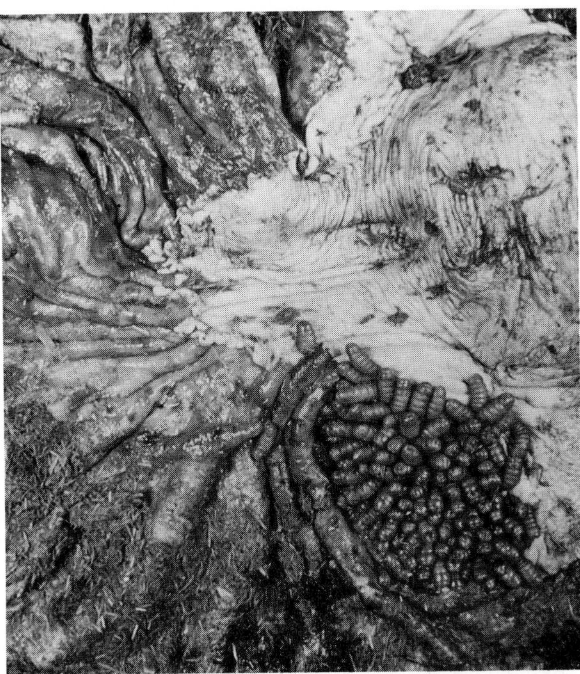

Figure 7–3

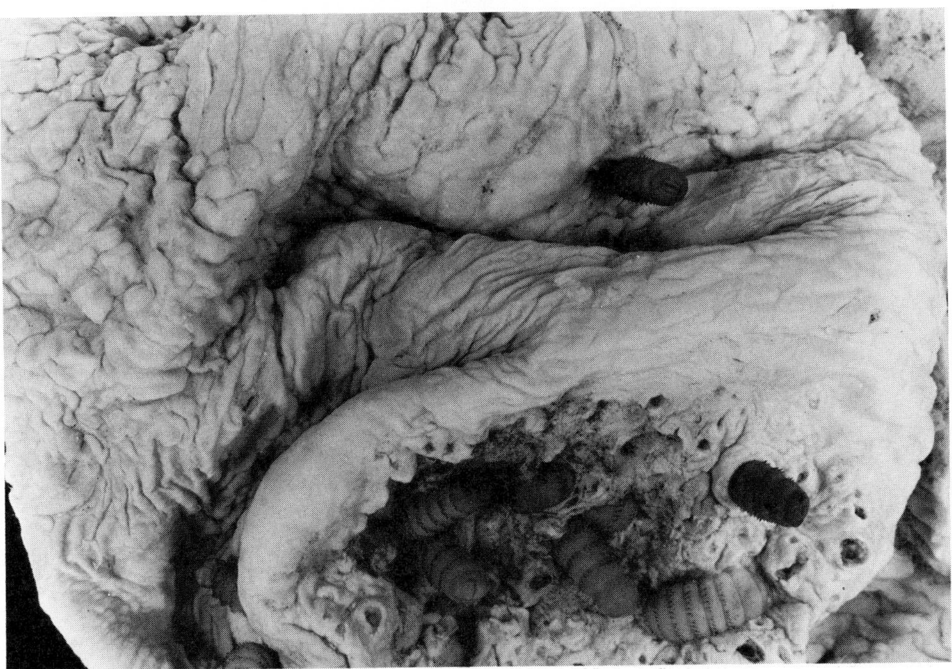

Figure 7–4

Figures 7–3 and 7–4. *Gastrophilus* larvae or bots in a horse's stomach (Fig. 7–3) and a close-up of a similar lesion (Fig. 7–4). (Museum specimen.) These are considered to be relatively nonpathogenic even though they cause ulcers, as seen in Figure 7–4.

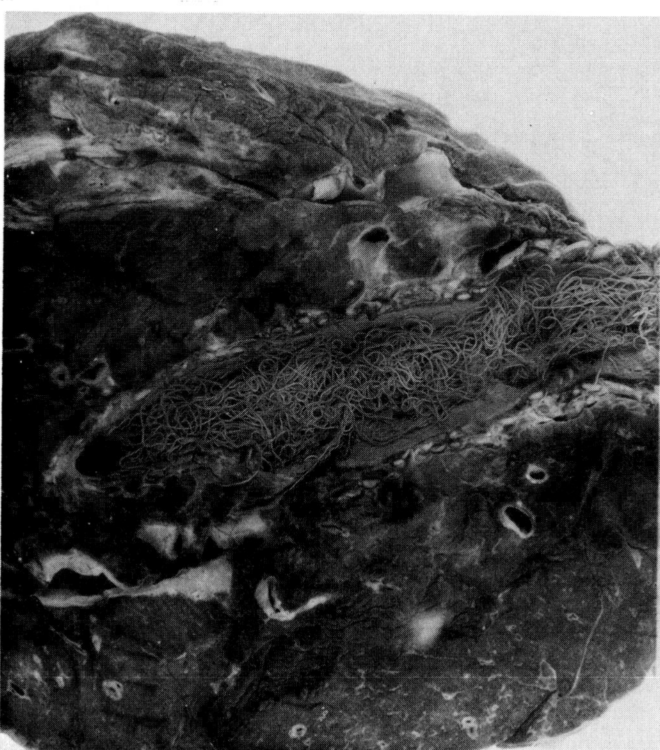

Figure 7–5. *Dictyocaulus filariae* lungworm in a sheep. Note the large number of worms in the bronchus with very little exudate. (Museum specimen.)

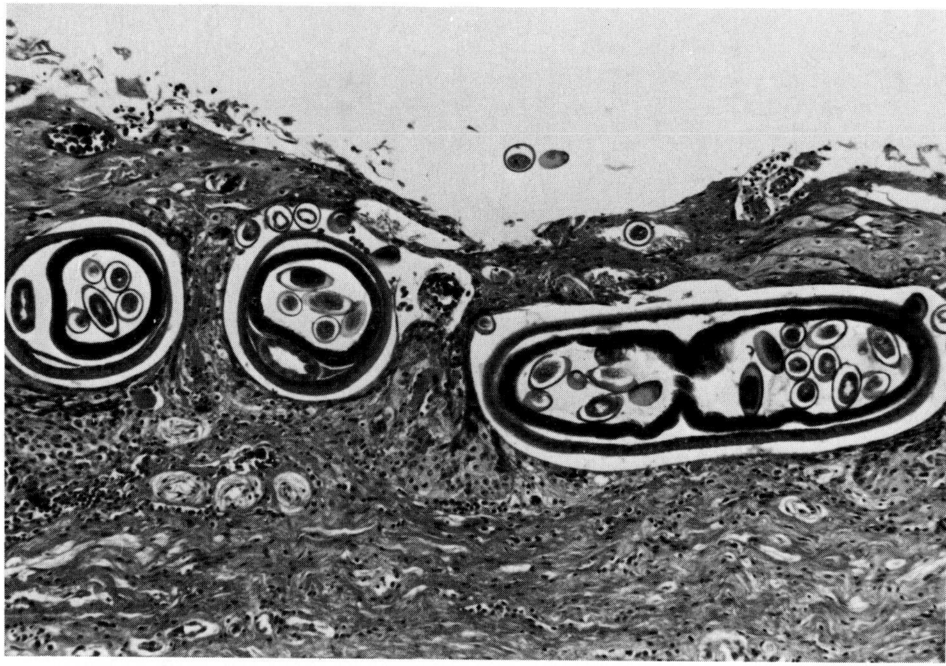

Figure 7–6. *Capillaria* worms in the esophagus of a bobwhite quail. These worms cause much damage as they penetrate into the mucosa and are quite pathogenic. Affected birds have great difficulty swallowing.

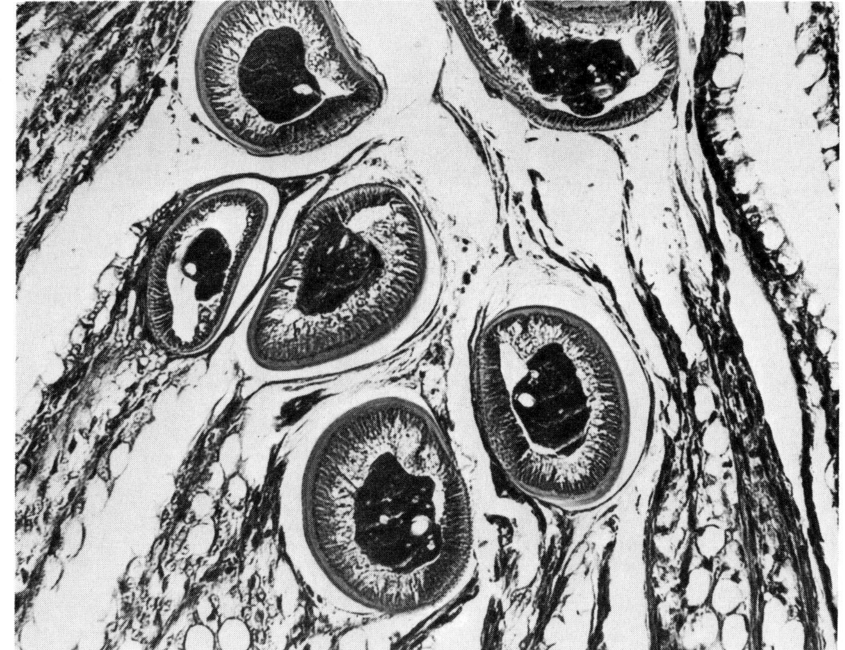

Figure 7–7. *Haemonchus contortus* worms in a sheep's abomasum. There is little tissue reaction, but the worms suck much blood and cause anemia.

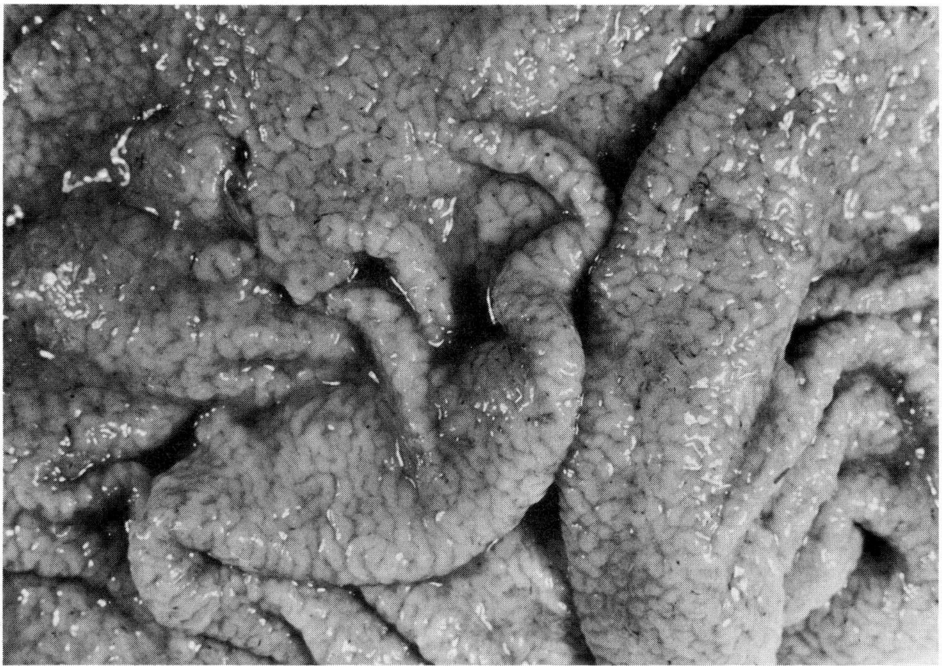

Figure 7–8. Thickened abomasal leaves in a calf with ostertagiasis. The appearance is called "Morocco leather."

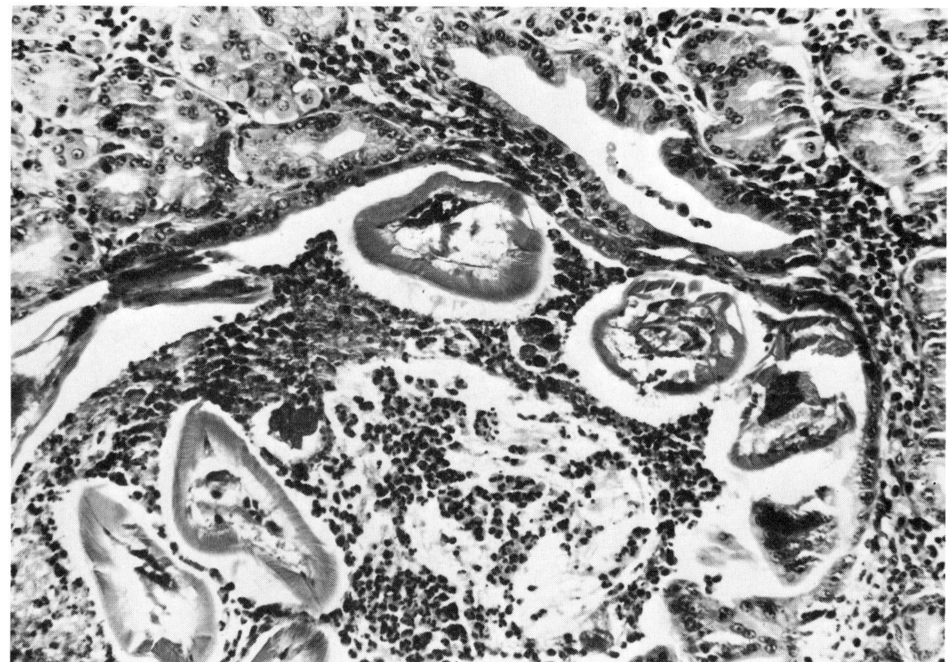

Figure 7–9. *Ostertagia* in the gastric mucosa, causing distention and obstruction of glands as well as necrosis of epithelium and inflammatory exudate.

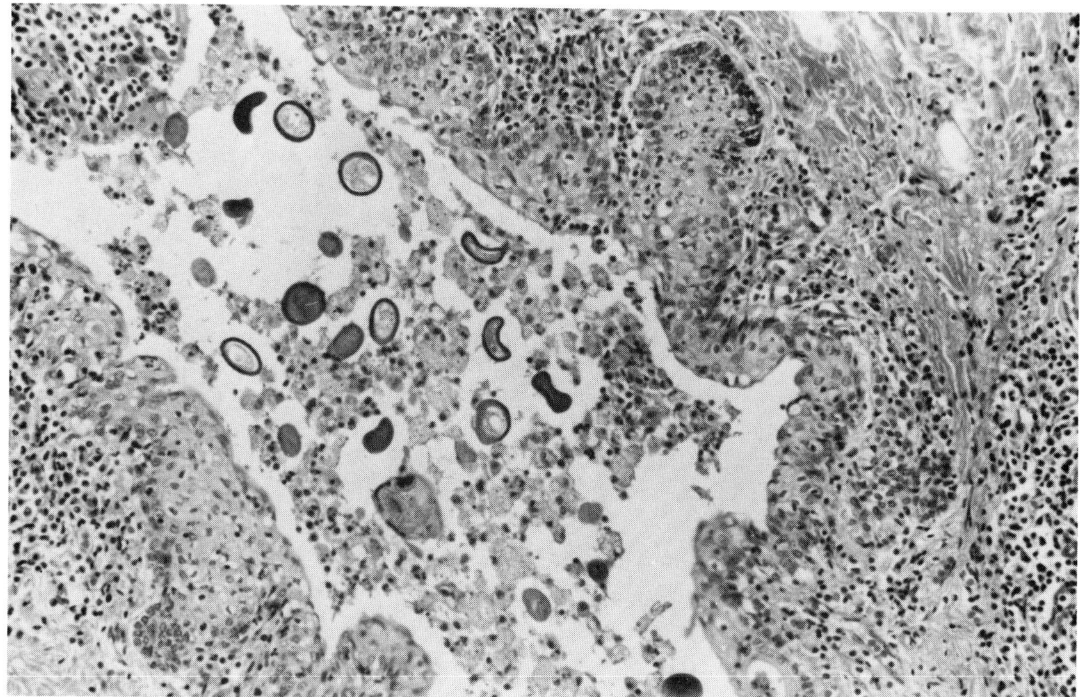

Figure 7–10. Eggs of *Crassicauda grampicola* in the mammary gland of a dolphin. Note the squamous metaplasia of ducts. These parasites cause involution of affected glands. (Courtesy of J. R. Geraci.)

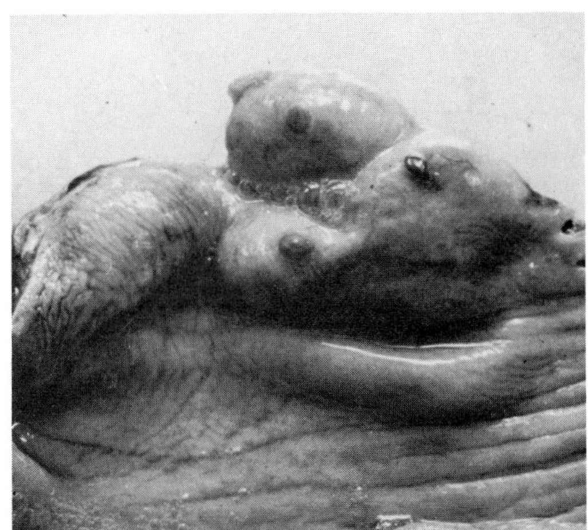

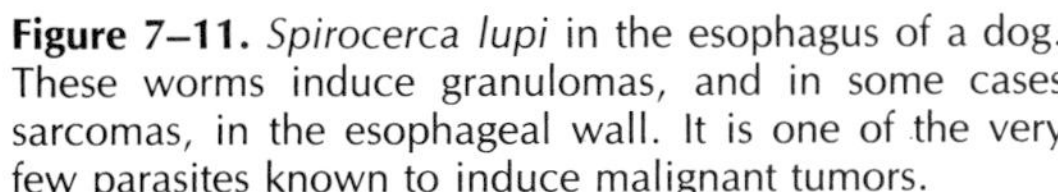

Figure 7–11. *Spirocerca lupi* in the esophagus of a dog. These worms induce granulomas, and in some cases sarcomas, in the esophageal wall. It is one of the very few parasites known to induce malignant tumors.

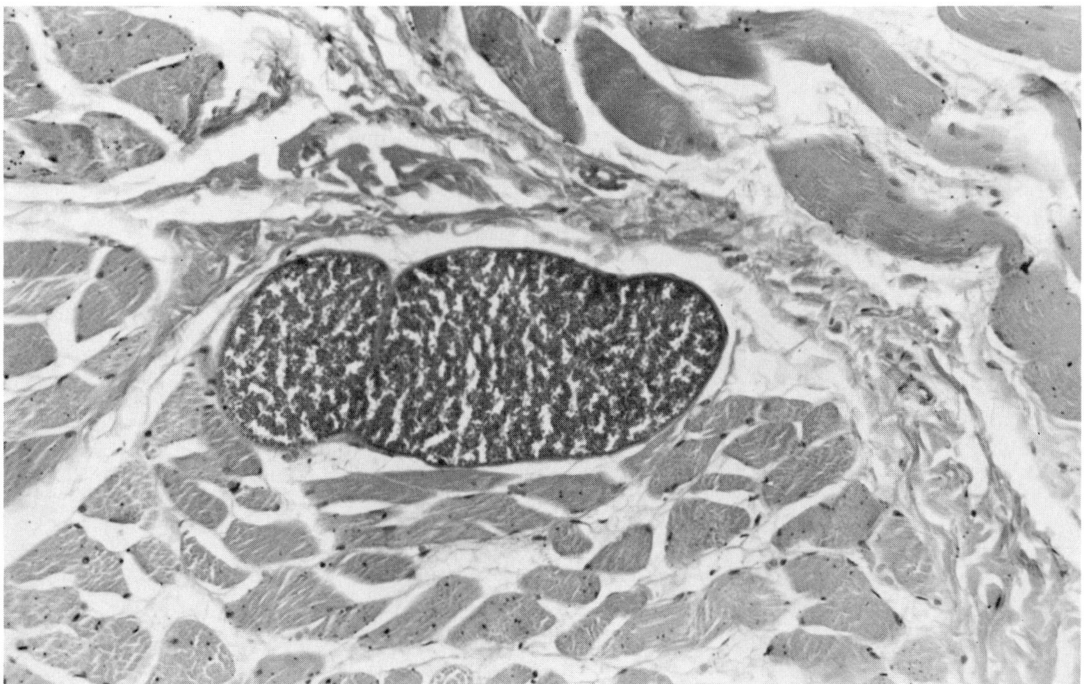

Figure 7–12. Large cyst of sarcosporidia in the muscle of a ringed seal. There is usually no reaction even when the organisms are very numerous. This infection is common in many species.

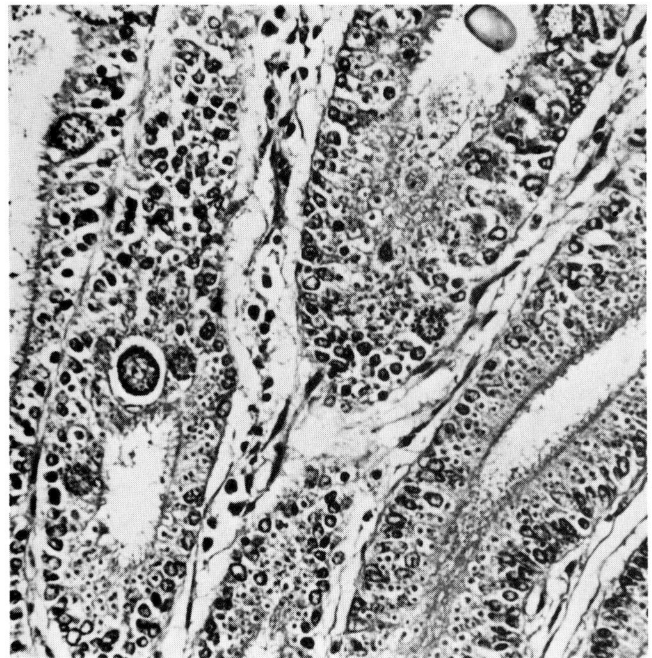

Figure 7–13. Coccidiosis in the intestinal mucosa. Various developmental stages are present, and almost all the epithelial cells are parasitized. The end result may be necrosis of much of the epithelial lining and a necrotizing enteritis.

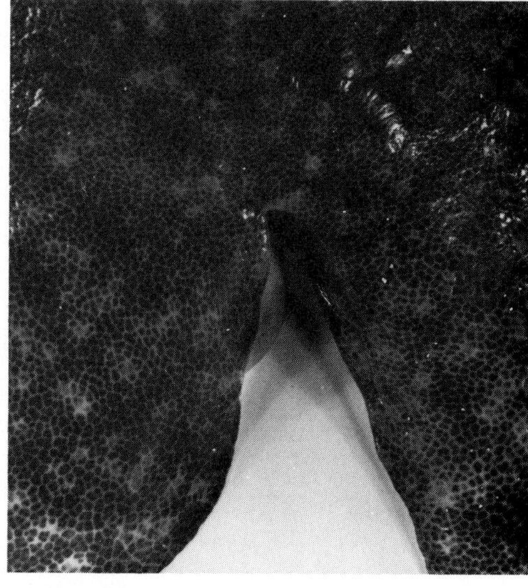

Figure 7–14. "Milk spots" on a porcine liver. The pale foci are areas of inflammation caused by migration of *Ascaris suum*.

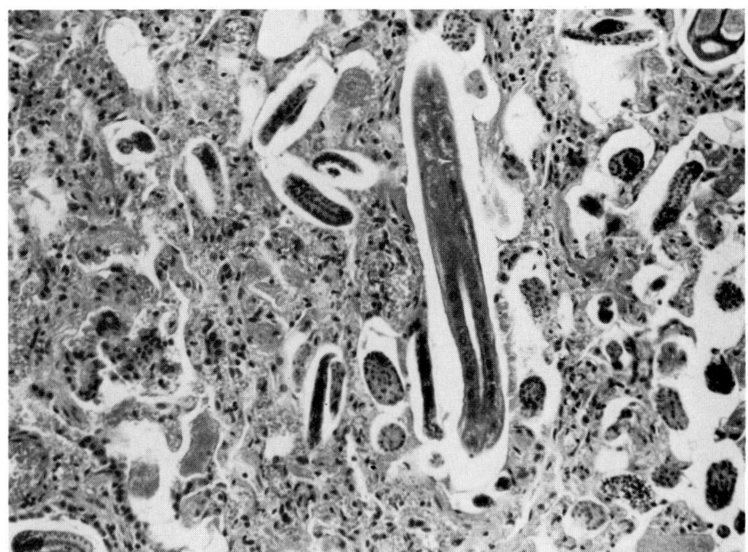

Figure 7–15. Müllerius lungworm and larvae in a sheep's lung. The lesions are usually very chronic and may contain calcified nodules. (Courtesy of B. Schiefer.)

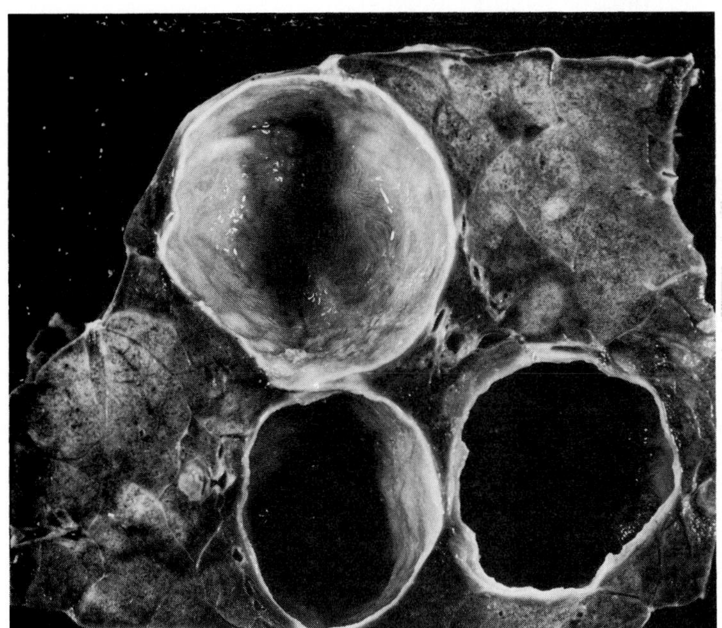

Figure 7–16. *Echinococcus* cysts in a bovine lung. (Courtesy of B. Schiefer.)

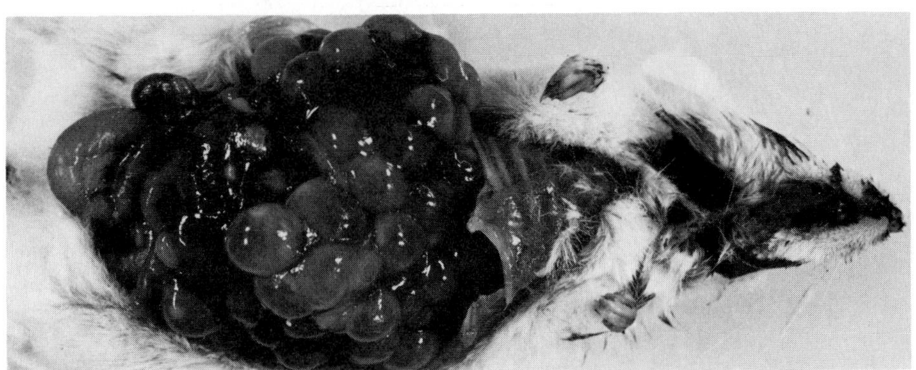

Figure 7–17. *Cysticercus fasciolaris* in a mouse. Note the large number of cysts.

Fungi

Fungal agents cause disease by three main methods: (1) ***invasion*** of living tissue by the fungus, (2) ***allergies*** resulting from contact with and development of hypersensitivity to fungal antigens and (3) ***toxicosis*** resulting from eating food containing toxic metabolites of fungi.

Disease production by fungal agents such as in blastomycosis and histoplasmosis results in granulomas in many organs. Ringworm is an example of a localized lesion. Many fungal infections seem to be opportunistic, such as aspergillosis of the air sacs in birds, and many are infections of body surfaces. In ruminants in particular, fungi seem to be nearby when ulceration of the mucosal surface of the digestive tract occurs. They invade tissue and have a remarkable ability to enter blood vessels and cause thrombosis. They spread in the circulation and also continue "cross-country" by invasion and result in extensive ischemic necrosis, as exemplified by mycotic rumenitis. Mycotic infections are characterized by their tenacity and rather sly habits.

A well-known allergic disease caused by fungi is farmer's lung, which is a hypersensitivity to ***Micropolyspora faeni,*** found in high levels in moldy hay. The disease occurs in humans and in cattle.

Aflatoxins occur after growth of ***Aspergillus flavus*** and ***A. parasiticus*** and are potent hepatotoxins best known as contaminants of ground nut meal. Moldy corn poisoning in pigs is due to ***Fusarium*** species. Facial eczema of sheep in New Zealand is a hepatotoxin that results in a photosensitization syndrome and is caused by ingestion of spores from ***Sporidesmium bakeri.*** A buildup of these occurs in the wet season after a dry period. Ergotism results in gangrene of the extremities when animals consume rye or other feed contaminated with ***Claviceps purpurea.*** Disease caused by fungal toxins is more common than generally realized and many types of fungi have been implicated as being toxic to animals.

Some mycotic lesions are illustrated in Figures 7–18 through 7–22.*

---

*The following figures also illustrate lesions caused by fungi:
Chapter 2: Figures 2–25, 2–87.
Chapter 4: Figures 4–81, 4–82, 4–94, 4–95.

Toxins

Toxic agents cause disease by ***direct contact*** or by ***absorption*** and strike at a particular vulnerable tissue. Direct contact by a potent toxin causes degeneration or necrosis, or a combination of the two, of the cells contacted. Absorption usually occurs through the skin and the respiratory and digestive tracts. Toxins have predilections for certain organs and types of cells. They cause either acute or chronic damage by derangement of the cell metabolism in subtle ways that take some time to develop or by outright destruction of organelles and necrosis of cells. Usually, their effects are ***dose-dependent,*** given the tissue and species sensitivities. The predilection sites and actions are discussed as a unit in Smith and co-workers (1982).

A toxic substance reacts adversely with some part or function in the living organism. The metabolism of toxic compounds is enzymic and occurs in two phases called I and II. ***The phase I reactions involve changes in the toxic compound, such as oxidations, reductions and hydrolysis, whereas the phase II reactions involve synthesis and are often called conjugation.*** In phase I the compound may develop reactive groups that allow it to proceed to phase II. Some compounds may go directly to phase II, and some may be essentially detoxified in phase I. The metabolism of foreign compounds occurs largely in the endoplasmic reticulum of the hepatocytes and mainly by oxidases through hydroxylation or oxygenation reactions. Some compounds may be metabolized in the gut by the normal bacterial flora.

Toxic compounds may be excreted in the urine in their original state or as the products of phase I and II reactions. The proportions of each will depend on the chemical nature of the compound, dose and route of administration, species, strain, age, sex, diet and environmental influences. The metabolic process generally converts toxic lipid-soluble foreign compounds, which tend to be reabsorbed by the renal tubules, ***into*** water-soluble polar products that are readily excreted. The products of phase I reactions may be less toxic or more toxic or may possess a different type of toxicity from that of their precursors. Phase II products are nontoxic or less toxic than the original compound. There are numerous examples of ***species susceptibility*** to toxic compounds, as well as ***age susceptibility.*** These differences must relate to the presence or absence of enzymes to detoxify the particular compound or the particular sensitivity of a key normal metabolic pathway to disruption by the toxic substance. It is therefore difficult to generalize about the specific actions of a toxic substance, since the action will vary with age, species and so forth. Chemical carcinogens are toxic compounds.

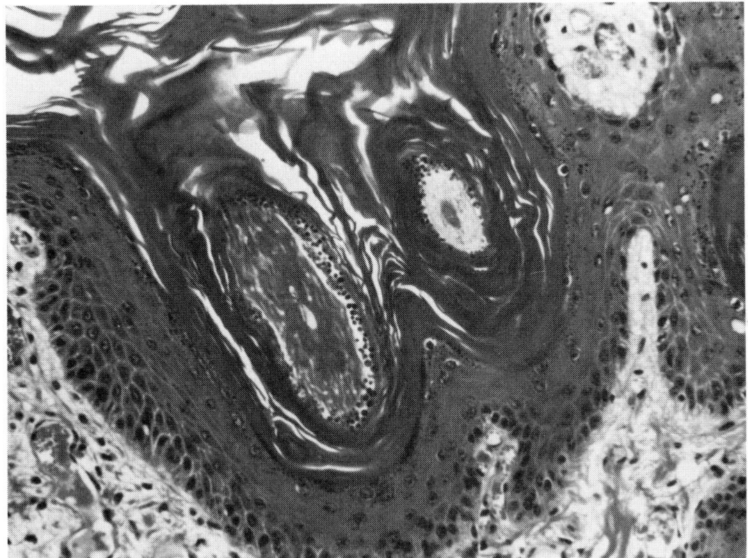

Figure 7–18

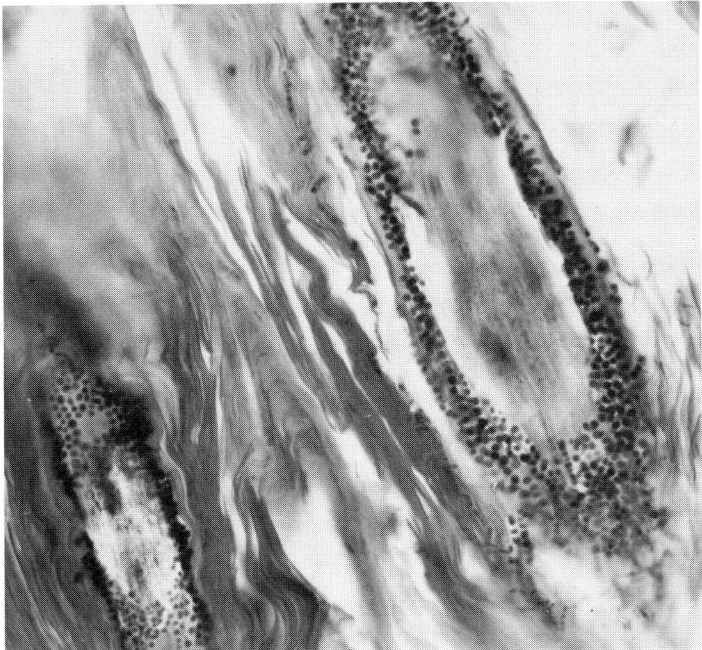

Figure 7–19

Figures 7–18 and 7–19. Spores of ringworm around hair follicles at different magnifications and planes of section.

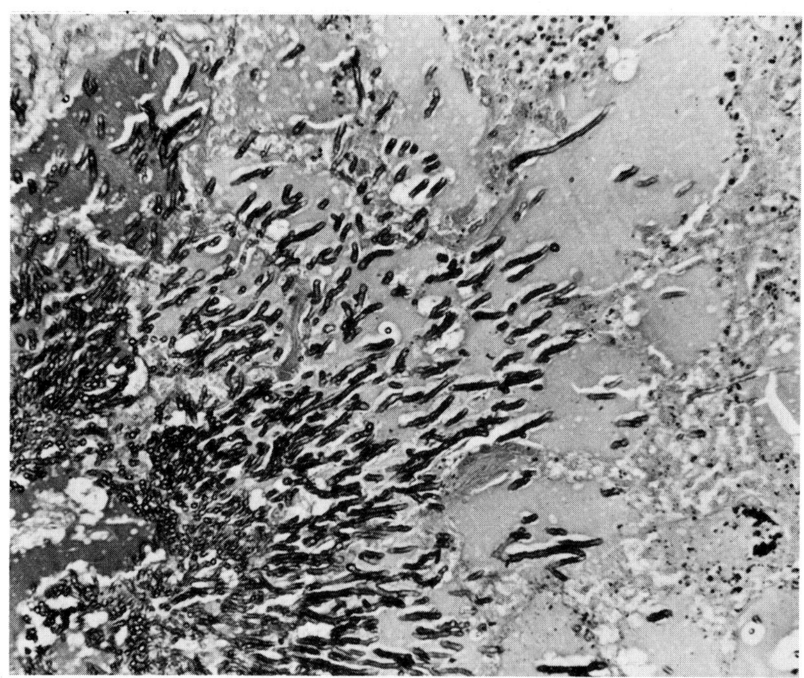

Figure 7–20

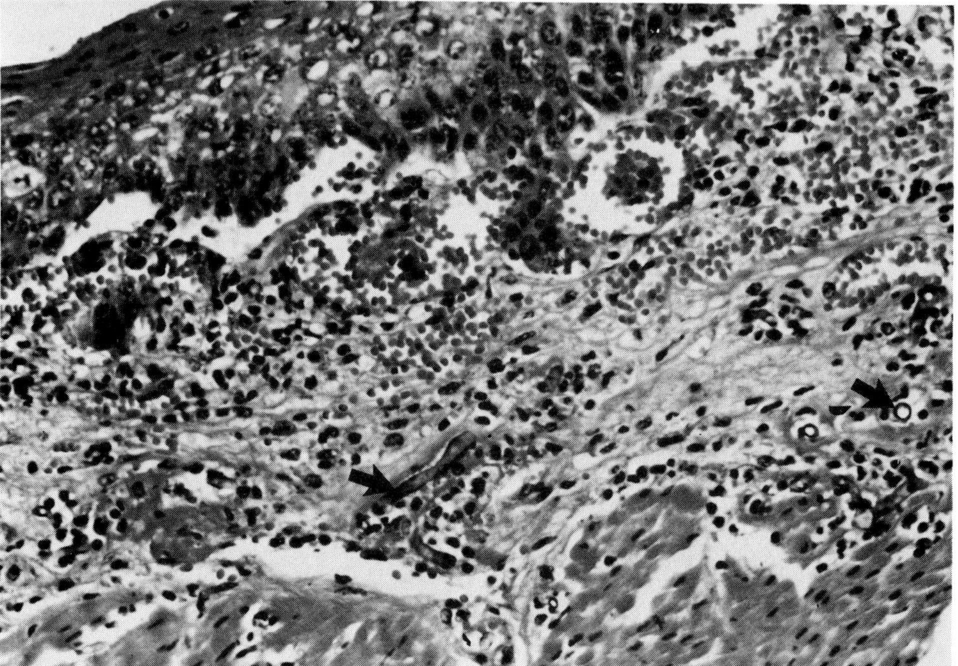

Figure 7–21

Figures 7–20 and 7–21. Fungal hyphae growing in a cow's lung (Fig. 7–20) (arrows) and in the submucosa of rumenal epithelium of a steer (Fig. 7–21). Each could be a sequel to mycotic rumenitis and grain overload (see Fig. 2–10).

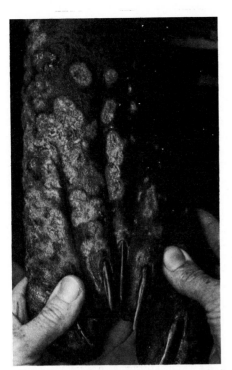

Figure 7–22. Chronic mycotic infection caused by Fusarium species on the flipper of a gray seal. (From Montali, R. J., et al.: Cyclic dermatitis associated with Fusarium sp. infection in pinnipeds. J. Am. Vet., Med. Assoc., *179*:1198, 1981. Reprinted by permission.)

The literature on environmental toxins is expanding rapidly.*

Many toxins cause minimal morphological lesions or induce quite nonspecific lesions. The history in a particular case may be essential in suggesting a toxin as a possible cause of death. Some toxins produce quite specific lesions that lead directly to a diagnosis. Often, local geographic or environmental influences account for diseases due to toxins.

Immune mechanisms involved in host-parasite disease mechanisms have been discussed in the chapter on inflammation (pages 229 to 249).

*The following figures illustrate lesions caused by or associated with toxins:

Chapter 2: Figures 2–10, 2–11, 2–68, 2–69, 2–86, 2–114, 2–119, 2–120.

Chapter 3: Figures 3–19, 3–39.

Chapter 4: Figures 4–151, 4–152.

Cause of Death

At the beginning of this book, reference was made to the difficulty of determining illness in that an individual may seem quite healthy with no signs of clinical disease, but in fact, may have a serious lesion which is close to being fatal. This point exemplifies the difficulty in making direct correlations between clinically apparent disease and serious disease in a tissue or organ that is life-threatening but not apparent. In food-producing animals the most serious diseases may be subclinical diseases that do not kill but which reduce growth rates and productivity. In some types of livestock, much greater economic loss occurs from feeding animals with subclinical disease than from losses caused by death from clinical disease. Producers often fail to appreciate this point and usually will not believe it until shown the calculations that substantiate the facts in dollar figures. In these circumstances the detection, treatment, and prevention of subclinical disease becomes the most important economic factor in increasing production and profit.

The difficulty in making clinical correlation with disease states in the live animal carries through to making direct correlations between clinical signs and lesions found during postmortem examination. Many times the correlations are excellent but still may be quite surprising from the standpoint of time. The massive pneumonic lesions in a steer with so-called shipping fever may be difficult to correlate with the animals *apparently* being clinically ill for one day or even found dead without clinical signs. Very often the lesions found in some diseases do not correlate well with clinical signs, and the lesions seem quite minor in relationship to the reported clinical signs. This situation is frustrating to the clinician. However, in time, both clinicians and pathologists recognize that this lack of correlation is reasonably common, and such situations should press both specialists to greater efforts in quantitating the degree of illness or lesions, finding better ways of evaluating illness and lesions, and learning more about disease processes.

Perhaps most important, the problems in correlations bring a much greater appreciation and respect for physiology, physiological adaptation and reserve, and the ability of compensatory mechanisms to protect the host. To the serious investigator or observer of disease, this appreciation increases steadily with time. It seems impossible that a dog with a small, severely atrophied, lumpy liver could have been clinically sick for only a week. A horse destroyed for chronic lameness has morphological lesions which seem insignificant, and another horse dead of colic with no history of lameness has impressive joint lesions which would be expected to result in serious clinical signs. This type of inconsistency is most apparent in the case of nervous system lesions. The difference is between the *expected* and the *observed* in relationship to the functional change, the gross lesions, and the microscopic lesions. There is an explanation, and an effort should be made to search for it.

Even the apparent lack of correlation between gross and microscopic lesions may be frustrating for the pathologist. This problem may be related to the lack of careful observation and recognition of gross lesions and the lack of appreciation of the pathogenesis and significance of microscopic lesions. However, given these limitations, some situations defy understanding. How could a particular animal be killed by what seems to be a very minor lesion or how could another possibly have lived so long with such massive lesions? Much more must be learned before these questions can be answered.

Disease → Etiology → Pathogenesis → Lesions → Diagnosis → Prognosis

SUGGESTIONS FOR FURTHER READING

General

Alexander, J. W.: Host defense mechanisms against infection. Surg. Clin. North Am., *52*:1367–1378, 1972.

Altura, B. M.: Reticuloendothelial cells and host defense. Adv. Microcirc., *9*:252–294, 1980.

Bellanti, J. A., and Dayton, D. H. (eds.): The Phagocytic Cell in Host Resistance. New York, Raven Press, 1975.

Cheville, N. F.: Environmental factors affecting the immune response of birds—a review. Avian Dis., *23*:308–314, 1979.

Donaldson, A. I.: Factors influencing the dispersal, survival, and deposition of airborne pathogens of farm animals. Vet. Bull., *48*:83–94, 1978.

Evans, A. S.: Causation and disease: the Henle-Koch postulates revisited. Yale J. Biol. Med., *49*:175–195, 1976.

Evans, A. S.: Causation and disease: a chronological journey. Am. J. Epidemiol., *108*:249–258, 1978.

Hutt, F. B.: Genetic Resistance to Disease in Domestic Animals. Ithaca, Cornell University Press (Comstock), 1958.

Kahrs, R. F., et al.: Diseases transmitted from pets to man: an evolving concern for veterinarians. Cornell Vet., *68*:442–459, 1978.

Keusch, G. T.: Specific membrane receptors: pathogenetic and therapeutic implications in infectious diseases. Rev. Inf. Dis., *1*:517–529, 1979.

Krakowa, S.: Transplacentally acquired microbial and parasitic diseases of dogs. J. Am. Vet. Med. Assoc., *171*:750–757, 1977.

Mackowiak, P. A.: Microbial synergism in human infection. N. Engl. J. Med., *298*:21–26, 83–87, 1978.

McGuire, T. C., et al.: An evaluation of contributions derived from investigation of equine immunodeficiencies. Vet. Imm. Immunopathol., *2*:101–110, 1981.

Mims, C. A.: The Pathogenesis of Infectious Disease. 2nd ed. New York, Academic Press, 1982.

Moulder, J. W.: Intracellular parasitism: life in an extreme environment. J. Infect. Dis., *130*:300–306, 1974.

Mudd, S. (ed.): Infectious Agents and Host Reactions. Philadelphia, W. B. Saunders Co., 1970.

Perryman, L. E.: Primary and secondary immune deficiencies of domestic animals. Adv. Vet. Sci. Comp. Med., *23*:23–52, 1979.

Peterson, P.: A perspective of infection and infectious disease. Perspect. Biol. Med., *23*:255–272, 1980.

Polk, H. C., et al.: Dissemination and causes of infection. Surg. Clin. North Am., *56*:817–829, 1976.

Roy, J. H. B.: Factors affecting susceptibility of calves to disease. J. Dairy Sci., *63*:650–664, 1980.

Sabin, A. B.: Overview and horizons in prevention of some human infectious diseases by vaccination. Am. J. Clin. Pathol., *70*:114–127, 1978.

Smith, H.: Microbial surfaces in relation to pathogenecity. Bacteriol. Rev., *41*:475–500, 1977.

Smith, H., and Pearce, J. H. (eds.): Microbial Pathogenicity in Man and Animals. Cambridge, The University Press, 1972.

Stevens, D. R., and Osburn, B. I.: Immune deficiency in a dog with distemper. J. Am. Vet. Med. Assoc., *168*:493–498, 1976.

Weinberg, E. G.: Iron and infection. Microbiol. Rev., *42*:45–66, 1978.

Weinstein, A. J., and Farkas, S.: Serologic tests in infectious diseases: Clinical utility and interpretation. Med. Clin. North Am., *62*:1099–1117, 1978.

Youmans, G. P., et al.: The Biologic and Clinical Basis of Infectious Diseases. Philadelphia, W. B. Saunders Company, 1975.

Bacterial Diseases

Adler, J.: The behavior of bacteria: on the mechanism of sensory transduction in bacterial chemotaxis. Johns Hopkins Med. J., *144*:121–126, 1979.

Aly, R., et al.: Bacterial adherence to nasal mucosal cells. Infect. Immun., *17*:546–549, 1977.

Arbuthnott, J. P.: Role of exotoxins in bacterial pathogenicity. J. Appl. Bacteriol., *44*:329–345, 1978.

Bailie, W. E., et al.: Aerobic bacterial flora of oral and nasal fluids of canines with reference to bacteria associated with bites. J. Clin. Microbiol., *7*:223–231, 1978.

Beachey, E. H.: Bacterial adherence: adhesin-receptor interactions mediating the attachment of bacteria to mucosal surfaces. J. Infect. Dis., *143*:325–345, 1981.

Berry, L. J.: Bacterial toxins. CRC Crit. Rev. Toxicol., *5*:239–318, 1977.

Boyd, A., and Simon, M.: Bacterial chemotaxis. Ann. Rev. Physiol., *44*:501–517, 1982.

Costerton, J. W., et al.: The role of bacterial surface structures in pathogenesis. CRC Crit. Rev. Microbiol., *8*:303–338, 1981.

Culbertson, R., and Osburn, B. I.: The biologic effects of bacterial endotoxin: a short review. Vet. Sci. Comm., *4*:3–14, 1980.

Deem, D. A.: Liver abscesses in cattle. Comp. Cont. Educ., *11*:12, S268–S274, 1980.

Dye, E. S., and Kapral, F..: Survival of *Staphylococcus aureus* in intraperitoneal abscesses. J. Med. Microbiol., *14*:185–194, 1981.

Garcia, M. M., et al.: Hepatic lesions and bacterial changes in mice during infection of *Fusobacterium necrophorum*. Can. J. Microbiol., *23*:1465–1477, 1977.

Gould, G. W.: Recent advances in the understanding of resistance and dormancy in bacterial spores. J. Appl. Bacteriol., *42*:297–309, 1977.

Hahn, H., and Kaufmann, S. H. E.: The role of cell-mediated immunity in bacterial infections. Rev. Inf. Dis., *3*:1221–1250, 1981.

Hirsch, D. C., et al.: Obligate anaerobes in clinical veterinary practice. J. Clin. Microbiol., *10*:188–191, 1979.

Johanson, W. G., et al.: Bacterial adherence to epithelial cells in bacillary colonization of the respiratory tract. Am. Rev. Resp. Dis., *121*:55–63, 1980.

Kannangara, D. W., et al.: Animal model for anaerobic lung abscess. Infect. Immun., *31*:592–597, 1981.

Kasper, D. K., and Finegold, S. M. (eds.): Virulence factors of anaerobic bacteria. Rev. Inf. Dis., *1*:245–400, 1979.

Kihlstrom, E., and Soderlung, G.: Endocytosis in mammalian nonprofessional phagocytes, with special reference to the pathogenesis of invasive micro-organisms. Monogr. Allergy, *17*:148–170, 1981.

Lindsey, J. R., et al.: Diseases due to mycoplasmas and rickettsias. *In* Benirschke, K., et al. (eds.): Pathology of Laboratory Animals. New York, Springer-Verlag, 1978, pp. 1481–1550.

MacNab, R. M.: Bacterial motility and chemotaxis: the molecular biology of a behavioral system. CRC Crit. Rev. Biochem., *5*:291–341, 1978.

Mandel, T. E., and Cheers, C.: Resistance and susceptibility of mice to bacterial infection: histopathology of listeriosis in resistant and susceptible strains. Infect. Immun., *30*:851–861, 1980.

Scott, D. W., et al.: Staphylococcal hypersensitivity in the dog. J. Am. Anim. Hosp. Assoc., *14*:766–779, 1978.

Tally, F. P., and Gorbach, S. L.: Clinical aspects of anaerobic infection. J. Infect., *1*:24–38, 1979.

Wing, E. J., and Young, J. B.: Acute starvation protects mice against *Listeria monocytogenes*. Infect. Immun., *28*:771–776, 1980.

Winter, A. J.: Mechanisms of immunity in bacterial infections. Adv. Vet. Sci. Comp. Med., *23*:53–69, 1979.

Viral Diseases

Allison, A. C.: Immunity and immunopathology in virus infections. Ann. Inst. Pasteur (Paris), *123*:585–608, 1972.

Cheville, N. F.: Cytopathology of Viral Diseases. Basel, S. Karger, 1975.

Cork, L. C., and Narayan, O.: The pathogenesis of viral leukoenceophalomyelitis-arthritis of goats. I. Persistent viral infection with progressive pathologic changes. Lab. Invest., *42*:596–602, 1980.

Dales, S.: Early events in cell-animal virus interactions. Bacteriol. Rev., *37*:103–135, 1973.

Dawson, M.: Maedi-visna: a review. Vet. Rec., *106*:212–216, 1980.

Hardy, W. D.: The feline leukemia virus. J. Am. Anim. Hosp. Assoc., *17*:954–980, 1981.

Hartley, W. J.: Post vaccinal inclusion body encephalitis in dogs. Vet. Pathol., *11*:301–312, 1974.

Hirsch, M. S., and Schwartz, M. N.: Antiviral agents. New Engl. J. Med., *302*:903–907, 949–953, 1980.

Hunt, R., et al.: Viral diseases. *In* Benirschke, K., et al. (eds.): Pathology of Laboratory Animals. New York, Springer-Verlag, 1978, pp. 1285–1366.

Jakab, G. J.: Mechanisms of virus-induced bacterial superinfections of the lung. Clin. Chest Med., *2*:59–66, 1981.

Kleinerman, E. S., et al.: Effects of virus infection on the inflammatory response. Am. J. Pathol., *85*:373–382, 1976.

Liggitt, H. D., and DeMartini, J. C.: The pathomorphology of malignant catarrhal fever. II. Multisystemic epithelial lesions. Vet. Pathol., *17*:73–83, 1980.

ter Meulen, V., and Hall, W. W.: Slow virus infections of the nervous system: virological, immunological, and pathogenetic considerations. J. Gen. Virol., *41*:1–25, 1978.

Mims, C. A.: General features of persistent virus infections. Postgrad. Med. J., *54*:581–586, 1978.

Mogensen, S. C.: Role of macrophages in natural resistance to virus infections. Microbiol. Rev., *43*:1–26, 1979.

Murphy, F. A.: Rabies pathogenesis. Arch Virol., *54*:279–297, 1977.

Notkins, A. L. (ed.): Viral Immunology and Immunopathology. New York, Academic Press, 1975.

Perryman, L. E.: Immunological mechanisms of injury in viral diseases. *In* Program of 31st Annual Meeting of American College of Veterinary Pathogists, New Orleans, December 1980, pp. 66–67.

Povey, C.: Viral diseases of cats: current concepts. Vet. Rec., *98*:293–299, 1976.

Rouse, B. T., and Babiuk, L. A.: Mechanisms of viral immunopathology. Adv. Vet. Sci. Comp. Med., *23*:104–137, 1979.

Shek, W. R., et al.: Natural and immune cytolysis of canine distemper virus infected target cells. Infect. Immun., *28*:724–734, 1980.

Weiss, R. C., and Scott, F. W.: Pathogenesis of feline infectious peritonitis: nature and development of viremia. Am. J. Vet. Res., *42*:382–390, 1981.

Weissman, R. M., and Droller, M. J.: Interferon: a perspective. Invest. Urol., *18*:189–196, 1980.

Parasitic Diseases

Anderson, R. M.: Depression of host population abundance by direct life cycle macroparasites. J. Theor. Biol., *82*:283–311, 1980.

Armour, J.: Bovine ostertagiasis: a review. Vet. Rec., *86*:184–190, 1970.

Bloom, B. R.: Games parasites play: how parasites evade immune surveillance. Nature, *279*:21–26, 1979.

Brasitus, T. A.: Parasites and malabsorption. Am. J. Med., *67*:1058–1065, 1979.

Crompton, D. W. T.: The sites occupied by some parasitic helminths in the alimentary tract of vertebrates. Biol. Rev., *48*:27–83, 1973.

Gaafar, S. M.: Pathology of Parasitic Diseases. Lafayette, Purdue University Studies, 1971.

Healey, M. C., and Gaafar, S. M.: Immunodeficiency in canine demodectic mange. I. Experimental production of lesions using antilymphocyte serum. Vet. Parasitol., *3*:121–131, 1977.

Lackie, A. M.: The activation of infective stages of endoparasites of vertebrates. Biol. Rev., *50*:285–323, 1975.

Michel, J. F.: Morphological changes in a parasitic nematode due to acquired resistance of the host. Nature, *215*:520–521, 1967.

Ogilvie, B. M.: Evasion of the immune response by parasites. Br. Med. Bull., *32*:177–181, 1976.

Poynter, D.: Some tissue reactions to the nematode parasites of animals. Adv. Parasitol., *4*:321–383, 1966.

Preston, J. M., and Allenby, E. W.: The influence of haemoglobin phenotype on the susceptibility of sheep to *Haemonchus contortus* infection in Kenya. Res. Vet. Sci., *26*:140–144, 1979.

Ristic, M.: Immunologic systems and protection in infections caused by intracellular blood protista. Vet. Parasitol., *2*:31–47, 1976.

Shadduck, J., and Pakes, S. P.: Protozoal and metazoal diseases. *In* Benirschke, et al. (eds.): Pathology of Laboratory Animals. New York, Springer-Verlag, 1978, pp. 1587–1696.

Sinclair, I. J.: The relationship between circulating antibodies and immunity to helminthic infections. Adv. Parasitol., *8*:97–138, 1970.

Soulsby, E. J. L.: Pathophysiology of Parasitic Infection. New York, Academic Press, 1976.

Soulsby, E. J. L.: The immune system and helminth infection in domestic animals. Adv. Vet. Sci. Comp. Med., *23*:71–103, 1979.

Toft, J. D., II, and Ekstrom, M. E.: Identification of metazoan parasites in tissue sections. *In* Montali, R. J., and Migaki, G. (eds.): The Comparative Pathology of Zoo Animals. Washington, Smithsonian Institution, 1980, pp. 369–378.

Fungal Diseases

Gravesen, S.: Fungi as a cause of allergic disease. Allergy, *34*:135–154, 1979.

Hayes, A. W.: Biological activities of mycotoxins. Mycopathologia, *65*:29–41, 1978.

Hayes, A. W.: Mycotoxins: a review of biological effects and their role in human diseases. Clin. Toxicol., *17*:45–83, 1980.

Jungerman, P. F., and Schwartzman, R. M.: Veterinary Medical Mycology. Philadelphia, Lea & Febiger, 1972.

Newberne, P. M., and Butler, W. H.: Acute and chronic effects of aflatoxin on the liver of domestic and laboratory animals. A Review. Cancer Res., *29*:236–250, 1969.

Pier, A. C.: Mycotoxins and animal health. Adv. Vet. Sci. Comp. Med., *25*:186–244, 1981.

Toxic Diseases

Aronson, A. L.: Chemical poisonings in small animal practice. Vet. Clin. North Am., *2*:379–395, 1972.

Barnes, J. M.: Mechanisms of toxicity: introduction. Br. Med. Bull., *25*:219–222, 1969.

Boyd, M. R.: Biochemical mechanisms in chemical-induced lung injury: roles of metabolic activation. CRC Crit. Rev. Toxicol., *8*:103–176, 1980.

Buck, W. B., et al.: Clinical and Diagnostic Veterinary Toxicology. Ames, Iowa State University Press, 1973.

Gerber, G. B., et al.: Toxicity, mutagenicity and teratogenicity of lead. Mutat. Res., *76*:115–141, 1980.

Gibson, J. R.: Monitoring methods and problems in aquatic and wildlife toxicology. *In* Gralla, E. J. (ed.): Scientific Considerations in Monitoring and Evaluating Toxicological Research. Washington, Hemisphere Publishing Corp., 1981.

Goldberg, L.: Toxicology: has a new era dawned? Pharmacol. Rev., *30*:351–370, 1979.

Humphreys, D. J.: A review of recent trends in animal poisoning. Br. Vet. J., *134*:128–145, 1978.

James, L. F., et al.: Plants Poisonous to Livestock in the Western States. U.S. Department of Agriculture Bull., No. 415, 1980.

Kingsbury, M.: Poisonous Plants of the United States and Canada. Englewood Cliffs, N.J., Prentice-Hall, Inc., 1964.

Koller, L. D.: Effects of environmental contaminants on the immune system. Adv. Vet. Sci. Comp. Med., *23*:267–295, 1979.

Krook, L., and Maylin, G. A.: Industrial fluoride pollution—chronic fluoride poisoning in Cornwall Island cattle. Cornell Vet., *69*(Suppl. 8):7–70, 1979.

Parke, D. V., and Williams, R. T.: Metabolism of toxic substances. Br. Med. Bull., *25*:256–262, 1969.

Rubin, E., and Lieber, C. S.: The effects of ethanol on the liver. Int. Rev. Exp. Pathol., *11*:177–232, 1972.

Smith, H. A., et al.: Veterinary Pathology. 5th ed. Philadelphia, Lea & Febiger, 1982.

Pritchard, J. B.: Toxic substances and cell membrane function. Fed. Proc., *38*:2220–2225, 1979.

APPENDIX I

PROCESSING AND HANDLING TISSUES; EXAMINATION AND NAMING OF LESIONS

Pieces of tissues should be collected as soon after death as possible. Each piece should be no more than 1 cm thick, which suggests that narrow slices of variable length and width should be selected. It is advisable to select tissues from most organs in order to have them available for examination in case they should be required. If not obtained at the time of necropsy, they cannot be used.

FIXATION

Fixation stops all enzymic processes in tissue, hardens the tissue for further processing and kills microorganisms. The volume of fixative should be 10 times that of the tissue. Nonprotein precipitants form additive compounds with tissue proteins. The best known of these is formalin. It is usually purchased as 37 per cent to 40 per cent formaldehyde, which is known as 100 per cent formalin. This solution should be diluted at the ratio of nine parts water to one part formalin for a 10 per cent solution and should be isotonic and buffered to prevent the distortion of cells and the formation of formalin pigment (100 ml formaldehyde, 900 ml tap water, 4 gm sodium monophosphate, 6.5 gm sodium diphosphate). Protein precipitating fixatives, such as Bouin's or Zenker's, are better fixatives but more expensive and take time to prepare. Most fixatives result in some degree of artifact, mostly shrinkage, which may be up to 25 per cent when formalin is used.

Tissues are fixed in 4 per cent glutaraldehyde for examination by electron microscopy, and the tissue must be cut into 1 mm cubes for proper fixation. These are embedded in resins and cut on an ultramicrotome. Fixatives are available that allow for processing for routine slide preparation as well as for electron microscopy. One of these is made as follows: 1.16 gm of NaH_2PO_4 in water; 0.27 gm of NaOH; 88 ml of H_2O; 10 ml of 40 per cent formaldehyde and 2 ml of 50 per cent glutaraldehyde.

PROCESSING

Once the tissue is fixed in formalin for 24 to 48 hours, small pieces 1 to 2 cm by 2 to 3 mm are selected for slide preparation. The tissues are passed through a series of alcohol solutions for complete dehydration and then through a clearing agent, such as xylol, before embedding in paraffin. Alcohol is not soluble in paraffin so xylol, which is soluble, must be used. Paraffin is used to hold the tissue for cutting very thin (5 to 6 micrometers) slices on a microtome. The thin slices of tissue are floated on water, picked up on slides and dried for staining.

STAINING

The routine stain for most purposes is hematoxylin and eosin. The eosin is an acid dye that stains the tissue red; the tissue is called acidophilic because it takes the acid stain. Hematoxylin is a basic stain and stains the basophilic nuclei bluish. The stains are actually neutral salts with polar radicals. Numerous special stains are available that selectively stain certain components of tissue for specific identification. All require positive controls for accurate interpretation. Lipid, iron, calcium, mucopolysaccharide, collagen, muscle, axons, myelin, astrocytes, bacteria, fungi and a host of other specific cells and components can be identified with special stains. For some purposes, their use requires the artist's touch. The manual from the Armed Forces Institute of Pathology outlines most stains and a book by Thompson (1966) discusses the reactions of stains in detail.

Some procedures require the use of fresh frozen tissues cut on a cryostat. Fluorescent antibody stains may be used to identify the specific antigens of microorganisms or the specific immunoglobulins in tissues. This procedure aids in rapid, specific identification of agents in tissues and is used particularly for viruses. Tissue sections are also used for autoradiographic localization of compounds in tissues. An animal is injected with a labeled isotope and the tissues are taken and cut into thin slices that are laid on film for development. The location of the labeled compound will be visible on the film overlay.

BIOPSY

Biopsy is the removal and examination of tissue from a live animal. Pieces may be selected for routine processing, but considerable information and often the specific diagnosis may be obtained by needle biopsy, touch imprint preparation or smears of spun down cells from fluids. Care and cleanliness are prerequisites for these procedures. Needle biopsy can be carried out with a 22 gauge needle; the content is smeared on slides, two slides are fixed in alcohol for Papanicolaou's stain and a duplicate slide is air-dried for Wright's stain. Impression smears may be prepared for staining in a similar manner.

QUANTITATION OF LESIONS

The two papers listed (Kapanci et al. [1969] and Striker et al. [1970]) provide ***examples*** of the degree of quantitation of the components of microscopic lesions that is possible, as well as the specific correlation of microscopic lesions with biochemical assessment of the functional abnormalities of the lesion. They illustrate what can be accomplished and will serve as a stimulus for other workers to do similar definitive work.

POSTMORTEM EXAMINATION

The books by Winter (1966) and Jones and Gleiser (1954) clearly describe and illustrate a method of postmortem procedure. Most laboratories have their own minor modifications. Rooney (1970) describes the procedures for horses and also describes the lesions commonly found in horses. This book should be available to those interested in horses, although not everyone would follow his method of opening a carcass.

For most domestic species, aside from horses, the carcass may be opened as follows. Lay the animal on its left side and make a ventral midline incision from the tip of the jaw to the pubis. Reflect the skin dorsally to the dorsal midline along with the front limb. Split the pelvis at the symphysis with a saw and open by pulling the right hind leg so as to apply pressure for splitting. The mandible is split to allow observation of the oral cavity. Remove the abdominal muscles along the ventral midline, the edge of the rib cage and the edge of the lumbar vertebrae. Pruning shears will break the ribs along the spine and at the xyphoid region and will allow the thoracic cavity to be opened. Skin the limbs well down and open several joints. All of the viscera should now be visible, and each part can be examined in detail. Look at the adrenals and pancreas before removing any viscera. The most important part is to open the carcass carefully so that all parts may be examined with ease. The brain is removed after ventral disarticulation of the atlantooccipital joint. Formalin, sterile plastic bags and swabs and sharp instruments should be available, as well as water, disinfectant, rubber gloves and a suitable location.

Submit well-fixed tissues of proper size in labeled bottles along with a clinical history and description of gross lesions. Frozen tissues for microbiological or toxicological examination may be required.

Much of the pathologist's time is concerned with performing autopsies, and the paper by King and Meehan (1973) is quite expressive regarding this function. The following quotation comes from their paper:

> It is a pernicious misconception that the mere performance of postmortem dissection leads to progress in medical science . . . progress depends not on the autopsy but on the person

who is examining the material. Those who believe that the more autopsies we perform, the more medical science will progress, are pleading not for more autopsies but for more persons who can profitably utilize the data of autopsies, persons who have imagination, originality, persistence, mental acuity, sound education and background, the indispensable "prepared mind" without which observations are quite sterile. It is a grave disservice to confuse the performance of autopsies with the spark of insight which the autopsy may trigger. We want the insight; and autopsies alone, no matter how numerous, are not the equivalent.

EXAMINATION AND NAMING OF LESIONS

DESCRIBING GROSS LESIONS

An accurate morphological description of a lesion will usually elicit what the lesion is. The usual features contained in a description are as follows:

Location. Precisely describe the location and extent of the lesion. For example, the anterior ventral one third of both lungs . . . entire caudal pole of the left kidney . . . ten centimeters above the ileocecal valve there is a small . . . both lungs are uniformly involved in a diffuse. . . .

Color. Most lesions are recognized by color changes. Many relate directly or indirectly to the circulatory system. Therefore, many descriptions involve the use of red, dark red, purple, black, bright red, pink, pale, white, etc. Masses of new abnormal tissue may be a variety of colors.

Size. Accurately state the size of lesions. Estimate the percentage of an organ or tissue which is abnormal. Discrete lesions can be measured accurately.

Shape. Lesions may be round, flat, irregular, oblong, pedunculated, discrete, diffuse, irregular, and so forth.

Consistency. Usual terms include comparisons with the normal texture of the tissue containing the lesion and include: rubbery, firm, hard, fluid, semisolid, and so forth.

Cut Surface. The cut surface of a lesion may be similar to the outer or visible surface, but many times it is quite different or may present several features that are not apparent from the outside. For example, a discrete mass visible on the surface may actually be an abscess or a tumor or a granuloma, according to the features visible on the cut surface.

NAMING OF GROSS LESIONS

An accurate gross description should lead to precise naming of a lesion by ***deduction*** from the characteristics and components of the lesion. Knowledge of the processes involved in ***general pathology*** includes the ability to recognize these processes in tissues. The task of describing lesions includes ***recognition of the components of the lesion*** such as the various types of inflammatory exudates, the appearance of degenerate or necrotic tissue, the appearance of hyperemic or congested tissue, the colors of abnormal pigments or the presence of abnormal masses of new tissue. The components tend to indicate the process.

ESTIMATING EXTENT AND SEVERITY OF GROSS LESIONS

Included in the naming of lesions is an estimate of the degree of ***severity,*** such as ***mild, moderate*** or ***severe,*** and also an indication of the ***age*** of the lesion, such as ***acute, subacute*** or ***chronic.*** The extent of lesions is defined by accurate measurement or an assessment of the percentage of the organ or tissue affected.

The following are examples of names of lesions:

moderate acute focal infarction
extensive multifocal caseous necrosis
diffuse mild congestion
diffuse extensive hyperemia
severe chronic passive congestion
diffuse moderate ecchymotic hemorrhage
severe acute hemorrhagic enteritis
moderate acute catarrhal enteritis
severe acute necrotizing tracheitis

moderate subacute catarrhal bronchopneumonia
extensive multifocal granulomatous dermatitis
moderate chronic purulent hepatitis
moderate chronic linear fibrosis
severe chronic diffuse renal fibrosis
moderate multifocal hepatic nodular hyperplasia
moderate diffuse thyroid atrophy
focal intestinal segmental aplasia
extensive diffuse metastatic pulmonary neoplasia
solitary large neoplastic mass
extensive metastatic implantation

NAMES OF COMMON LESIONS WITHIN VARIOUS BODY SYSTEMS

The following are names of some lesions that occur in the various body systems of animals. The "qualifiers" of time and extent are not included, but would be required for accurate naming. The purpose of the list is to provide an introduction to the names used in *special pathology* of body systems and to emphasize that the terminology of *general pathology* applies to most of the terms. The list is not complete but includes many of the most common lesions.

Respiratory System

atelectasis
bronchopneumonia
embolic pneumonia
emphysema
empyema
fibrinous pneumonia
gangrenous pneumonia
granulomatous pneumonia
interstitial pneumonia
metastatic pulmonary neoplasia
necrotizing bronchiolitis
necrotizing laryngitis
necrotizing tracheitis
pleuritis
pulmonary abscess
pulmonary carcinoma
pulmonary congestion
pulmonary edema
pulmonary hemorrhage
purulent rhinitis
purulent sinusitis

Digestive System

abomasitis
bloat
catarrhal enteritis
dental tartar
diphtheritic enteritis
esophagitis
fibrinous enteritis
gastric mucosal infarction
gastric torsion
gastric ulceration
gastritis
glossitis
granulomatous enteritis
hemorrhagic enteritis
intestinal carcinoma
intestinal infarction
intestinal torsion
intussusception
periodontitis
pharyngitis
rumenitis
stomatitis
tonsillitis

Urinary System

amyloidosis
calcification
congenital cysts
cystitis
glomerulonephritis
granulomatous nephritis
hemoglobinuria
hydronephrosis
interstitial nephritis
nephrosis
purulent nephritis
pyelonephritis
renal calculus
renal carcinoma
renal cortical necrosis
renal dysplasia
renal hypoplasia
renal infarction
transitional cell carcinoma
urethritis

Integumentary System

acanthosis
alopecia
atrophy
basal cell tumor
crusts
dermatitis
epitheliogenesis imperfecta
fissure
folliculitis
gangrene
histiocytoma
hyperkeratosis
hypotrichosis
inclusion cyst
macule
mast cell tumor
melanoma
necrosis
papilloma
papule
parakeratosis
perianal gland adenoma
pustule
scales
seborrhea
squamous cell carcinoma
vesicle
wheal

Female Genital System

abortion
cervicitis
congenital cysts

cystic corpus luteum
cystic graafian follicle
cystic uterine hyperplasia
endometritis
granulosa cell tumor
intersex
luteinized cyst
mammary dysplasia
mammary neoplasia
mastitis
metritis
ovarian carcinoma
ovarian hypoplasia
parovarian cysts
placentitis
pyometra
salpingitis
segmental uterine aplasia
uterine carcinoma
uterine leiomyoma
vaginitis

Male Genital System

balanoposthitis
canine venereal tumor
carcinoma of the penis
epididymal segmental aplasia
epididymitis
interstitial cell tumor
orchitis
penile fibroma
prostatitis
prostatic carcinoma
seminal vesiculitis
seminoma
Sertoli cell tumor
sperm granuloma
testicular degeneration
testicular hypoplasia

Liver

atrophy
bile duct carcinoma
cholangiohepatitis
diffuse hepatitis
focal hepatic necrosis
granulomatous hepatitis
hepatocellular carcinoma
lipidosis
massive necrosis
nodular hyperplasia
passive congestion
periacinar necrosis
purulent hepatitis

Pancreas

atrophy
carcinoma
diabetes
nodular hyperplasia
pancreatitis

Peritoneum

ascites
fat necrosis
mesothelioma
metastatic neoplasia
peritonitis

Circulatory System

arteriosclerosis
arteritis
atherosclerosis
dilated heart
endocarditis
endocardiosis
fibrinoid necrosis
hemangioma
hemangiopericytoma
hemangiosarcoma
infarction
lymphangiectasia
lymphangitis
myocardial degeneration
myocardial hypertrophy
myocarditis
phlebitis
thrombosis

Bones and Joints

arthritis
chondrodystrophy
chondrosarcoma
degenerative arthropathy
fluorine toxicity
osteodystrophia fibrosa
osteitis
osteogenic sarcoma
osteomalacia
osteomyelitis
osteophyte
osteoporosis
osteosis
prolapsed intervertebral disc
rickets
skeletal dysplasia
spondylosis
tenovaginitis

Hematopoietic System

anemia
caseous lymphadenitis
granulomatous lymphadenitis
purulent lymphadenitis
hemorrhagic diathesis
hemorrhagic splenitis
lymphadenitis
lymphosarcoma and related tumors
marrow dysplasia
myelogenous leukemia
purpura
purulent lymphadenitis
reticuloendothelial hyperplasia
splenic nodular hyperplasia
splenic siderotic nodules
splenic torsion
splenitis
splenomegaly
thymic atrophy

Endocrine System

adrenal cortical adenoma
atrophy
congenital cysts
goiter
hyperplasia
nodular hyperplasia
pheochromocytoma
pituitary abscess
pituitary adenoma
thyroid carcinoma
thyroiditis

Muscle

arthrogryposis
atrophy
calcification

degeneration
dystrophy
eosinophilic myositis
gangrenous myositis
hemorrhage
myonecrosis
myositis
tendinitis

Nervous System

astrocytoma
cerebellar hypoplasia
cerebral edema
demyelination
encephalitis
encephalomalacia
encephalomyelitis
ependymoma
ganglionitis
gliosis
hemorrhage
hydranencephaly
hydrocephalus
hypomyelinogenesis
infarction
meningioma
meningitis
myelitis
myelodysplasia
neurofibroma
neuronolipidosis
oligodendroglioma
syringomyelia

Eye

anophthalmia
cataract
choroiditis
coloboma
conjunctivitis
corneal edema
epidermoid carcinoma
glaucoma
hypoplasia of the optic nerve
keratitis
microphthalmia
ophthalmitis
pannus
retinal atrophy
retinitis
uveitis

Ear

otitis externa
otitis media
hypoplasia

SUGGESTIONS FOR FURTHER READING

Technical Procedures

A debate on the autopsy: its quality control function in medicine. Hum. Pathol., *5*:605–618, 1974.

Armed Forces Institute of Pathology: Manual of Histologic and Special Staining Techniques. 2nd ed. New York, McGraw-Hill Book Company, 1960.

DeRoy, A. K: The autopsy as a teaching-learning tool for medical undergraduates. J. Med. Educ., *51*:1016–1018, 1976.

Jones, T. C., and C. A. Gleiser (eds.): Veterinary Necropsy Procedures. Philadelphia, J. B. Lippincott Co., 1954.

Kapanci, Y., et al.: Pathogenesis and reversibility of the pulmonary lesions of oxygen toxicity in monkeys. II. Ultrastructural and morphometric studies. Lab. Invest., *20*:101–118, 1969.

King, L. S., and Meehan, M. C.: A history of the autopsy. Am. J. Pathol. *73*:514–544, 1973.

Rooney, J. R.: Autopsy of the Horse—Technique & Interpretation. Baltimore, The Williams & Wilkins Co., 1970.

Schlumberger, H. G.: Manual of experiments in pathology. Lab. Invest., *8*(Suppl):1017–1145, 1959.

Striker, G. E., et al.: Structural-functional correlations in renal disease. Part I: A method for assaying and classifying histopathologic changes in renal disease. Hum. Pathol., *1*:615–641, 1970.

Thompson, S. W.: Selected Histochemical and Histopathological Methods. Springfield, Illinois, Charles C Thomas, 1966.

Thompson, S. W., and Luna, L. C.: An Atlas of Artifacts: Encountered in Preparation of Microscopic Tissue Sections. Springfield, Illinois, Charles C Thomas, 1977.

Winter, H.: Post Mortem Examination of Ruminants. St. Lucia, Queensland, Australia, University of Queensland Press, 1966.

APPENDIX II

HISTORICAL ASPECTS OF PATHOLOGY

A History of Pathology by E. R. Long is a must for anyone with a keen interest in pathology. It is a delightfully readable but short and imaginative book that covers the major civilizations up to modern times. Long explains the basics of ***humoral pathology,*** the four humors from Hippocrates and the works of Celsus and Galen and goes into detail about the influence of the Renaissance on the understanding of disease. It is interesting to follow the identification of lesions from organs to tissues to cells, culminating in the profound influence of Virchow on the ***cellular basis of disease.*** Long also wrote ***A History of American Pathology,*** in which veterinary pathology is mentioned. Leon Saunders has a specific interest in the history of veterinary pathology and has written several papers and a book on this topic; it is hoped that he will publish other articles on the subject.

There are a number of books and papers on the historical aspects of pathology, and a few references are included here to whet the appetite of interested persons. ***Diseases in Antiquity*** (Brothwell and Sandison) is highly recommended. The discipline of pathology has passed through an evolutionary process that still continues. A few references are included for those interested in recent changes. There is an Institute of the History of Medicine at the Medical School of Johns Hopkins University.

A glimpse of some historical aspects is appropriate here.

The oldest civilized people, the Chinese, Indians and Egyptians, believed in the demoniac nature of disease. The cause of disease was considered to be the displeasure of evil spirits with the individual in question, and the measures taken by the primitive medical man were directed toward appeasing these evil spirits.

> In the 5,000 years of shifting Egyptian dynasty before the Arabs swept across the banks of the Nile, three-quarters of a billion human bodies with all the ills to which flesh is heir passed under the hands of Egyptian embalmers. A large portion of these were opened in the process and countless of thousands of diseased hearts, shrunken, abscessed and tuberculous lungs, cirrhotic livers, enlarged and atrophied spleens, infected kidneys, hardened arteries and clotted veins in gigantic solemn procession must have been seen, handled, concealed in jars or thrown away. Of all the pathological knowledge that must have been occasionally, if momentarily obtained in these 50 centuries of monotonous and ruthless coarse dissection, scarcely a trace has survived in written records. (Long [1928])

With the arrival of Greek culture, a scientific study of medicine began and repudiation of demon worship occurred. From Hippocrates to Virchow, pathology was considered to be humoral. The introduction of ***humoral pathology*** is credited to Hippocrates of Cos who has, for this and other reasons, been honored with the name the Father of Medicine.

Humoral pathology taught that health was due to a correct mixture, a eucrasia (G. eu = well and krasis = mixing), of the four fluids of the body and that disease was due to an incorrect mixture, dyscrasia (G. dys = bad). The four elements of Greek philosophy, air, water, fire and earth, and the four qualities, moisture, cold, warmth and dryness, found their analogues in the four humors of the body: the ***blood,*** which was warm and moist like air; the ***phlegm,*** which was cold and moist like water; the ***yellow bile,*** which was warm and dry like fire; and the ***black bile,*** which was cold and dry like earth. The source of these humors was defined: for the blood, the heart; for the phlegm, the brain; for the yellow bile, the liver; and for the black bile, the spleen.

Humoral pathology was supported by three essential observations: 1. Diseases were often characterized by increased discharge of fluid, perspiration and fever, vomition, diarrhea, catarrhal discharge, exudation and transudation to the body cavities and so forth. 2. Blood was the vital tissue, and the individual died if exsanguinated. 3. The coagulation of blood was different in healthy and sick individuals. What was called phlegm by the pathologists is the same as our fibrin, a question of nomenclature only. The interpretation, however, was different. What nowadays is considered to be the *effect* of the disease was considered by the humoral pathologists to be the *cause.*

The role of the four humors in health and disease was summarized by one of the pupils of Hippocrates as follows (Long): "The body consists of blood, phlegm, the black bile and the yellow bile and that is its real nature in the fundament of health and disease. The body is then in the midst of health when a well balanced proportion exists between the four humors; on the other hand, the body suffers if one of these humors occurs too little or too late, or if it is separated from the other three." Too much phlegm in an organ, for instance, resulted from phlegm overfilling the brain and being transported to the organ in question and could result in widely varying diseases. Too much phlegm in the lungs caused pneumonia; too much in the abdominal cavity caused ascites; too much in the rectum caused hemorrhoids; and so on. In mild cases, the phlegm simply poured out through the natural tap of the brain, the nose, thus resulting in nasal catarrh. The black bile, however, was most feared as the greatest power of evil.

According to the Hippocratic concept, disease tended to pass through three stages: a raw preliminary stage, a ripening stage called the stage of coction or pepsis and finally a stage of crisis in which elimination of the superfluous humor or abnormal mixture of humors occurred. According to this doctrine, in the firmly grounded Hippocratic belief in the normal tendency of the body towards self-cure, certain symptoms of disease, such as fever, represented the effort of the body to preserve life through coction or cooking of the altered fluid, while others, the cough, vomition, diarrhea, sweating, ulceration and so on, signified the crises in which the excremental humors, formed through the process of coction, were expelled. Should the body be unable to accomplish coction or sustain crises the patient might die.

Postmortem examination of humans was not permitted during the early days of humoral pathology, and the pathologists had, therefore, very confused conceptions of normal anatomy in the morphological background of diseases. This did not prevent them from having very decided opinions concerning the organs and their functions, which no one could verify or deny.

There were several opponents to the Hippocratic theories in the early days. One such opposing theory was based on the belief that the arteries contained air and the veins contained blood and therefore two different circulatory systems were recognized—one for blood from the heart and the other for air from the lungs.

A great deal of history of the early humoral pathologists was recorded in the work of ***Celsus*** (30 BC to AD 30). His work, however, was not discovered and read until AD 1440. A great number of the conditions that are recognized today are well described in the work of Celsus but probably appear with somewhat different nomenclature.

Humoral pathology was brought to its height and most extreme development by Claudius ***Galen*** (AD 129–201), of Pergamos in Asia Minor, who lived most of his life in Rome. Long has made the statement that Galen is perhaps the greatest medical figure of all times. Through his eighty works, Galen held despotic authority over European medicine for thirteen centuries after his death, with all their errors and truths accepted as medical gospel. Galen's contributions to pathology must be judged from his having had no opportunities to perform postmortem examinations. Had Roman traditions licensed autopsy, there is no limit to what he might have learned. No man who ever lived would have made more of the opportunity.

With the passing of Galen, medicine entered into its long period of nonproductivity. The Middle Ages made few contributions to medicine, and in many respects, this period meant a return to the idol worshipping and theistic medicine of antiquity.

As with so many other fields of knowledge, the Renaissance brought forth great changes in medicine and pathology. The works of Galen were questioned and new investigations were made. One of the early names in this period is Antonio Benivieni of Florence, who lived about 1500. Benivieni was one of the first to publish autopsy records and, in fact, to request permission for autopsies and perform them. The 16th century is often called the century of anatomy. What is generally unappreciated is that it was only slightly less a century of pathological anatomy. The great anatomists Vesalius and Eustachius were all pathological anatomists as well.

One of the great men in the history of medicine from France was ***Fernel*** (1497–1558). He wrote textbooks on physiology, pathology and therapeutics. He was one of the first to write and describe diseases ***according to organs or parts of the body.*** He generally divided his diseases into those affecting parts above the diaphragm, those involving the parts below and external diseases. One of his books, entitled ***Pathologiae Libri,*** was the first medical work to be called a text of pathology. He described diseases of the stomach, liver, gallbladder, spleen, mesentery, pancreas, intestines, kidneys and the organs of the reproductive tract.

One of the great events in medicine and in pathology came in 1628 when William ***Harvey*** published his book that showed for the first time ***the circulation of the blood*** and the proper function of the heart. Until the work of Harvey was published, it was generally believed that the circulation of the blood was a simple ebb and flow in the arteries and veins. Probably no single discovery has been of more far-reaching effect in medicine or pathology.

Malpighi extended Harvey's work and discovered the capillaries and erythrocytes and made masterly microscopic descriptions of the kidney, lungs and spleen. Also of great significance during these times was the invention of the ***microscope*** by Hans and Zacharias Jannsen in Holland. Cornelius Drebbel, also of Holland, made a better microscope and the credit for the introduction of the instrument is really his. Another Dutchman, Leeuwenhoek, accomplished its ultimate popularization.

Modern pathology is said to have begun with ***Morgagni.*** During the 17th and 18th centuries, the chair of anatomy at Padua was held by three of the greatest men of anatomy and pathological anatomy—Malpighi, Valsalva and Morgagni. The work of Morgagni led to immediate abandonment of all preceding dissertations on pathological anatomy. The reason for this was the extraordinary completeness of ***correlation between clinical detail and postmortem revelations.*** Morgagni's inestimable service to the science of pathology was the emphasis on detail and thoroughness. He introduced nothing new in the way of method and made few discoveries. In no way did he revolutionize pathology, as Bichat and Virchow did, but he improved existing knowledge in every field he touched. After Morgagni, pathological anatomy could never again be slipshod or cursory; the new standards were too high.

The next major change in pathology was the emphasis on disease in ***specific organs*** and not just in the fluids of the body. Xavier ***Bichat*** (1771–1802) went beyond dealing with just organs. From his dissections, he pointed out that not just the organs but ***specific tissues within the organ*** could be involved separately. Bichat identified 21 different tissues, all without the use of a microscope.

Up to the 19th century, pathological anatomy had seen its greatest men in Italy (Benivieni, Malpighi, Valsalva, Morgagni), in France (Fernel, Bichat) and in England (Harvey, John Hunter). In the 19th century, the dominance changed to Germany. The last great humoral pathologist was Carl ***Rokitansky,*** who was a contemporary of Virchow's. He explained practically all diseases as a result of blood anomalies. In spite of this, he was considered to be the ablest descriptive pathologist of his or any day.

Pathology was completely reformed by the ***cellular teachings*** born in Germany. The inspiration for this development came from a remarkable man, Johannes ***Muller.*** As a preceptor of Schwann, Henle and Virchow, he was the source for both modern histology and cellular pathology.

Virchow went to great lengths in order to disprove the theory of ***spontaneous generation*** of cells. Long writes the following about Virchow:

> He proceeded to ***rebuild pathology on his true conception of the human body as an organized cell state,*** a social system of continuous development in which each microscopic unit performs its part. All fields of pathology were cleared by new knowledge. Inflammation, tumor growths, the degenerations etc. were to be thought of in

these cellular relations and in each of these fields Virchow himself led the way in bringing about the change. He deserves the title of "the father of pathology."

Virchow not only emphasized cells in pathology but also recognized that the biochemical changes in tissues and fluids were very significant, and he clearly forecast the development of ***clinical pathology.*** After 1860, Virchow turned his main interest in other directions—to anthropology and politics. He was the Liberal leader in the German parliament and as such was Bismark's strongest opponent.

Many of the technical procedures used in pathology today were developed in the late 1800's. Some of these were the following: freezing tissues for sectioning; the invention of the microtome; paraffin embedding; various fixatives, including formalin; and a great deal of work on staining procedures.

Not too distant from proceedings in pathology were the developments made in bacteriology and immunology. Such names as Jenner, Bassi, Henle, Pasteur, Lister, Koch, Klebs and many others produced a revolutionary change in microbiology.

Thus, the history of pathology passed through the ***theistic*** and ***humoral phases*** and is now in the ***cellular phase.*** A perusal of the literature, however, would make one wonder today if pathology is not again going somewhat in the direction of humoral pathology. Many diseases are being explained by the effects of the endocrine glands and by antigen-antibody reactions, all of which are manifestations of products carried in the blood stream.

SUGGESTIONS FOR FURTHER READING

Historical Aspects of Pathology

Brothwell, D., and Sandison, A. T.: Diseases in Antiquity. Springfield, Illinois, Charles C Thomas, 1967.

Cartwright, F. F.: Disease and History. London, Hard-Davis MacGibbon, 1972.

Cockburn, T. A.: Death and disease in ancient Egypt. Science, *181*:470–471, 1973.

Harcourt, R. A.: The paleopathology of animal skeletal remains. Vet. Rec., *89*:267–272, 1971.

Hippocrates: The Theory and Practice of Medicine. New York, The Citadel Press, 1964.

King, L. S.: A history of the autopsy. Am. J. Pathol., *73*:513–544, 1973.

Long, E. R.: A History of American Pathology. Springfield, Illinois, Charles C Thomas, 1962.

Long, E. R.: A History of Pathology. Baltimore, Williams and Wilkins Co., 1928.

Long, E. R.: Selected Readings in Pathology from Hippocrates to Virchow. Springfield, Illinois, Charles C Thomas, 1929.

Majno, G.: The Healing Hand: Man and Wound in the Ancient World. Cambridge, Harvard University Press, 1975.

Majno, G., and Joris, I.: The microscope in the history of pathology. Virchows Arch. [Pathol. Anat.], *360*:273–286, 1973.

Miller, G.: Bibliography of the history of medicine of the U.S. and Canada—1963. Bull. Hist. Med., *38*:538–577, 1964.

Moodie, R. L.: Paleopathology. Urbana, University of Illinois, 1923.

Rather, L. J.: Rudolph Virchow's views on pathology, pathological anatomy and cellular pathology. Arch. Pathol., *82*:197–204, 1966.

Reasoner, M. A.: Prehistoric and ancient disease. The Military Surgeon, *65*:339–363, 1929.

Reyman, T. A., Barraco, R., and Cockburn, A.: Histopathological examination of an Egyptian mummy. Bull. N. Y. Acad. Med., *52*:506–516, 1976.

Saunders, L. Z.: Some pioneers in comparative medicine. Can. Vet. J., *14*:27–35, 1973.

Saunders, L. Z.: William H. Feldman—1892–1974. Vet. Pathol., *11*:198–202, 1974.

Saunders, L. Z., and Barron, C. N.: A century of veterinary pathology at the A.F.I.P. 1870–1970. Dr. Woodward on bovine pleuropneumonia. Pathol. Vet., *7*:193–224, 1970.

Skinsnes, O. K.: Postmortem examination and inquest in old China. Arch. Pathol., *74*:304–312, 1962.

Tedeschi, C. G.: The pathology of Bonet and Morgagni. (A historical introduction to the autopsy.) Hum. Pathol., *5*:601–603, 1974.

Thorwald, J.: Science and Secrets of Early Medicine. Egypt, Mesopotamia, India, China, Mexico, Peru. London, Thames and Hudson Ltd., 1962.

Virchow, R. (trans. L. J. Rather): Disease, Life, and Man, Selected Essays. Stanford, Stanford University Press, 1958.

Zeuner, F. E.: A History of Domesticated Animals. London, Hutchinson of London, 1963

APPENDIX III

SOME GREEK AND LATIN ROOTS AND AFFIXES*

a-, an-: Gk. = not, without. *atrophy, anaemia, anoxia, aplasia, avascular, amorphous, asepsis*

aden: Gk. = a gland. *adenitis, adenoma, adenosis*

angeion: Gk. = a vessel. *angioma, lymphangitis, cholangitis*

anthrax: Gk. = coal. *anthrax, anthracosis*

anti-: Gk. = against, opposite. *antibody, antigen, antitoxin, antidote, antisepsis*

arthron: Gk. = a joint. *arthrology, arthritis*

autos: Gk. = self. *autolysis, autopsy, autonomy, autogenous*

blastos: Gk. = a sprout, hence something immature. *fibroblast, erythroblast, myeloblast, neuroblastoma, retinoblastoma*

bolos: Gk. = a lump. *bolus, embolus*

carcino: Gk. **karkinos** = a crab or cancer. *carcinoma, carcinogenic*

cele: Gk. **kele** = a swelling. *hydrocele, hematocele, mucocele, cystocele, meningocele, encephalocele*

chrom: Gk. **khromos** = color. *cytochrome, chromaffin, chromatolysis, chromium*

chym: Gk. **khumos** = juice. *chyme, parenchyma, mesenchyme, ecchymosis*

coll: Gk. **kolla** = glue. *collagen, colloid*

cyst: Gk. **kustis** = a bladder. *cyst, cystitis, cholecystitis*

cyt: Gk. **kutos** = a cell or vessel. *cytology, leucocyte, erythrocyte, cytoplasm, syncytia, cytolysis*

derma: Gk. = skin. *dermis, epidermis, dermatology, dermatitis*

dia-: Gk. = through, across. *diarrhea, diabetes, diuresis, dialysis, diapedesis, diagnosis, diaphragm*

dys: Gk. = bad. *dyspepsia, dysentery, dysphagia, dyspnoea, dysplasia*

ectasis: Gk. = expansion. *bronchiectasis, telangiectasis, lymphangiectasis*

-ectomy: Gk. = a cutting out or excision. *appendectomy, lymphadenectomy*

em-, en-: Gk. and Lat. = in, into. *embolism, empyema, encyst, endemic*

-emia: Gk. **haima** = blood. *anemia, hyperemia, ischemia, pyemia, uremia*

endo-: Gk. = within. *endocardium, endometrium, endarteritis, endogenous*

enteron: Gk. = the bowel. *enteritis, enterolith, dysentery*

epi-: Gk. = upon. *epicardium, epiphysis, epithelium*

erythros: Gk. = red. *erythrocyte, erythropoiesis, erythema*

gaster: Gk. = stomach. *gastritis, gastrostomy*

gen, genesis: from Lat. and Gk. = birth, origin, begetting. *gene, genetics, genital, histogenesis, carcinogenesis, fibrinogen, androgen, estrogen*

---

*Adapted from R. A. Willis: Principles of Pathology. Philadelphia, F. A. Davis Company (Butterworth), 1961.

gnosis: Gk. = knowledge. *diagnosis, prognosis*

hem: Gk. **haima** = blood. *hemorrhage, hemoglobin, hemoptysis, hematuria, hematocele, hemopoiesis*

heteros: Gk. = other, different. *heterotopia, heterologous*

homos: Gk. = same. *homology, homozygous*

hyalos: Gk. = glass. *hyaline, keratohyalin, hyaluronic acid*

hydr, hygr: from Gk. = water, wet. *hydronephrosis, hydrocephalus, hydrophobia, hydrocele, hydatid, hygroma, hygroscopic*

hyper-: Gk. = over, excessive. *hyperplasia, hypertrophy, hyperemia, hyperostosis, hyperglycemia*

hypo-: Gk. = under, deficient. *hypoplasia, hypoglycemia, hypotonus, hypodermic*

idio-: Gk. = one's own. *idiopathic, idiosyncrasy*

-itis: Gk. suffix = inflammation. *appendicitis, tonsillitis, hepatitis*

lapsus: Lat. = a slip. *prolapse, relapse, collapse*

leukos: Gk. = white. *leucocyte, leucoplakia, leukemia, leukorrhea*

lipos: Gk. = fat. *lipoid, lipase, lipoma*

lithos: Gk. = a stone. *cholelithiasis, nephrolithiasis, enterolith*

lysis: Gk. = loosening or solution. *lysis, hemolysis, autolysis, paralysis, analysis*

macro-: Gk. makros = large. *macrocyte, macrophage*

malakos: Gk. = softening. *osteomalacia, myomalacia*

mastos: Gk. = breast. *mastitis*

mega-, megalo-: from Gk. **megos** = great. *megacolon, megaloblast, megakaryocyte, acromegaly, splenomegaly*

melan-: from Gk. **melas, melanos** = black. *melanin, melanoma, melancholia*

mesos: Gk. = middle, intermediate. *mesoderm, mesenchyme, mesentery*

mikros: Gk. = small. *microscope, microcephaly*

monos: Gk. = alone, single. *mononuclear, monoxide, monogamy*

morphe: Gk. = form, shape. *polymorphonuclear, morphology, pleomorphism, amorphous*

myc: from Gk. **mukes** = a mushroom, hence a fungus. *mycology, actinomyces, blastomyces, mycelium, mycetoma*

myelos: Gk. = marrow. *myelitis, osteomyelitis*

my-, myo-: from Gk. **mus** = muscle. *myositis, myoma*

nekros: Gk. = a corpse. *necropsy, necrosis, necropolis*

nephros: Gk. = a kidney. *nephritis, nephroblastoma*

neuron: Gk. = a nerve. *neuron, neuritis, neurolemma*

-oid, -ode: Lat. and Gk. suffix = like. *deltoid, mastoid, amyloid, fibroid*

oligos: Gk. = scanty. *oligemia, oliguria, oligohydramnios*

-oma, -ome: Gk. suffix, **-ma, -me,** expressing result of an action, used in pathology mainly for tumors. *adenoma, carcinoma, sarcoma,* etc.; *atheroma, coloboma, granuloma*

orthos: Gk. = straight. *orthopedics, orthodox*

-osis, -asis: Gk. suffix = a process or condition. *tuberculosis, pneumoconiosis, necrosis, scoliosis, exostosis, fibrosis*

para-: Gk. = beside. *parovarium, parametrium, paratyphoid fever, paralysis, parasite*

pathos: Gk. = suffering. *pathology, pathogenic, encephalopathy, osteoarthropathy*

peri-: Gk. = around. *pericardium, periosteum*

phagos: Gk. = eating. *phagocyte, macrophage, bacteriophage, dysphagia*

philos: Gk. = friend, lover. *eosinophil, basophil, philosophy*

phlebos: Gk. = a vein. *phlebitis, phlebolith, phlebotomy*

phobos: Gk. = fear. *phobia, hydrophobia, photophobia, claustrophobia, chromophobe*

physa: Gk. = a puff of wind. *emphysema*

physis: Gk. = nature. *physics, physiology, physician*

phyton: Gk. = a plant; also **physis** = a growth. *osteophyte, chondrophyte, saprophyte, diaphysis, epiphysis*

plast, plasia, plasm: from Gk. **plastos** = molded. *plastic, protoplasm, plasmodium, aplasia, hyperplasia, metaplasia, anaplasia*

pleo-: Gk. = more. *pleomorphism, pleocytosis*

pneumon: Gk. = lung; related to **pneuma** = air, and **pneo** = breathe. *pneumonia, pneumothorax, dyspnea, apnea, hyperpnea*

polios: Gk. = gray. *poliomyelitis*

poly-: Gk. = many. *polymorphism, polymorphonuclear*

pseudo: Gk. = false. *pseudopodia, pseudohermaphrodite*

pyon: Gk. = pus. *pyogenic, pyemia, empyema*

rhinos: Gk. = nose. *rhinitis*

-rrhea: from Gk. **rhoia** = a flow. *diarrhea*

sarkos: Gk. = flesh. *sarcolemma, sarcoma*

skleros: Gk. = hard. *sclera, sclerosis, scleroderma*

septikos: Gk. = putrid. *septic, asepsis, antisepsis, septicemia, Cl. septicum*

stasis: Gk. = a standing, state. *stasis, hemostasis, metastasis*

teratos: Gk. = a monster, deformity. *teratology, teratoma, teratogenic*

thesis: Gk. = thing laid down. *thesis, hypothesis, synthesis*

thrombos: Gk. = a lump, clot. *thrombus, thrombin, thrombocyte, thombosis*

topos: Gk. = a place. *ectopia, heterotopia*

trope: Gk. = a turning. *tropism, chemotropic, lipotropic, gonadotropic*

trophe: Gk. = food, nutrition. *trophic, atrophy, hypertrophy, dystrophy*

zoon: Gk. = an animal. *protozoa, metazoa, spermatozoan, merozoite*

APPENDIX IV

LEARNING REQUIREMENTS AND OBJECTIVES FOR GENERAL PATHOLOGY

Dr. Billy Ward of Mississippi State University directed the development of "Content Analysis of Veterinary Pathology" as a model National Program for Instructional Development, a project funded by the National Institutes of Health. The content attempted to explicitly describe the ***learning requirements*** for veterinary pathology expected from a graduating veterinarian. Specific ***behavioral objectives*** were established to develop ***skills*** directed toward problem solving in case oriented situations.

Parts of the Content Analysis and the general format are used here to provide the student with an indication of ***what is expected in terms of knowledge and skills.*** Dr. Ward has given permission for parts of the material to be used. Deviations from the Content Analysis occur mainly to conform with the format and objectives of this book.

CHAPTER 1: INTRODUCTION

Define, spell, pronounce and ***use*** the following terms:

- Clinical sign
- Diagnosis
- Disease
- Etiological diagnosis
- Etiology
- General pathology
- Lesion
- Morphological diagnosis
- Pathogenesis
- Pathologist
- Pathology
- Prognosis
- Special Pathology
- Symptom

Explain the meaning and ***discuss*** the importance of the following:

- Clinical sign
- Diagnosis
- Etiology
- Lesion
- Pathogenesis
- Pathology
- Prognosis
- Symptom

CHAPTER 2: DEGENERATION AND NECROSIS

Degeneration

Describe gross, light microscopic and electron microscopic changes associated with cell swelling.
List the causes and mechanisms of cell degeneration.
Discuss the range of homeostatic adaptability in relation to cell injury.
Outline the morphological and functional changes that occur in injury to the following structures:

- Cell membrane
- Endoplasmic reticulum
- Lysosomes
- Mitochondria
- Nucleus
- Ribosomes

Identify and ***describe*** fatty change at the gross and microscopic level.
State the tissues in which fatty change is most frequently recognized grossly.
Discuss causes of fatty change.
Outline the pathogenesis of fatty change in the liver.

Predict the fate of cells that have undergone fatty degeneration if the inciting agent is removed or neutralized.
Discuss the pathogenesis, etiology and lesions associated with amyloidosis.

Necrosis, Necrobiosis

Contrast the morphological features (gross and light microscopic) of necrotic tissue with those of living tissue.
State the basic differences among necrosis, necrobiosis, somatic death and degeneration.
Compare causes and mechanisms of cell death to cell degeneration.
Discuss the following types of necrosis in terms of

Morphologic features (gross and microscopic)
Situations under which they commonly occur (tissues and cause)
Pathogenesis
Fate, if the cause persists or is removed or neutralized:

Coagulation necrosis
Caseous necrosis
Fat necrosis
Liquefaction necrosis
Gangrenous necrosis

Postmortem Changes

Compare the morphological (gross and microscopic) similarities and differences between ***antemortem lesions*** and ***postmortem changes***, particularly between autolysis and necrosis.
Outline the pathogenesis of autolysis.
Identify and *describe* the gross appearance or characteristics of:

Algor mortis
Autolysis
Focal putrefaction
Hypostatic congestion
Imbibition of bile
Imbibition of hemoglobin
Livor mortis
Postmortem emphysema
Postmortem tympany
Pseudomelanosis
Rigor mortis

Explain the effect of the following on postmortem changes:

Ambient temperature
Amount of body fat
Body temperature at time of death
Physical condition of animal prior to death

Calcification and Pigmentation

Compare dystrophic and metastatic calcification in terms of

Cause
Pathogenesis
Sites of occurrence
Gross and microscopic appearance

Discuss the fate of calcific lesions.
Discuss the following pigments in terms of

Gross and microscopic identification and description
Causes
Sites of occurrence
Pathogenesis
Effects on the host
Ultimate fate:
Bilirubin
Carbon
Carotene
Ceroid
Hemosiderin
Lipofuscin
Melanin
Porphyrins

Outline the principal chemical steps in the formation of hemosiderin and bilirubin and *name* the tissue and cellular site where these events occur.

General

Recognize, describe and *explain* the significance of

Anthracosis
Calcinosis
Caseous necrosis
Ceroid
Cholesterol clefts
Chromatolysis
Cloudy swelling
Coagulation necrosis
Corpora amylacea
Erosion
Fat necrosis

Fatty infiltration
Fibrinoid
Focal necrosis
Gangrene
Gout
Heart failure cells
Hematin
Hemosiderosis
Hyaline casts
Hyaline droplets
Hydropic degeneration
Inclusion bodies
Jaundice (icterus)
Karyolysis
Karyorrhexis
Lipofuscin
Malacia
Melanosis
Microvesicle
Nuclear debris
Phagosome
Photosensitization
Pneumoconiosis
Porphyria
Pyknosis
Sequestration
Slough
Steatitis
Storage disease
Ulcer

CHAPTER 3: CIRCULATORY DISTURBANCES

Outline the pathogenesis of hyperemia and congestion.
Distinguish hyperemia and congestion from hemorrhage.
Recognize and ***describe*** the following:
Congestion
Edema
Hematoma
Hemorrhage
Hyperemia
Outline the pathogenesis of chronic passive congestion and ***describe*** the gross and microscopic lesions associated with the condition.
Explain the etiological factors, pathogenesis and fate of various types of hemorrhage.
List the causes of edema.
Explain the fate of edema.
List and ***recognize*** the types of local and general edema.
Distinguish between edematous swellings and those swellings caused by hemorrhage or inflammation.
Explain the pathogenesis of ascites.
Describe the main mechanisms of hemostasis.
Explain the pathogenesis of thrombosis and ***recognize*** various types of thrombi.
List factors predisposing to thrombosis.
Outline the pathogenesis of the embolic process.
Recognize and ***describe*** infarcts in the kidneys, heart, lungs and brain and ***evaluate*** the age of infarcts.
Differentiate between the following:
Mural and valvular thrombi
Red, white and mixed thrombi
Septic and nonseptic thrombi
A thrombus and a clot
A thrombus and a chicken fat clot
Explain the pathogenesis and significance of
Acidosis
Alkylosis
Congestive atelectasis
Dehydration
Disseminated intravascular coagulation
Renal tubular necrosis
Shock
Sludging
Visceral pooling
Define, spell, pronounce and ***use*** the following terms:
Anasarca
Anoxia
Bruise
Cyanosis
Diapedesis
Ecchymosis
Embolus
Extrinsic system
Fibrinolysis
Hageman factor
Hemopericardium
Hemoperitoneum
Hemorrhagic diathesis
Hemothorax
Hyalin thrombus
Hydropericardium
Hydrothorax
Hyperemic
Hypoproteinemia
Hypoxia
Infarct
Intrinsic system
Ischemia

Organized thrombus
Petechia
Plasmin
Purpura
Recanalized thrombus
Saddle thrombus
Thrombocytopenia
Thromboplastin
Transudate

CHAPTER 4: INFLAMMATION AND REPAIR

Outline the sequence of events that occur in an area of acute inflammation.
List the chemical mediators of acute inflammation and ***describe*** their source and function in the reaction.
List the cells of an acute inflammatory lesion and ***describe*** their source, function and fate.
List the chemical mediators of chronic inflammation and ***describe*** their source and function in the reaction.
List the cells of a chronic inflammatory lesion and ***describe*** their source, function and fate.
Explain chemotaxis and ***list*** substances that are chemotactic.
For each of the following
- ***Recognize*** and ***describe*** the gross and microscopic features
- ***Outline*** the pathogenesis
- ***List*** the most likely location
- ***List*** the most likely etiological agents
- ***Distinguish*** between and identify
- ***Predict*** the fate:
  - Serous inflammation
  - Catarrhal inflammation
  - Fibrinous inflammation
  - Purulent inflammation
  - Hemorrhagic inflammation
  - Granulomatous inflammation

Discuss the role of immune mechanisms in the inflammatory response.
Recognize and ***explain*** the development of the following:
- Abscess
- Adhesion
- Diphtheritic membrane
- Granuloma

Define, spell, pronounce and ***use*** the following terms as they relate to inflammation, injury and healing:

Abrasion
Abscess
Acute
Adhesion
Anaphylaxis
Antibody
Antigen
Arthus reaction
Autoimmune disease
Blast
Cellulitis
Chalone
Chemotaxis
Chronic
Cicatrix
Club colony
Collagenolysis
Complement
Concussion
Contusion
Corticosteroid
Croupous
Delayed hypersensitivity
Diphtheritic membrane
Empyema
Exudate
Fever
Fibrin
Fibrin cast
Fibrosis
First intention healing
Granulation tissue
Granuloma
Heterophil
Histamine
Hypersensitivity
Inflammation
Immune complex
Kallikrein
Keloid
Kinin
Laceration
Leukocytosis
Leukopenia
Lymphokine
Microabscess
Mitogen
Myeloperoxidase
Myofibroblast
Opsonin
Phagocytosis
Phagolysosome
Phagosome
Phlegmon
Prostaglandin
Proud flesh
Pus
Pustule
Pyogenic

Pyogenic membrane
Pyrogen
Regeneration
Resolution
Scab
Scar
Scirrhous
Second intention healing
Serum sickness
Sinus tract
Subacute
Suppuration
Trauma

Discuss and ***explain*** the process of healing in a tissue following necrosis and inflammation.

Describe the formation of granulation tissue and ***explain*** the mechanisms involved.

Describe and ***explain*** the mechanisms and limitations involved in regeneration of tissues.

Discuss factors that influence healing and ***indicate*** their specific influence.

Discuss the regenerative and reparative capabilities of the following tissue components:

Adrenal
Blood
Blood vessels
Bone
Brain
Bronchus
Cartilage
Connective tissue
Ear
Eye
Fat
Heart muscle
Intestine
Kidney
Ligament
Liver
Mammary gland
Nerve
Ovary
Pancreas
Pituitary
Prostate
Skeletal muscle
Skin
Smooth muscle
Stomach
Tendon
Testis
Thyroid
Trachea
Ureter
Uterus

CHAPTER 5: DISTURBANCES OF GROWTH

For each of the following:

Recognize and ***identify*** an example
Explain the pathogenesis and significance and ***discuss*** the causes:

Agenesis
Aplasia
Atresia
Atrophy
Callus
Cystic hyperplasia
Denervation atrophy
Disuse atrophy
Dysplasia
Hyperplasia
Hypertrophy
Hypoplasia
Involution
Metaplasia
Nodular hyperplasia
Pressure atrophy
Squamous metaplasia

Differentiate

Atrophy from hyperplasia, aplasia and agenesis
Hypertrophy from hyperplasia
Metaplasia from anaplasia and dysplasia

Outline the causes of aging.

Define, spell, pronounce and ***use*** the following terms:

Anaplasia
Anomaly
Chimera
Congenital
Cyst
Euplasia
Hamartoma
Iatrogenic
Karyotype
Mosaicism
Proplasia
Retroplasia
Teratology

CHAPTER 6: NEOPLASIA

Define, spell, pronounce and ***use*** the following terms:

Adenocarcinoma
Adenoma
Alpha fetal globulin
Benign
Biological behavior
Cancer

Carcinoma
Carcinoma in situ
Carcinoembryonic antigen
Clone
Contact inhibition
Derepression
Differentiation
Embryonic tumor
Exfoliative cytology
Histogenesis
Hyperchromatism
Implantation
Impression smear
Initiation
Leukemia
Malignant
Metastasis
Mitotic index
Needle biopsy
Neoplasia
Oncogene theory
Oncogenesis
Oncogenic
Oncology
Oncornavirus
Polyp
Papova
Precancerous lesion
Promotion
Protovirus theory
Sarcoma
Teratoma
Transformation
Tumor

Explain the basis of classification of tumors.
Differentiate between benign and malignant tumors in terms of
Structure
Growth
Differentiation
Metastatic properties
Prognosis

Name the main tumors of each organ in the body.
Explain the means by which tumors are identified and differentiated from other biological abnormalities in tissues.
List the distinctive tissue and cellular features that are characteristic of tumors.
List the cytological features that are characteristic of malignancy.
Explain the means by which tumors metastasize.
Explain the means of microscopic grading of tumors.
Explain the criteria used in the evaluation of the prognosis of a tumor.
List the various types of therapy for tumors and ***explain*** the basis of their actions.
Explain the mechanisms by which viruses and chemicals transform cells.
Explain the pathogenetic mechanisms by which irradiation, chemicals and viruses cause cancer, including common features.
List common tumors in each of the following: cat, chicken, cow, dog, horse, pig, sheep.

CHAPTER 7: HOST-PARASITE RELATIONSHIPS

Define, spell, pronounce and ***use*** the following terms:
Age resistance
Aggressin
Clinical disease
Commensalism
Cytolytic
Enzootic
Epizootic
Immune resistance
Integrated infection
Latent infection
Mycotoxin
Natural resistance
Parasitism
Pathogenicity
Subclinical disease
Symbiosis
Tissue affinity
Tropism
Virulence

Explain the means by which the following agents cause tissue injury:
Bacteria
Fungus
Parasite
Toxin
Virus

Discuss significant factors that protect the host from injury.
Explain the influence of environment on infectious disease.
Explain the features that some agents have that allow them to survive and cause disease.

Index

Note: Page numbers in *italic* refer to illustrations; references to tables are indicated by *t*.